Image-Guided Therapy Systems

Artech House Series
Engineering in Medicine & Biology

Series Editors

Martin L. Yarmush, Harvard Medical School
Christopher J. James, University of Southampton

Advanced Methods and Tools for ECG Data Analysis, Gari D. Clifford, Francisco Azuaje, and Patrick E. McSharry, editors

Advances in Photodynamic Therapy: Basic, Translational, and Clinical, Michael Hamblin and Pawel Mroz, editors

Biological Database Modeling, Jake Chen and Amandeep S. Sidhu, editors

Biomedical Informatics in Translational Research, Hai Hu, Michael Liebman, and Richard Mural

Biomedical Surfaces, Jeremy Ramsden

Genome Sequencing Technology and Algorithms, Sun Kim, Haixu Tang, and Elaine R. Mardis, editors

Image-Guided Therapy Systems, Shahram Vaezy and Vesna Zderic, editors

Inorganic Nanoprobes for Biological Sensing and Imaging, Hedi Mattoussi and Jinwoo Cheon, editors

Intelligent Systems Modeling and Decision Support in Bioengineering, Mahdi Mahfouf

Life Science Automation Fundamentals and Applications, Mingjun Zhang, Bradley Nelson, and Robin Felder, editors

Microscopic Image Analysis for Life Science Applications, Jens Rittscher, Stephen T. C. Wong, and Raghu Machiraju, editors

Next Generation Artificial Vision Systems: Reverse Engineering the Human Visual System, Maria Petrou and Anil Bharath, editors

Quantitative EEG Analysis Methods and Clinical Applications Shanbao Tong and Nitish V. Thakor, editors

Systems Bioinformatics: An Engineering Case-Based Approach, Gil Alterovitz and Marco F. Ramoni, editors

Systems Engineering Approach to Medical Automation, Robin Felder

Translational Approaches in Tissue Engineering and Regenerative Medicine, Jeremy Mao, Gordana Vunjak-Novakovic, Antonios G. Mikos, and Anthony Atala, editors

Image-Guided Therapy Systems

Shahram Vaezy
Vesna Zderic

Editors

ARTECH
HOUSE

BOSTON | LONDON
artechhouse.com

Library of Congress Cataloging-in-Publication Data
A catalog record for this book is available from the U.S. Library of Congress.

British Library Cataloguing in Publication Data
A catalog record for this book is available from the British Library.

ISBN-13: 978-1-59693-109-1

Cover design by Yekaterina Ratner

685 Canton Street
Norwood, MA 02062

DISCLAIMER OF WARRANTY

The technical descriptions, procedures, and computer programs in this book have been developed with the greatest of care and they have been useful to the author in a broad range of applications; however, they are provided as is, without warranty of any kind. Artech House, Inc. and the authors and editors of the book titled *Image-Guided Therapy Systems* make no warranties, expressed or implied, that the equations, programs, and procedures in this book or its associated software are free of error, or are consistent with any particular standard of merchantability, or will meet your requirements for any particular application. They should not be relied upon for solving a problem whose incorrect solution could result in injury to a person or loss of property. Any use of the programs or procedures in such a manner is at the user's own risk. The editors, author, and publisher disclaim all liability for direct, incidental, or consequent damages resulting from use of the programs or procedures in this book or the associated software.

10 9 8 7 6 5 4 3 2 1

Contents

CHAPTER 18

CHAPTER 19

Preface

The movie *Fantastic Voyage*, where a microscopic submarine with an even smaller-sized crew goes inside a human body to treat a blood clot in the brain, was a fantasy, but it had a clear message. The need for visualization of internal organs and tissues for subsequent therapy using innovative treatment tools is a real need if we want to go beyond traditional medicine of "take a pill and call me in the morning." In fact, today's medicine has embarked on a fantastic voyage of its own in developing tools that can do exactly what the movie envisioned. These tools would help visualize biological structures with increasing resolution, down to the cell level, and apply local, specific therapies with increasing diversity in their capabilities. The engineering integration of imaging and therapy modalities to allow the fantasy-like treatments deep in the body has resulted in a new field in medicine, dubbed image-guided therapy. This book provides a survey of this field from a systems engineering perspective.

The structure of this book is simple, and builds upon basic concepts. There are three parts, each reviewing a fundamental block in our survey of image-guided therapy systems. In each part, chapters provide details relevant to the section. Part I is about where our voyage begins, and where it's going. A historical view of interventional medicine and the time-tested conventional surgery, as well as some future directions is presented in Part I. Part II is about therapy. Chapters on various therapeutic modalities such as lasers, radio frequency ablation, cryotherapy, and so forth provide a perspective of the current capabilities of therapy. Part III is on integration of imaging and therapy to develop image-guided therapy systems. Important issues in the integration of these modalities to achieve high degrees of specificity and sensitivity are presented in the chapters of Part III.

The CD accompanying this book provides high-quality or color versions of some of the images presented in the text. These images are intended for you to see details that might be otherwise hard to distinguish in low-resolution or black-and-white images. A picture is worth a thousand words.

We are indebted to our coauthors for their expert and generous contribution of their chapters. They have written this book. Each chapter provides a gateway to the field it represents. Keep in mind that each field is prospering with advancements and innovations that the workers in the field are achieving with their cutting edge research. Our authors have provided the starting point for the readers to look into the field, become equipped with the language and terminology, and be able to pursue that area if they so choose. We thank our authors for this introduction.

We would like to thank Wayne Yuhasz of Artech House Publishers for his vision and tireless support of this project. Our hope is that projects like this provide a continuous stream of knowledge for students, engineers, and clinicians who are working in the field.

Shahram Vaezy
Seattle, Washington
Vesna Zderic
Washington, D.C.
Editors
June 2009

PART I

Introduction: Diagnosis and Therapy

CHAPTER 1

Diagnosis and Therapy: History, Current Status, and Future Directions

Vesna Zderic and Shahram Vaezy

1.1 Ancient Times

Surgery was known to mankind probably since the beginning of civilization [1]. The first surgeries included fairly simple procedures such as wound stitching and circumcision, but also surprisingly complex operations such as removal of bladder stones and skull trephination. Before any surgery instruments were available, wounds may have been stitched together by thorns and sutured with a plant fiber, as still done today by Masai in East Africa. An even more convenient solution was developed by tribes in India and South America. They encouraged termites to bite across the wound held by a healer. After the bite, the termite was decapitated leaving the jaws tightly stitching the wound, quite similar to metal clips used in modern surgery. Circumcision was likely the first elective surgery performed by humans. It has been practiced in ancient Egypt by priests and the royal family, as shown on the tomb carvings dating back to 2400–3000 B.C. (Figure 1.1), and also throughout the rest of the ancient world such as in Australia, equatorial Africa, South America, and the Pacific islands. The origins of this procedure are religious or possibly due to hygienic reasons [2]. Operations to remove bladder stones via the perineum were performed by Hindu, Greek, Roman, and Arab surgeons. They often wrote detailed descriptions of the surgery, including preoperative and postoperative care and management. Historically, bladder stones were a disease affecting young boys; however, in the today's developed world they are most common among men over 50 years of age.

Trephination of the skull, defined as a surgical opening of the skull using primitive tools, probably originates from Neolithic times 7,000 to 10,000 years ago, and was performed in various parts of the world (i.e., Europe, North Africa, the west coast of America, New Guinea, and Peru). It is still performed today in some parts of Africa, South America, and Melanesia [2]. The trephination instruments initially consisted of a piece of a stone with a wooden handle, and were later replaced by a copper or bronze blade. Several holes or squares were usually produced (Figure 1.2), with a very good survival rate (as observed by the healing occurring around the trephined holes). In most cases, it appears that the trephination was carried out following the head injury, thus likely saving the patients from death due to brain swelling. However, there are only speculations about the reasons of trephinations of

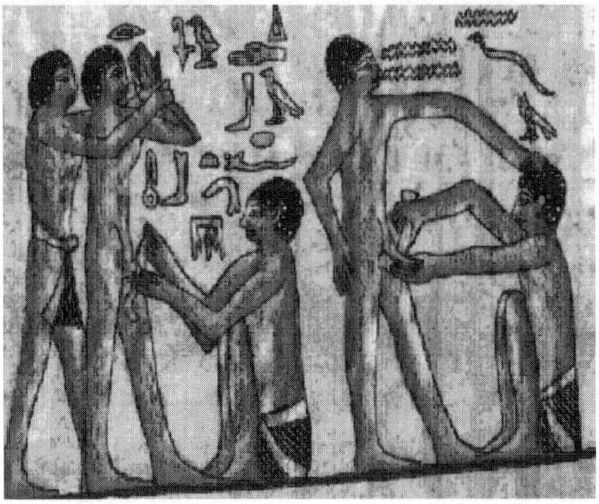

Figure 1.1 Picture from the wall of an ancient Egyptian pyramid showing circumcision done on two patients. One of them had to be restrained, while some type of topical anesthetic ointment may have been used on the other patient.

the skulls with no obvious head injury, some of them include healing of intractable headaches and epilepsy, or attempts to give the patient magical powers.

By 2000–4000 B.C., the laws that regulated the practice of surgery were starting to form. King Hammurabi of Mesopotamia imposed strict laws punishing any malpractice, thus making the vocation of a surgeon a fairly dangerous one. For example, if during an eye operation, the surgeon destroyed the eye, the punishment was cutting of both of the surgeon's hands. The laws were followed by an oath written by Greek physician Hippocrates in ~400 B.C., a pledge still taken by physicians today to perform to the best of their ability. Initially, surgeons were mostly focusing

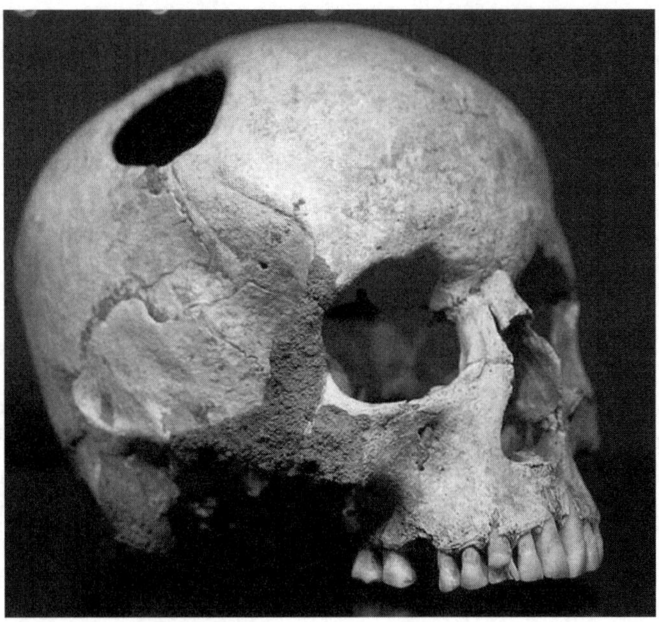

Figure 1.2 Neolitic girl skull; the girl survived. (*Source:* Natural History Museum, Lausanne.)

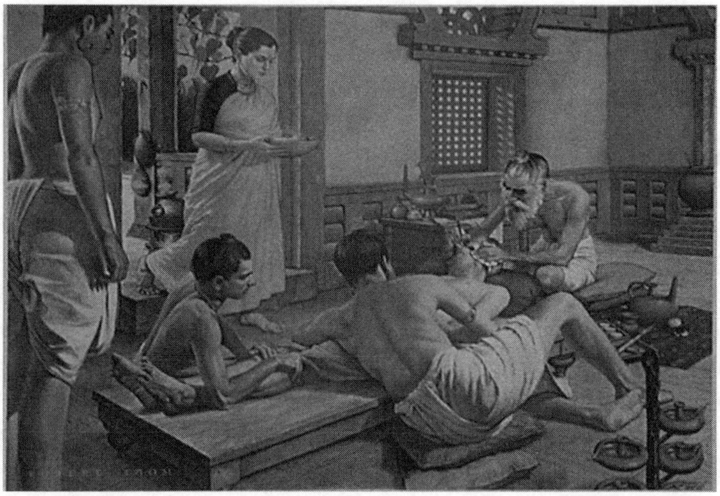

Figure 1.3 Painting of Sushruta performing cataract surgery. (*From:* [3]. © 2007 Sanjay Saraf. Reprinted with permission.)

on healing of wounds, fractures, and abscesses. However, in the next few thousands of years a variety of novel surgical procedures developed. These procedures are described in great detail in the manuscripts written by an Indian surgeon Sushruta. For example, he described the cataract removal surgeries (Figure 1.3), in which the opaque lens of the eye was mobilized with a scalpel and pushed away from the field of view. He also described one of the first cosmetic surgery operations for restoration of an amputated nose, by using a skin graft from the forehead. The demand for this operation was fairly high since this was a standard punishment for adultery in those days. This cosmetic surgery procedure remained in practice for hundreds of years, and was used as late as the nineteenth century.

The development of novel surgical procedures was accompanied by a development of a variety of surgical instruments. Roman surgical instruments resembled to a great degree today's tools including variety of scalpels, forceps, hooks, drills, and even speculum for gynecological procedures (Figure 1.4). Also, heating of the metal instruments was discovered as early as in ancient Egypt for the purpose of wound cauterization. For this, a knife, heated till it turned red, was used to produce cut and seal the blood vessels at the same time, thus reducing bleeding. By the time

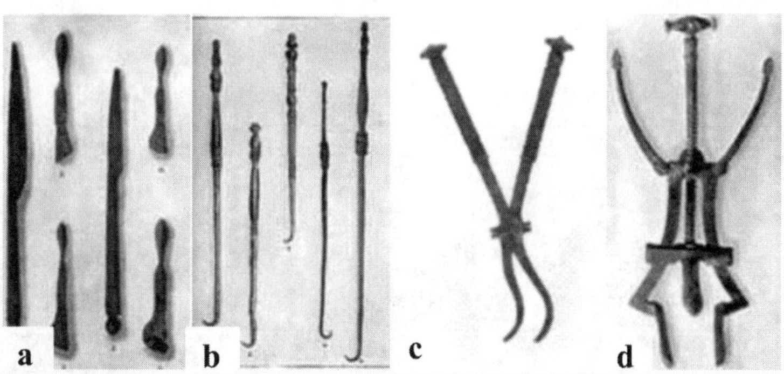

Figure 1.4 Surgical instruments used in ancient Rome: (a) scalpels; (b) hooks; (c) forceps; and (d) speculum. (Images obtained from [4].)

of Roman Empire, the cautery appeared to be a fairly popular tool used for both hemostasis and tumor coagulation.

1.2 Renaissance

Renaissance renewed the interest in medicine and the further development of surgery. For example, at this time a French surgeon Lanfranchi (1315) provided a detail description of hemorrhage control, successfully differentiating among arterial, venous, and capillary bleeding. He introduced the first type of tissue glue for hemorrhage control: recommending soaking of a bandage into an egg white before placing it over the wound. He also recommended applying manual pressure over the injured blood vessel for over an hour until a permanent clot is produced; a procedure that is still in use today following the femoral artery catheterizations. If the clotting does not occur in this time, the surgeon was recommended to pull out the end of the blood vessel in order to twist it or to tie it using a silk thread or otherwise seal it with cautery. Lanfranchi also recognized the nerve injury as a reason for loss of feeling and mobility in the limb. For this, he advised applying sutures in order to approximate the nerve endings.

Possibly the most famous European surgeon was Johannes Schultes (known as Scultetus) (1595–1645) born in Ulm. He wrote *Armamentarium Chirurgicum*, which contained a complete catalog of all surgical instruments known at the time, methods of bandaging and splinting, and descriptions of a large number of operative procedures with illustrations, just to name a few shown here: tracheotomy (Figure 1.5), amputation (Figure 1.6), cesarean section (Figure 1.7), and mastectomy for breast cancer (Figure 1.8). In general, all these procedures were designed such that they could be performed as fast as possible since no anesthesia was applied, and patients usually had to be kept still by the force.

1.3 Open Surgery in Modern Times

Operation of abdominal solid organs was introduced to surgery practice in the nineteenth century. For example, the first successful elective laparotomy was performed in 1809 by a Kentucky surgeon, Dr. McDowell. He operated on a 44-year

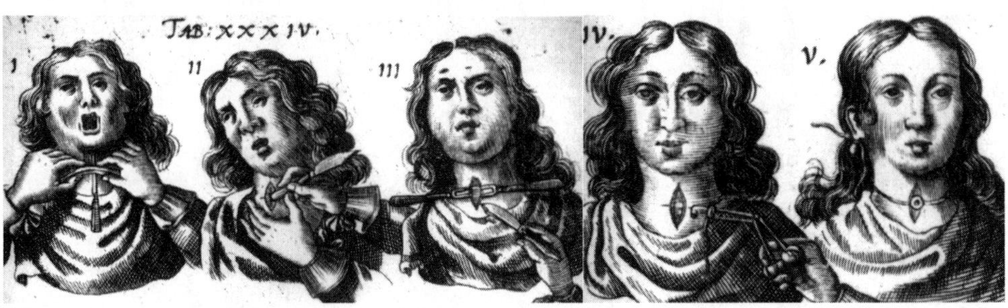

Figure 1.5 Tracheotomy procedure, performed in sixteenth century. Similar procedure is performed today in emergency situations. (*Source: Armamentarium Chirurgicum.*)

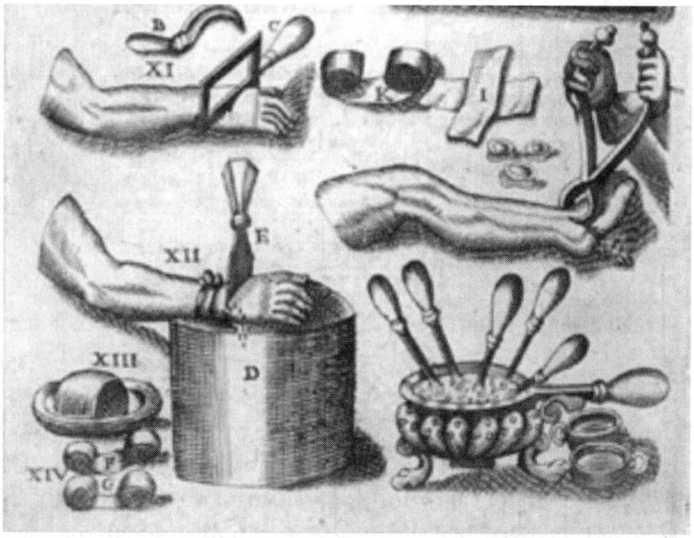

Figure 1.6 Illustration of amputation procedures. After the limb was amputated with a sharp metal object (i.e., saw) the bleeding was stopped with a cauterizing iron. (*Source: Armamentarium Chirurgicum.*)

old patient to remove a large ovarian tumor. About 10 kg of tumor was removed, and the patients recovered and lived to be 78. The first successful splenectomy was performed in 1893 by Dr. Riegner, a chief surgeon at the All Saints Hospital in Breslau. This operation was performed on a 14-year-old worker who fell down from the height of two floors. This boy would most probably have died due to a severed spleen if Dr. Riegner had not managed to completely tie off his splenic vessels (there had already been 1.5 liters of blood pooled in the boy's abdomen at the time of operation). In 1897, the first surgery of the beating heart was performed by

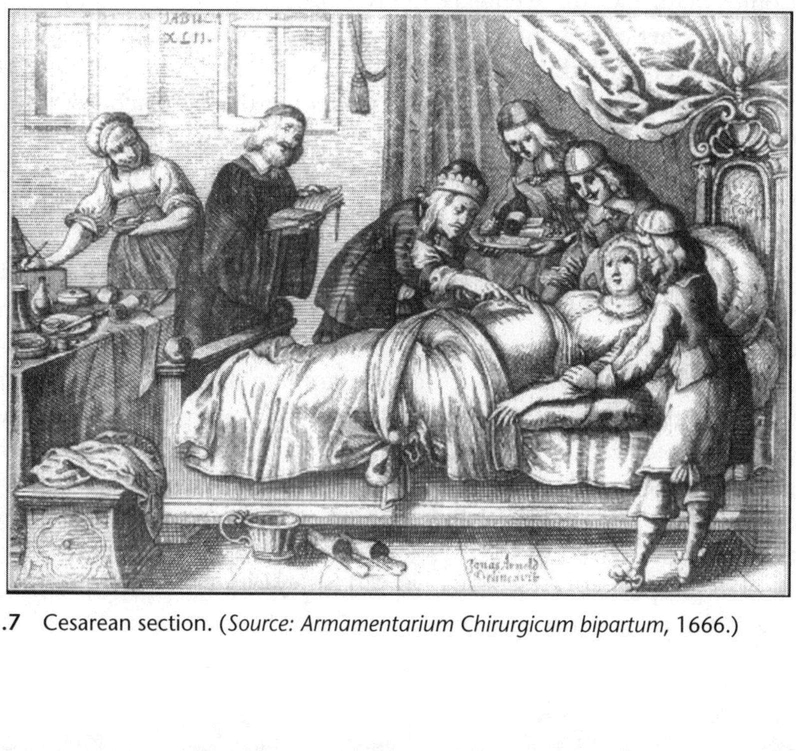

Figure 1.7 Cesarean section. (*Source: Armamentarium Chirurgicum bipartum*, 1666.)

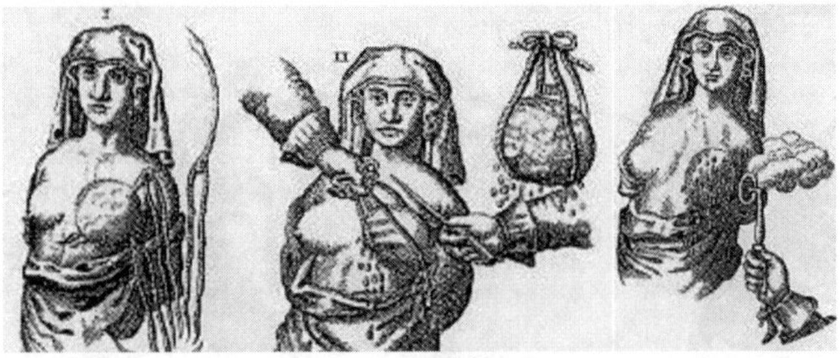

Figure 1.8 Mastectomy procedure. The instrument constricted the base of the breast, which was then amputated with a blade. The cautery was used to stop the bleeding. (*Source: Armamentarium Chirurgicum.*)

Dr. Rehn from Frankfurt. He wanted to save a young man who was stabbed with a knife into his left chest. After cutting through the interspace, Dr. Rehn resected the fifth rib, opened the pericardium and sutured the wound in the right ventricle, and finally packed the pericardial cavity. Amazingly, the patient survived and eventually fully recovered.

The most important developments of the nineteenth century were the introduction of anesthesia into everyday practice and the development of antiseptic and aseptic surgery procedures. Some form of anesthesia was likely applied from the earliest days in an attempt to reduce the pain of injury and surgical procedures. For anesthesia purpose, poppies were occasionally mentioned in Egyptian medicine, while the extract of the coca plant was used by South American practitioners. Large doses of alcohol, opium, or mandragora were also utilized to make patients oblivious to the horror of the performed procedures. Inhaling nitrous oxide (laughing gas) was apparently popular as a party drug in the eighteenth century, and it was accidentally discovered by a chemist Humphry Davy (1778–1829) as capable of diminishing physical pain. However almost a century passed until a dentist from Connecticut, Horace Wells (1815–1848), was the first to apply nitrous oxide gas as an anesthetic, to achieve painless tooth removal. The gas was administered from an animal bladder through a wooden tube placed in the mouth of the patient. Dr. Wells went to Boston to show his discovery at the Massachusetts General Hospital in 1845. His experiment failed miserably but he continued to use nitrous oxide in his own practice. At the same time, Dr. Morton, also a dentist, happened to observe Dr. Wells failed demonstration and decided to use ether during dental extractions, with complete success. Dr. Morton offered his anesthesia method to Massachusetts General Hospital and it was first applied there during surgery in 1846. The patient was a 21-year-old servant girl undergoing leg amputation due to the tuberculosis of the knee joint. Before the amputation, she was exposed to gas utilizing an ether inhaler developed by Dr. Morton. The amputation was completely painless (when the patient recovered from anesthesia she was not aware that her leg was already cut off). This event marked the end of a long era of horrible sufferings of surgery patients (at least in Western civilization) who had little to count on during the procedures but prayers and the surgeon's speed. The surgeons of these times had to be trained to be able to amputate a leg in less than 30 seconds.

Dr. Joseph Lister, Professor of Surgery at Glasgow Royal Infirmary, is considered a father of antiseptic surgery. In 1865, he applied undiluted carbolic acid on the compound fracture wounds in the leg of an 11-year-old boy [5]. The wound started to heal without the usual infection, and the patient walked out of a hospital in 6 weeks, which was quite a miracle. Before Lister's discovery, the infections encountered after injury or surgery often led to limb amputation or death. The late nineteenth century also represents the start of aseptic surgery, which was developed by German surgeons Dr. Neuber, Dr. Schimmelbush, and Dr. von Bergman. To diminish the exposure of open wounds to infectious agents, they introduced the use of steam sterilization of instruments, air filtration, and wearing of surgical gowns, masks, caps, and gloves. Before this development, the surgeons may have worn a gown to protect their clothes but no other protection (Figure 1.9).

The twentieth century brought many exciting new developments that made possible saving or prolonging the life of patients who previously had no chance of survival. These developments included organ transplantations, introduction of artificial organs, and significant advancements in heart surgery. The first successful kidney transplantation between identical twins took place in 1954 in Brigham Hospital in Boston. However, it took a few more decades to work out the challenging problem of immuno-induced organ rejection of the organs obtained from nonidentical donors. At a similar time, another approach was developed to save patients from dying from kidney failure. Artificial organs such as limbs, hands, and eyes were used for centuries to facilitate locomotion and for aesthetic reasons. However, the first artificial organ that could perform a complex functional task was an artificial kidney, a dialysis machine originally developed by Willem Kolff in the Netherlands in the late 1930s. This machine was able to filter blood impurities using a permeable cellophane membrane (Figure 1.10). By the 1950s, the importance of this discovery was recognized by Dr. Page from the Cleveland Clinic, and the company Travenol started to commercially manufacture artificial kidneys in 1956. Initially, dialysis was mostly used in acute cases of kidney failures (due to intoxication,

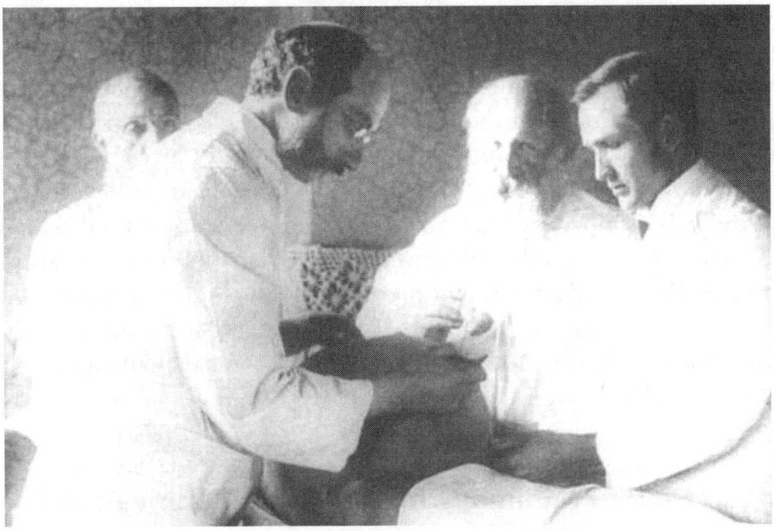

Figure 1.9 Surgeons performing a tumor operation at Terre Haute Sanitarium, Indiana, in 1893. Note the absence of gloves and surgical masks. (Image obtained from *Wabash Valley Magazine*, September/October 1992.)

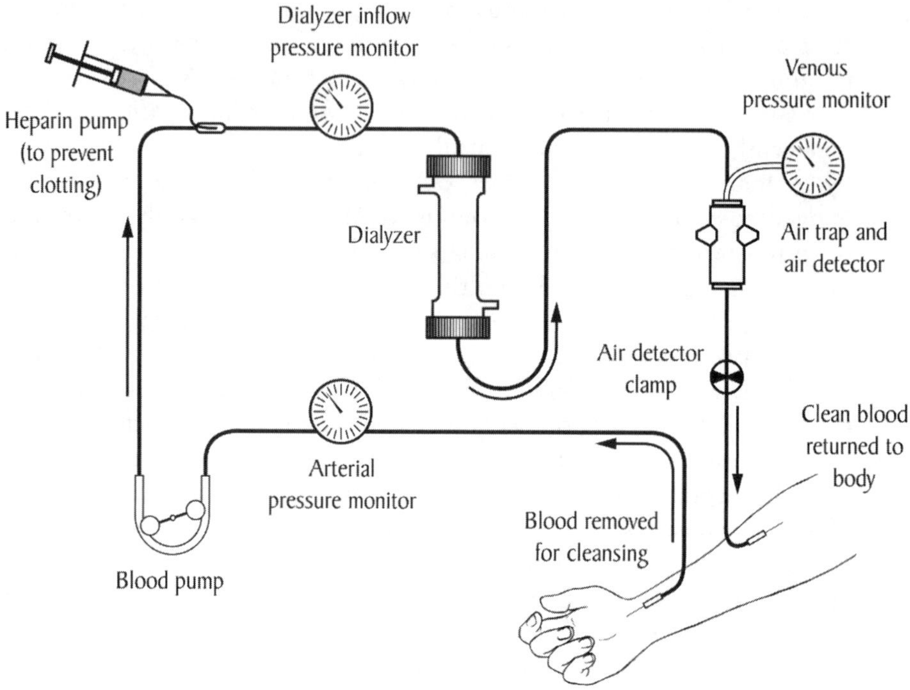

Figure 1.10 Artificial kidney. A schematic of the dialysis process. (Image obtained from the National Institute of Diabetes and Digestive and Kidney Diseases of the National Institutes of Health and the U.S. Department of Health and Human Services.)

burns, and so forth) in patients that could hopefully restore normal function, but was soon adopted as a method of prolonging life of patients suffering from end-stage renal disease.

Another exciting development occurred in 1952 when University of Minnesota surgeons, Drs. Lillehei and Lewis, performed the first successful open heart surgery in a 5-year-old girl born with a hole in her heart. This operation was made possible by the work of a Canadian surgeon Dr. Bigelow, who showed that at lower temperatures, the tissues of the body and brain needed less oxygen, and could survive without oxygenated blood for longer (10 minutes as opposed to 4 minutes). The girl was therefore cooled down to 27.2°C, her heart was opened after the blood inflow was stopped by clamping, and the hole was sutured. However, this hypothermic approach could only be performed for surgeries of heart defects that were not complex, since even a hypothermic person could not survive with no heart beat for long. The solution to this problem was heart-lung machine, which was finally ready for patient use in 1958 after various technical challenges (such as production of air embolisms) were solved.

1.4 Image-Guided Minimally Invasive and Noninvasive Therapies

Maybe the most important advancements occurring in the twentieth century were in the areas of minimally invasive surgery procedures. These advancements were predominantly made possible by a development of novel imaging modalities, which were usually very quickly adopted by surgeons and combined with appropriate therapy procedures. For example, the discovery of X-rays by Roentgen in 1895 was followed soon by their application in localization of foreign bodies and diagnosis of fractures, published in the *Lancet* in 1896. These early radiological procedures were fairly unsophisticated, as compared to today's standards (Figure 1.11). The image resolution was low and the procedure required about 10 minutes of exposure time, resulting in dangerously high delivered doses of radiation. However, these images provided the first exciting opportunity to observe the insides of the body for a more definitive diagnosis. Diagnostic applications of X-rays were soon followed by their applications in therapy. Radiation therapy in the treatment of early breast cancer was pioneered at the Curie Institute in Paris around 1936. The subsequent studies showed that local extraction of tumors combined with radiotherapy had comparable results with mastectomy, with similar survival rates. Figure 1.12 shows a painting of a radiologist performing radiation of a breast cancer. Note that he wears no protection, since the deleterious effects of X-rays were not really known at the time. Unfortunately, many of the early X-rays researchers (including Maria and Pierre Curie) developed terminal diseases as a result of excessive exposure to X-rays.

As another example, almost as soon as the electrical bulb was miniaturized into an electric cytoscope in 1879, it was utilized in providing illumination during examinations of the bladder interior. In 1901, Georg Kelling from Dresden placed a cytoscope into the peritoneal cavity to observe the effect of increased pneumoperitoneal pressures on the small bowel, which was one of the first diagnostic laparoscopy procedures. In 1937, Hope described the use of peritoneoscopy as a method for diagnosing of ectopic pregnancy. By the 1930s, the laparoscopy procedures were not performed just for diagnosis but also for therapy. In 1933, the first lysis of adhesions was described, followed by a report in 1936 on the tubal ligation with electrocoagulation. Around this time, laparoscopy also became a method for obtaining intraperitoneal biopsies and draining of ascites. Burns and the risk of electrocution presented a serious problem in these early days of laparoscopy. The major

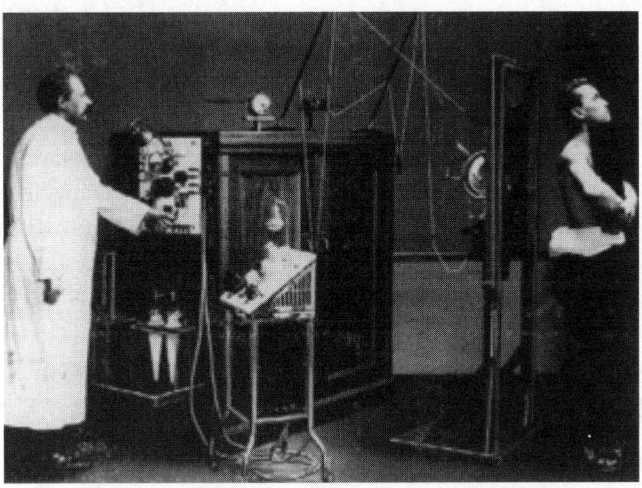

Figure 1.11 The original X-ray system for observation of patient lungs. Note that the patient has to hold the imaging cassette.

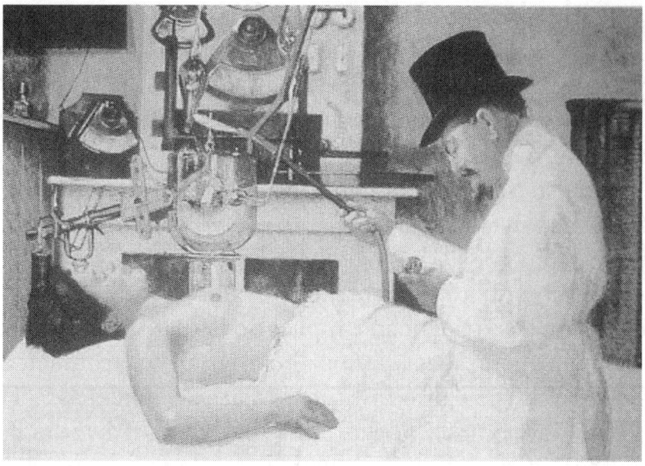

Figure 1.12 Painting of breast cancer irradiation circa 1908.

technology advances in the early 1950s allowed further development of laparoscopy techniques. The first was the discovery of cold light by Forestier in 1952. This was based on the fiberglass illumination technology that produced an intense light at low temperatures, reducing the chances of intraperitoneal burns and improving the image quality. The other major advance came in 1953 by a development of a rod lens system which doubled the light carrying capacity of the laparoscope, allowing production of a bright, true color image. Modern laparoscope consists of a rod lens system that is usually connected to a video camera and monitor, and a fiber optic cable connected to a cold light source (halogen or xenon) inserted into the body via canula through a small incision, to illuminate the operative field. Additional various specialized surgical instruments can be introduced through side ports to perform the surgery (Figure 1.13).

Today, diagnostic laparoscopy is often used in gynecology to determine causes of persistent pelvic pain and also for staging of the malignancy of abdominal organs to determine whether palliative or curative approaches should be taken. Even very high resolution imaging techniques such as CT and MRI, often fail to detect small metastases in the peritoneal cavity or on the surface of the liver, which can be observed easily during laparoscopic procedures. The therapeutic laparoscopic applications are also numerous. In 1985, a German physician Dr. Muhe performed the first laparoscopy cholecystetomy (removal of a gallbladder), which is one of the most common laparoscopic procedures today. Other applications include removal of tumors in the liver and bowels, appendectomy, removal of adrenal glands, and gastric bypass surgery in obese patients. Also, robotic-assisted surgery has been implemented for operations in which fine movements and precision are critical (Figure 1.14). So far these robot-assisted surgical devices (e.g., da Vinci Surgical System) have been used for the positioning of endoscope, and in general, urologic, gynecologic, and cardiothoracic procedures. The eventual goal is to design a robot that can perform truly challenging procedures, for example, a closed-chest beating-heart surgery.

Similar to laparoscopy, catheter angiographic procedure started as a purely diagnostic method and is now extensively used in therapy. The first attempts at

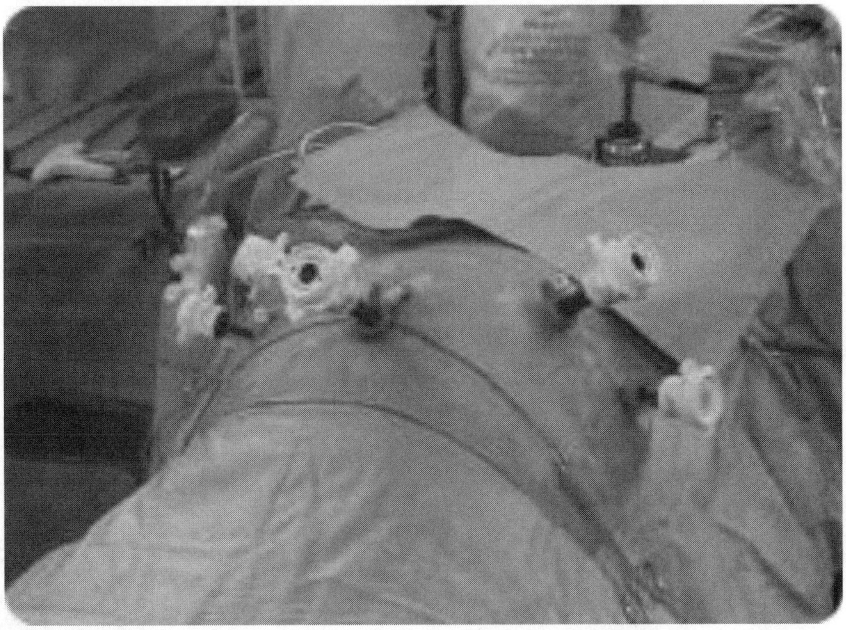

Figure 1.13 An example of a laparoscopy setup. (*Source:* http://www.laparoscopicurology.co.uk/. Reprinted with permission.)

cardiac catheterization and angiocariodgraphy were performed by Dr. Forsmann in 1929, who introduced urologic catheter from brachial vein into right atrium of his own heart, and observed it with X-rays [6]. By the 1940s this approach was used for measurements of heart pressures in normal and diseased hearts. The therapeutic breakthrough happened in 1977, when Gruentzig and Hoff designed a balloon dilation catheter for use in the coronary arteries, thus providing a life-saving treatment for the patients with ischemic heart disease. In this method, under real-time X-ray guidance (i.e., fluoroscopy), a catheter is directed into an obstructed coronary artery, and a guide wire is placed across obstructed area (i.e., atherosclerosic lesion).

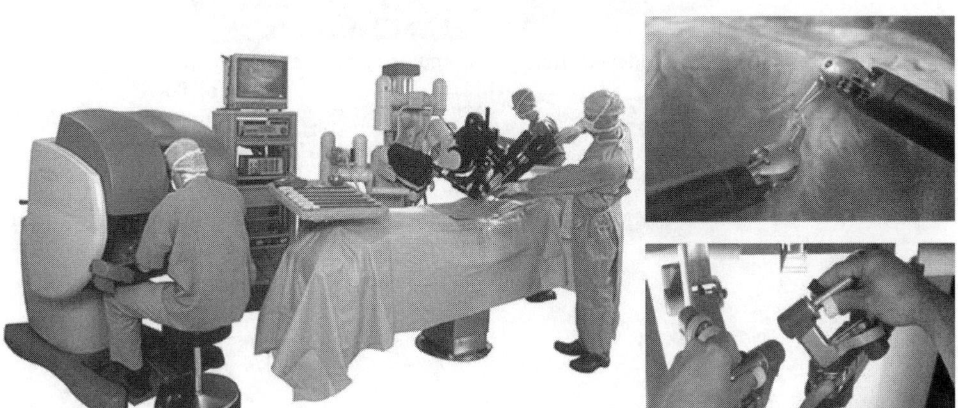

Figure 1.14 Robotic-assisted surgery. The surgeon's hands movements are translated into robotic movements that have finer control and less tremor. (Photos courtesy of Intuitive Surgical, Inc., 2009.)

A balloon catheter is then passed over the guide wire and inflated to reduce the degree of coronary obstruction (Figure 1.15). This treatment is currently performed in more than 400,000 patients per year in the United States [7].

Imaging developments of the 1950s through the 1970s introduced to the medical field diagnostic ultrasound, radionuclide imaging techniques, magnetic resonance imaging (MRI), and computed tomography (CT). All of these methods keep being improved to date, thus allowing better resolution, better contrast, and easier observation of the pathological changes in the tissue, even when these changes are still very small (of a millimeter in size). The diagnostic developments were followed by the development of novel therapeutic methods, such as lasers, argon beam co-

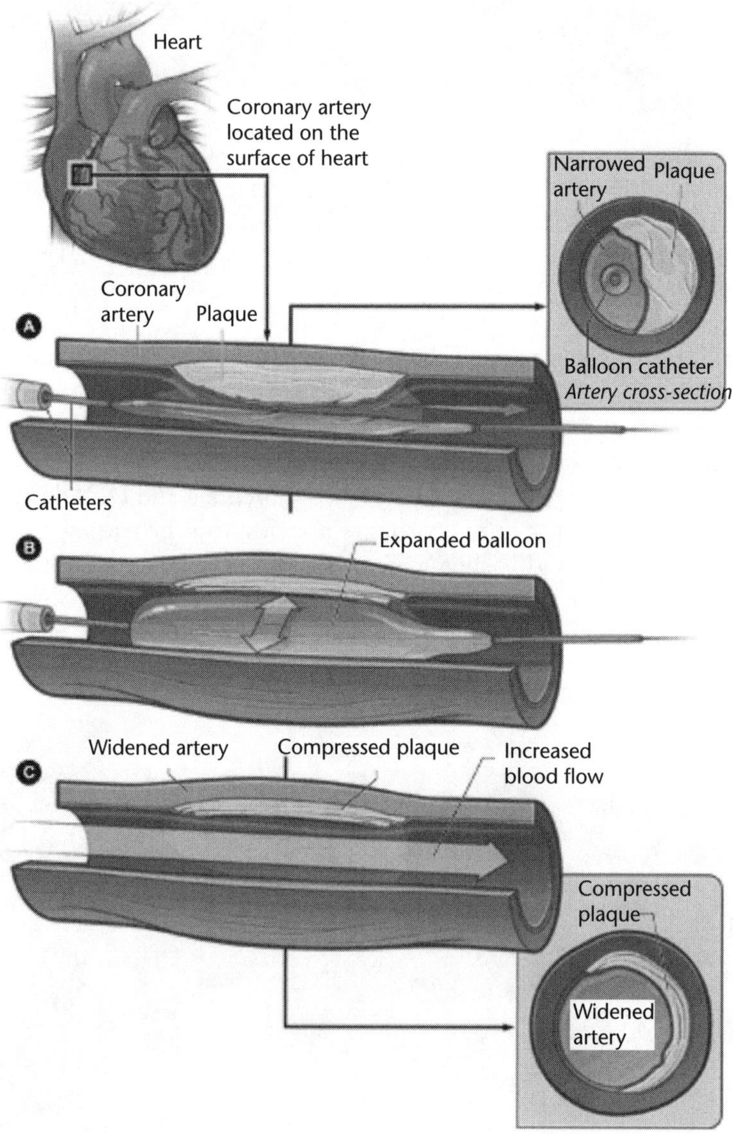

Figure 1.15 Angioplasty of a narrowed coronary artery. (Image obtained from the National Heart, Lung, and Blood Institute of the National Institutes of Health and the U.S. Department of Health and Human Services.)

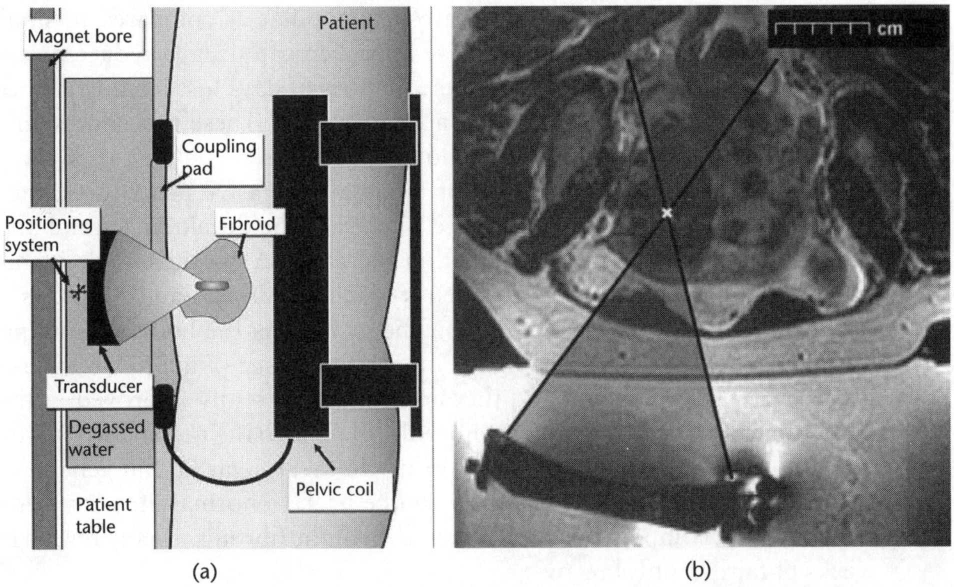

Figure 1.16 MRI-guided HIFU treatment of uterine fibroids: (a) tumor is treated noninvasively using focused ultrasound waves; and (b) treatment is guided using MRI imaging, which allows excellent observation of the anatomy and temperature measurements at the treatment site. (*From:* [8]. © 2003 Radiological Society of North America. Reprinted with permission.)

agulator, RF ablation, and gamma knife. Currently an amazingly large number of minimally invasive procedures are offered in the hospitals of the developed world. Just to name a few: cardiovascular procedures (e.g., restoration of heart valves and patent foramen ovale), gastroenterologic and colon surgery (e.g., laparoscopic treatment of inflammatory bowel disease), gynecological procedures (e.g., uterine artery embolization for fibroids, removal of benign ovarian cysts), and neurosurgery (e.g., volumetric stereotactic resection of brain tumors, gamma knife sterotac-

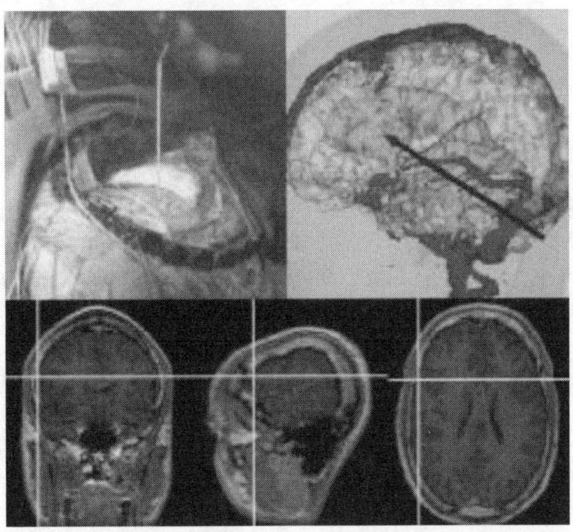

Figure 1.17 Brain surgery research done at the MIT CSAIL Lab and Brigham and Women's Hospital. A 3D functional MRI model is used to evaluate the location and size of the tumor. Custom-made software is used to perform the surgery planning; that is, find the path that a surgical tool should follow to extract the tumor with minimal damage to important brain regions.

tic radiosurgery). Such procedures are very popular as compared to similar open surgeries, since the minimally invasive approach can usually reduce postoperative pain, speed up recovery and reduce the number of days lost from work, reduce the potential complications, and result in smaller scars. These procedures will be covered in much greater detail in the following chapters.

As a follow-up to the success of minimally invasive procedures, the twenty-first century has brought an increased interest in the development and application of completely noninvasive nonradiation therapies. A good example is the current popularity of image-guided high-intensity focused ultrasound (HIFU), as a modality capable of delivering cauterization energy deep in the body without producing any cuts in the skin or damaging the intervening tissue (Figure 1.16). This therapy, guided with MRI imaging and thermometry, is currently approved in the United States for the treatment of uterine fibroids [8]. Due to the noninvasive nature of this method, patients are only sedated during the treatment, and in general can leave the hospital immediately afterwards and be back to normal life activities within a day or two. In comparison, surgical removal of the fibroids usually results in several weeks of fairly painful recovery.

The future will likely bring improvements in both diagnosis and therapy. Examples of further developments include: image fusion of CT, MRI, and PET images to obtain complete anatomical and metabolic information about tumors as well as healthy sensitive structures that should not be damaged during the procedure (Figure 1.17), real-time 3D imaging, real-time integration of imaging with various treatment modalities, overlaying tissue depth imaging information over the surgeon's visual field for easy access to treatment areas, and real-time instrument tracking to allow their correct placement deep under the organ surface. The final goal is to make even major surgical operations fast and minimally disruptive to the patient's daily life, while still keeping the high safety of such procedures.

References

[1] Magner, L. N., *A History of Medicine*, 2nd ed., New York: Taylor and Francis Group, 2005.

[2] Ellis, H., *A History of Surgery*, Greenwich Medical Media, Cambridge University Press, 2002.

[3] Saraf, S., and R. S. Parihar, "Sushruta: The First Plastic Surgeon in 600 B.C.," *The Internet Journal of Plastic Surgery*, Vol. 4, No. 2, 2007.

[4] Milne, J. S., *Surgical Instruments in Greek and Roman Times*, Oxford, U.K.: Claredon Press, 1907.

[5] Ellis, H., *Operations That Made History*, Greenwich Medical Media, Cambridge University Press, 1996.

[6] Wilms, G., and A. L. Baert, "The History of Angiography," *J. Belge. Radiol.*, Vol. 78, 1995, pp. 299–302.

[7] LeBoutillier, M., III, and V. J. DiSesa, "Ischemic Heart Disease," in M.W. Mulholland et al., (eds.), *Greenfield's Surgery: Scientific Principles and Practice*, 4th ed., Philadelphia, PA: Lippincott Williams & Wilkins, 2006, pp. 1477–1496.

[8] Tempany, C. M. C., et al., "MR Imaging–Guided Focused Ultrasound Surgery of Uterine Leiomyomas: A Feasibility Study," *Radiology*, Vol. 226, 2003, p. 897.

CHAPTER 2

Medical Imaging

Orpheus Kolokythas, Dean K. Shibata, and Theodore J. Dubinsky

Medical imaging has undergone tremendous changes since the discovery of X-rays in 1895 by Wilhelm C. Röntgen. Depending on the organ of interest, lesion location, size, availability of imaging systems, and operators' expertise, a plethora of imaging techniques now exists to guide diagnostic and therapeutic procedures. With the advent of flexible fiber optics, endoscopy has now largely replaced fluoroscopic radiographic techniques for the exploration of hollow organs and cavities of the body. Cross-sectional imaging modalities such as ultrasound, computed tomography (CT), and magnetic resonance imaging (MRI) are predominately used for the evaluation of parenchymal organs, such as the brain, musculoskeletal system, liver, pancreas, kidneys, and spleen, which are not otherwise accessible without invasive approaches. These methods are even beginning to play a significant role in the evaluation of hollow organs, because they are less invasive compared with endoscopic methods and offer visual as well as functional information. In some organs such as the small bowel or bone marrow the desired information cannot be obtained with any other modalities.

However, cross-sectional imaging techniques have limitations: they do not offer real color information about inflamed or malignant epithelial surfaces as endoscopy does, and the clinical information needed often depends on the administration of intravenous contrast or tracer materials, which carry the potential for adverse side effects. Another limitation in comparison to endoscopic methods is the lack of immediate access for obtaining tissue specimens. However, ultrasound, CT, and MR can be used to guide diagnostic procedures such as aspirations and biopsies, and therapies such as drainage of fluid collections, nerve blockages, and tumor ablations. A combination of imaging methods is indicated in specific situations: endoscopic retrograde cholangio-pancreatography (ERCP) is the classical imaging method that combines real-time fluoroscopy with endoscopy. It is used to visualize the duodenal papilla and to obtain morphologic and tissue information from the biliary and pancreatic ducts. For CT myelography a contrast agent is injected into the arachnoidal space and for MR arthrography contrast is injected into a joint; both methods are using real-time fluoroscopy to guide the injection needle safely and accurately into the target. Using this combination technique both modalities provide better information about the cavities and bordering structures they are intended to visualize than CT or MR alone.

Fusion imaging of two cross-sectional imaging modalities coregisters CT or MR data sets with real-time sonography or with one another and has been recently introduced to achieve percutaneous access to targets in the body that cannot be approached by one imaging method alone [1, 2].

This chapter will give an overview over the various modern imaging modalities that exist; it will focus on the methods that can also be used to guide diagnostic and therapeutic procedures of any desired organ or target within the body. The technology behind the most common imaging methods will be discussed in more detail in the subsequent chapters.

2.1 Ultrasound

Ultrasound is widely available and is the only method that is portable, which allows it to be used at the patient's bedside. This is a key advantage for critically ill patients who would be at risk if moved to another examination room. Even though ultrasound is the primary modality for image-guided procedures in the operating room (OR), OR compatible MR guidance systems have been developed [3–7].

Ultrasonography provides imaging and guidance without exposing the patient or personnel to ionizing radiation as does CT or to significant electromagnetic fields as does MR.

Beyond these technical advantages, ultrasound is also the most cost efficient guidance tool [8]. There are, however, significant technical challenges with ultrasound: lesions located behind gas containing structures such as the lung, stomach, or bowel, or behind bones cannot be visualized. Also, lesions located in central anatomic locations of the body such as the pancreas, retroperitoneal lymph nodes, and pelvic masses will often not be accessible to ultrasound. Since ultrasound is based on the visualization of tissue interfaces, highly reflecting parenchymal organs such as fatty livers may decrease the acoustic penetration. In ultrasound-guided procedures such as percutaneous biopsies of tumor ablations this may be the case even to a degree that either the target or the probe or both are not visualized to the extent needed to enable a confident and safe execution of the intervention. Also, the fact that a certain angle would have to be used to visualize the needle device—with or without a physical guiding device—may pose an obstacle since interleaving structures such as bones, hollow organs, the gallbladder, bile ducts in the liver, and vessels may be in the planned biopsy path. In these cases CT guidance may be used allowing other options for needle angulation to the target (Figure 2.1).

Depending on the operator's expertise, however, trajectories through the small bowel using fine needle techniques are possible to achieve access to deeply located biopsy targets [9].

2.1.1 Fundamental Ultrasound

Ultrasound offers unique advantages over all other imaging modalities: In fundamental mode (so called B-mode) it allows real-time guidance at imaging frame rates over 50 Hz at a high spatial resolution. Depending on the transducers used, frequency, depth of scan, specific organ, and other parameters, the resolution of ultrasound may be in the order of 0.5 mm with a curvilinear transducer, and 0.2 mm with a linear transducer. However, almost all real-time guidance can now be

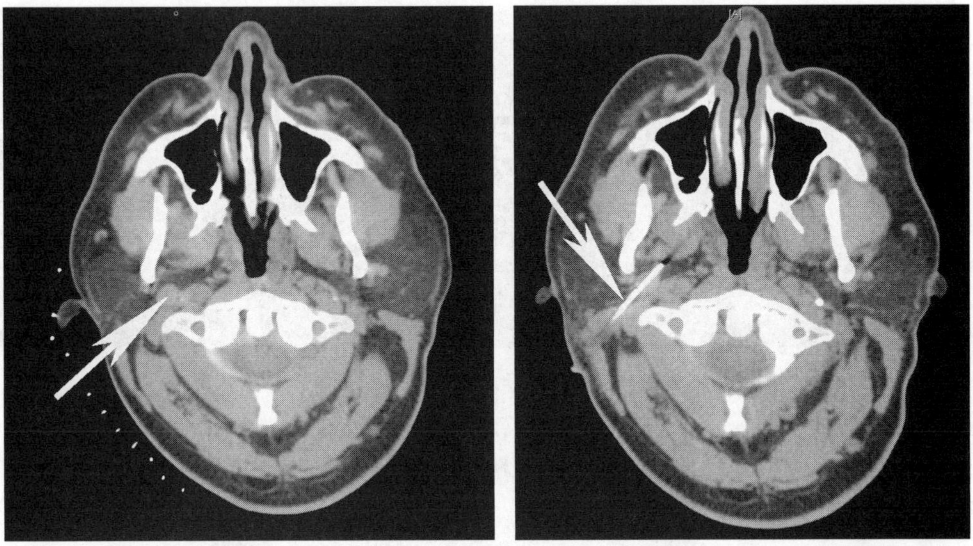

(a) (b)

Figure 2.1 (a) CT-guided parotid tumor pre biopsy. On this noncontrast axial CT scan through the face, there is a small 5-mm soft tissue mass (arrow) within the deep lobe of the right parotid gland in this patient with prior tumor resection superficially and concern for recurrence on follow-up imaging. (b) CT-guided parotid tumor needle biopsy. Now a 20 gauge needle is seen directed with CT guidance via a posterior lateral approach into the small mass to obtain a fine needle aspiration. Cytology revealed pleomorphic adenoma.

achieved with CT fluoroscopy at frame rates in the range of six frames per second and MRI at a range of 10 to 20 frames per second, both at millimeter or less resolution [10, 11]. Real-time guidance is useful and often indispensable to increase the safety and decrease the duration of a procedure (Figure 2.2).

Contrast resolution of ultrasound, however, may be lower than CT or MR in some instances, sometimes resulting in nonvisualization of the target. This possible limitation is now in many situations alleviated by the administration of intravenous sonographic contrast agents when available (see Section 2.1.3).

2.1.2 Doppler Ultrasound

Doppler ultrasound is the sonographic quantification and visualization of flow. Color-coded Doppler ultrasound displays both blood flow and direction. This may be helpful when guiding percutaneous instruments such as biopsy or ablation probes into organs, which have multiple blood vessels within or overlying the lesion of interest. Color Doppler ultrasound may be helpful in identifying those vessels, which provides useful information for planning and executing a percutaneous or intraoperative procedure safely. Damage to blood vessels may otherwise result in significant complications. Such complications include penetration trauma to blood vessels with the introducing device resulting in bleeding, arterio-venous fistulas, and unintended thrombosis of vessels due to therapeutic procedures such as radiofrequency ablation of tumors.

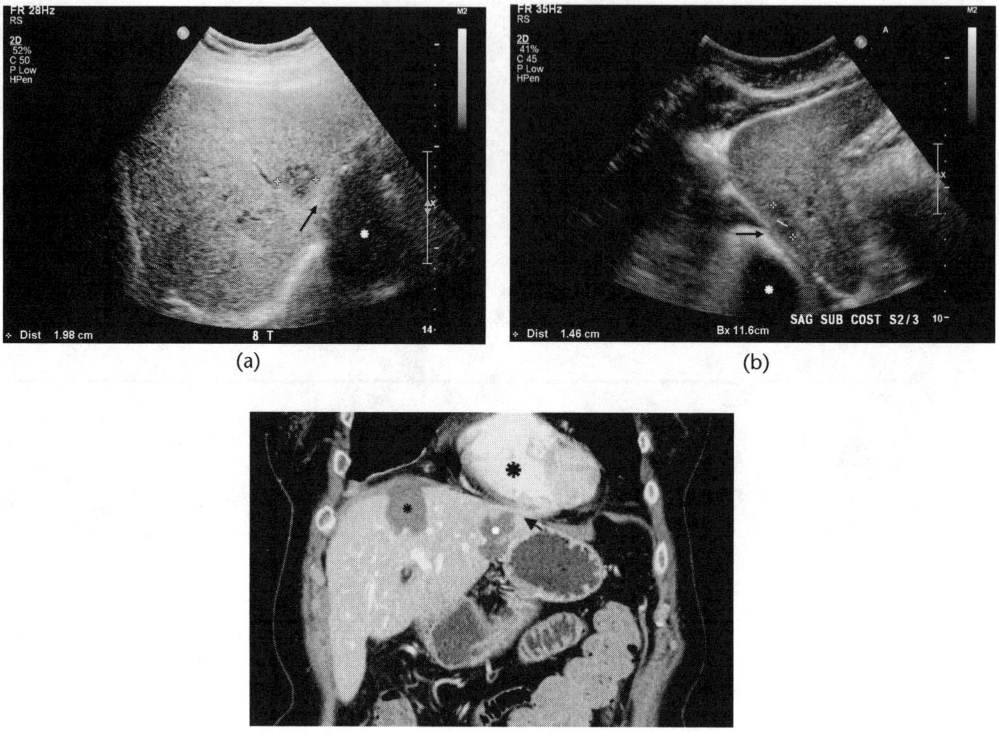

(c)

Figure 2.2 Ultrasound-guided percutaneous radiofrequency ablation (RFA) of a colorectal metastasis in the left lobe of the liver adjacent to the heart. Ultrasound of the liver in (a) transverse and (b) sagittal orientation previous to the RFA demonstrates small hypoechoic mass (++) in close proximity to the heart (large black ✱) and abutting the diaphragm (arrow). Dotted line in (b) represents the planned trajectory of the RFA probe. Close proximity of the mass to the right ventricle required precise positioning of the RFA probe in breath hold with real-time guidance, precluding CT as a guidance tool. (c) Contrast enhanced CT taken 2 months later demonstrates complete ablation of tumor site (white small asterix) abutting the diaphragm (arrow). Black small asterisk indicates second site of successful tumor ablation (black large asterisk over the right ventricle of the heart).

2.1.3 Contrast Enhanced Ultrasound

Contrast enhanced ultrasound (CEUS) is a method using a suspension of microspheres as a reflective agent to enhance the reflected transmit pulse. While this can be used to visualize fluids in the genitourinary system or cavities in the gastro-intestinal system, by far the widest application is intravenous administration to enhance organs, blood vessels, and tumors. Ultrasound contrast agents undergo specific interactions when exposed to the acoustic pulse, resulting in a harmonic signal [12]. They contain microscopic bubbles in the range of 5 to 10 micrometers and are thus smaller than red blood cells; this allows them to pass safely through the capillary vessels without causing occluding side effects. Depending on the mechanical index chosen and based on the nature of the agent's membrane, the reflected signal may be a result of the destruction of the bubble, or may be the result of an oscillating movement of its shell.

The first generation contrast agents were made out of a more rigid capsule, which would be destroyed when exposed to the ultrasound pulse [13]. The result is a bright, very short reflection. The advantage of this mechanism lies in the intensity of the reflected signal, making it a very sensitive method for bubble detection. However, the major disadvantage of these agents is the inability to be visualized in the same imaging plane for longer than a few frames since the microspheres would be immediately destroyed after exposure to the first acoustic pulse.

The microspheres of the second generation contrast agents are made of a different, more flexible shell; this results in an oscillating reaction to the sonographic beam if a low enough mechanical index, usually below 0.2, is chosen. Since the agent is not destroyed when exposed to the pulse, it can be visualized for a longer period of time in the same imaging session. This property is key to the ability to evaluate contrast kinetics of an organ or mass. However, it requires specific measures to detect the agents, since the low mechanical index, which is mandatory for a nondestructive imaging mode, results in significantly reduced image quality and sensitivity for contrast detection. Tissue cancellation techniques such as pulse inversion or power modulation have been developed to filter out the specific harmonic signal emanating from the acoustic interaction with the contrast agents [12, 14, 15].

CEUS has been shown to be more sensitive and specific in the detection and characterization of a variety of lesions, mostly masses within the liver, than fundamental ultrasound [16–18]. This is also the case for its intraoperative use, where a higher detection rate of metastases in the liver has been shown to change management in over 30% of patients [19].

CEUS as a guidance tool for percutaneous procedures has its place when the target cannot be seen or not seen well enough with conventional ultrasound. Lesions that would have been amenable to biopsy or procedure, otherwise only by more expensive and resource intensive methods such as CT or MR, may be visible by the use of ultrasound contrast agents even within the interventional suite. CEUS adds the advantage of high spatial and temporal resolution over CT and MR guidance for lesions difficult to reach, for example, when percutaneous tumor ablation is planned on tumors located in the dome of the liver or close to diaphragm, lungs, and heart (Figure 2.3).

Its cost effectiveness over CT and MR has been shown recently [20]. Other major advantages over iodine or gadolinium contrast agents are repeatable injectability, which is crucial for procedure guidance, decreased nephro-toxicity, and minimal allergic potential.

With the advent of transducers capable of three- and four-dimensional ultrasound contrast imaging, dynamic bolus analyses and dedicated display options are available to detect, characterize, and display vascular and pathologic structures, similar to other volumetric imaging methods. This may be advantageous when interventional procedures such as tumor ablations are planned on lesions that are not or not well seen on conventional ultrasound and that cannot be performed with CT or MR guidance (Figure 2.4).

One limitation of CEUS, however, is its limited availability: while it is widely used for a variety of indications and organs in European and Asian countries, ultrasound contrast agents are not approved by regulatory bodies in the United States for other than the diagnostic evaluation of the left cardiac ventricle. Also, CEUS is subject to some of the same technical limitations as is conventional ultrasound; and furthermore, higher costs, a stronger dependence on acoustic penetration, and

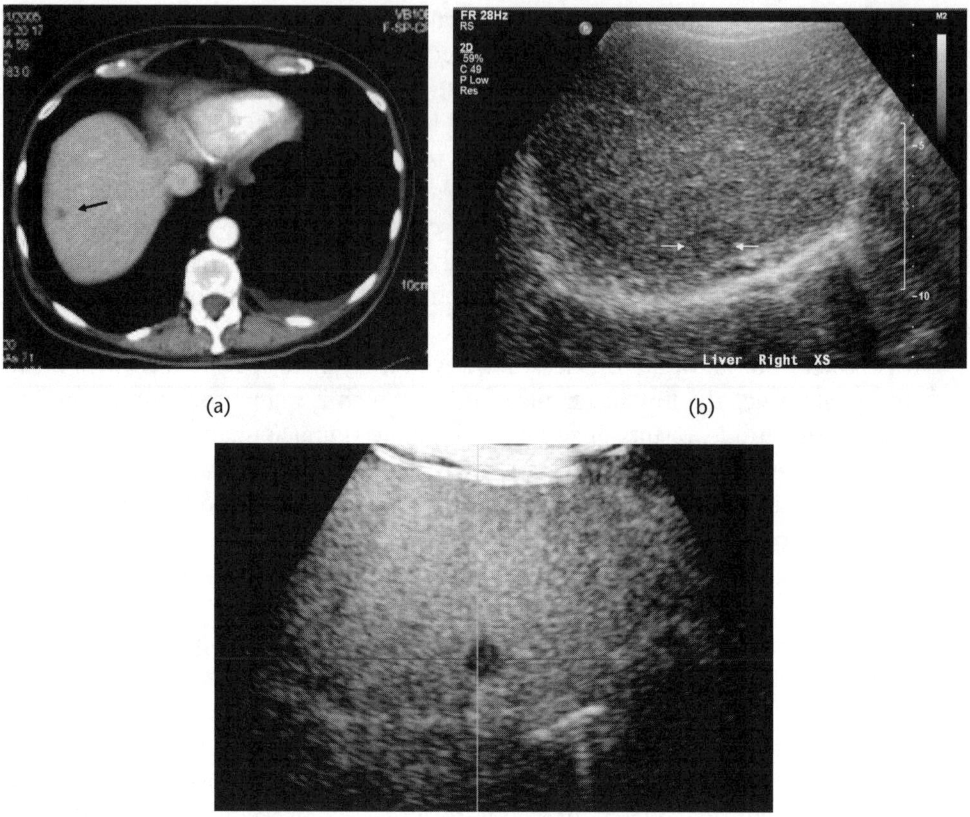

(a) (b)

(c)

Figure 2.3 Patient with small colorectal metastasis on the dome of the liver. (a) Contrast enhanced CT demonstrates a small hypodense metastasis in the right lobe of the liver. (b) Fundamental ultrasound shows a vague, small isoechoic lesion in similar location, suspicious for the metastasis. However, since the lesion was difficult to find and was not confidently seen in other orientations than the axial scanning direction, CEUS was performed to confirm the diagnosis prior to percutaneous tumor ablation. (c) CEUS clearly demonstrates hypoechoic mass (cross hair) in the portal-venous contrast phase, corresponding well to the lesion on CT and to the suspicious area previously suggested on fundamental ultrasound. CEUS increased the confidence of the operator and allowed visualization in multiple imaging planes. Mass was treated successfully with uncomplicated percutaneous radiofrequency ablation.

specific hardware and software requirements as well as operator and interpretation expertise are involved in the application of this method.

2.1.4 New Technologies for Guidance

New transducer technology such as real-time 3D (4D) using a matrix probe design opens new pathways to visualize the interventional needle in another plane simultaneously to the primary plane at a higher temporal resolution than mechanically driven oscillating 3D/4D probes. This may overcome partial volume effects in the primary imaging plane, which sometimes may compromise the conspicuity of the needle tip. Biplane ultrasound may allow real-time visualization of organs or structures in close proximity to the target that are otherwise only seen by sweeping in and out of the needle plane or by choosing a different image orientation (Figure 2.5).

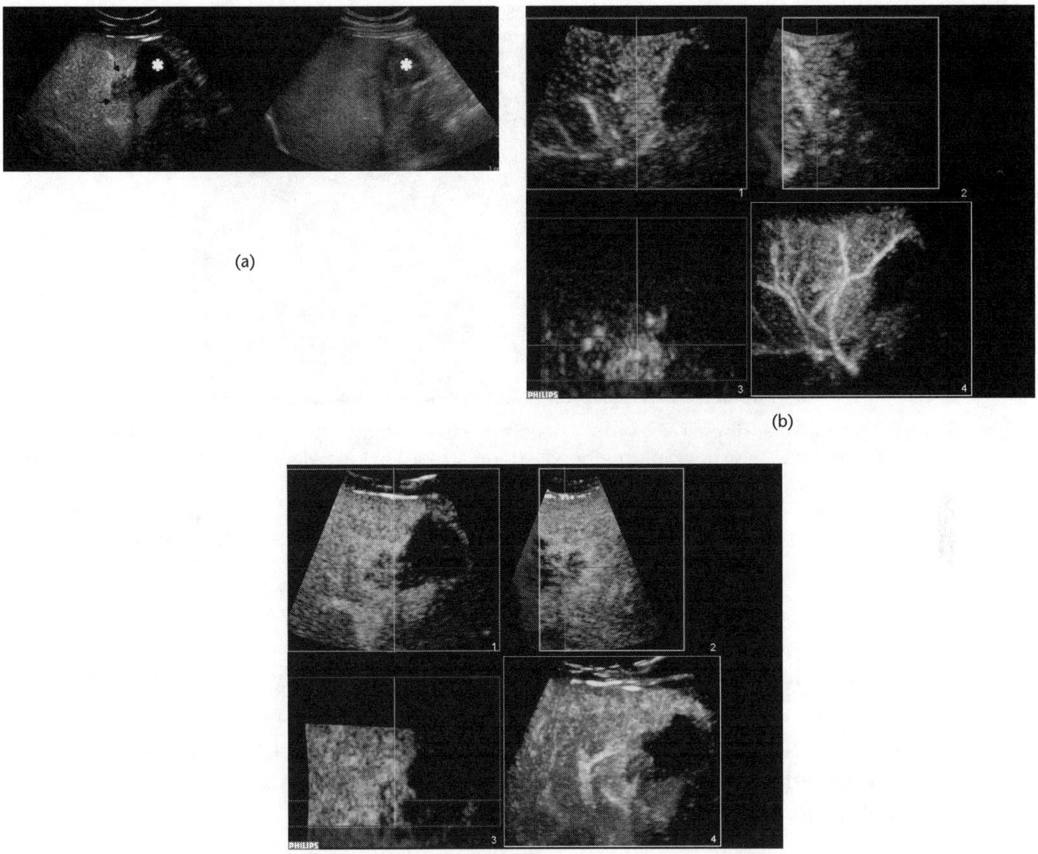

(a) (b) (c)

Figure 2.4 Contrast enhanced ultrasound in a patient with locally recurrent colorectal metastasis, previously treated with percutaneous radiofrequency ablation and now referred for repeated percutaneous tumor ablation. (a) Two-dimensional intercostally obtained ultrasound of the liver: side-by-side display demonstrates CEUS on the left and simultaneous conventional ultrasound on the right. Note that CEUS demonstrates an enhancing mass (arrows), clearly distinguishing the metastasis from the adjacent nonenhancing previous RFA site (✱), while conventional ultrasound does not allow precise distinction and characterization of the recurrent mass from the RFA site. (b) Four-dimensional volumetric acquisition of different contrast phases using a mechanically steered oscillating curved array transducer: 4D mode obtained through the same narrow acoustic window (intercostal space) allows multiplanar display of one volume at high temporal resolution and in various imaging planes that cannot be obtained due to anatomic obstacles such as ribs and bowl gas: 1 = scanning plane (axial); 2 = nonobtainable sagittal; 3 = nonobtainable coronal plane, all demonstrating that the mass is actually hypervascular on arterial phase (cross hair), typical for metastasis; and 4 = three-dimensional rendition allowing analysis of spatial relationship of the recurrent mass to surrounding arteries. (c) 4D of the same volume obtained a few seconds later in the portalvenous phase: previously hypervascular metastasis now is hypovascular (cross hair), consistent with "wash-out" contrast kinetics, characteristic for a malignant mass. Again, vessels and their spatial relation to the mass can be analyzed in multiplanar 2D reformations (1–3) or in the three-dimensional rendition (4). This frame is focusing on the portal and hepatic veins.

This novel method has not been investigated thoroughly and it remains to be seen if it proves to be a problem solving method for challenging targets or if it may serve as a tool to increase safety of the procedure and the confidence level of the operator.

Tissue Doppler imaging has been recently introduced to increase needle conspicuity in the deep locations or within tissue with poor acoustic penetration such as

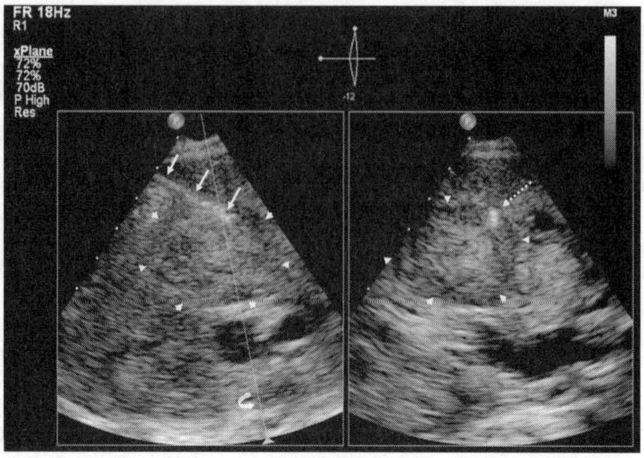

Figure 2.5 Biplanar display of a biopsy needle in a liver metastasis using a matrix probe (3-1 MHz). Left part of the displays shows biopsy needle (long arrows) in long view located in the upper portion of the concentrically hyper- and hypoechoic mass (arrow heads). Thin line (curved arrow) represents reference plane, which can be adjusted using a trackball. Right side of the image displays secondary imaging plane in real time, orthogonal to the primary guidance plane. Biopsy needle is seen as a small dot (dotted arrow).

fatty livers [21]. This method takes advantage of the sensitivity towards motion that is inherent to ultrasound Doppler and labels the moving needle as long as it is in motion and included in the imaging plane. The method is limited, however, by the acoustic penetration capabilities of the transducer, and has also not been evaluated for its clinical value (Figure 2.6).

2.2 Imaging Methods Using Ionizing Radiation

The utilization of ionizing radiation is the oldest form of medical imaging. Since the discovery of X-rays, a variety of methods have been developed in the field of medicine to utilize electromagnetic ionizing radiation for imaging purposes. They all are based on the principle that an image is generated when ionizing photons experience variable attenuation when passing through different substances before they cause a trace on the detector.

Radiographic methods producing an image without the need of a radioactive substance and nuclear modalities, depending on an injectable tracer, are being distinguished.

Two specific imaging principles within the nonnuclear imaging modalities have been developed: conventional radiography and radiodensitometry. Conventional radiography produces images based on differences in tissue density utilizing photons with a large spectrum of photon peak absorption coefficients. This results in the delivery of a large spectrum of grey scales in one image, which may provide very detailed anatomic spatial information. However, this method is not specific for the analysis of tissue quality, since the delivered image is a projected compound of the attenuation of photons of different energy spectrums passing though different tissues.

Radiodensitometry (=absorptiometry) utilizes photons of only one, or now sometimes two, known energy spectra (dual energy X-ray absorptiometry; DEXA).

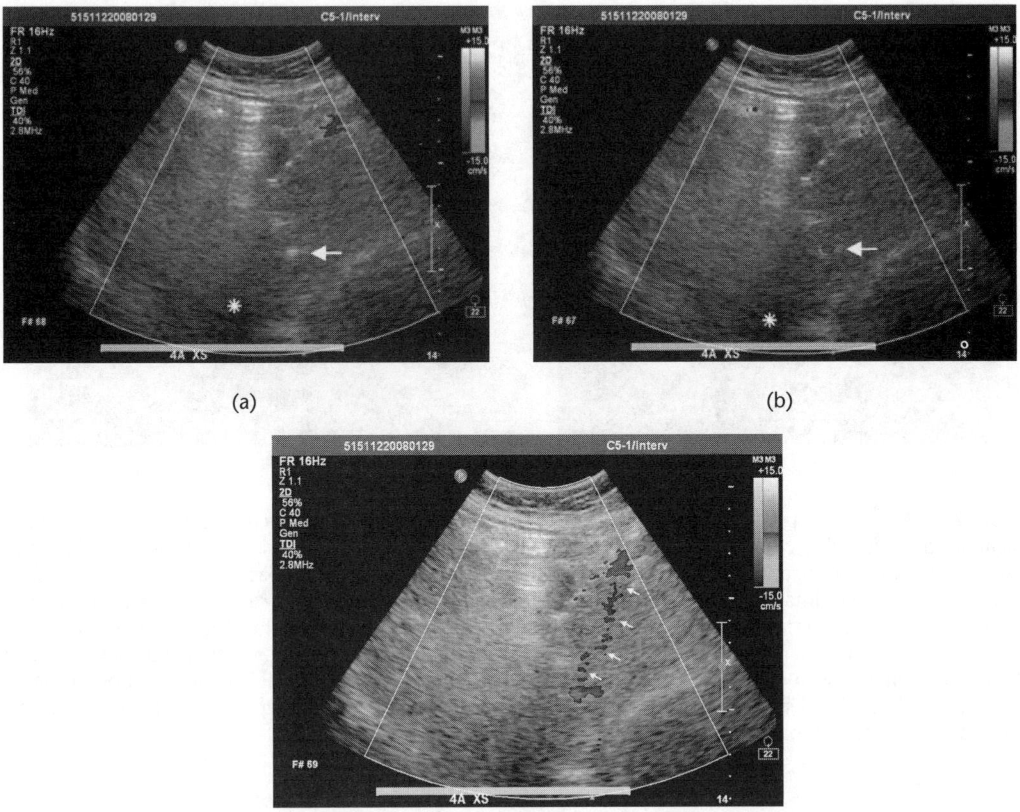

(c)

Figure 2.6 Needle guidance with sonographic tissue Doppler imaging (TDI) for tumor ablation in a patient with a poorly visualized tumor (✱). (a) Vaguely seen hypoechoic hepatocellular carcinoma in the left lobe of the liver. Echogenic needle tip is highlighted by the arrow. (b) Once the needle is moved slightly, a color dot is created at the needle tip (arrow). (c) Further movement of the needle results in colorful reflection along the entire needle shaft (arrows).

Any attenuation of energy in this modality can be attributed to the tissue qualities of the target tissues defined before, for example bone densitometry [22]. Conventional absorptiometry, however, has no role in image guidance; its cross-sectional equivalent imaging method Dual Energy CT (DE-CT) is a new modality and still has to be evaluated for its role as a diagnostic or guidance tool (see Section 2.2.2.1).

2.2.1 Conventional Radiography

2.2.1.1 Plain Film Radiography

Plain film radiography as a guidance tool is used in only a few selected instances. In contrast to fluoroscopy, radiography is a static imaging modality, hence the term "guidance" is probably not accurate; instead "plain film monitored" exam would be more precise.

The main indication for a procedure that is monitored by plain film is wire localization for operative excision of a lesion in the breast. These abnormalities

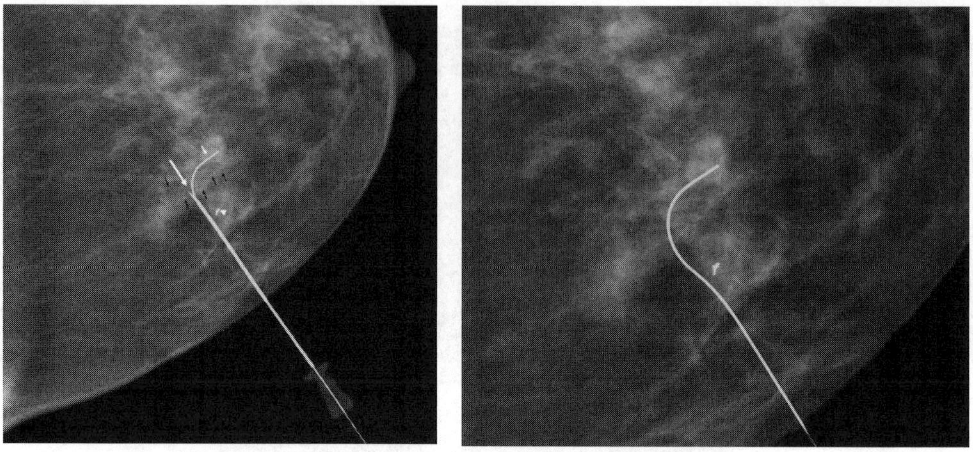

(a) (b)

Figure 2.7 Mammographic-guided wire localization of a group of microcalcifications in the breast. Fine calcifications are not visible with ultrasound or MRI. A marker clip was inserted during prior stereotactic vacuum assisted biopsy [arrow head in (a)]. Pathology revealed atypical ductal hyperplasia, which is associated with malignancy in approximately 20% of cases. Therefore, surgical excision was recommended. (a) Plain film mammogram demonstrates introducer needle (long arrow) through which the localization wire (short arrow) is advanced into the area of microcalcifications (black arrows). (b) The introducer needle has been removed. The localization wire is in ideal position marking the location of the microcalcifications. A portion of the wire extends out of the skin. Final histology of excised area revealed benign focal atypical ductal hyperplasia, sclerosing adenosis, papillomas, and no associated malignancy.

may be mass-like opacifications of the plain film or microcalcifications or both. Microcalcifications can only be seen confidently and reproducibly by high-resolution plain film radiography.

Under intermittent plain film control, a thin flexible wire is percutaneously inserted into the target with the help of a coaxial needle and a stereotactic reference system such as a radio-opaque grid placed on the examination table. The introducing needle is then removed and the wire remains within the target due to the hook like configuration of its tip (Figure 2.7). Various configurations of wire tips are available.

2.2.1.2 Fluoroscopy

Conventional fluoroscopy has been the classical method to evaluate dynamic processes and kinetics in the body. To name only the most common indications, localizing a nodule in the lung, identifying foreign bodies in the gastro-intestinal tract, and monitoring the excursion of the diaphragm have been traditional indications for fluoroscopy. With the administration of oral, rectal, or intravenous contrast, fluoroscopy became the most commonly used method to evaluate hollow organs and vessels before the introduction of endoscopy and CT or MR angiography. Conventional fluoroscopy is still the most important and most commonly used modality to steer catheter based percutaneous angiographic, pancreato-biliary, gastrointestinal, genito-urinary, and musculoskeletal diagnostic and therapeutic procedures (Figures 2.8 and 2.9).

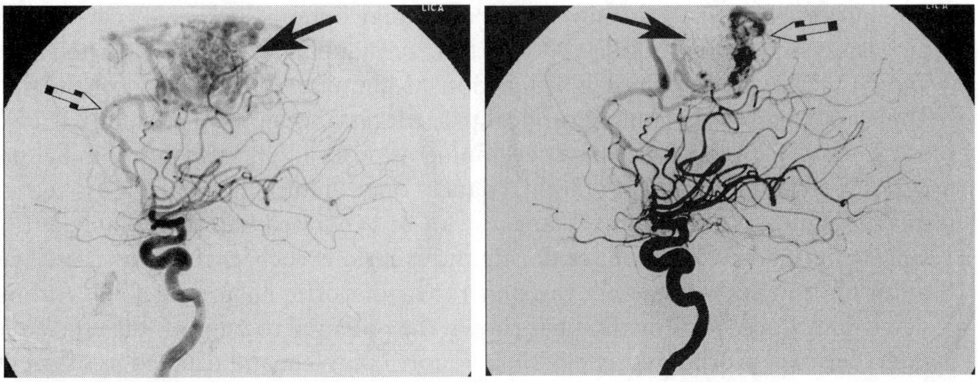

(a) (b)

Figure 2.8 (a) Frontal AVM pre-treatment. Lateral view of left internal carotid cerebral angiogram during late arterial phase shows a tangle of abnormal vessels (dark arrow) within the medial frontal lobe consistent with an arterio-venous malformation (AVM). Note enlarged feeding arteries, most prominently the callosal marginal branch (open arrow) of the anterior cerebral artery. (b) Frontal AVM post-treatment. Similar lateral view shows Onyx liquid embolization material (dark arrow) deposited via branches of the anterior cerebral artery occluding the anterior and middle portions of the AVM. There is residual nidus posteriorly (open arrow) which will be subject to further embolization prior to surgical resection.

It also is the most commonly used portable imaging method in the operating room for guiding surgery of the musculoskeletal system. When configured in a C-arm system, digital fluoroscopy offers maximum flexibility while allowing virtually infinite angulations, over- and under-table modes, multiple guidance options such as roadmap views and various filtering settings, and pulse fluoroscopy modes to decrease the exposure to radiation. Newer developments in tube technology and

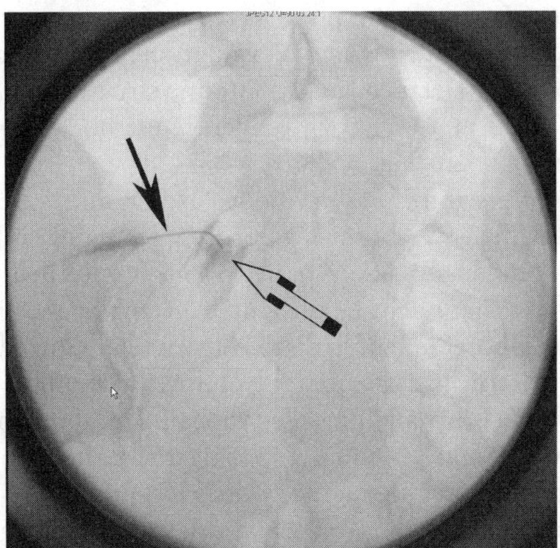

Figure 2.9 Fluoro-guided sacral epidural injection. Posterior view shows 22 gauge spinal needle (dark arrow) directed at the left S1 nerve root. A mixture of iodinated contrast, a short acting local anesthetic and an anti-inflammatory long acting drug are injected epidurally (open arrow) along the S1 nerve root to provide relief often up to several months for patients with chronic radicular pain.

post-processing software allow expanded display options such as 3D rotational angiography and tomosynthesis. Both methods result in a single reconstructed 3D image synthesized from multiple acquisitions. Mammographic, musculoskeletal, and applications around planning surgical procedures have been suggested [23, 24].

Dyna-CT is one of the latest developments resulting from advances in flat panel detector technology. When rotational data of one volume is acquired, cross-sectional image renditions similar to CT images can be generated within the interventional suite, offering new capabilities during interventions such as the immediate evaluation for endoleak after endovascular repair of aortic aneurysms [25]. Although newly introduced, this method has shown the potential to improve the efficiency of interventional procedures by enabling a more complete and detailed assessment of treatment than conventional fluoroscopy.

2.2.2 Computed Tomography

2.2.2.1 Multidetector Computed Tomography

Computed tomography (CT) is one of the most commonly used imaging modalities in modern medicine. Its wide availability, rapid image acquisition, high spatial resolution, limited dependence on patients' body habitus, and its high degree of reproducibility has allowed CT to be the imaging modality of choice for a large number of clinical questions across the medical field. The invention of CT in 1973 by Sir Godfrey N. Hounsfield introduced a cross-sectional imaging modality to the spectrum of diagnostic imaging tools utilizing X-rays which allowed insights into the human body free of superimposition.

Multidetector CT (MDCT) represents another quantum leap to the development of CT technology, allowing rapid and simultaneous acquisition of more than one slice at a time. Along with the exponential development of computing power, this new technology has enabled volume coverage of entire organ systems such as the chest, the GI tract, or the vascular system in one breath hold if necessary and has opened the door to new dynamic evaluations of moving targets such as the heart at high resolution. Detailed small anatomic structures such as the coronary arteries can be visualized in a variety of rendering methods allowing noninvasive insights into the beating heart (Figure 2.10).

MDCT offers information about cardiac and vascular anatomy that is not available with invasive coronary fluoroscopic angiography. While fluoroscopic angiography offers unsurpassed spatial resolution in the range of 0.2 mm, extravascular structures that might be of significant importance for the diagnosis such as a partially thrombosed aneurysm are often not visualized using this method alone. ECG-gated CT coronary angiography allows motionless depiction of anatomy and pathology of the heart and provides virtually unlimited perspectives of one and the same anatomic region without exposing the patient to additional radiation like conventional coronary angiography does (Figure 2.11).

Other advantages of MDCT, but also of other imaging modalities such as ultrasound, MR, or PET which allow the acquisition of entire organ volumes, are the capability for volumetric organ assessment, volumetric display in various modes such as 2D and 3D renditions including virtual flights through hollow organ systems such as the cerebral ventricles, bronchi, or the colon and a variety of display

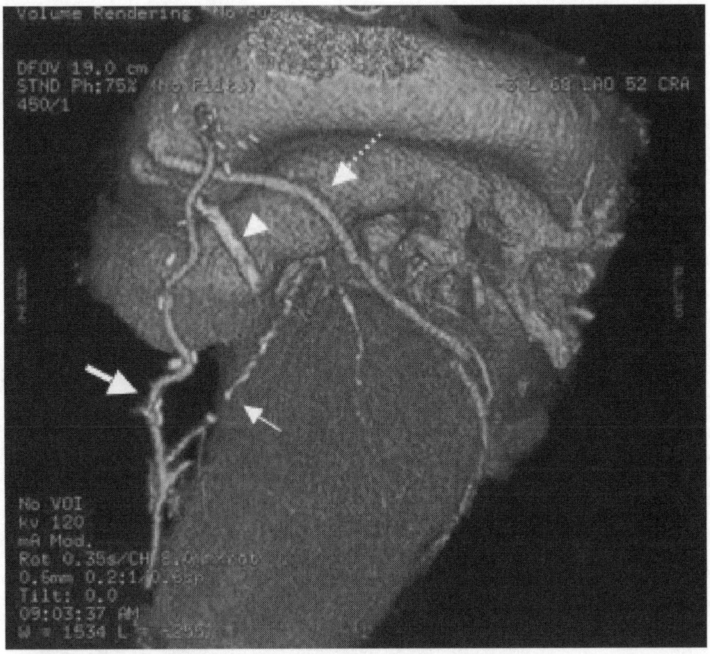

(a)

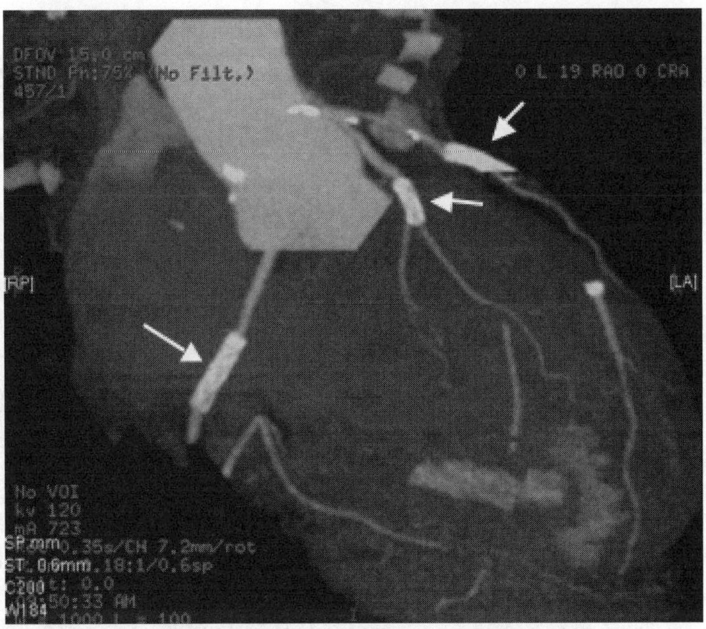

(b)

Figure 2.10 ECG-gated CT coronary angiogram of the heart: different postprocessing methods display various complex findings. (a–c) Different reconstruction methods on three different patients. (a) 3D rendition (volume rendering) of the coronary arteries following surgery: left internal mammary artery bypass (thick arrow) bridging the calcified and occluded left anterior descending artery (thin arrow). Patient also had saphenous venous graft (dotted arrow). Note metal stent (arrow head) with absent contrast filling representing occlusion. (b) Maximum intensity projection (MIP) of the heart with three vascular stents (arrows) in the coronary arteries.

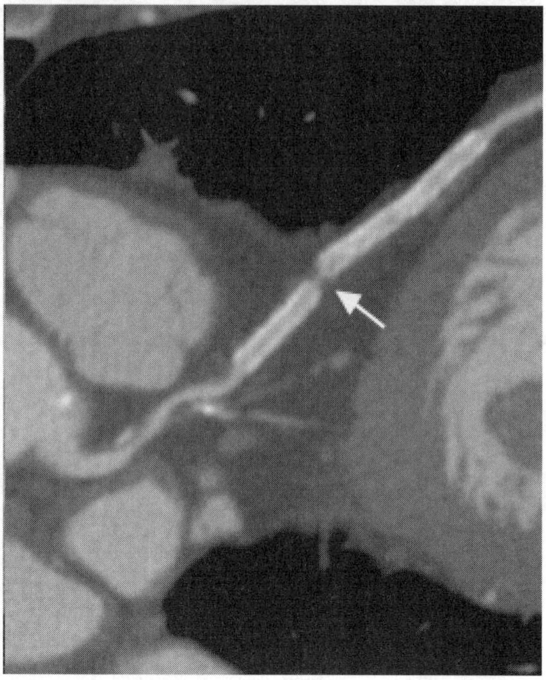

(c)

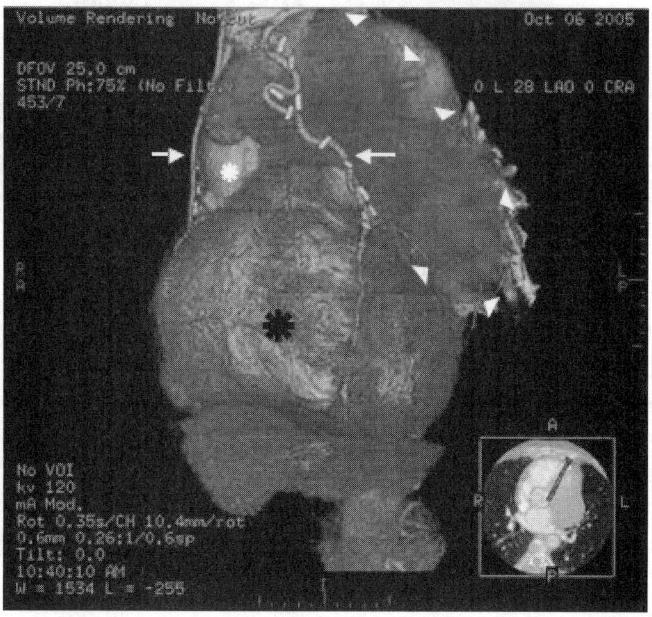

(d)

Figure 2.10 (*continued*) (c) Curved 2D multiplanar reformation along a coronary artery with two stents next to each other and a stenotic segment in between the stents (arrow). (d–e) One patient with a large pseudoaneurysm of a left internal mammary artery graft, normal right internal mammary artery graft, and saphenous venous graft. (d) 3D volume rendering shows overview over the aortic root (small ✱), right and left internal mammary coronary artery bypasses (arrows), myocardium (large ✱), and pseudoaneurysm (arrow heads).

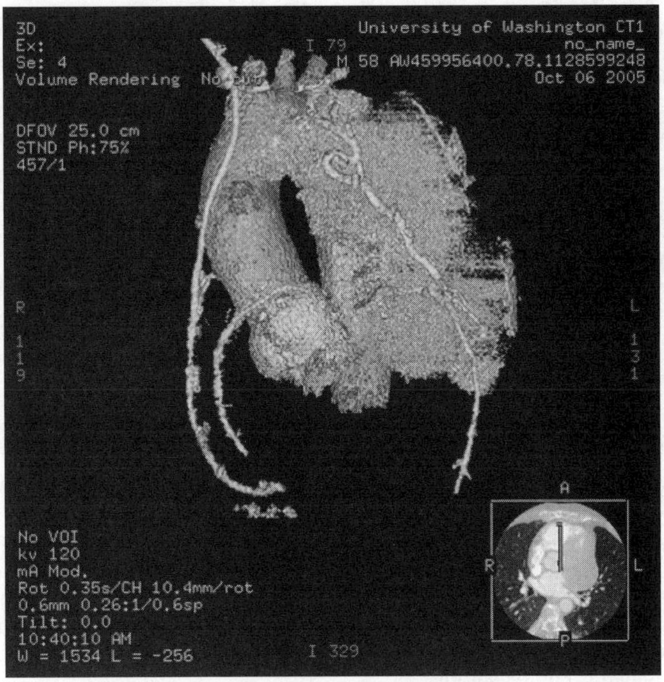

(e)

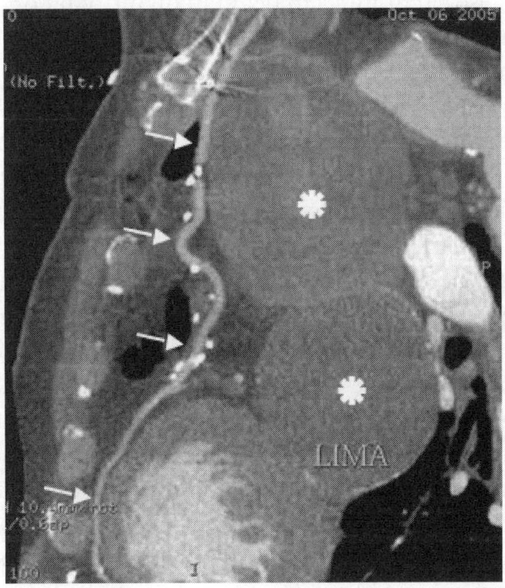

(f)

Figure 2.10 (*continued*) (e) Differently chosen opacificities of volume rendered view displaying selectively the aortic root, and the three coronary artery bypass grafts (white) and the pseudoaneurysm in different colors. (f) Curved multiplanar reformations along the left internal mammarian artery (LIMA) bypass (arrows), showing its spatial relationship to the entire craniocaudal extension of the pseudoanurysm (✱).

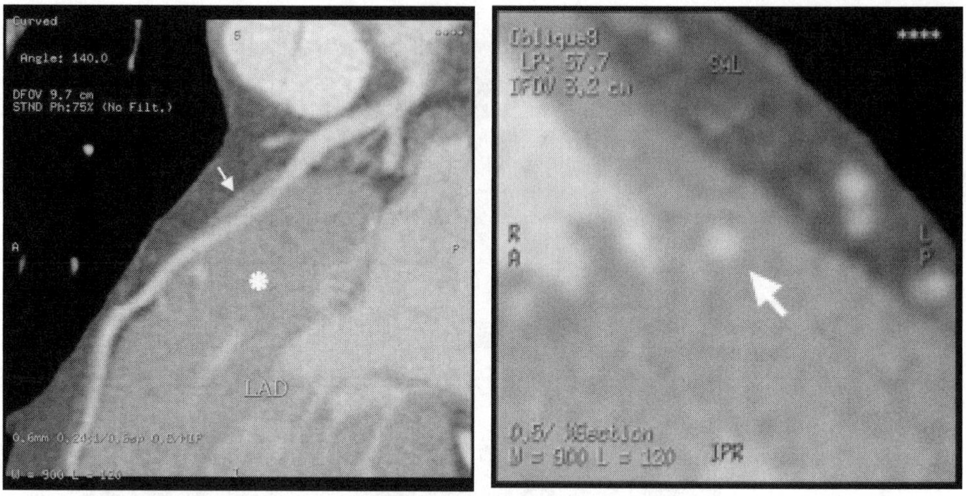

(a) (b)

Figure 2.11 ECG-gated coronary CT angiogram. 2D reformations of the left anterior descending coronary artery demonstrate that a short proximal segment of the artery describes an intramuscular course, while the more distal segment is located on the surface of the myocardium: (a) reformation along the long axis of the vessel, arrow pointing to the intramuscular segment (✱=myocardium); (b) transverse view of the coronary artery through the intramuscular segment demonstrates that the artery is completely surrounded by myocardium, which is a variant of normal that may result in critical ischemic complications.

methods such as virtual bronchography or colonoscopy simulating traditional techniques. All these capabilities may aid in quantifying organ sizes and tumor volumes by segmentation algorithms (Figure 2.12) or may just target a more intuitive and comprehensive display of complex anatomic structures (Figures 2.13 and 2.14).

The latest developments in CT technology focus on more rapid image acquisitions and tissue analysis, achievable with the introduction of Dual Source CT (DS-CT) or Dual Energy CT (DE-CT). While DS-CT takes advantage of utilizing two separate X-ray tubes, which allows improvement in temporal resolution to 42 msec [26, 27], DE-CT generates two images of the same slice location by rapidly switching the tube voltage of one source. The latter technique allows analysis of tissue composition in the same way DS-CT does, but lacks the additional speed enabled by the second tube [28, 29]. Advantages of more rapid image acquisition below 180 msec per slice are mostly centered around cardiovascular applications, mainly focusing on imaging of the coronary arteries and small vessels. Tissue composition analysis independent from image acquisition speed offers new clinical applications such as the evaluation of kidney stones, stent lumen patency, and bone mineralization. The separation of iodine contrast, of calcified vascular plaques, soft tissue and osseous structures represent other targets of research around this new technical development [29, 30].

CT is the modality of choice for needle guidance where ultrasound is challenged as long as the procedure can be performed outside the operating room: Lesions located deep in the body such as the mediastinum, retroperitoneum, lungs or skeleton are typical targets for percutaneous procedures. Sometimes it is also used in more superficial locations such as the neck, subcutaneous tissues, or musculature where

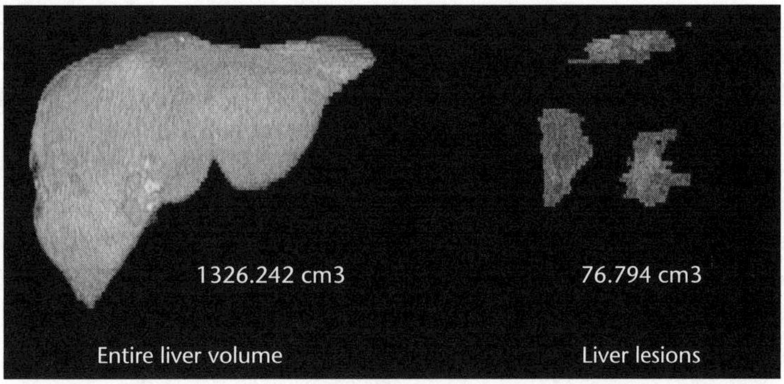

Figure 2.12 Computer assisted volumetric calculation of liver and tumor volumes in a patient with colorectal metastases to the liver of a contrast enhanced CT dataset: (left) manual segmentation of the liver based on axial images with resulting 3D rendition (volume rendering) and computer assisted calculation of the entire organ volume; (right) same method applied to the multiple tumors within the liver with segmentation of metastases and total calculated tumor volume. Ratio of the tumor-to-liver volume is used to aid in the dose calculation for Y^{90} embolotherapy of liver metastases. The method is also used to calculate residual liver volume prior to partial liver resection, which is a prognostic parameter for the surgical outcome.

sonographic access would be possible but not ideal or where small anatomic variations would pose an obstacle to ultrasound guidance (Figure 2.1). The choice of which guidance method to use may be dependent on availability and the operator's experience, expertise, and school of training. Another advantage of CT is that the procedure may be well documented since the stored images are more reproducible than ultrasound sometimes may be.

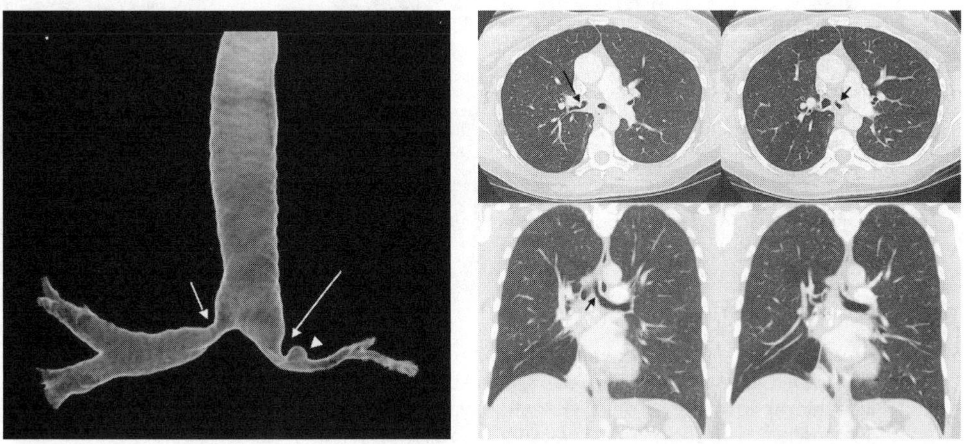

(a) (b)

Figure 2.13 Transparent 3D volume rendering (virtual bronchography) of the bronchial tree of a patient with bilateral bronchial stenoses. The rendition can be rotated in any direction; viewed from posteriorly both the high grade stenosis of the right main bronchus (long arrow) and moderate stenosis of the left main bronchus (short arrow) are seen in one view. Note that the complex configuration of the two stenotic segments as well as a post-stenotic bronchial dilatation (arrow head) are easier appreciated on the virtual bronchogram (a) when compared to the axial and coronal 2D reformations (b), where even four representative images are not sufficient to display the pathology in its full extent.

Major disadvantages are the lack of real-time guidance and exposure to ionizing radiation for the patient. CT fluoroscopy increases exposure to radiation for the operator and is limited to patients whose body habitus is small enough to accommodate the percutaneous device in the scanning plane while scanning.

CT may also be the only method to visualize a lesion within an otherwise easily accessible organ, such as the liver, such as when a lesion is not detected with the low contrast resolution of ultrasound. In this case the target may be seen without intravenous contrast administration or IV contrast would be necessary to identify the target. Contrast administration, if mandatory to visualize the target, however, may complicate a CT-guided procedure, since patients' renal function and potential for an allergic reaction to iodine contrast have to be considered. Other indications for IV contrast administration on CT-guided interventions are visualization of structures with adjacent structures at risk such as blood vessels, the renal collecting

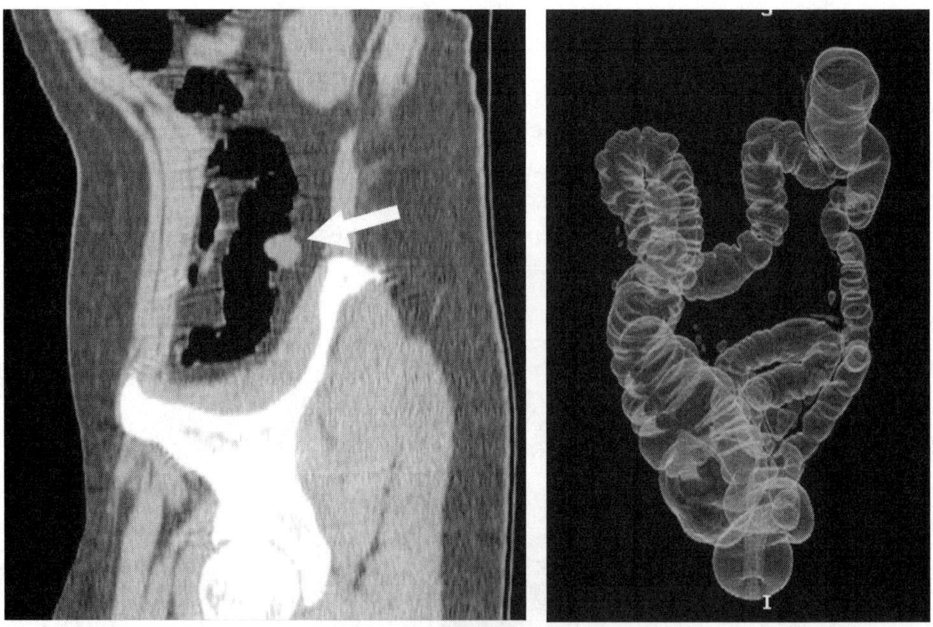

(a) (b)

Figure 2.14 (a–d) Patient with a submucosal gastrointestinal stromatumor (GIST) of the descending colon. Different display modes rendered from one eight-channel MDCT dataset with 1.25-mm slice thickness, following rectal distention with a CO_2 insufflator. (a) 2D sagittal reconstruction of the descending colon shows small oval submucosal mass (arrow). (b) Rendition in "virtual enema" mode simulating double contrast barium study. Adequate distention of colon allows good overview of the entire colon, but superimposed bowel loops preclude evaluation of the mass, which is not seen in this projection. (c) Virtual enema rendition rotated and magnified to the area of interest now demonstrates the mucosal impression caused by the submucosal GIST. White arrow highlights pseudo-impression caused by adherent stool, simulating presence of a second mass. (d) "Virtual flight" mode through the same segment of the descending colon demonstrates mucosal elevation caused by the underlying mass. Note mild degradation of image quality due to large zoom factor, enhancing the stair step artifacts resulting from 1.25-mm slice thickness. [Images (a–d) are courtesy of Dr. Carlos Cuevas, University of Washington, Seattle, Washington, Body Imaging.] (e) VR colonoscopy of a different patient than in (a–d) obtained with a 64-channel MDCT and a slice thickness of 0.625 mm: normal transverse colon; note better image quality than (a–d) due to isotropic voxel size (✱).

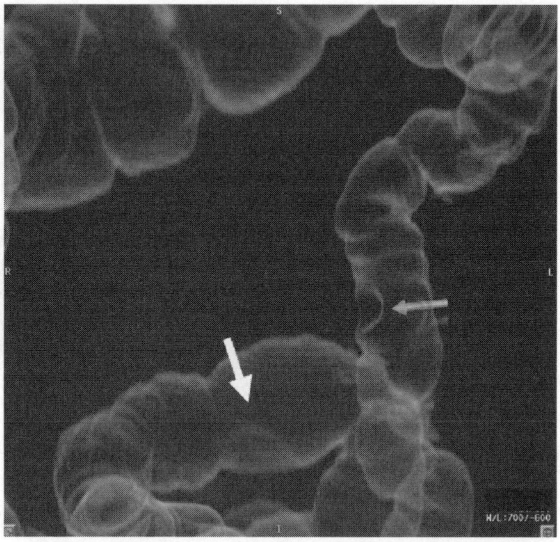

(c)

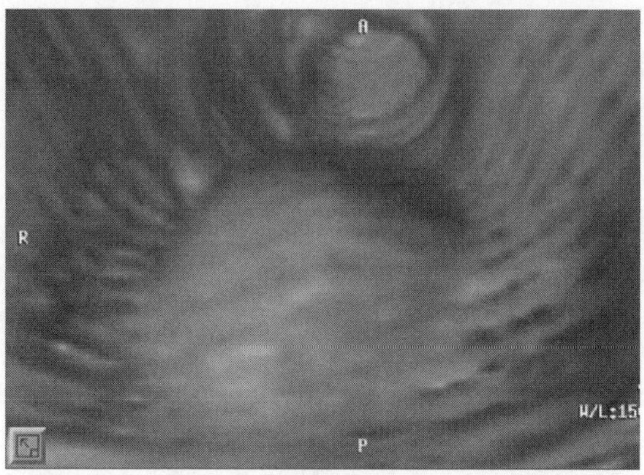

(d)

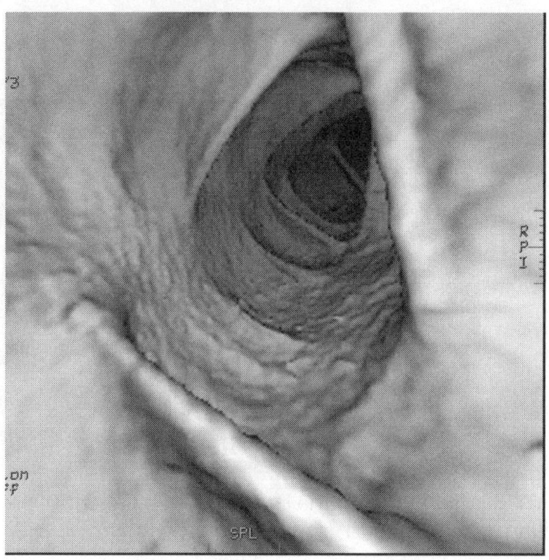

(e)

Figure 2.14 (*continued*)

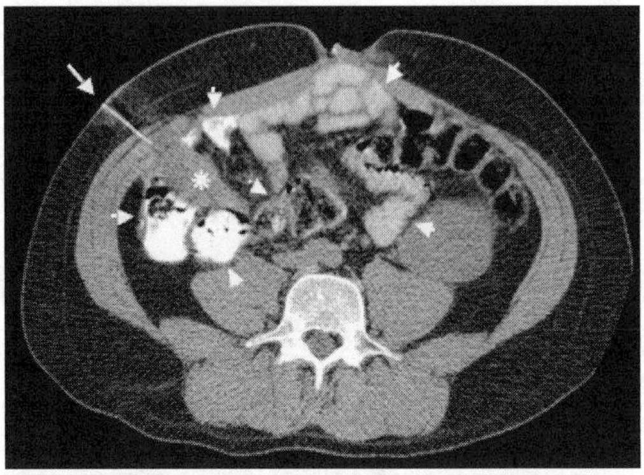

Figure 2.15 CT-guided percutaneous biopsy of pancreas transplant for questionable graft rejection. Bowel loops (arrow heads) around the transplanted pancreas (✱), which is located in the lower abdomen, are opacified with positive oral contrast, allowing for better delineation of the graft. The biopsy needle (arrow) is being safely advanced towards the pancreas without transgressing bowel loops.

system or the ureters. Oral positive contrast may be given for opacification of bowel loops, if they need to be clearly visualized in order to be avoided, for example for transperitoneal biopsies or deep abdominal or pelvic targets such pancreas transplants or mesenteric masses (Figure 2.15).

CT guidance is usually also the first choice for procedures on the skeleton. Biopsies, nerve blocks, or radiofrequency ablations of bone tumors are usually performed without the need for contrast agents thanks to the inherent high contrast of bone and their lesions (Figures 2.16 and 2.17).

CT furthermore offers the advantage of immediate documentation of possible complications such as pneumothorax and hemorrhage as a result of the procedure or of pathologies and alterations that might have occurred since the last imaging

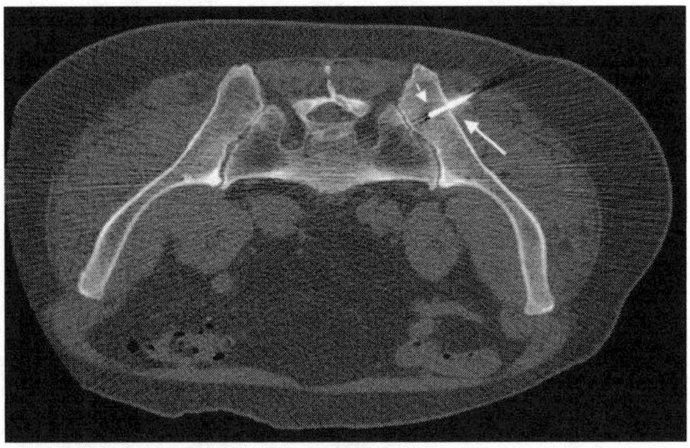

Figure 2.16 CT-guided biopsy of the iliac bone on a patient in prone position with suspected metastasis from lung cancer: coaxial biopsy needle (long arrow) within the subtle lucent mass (short arrow).

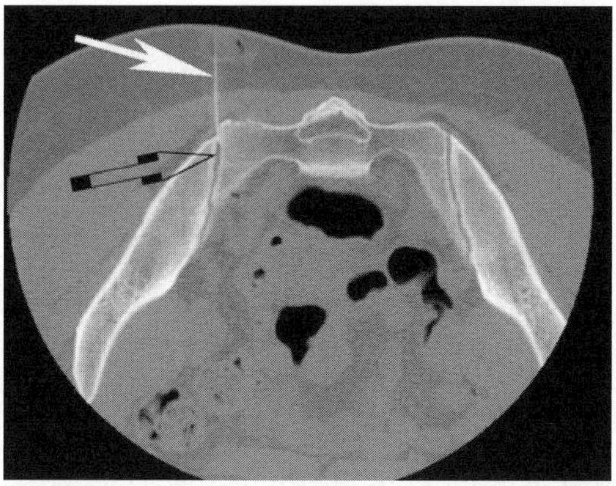

Figure 2.17 CT-guided sacroiliac joint injection. This CT scan though the pelvis with the patient in prone position shows a 22 gauge spinal needle (white arrow) directed anteriorly into the sacroiliac joint (open arrow). A combination of an anti-inflammatory drug and local anesthetic was injected with relief of this patient's arthritic pelvic pain.

exam; these findings might change the patients' clinical management as much as the biopsy result itself.

2.2.2.2 CT Fluoroscopy

CT fluoroscopy is now built into nearly all MDCT systems. It is designed to allow faster incremental control of needle position or even almost real-time in-plane guidance or percutaneous procedures. In-plane CT-fluoro mode poses smaller exposure to ionizing radiation for the patient and may significantly speed up the procedure, but translates into greater radiation to the operator. The operator is acting immediately next to the patient and to the gantry where scattered radiation is the highest in the examination room.

Specific instances which may take advantage of the real-time guidance of fluoro CT include targeting small mobile lesions such as pulmonary nodules for biopsy which move during breathing [31].

The choice of which method of CT to use—static, incremental, or CT fluoro guidance—depends on the operators' preference and may also depend on ease of use offered by the operating system.

Future developments in the fields of CT will focus on reconstruction methods, flat-panel CT, dual and multisource CT, new scanning modes, energy-sensitive CT, nano-CT, phase-contrast CT, and others [28].

2.2.3 Nuclear Medicine

Nuclear medicine is the imaging discipline using scintigraphic systems to detect ionizing radiating agents inserted into the body. In contrast to other radiographic methods it always depends on the presence of an administered radiation source.

The other fundamental difference to other imaging methods is that it mainly displays functional information of body systems.

A large variety of scintigraphic methods and tracers exist to answer clinical questions of very different nature.

Positron emission tomography (PET) as: (1) the currently most important cross-sectional nuclear imaging modality for detection of malignancies and lymphangiography for sentinel lymph node detection, and as (2) a conventional scintigraphic guidance tool are introduced in the following two sections.

2.2.3.1 Positron Emission Tomography

Similar to other scintigraphic methods, PET is a cross-sectional imaging method that uses labeled injectable tracers to study and display functional processes. The unique feature compared with other techniques is that PET detects pairs of photons indirectly emitted by the positrons which are emitted by the injected radionuclide (e.g., F-18). Depending on the nature of the radioisotope, a metabolic process is detected in three dimensions and may be reconstructed in a variety of displays. Modern scanners use a built-in CT to correct for the attenuation the emitted signals undergo and to facilitate correlation with anatomic registration (PET-CT). This represents one of the modality fusion techniques, which has already entered daily practice. The functional processes can also be quantified.

The most common radionuclide used in PET is fluorodeoxyglucose (FDG), an analog of sugar (glucose), which metabolizes quickly in tissues and can be detected within an hour after injection. Its role is to detect abnormal metabolic features associated with malignancy that often precede morphologic findings [32–35]. It has also the potential to distinguish between tumor cell populations that respond to treatment from the ones that do not and may thus modify treatment decisions where morphologic methods demonstrate no difference between active and treated tumors (Figure 2.18). A number of other PET tracers are available that help study other cellular functions and microenvironments [32, 33, 36].

2.2.3.2 Sentinel Lymph Node Lymphangiography

Lymphscintigraphy uses tracers such as Tc-99m sulphur colloid to trace lymphatic drainage pathways and lymph nodes. The concept of sentinel lymph node lymphangiography is based on the principle that lymph nodes closest to a malignant tumor are the first filter (sentinel lymph nodes) for metastatic tumor cells. If this or these lymph nodes are free of tumor metastases, it can be assumed that more remote lymph nodes are also not invaded by metastases, which may spare the patient from a diagnostic lymph node dissection. This concept is used for breast cancer staging and other tumors such as melanoma.

The location of the tumor is known by palpation or imaging. The subcutaneous skin immediately around the tumor is injected with the radioactive substance, which is then taken up by lymphatic tracts and lymph nodes. After a certain delay a scintigraphic camera maps the radioactivity over the area of interest. The spots with the highest count are being confirmed with a handheld probe, and labeled

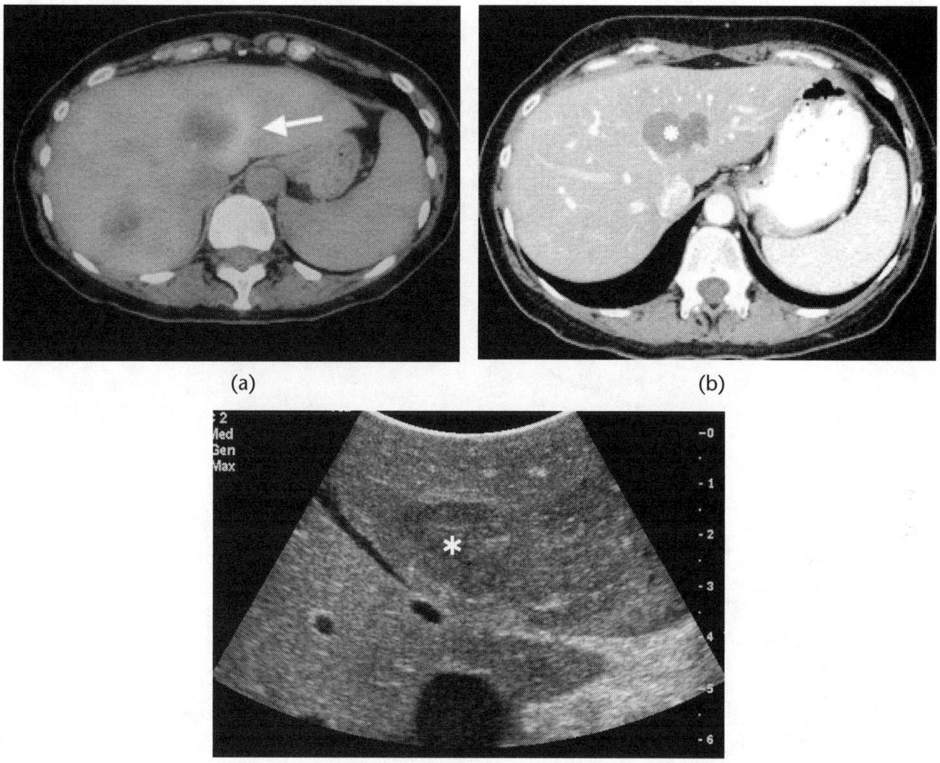

(a) (b) (c)

Figure 2.18 Metastasis from colon cancer in the left lobe of the liver after chemotherapy. (a) FDG-PET-CT clearly demonstrates increased uptake of radioactive tracer at the lateral margin of the tumor (arrow), while (b) contrast enhanced CT and (c) intraoperative ultrasound do not show a difference between the treated part of the metastasis and residual tumor (both tumor portions are hypodense, hypoechoic respectively on CT and US). The FDG avid tumor portion was targeted for intraoperative radiofrequency ablation using anatomic landmarks.

on the skin, thus prepared for the surgeon to be excised for histologic evaluation. The degree of accumulated radioactivity in the lymph node does not correlate with metastatic involvement, but the objective of this modality is to mark the sentinel lymph node for excision (Figure 2.19).

2.3 Magnetic Resonance Imaging

Magnetic resonance imaging (MRI) is an imaging modality that displays chemical information emanating from protons. The most commonly targeted proton in medical MR imaging is hydrogen (H). Since the human body is about 60% water (H_2O), as well as 5% to 25% fat, MRI is capable of visualizing anatomic details with an unsurpassed soft tissue contrast and spatial resolution not seen with any other method. The traditional in vitro application of MR has been spectroscopy for chemical analysis, but engineering efforts mainly related to signal localization introduced MR as a medical imaging modality in 1973. Modern MR scanners have

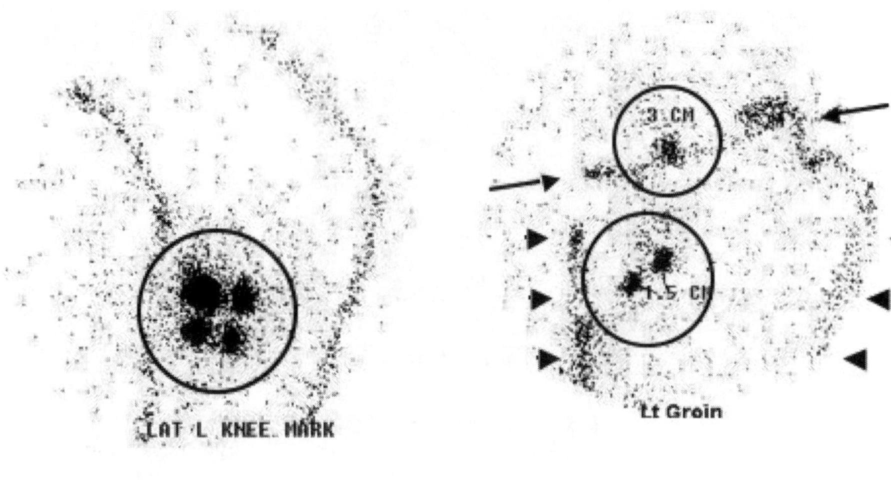

(a) (b)

Figure 2.19 Lymphscintigraphy of the left lower extremity for identification of sentinel lymph node in a patient with malignant melanoma below the left knee. (a) Subcutaneous injection of 1 mCi Tc-99m sulfur colloid (circle) below the left knee laterally in four sites around the surgical site of the primary tumor. (b) Focal uptake of activity (circles) in the groin is suggestive of sentinel lymph nodes (SLN). Following identification on the lymphoscintigram, the location of SLN is marked on the skin, which was outlined by a radioactive pen (arrow heads), over the lymph nodes for surgical sampling after being localized with a scintigraphic hand probe (not shown). Arrows indicate location of the inguinal ligament. (Courtesy Dr. Carrie Marder, University of Washington, Seattle, Washington, Radiology.)

the capability of performing in vivo spectroscopy, thus enabling chemical analysis of lesions or abnormal physiology noninvasively.

2.3.1 Conventional MRI

Conventional MRI provides detailed spatial information of virtually any part in the body. Its main advantage is in the imaging of nonaerated and nonosseous structures, including bone marrow. However, newer developments have successfully targeted functional analysis of the lungs using hyperpolarized noble gases such as He^3 or Xe^{129} [37, 38]. While the spin echo imaging technique offers high-resolution images of acquisition times too long to be performed in one breath hold, gradient echo sequences have been in use for a number of years that allow rapid image acquisition with an excellent spatial and soft tissue resolution [39].

The development of specific techniques that image blood flow without or with the help of intravenous contrast agents is called magnetic resonance angiography (MRA). MRA offers high-resolution images of vessels close to the spatial resolution generated by conventional catheter based angiography, but without the risks of complications such as strokes or vessel injury. Diagnostic MRA noninvasively provides a plethora of anatomic and functional information about complex vascular disorders which can aid in the planning and execution of surgical or percutaneous catheter based treatment such as stent placements over stenotic arteries and veins, and occlusions of bleeding sources, tumors, aneurysms, and arterio-venous malformations (Figure 2.20).

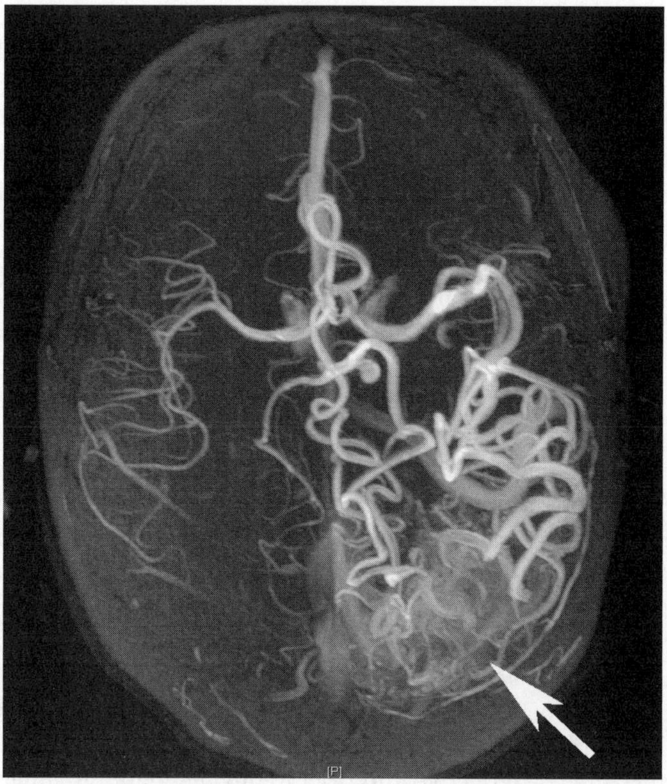

Figure 2.20 Cerebral MR angiogram (MRA). In this collapsed axial projection maximum intensity projection image from a 3D time of flight MRA, there is an AVM in the left occipital lobe (arrow). In this noncontrast technique, moving water protons entering the brain from arteries in the neck appear hyperintense. Feeding the AVM anteriorly are multiple enlarged arteries.

MRI has been investigated for its potential as an interventional guidance tool for more than 20 years. It can be used as a guidance modality for lesions occult to ultrasound and CT [40]. This is specifically true for masses in the brain [6, 41] and the female breast [39, 42–44]. Other applications in the head and neck, abdomen, and pelvis have been described [4, 40, 45–47]. Improvements of pulse sequences, coil designs, and other hardware have made real-time MR-guided aspirations and biopsies possible in both open and closed bore systems [6, 7, 48–50].

Independent from the target organ, MR-guided interventions require specific arrangements of hardware and software implementations [4]. Several requirements need to be considered to safely conduct MR-guided interventions: visualization of the target as well as the needle device, physical access to the patient, pulse sequences that allow rapid image acquisition and display, and MR compatibility of the interventional devices and their support systems [4]. Depending on the demands of the procedure and on availability, a conventional cylindrical scanner, as it is being used for diagnostic purposes or an open scanner configuration may be chosen [4]. Various system configurations and designs have been developed to allow access to the operating field at minimal degradation of image quality [4].

MRI has been used in open systems to guide devices in almost real time to the target [51]. Degradation of image quality due the lower strength of the magnetic field must be accepted, but adequate rather than perfect image quality is acceptable, as long as imaging at real-time or almost-real-time speed is achieved. Applications in the head and neck area as well as the spine, musculoskeletal, hepato-pancreato-biliary system, and genitourinary system have been reported [47, 52–56]. However, significantly higher costs compared with ultrasound and CT and the additional expense of MRI compatible materials and biopsy devices, and the difficulty of engineering a truly open scanner configuration have limited the use of MRI for guidance purposes to dedicated imaging centers and to selected indications.

New approaches combining the image quality of a high field conventional system and the real-time MR-fluoroscopy capabilities of an open system include short wide bore systems recently available at 1.5 Tesla [48].

More commonly, MR-guided placement of localization wires within breast lesions can be performed in conventional MR systems using contrast enhanced T1 weighted gradient echo sequences. For this purpose the patient may be positioned supine or prone on the MR scanner, although the prone position is preferred. The breast is immobilized for the procedure on a dedicated table, designed to accommodate free access to the organ [44]. An MR compatible localization wire is inserted under intermittent imaging guidance outside the gantry in a similar manner as plain film radiography or with CT guidance is used for other organs (Figure 2.21).

An obvious disadvantage of this technique is the absence of real-time guidance, which may increase the overall time of the procedure. However, it still has a role in lesions with poor soft tissue contrast since 1.5T standard field systems are more available and cost effective and because image quality is superior to open low field scanners [4, 44].

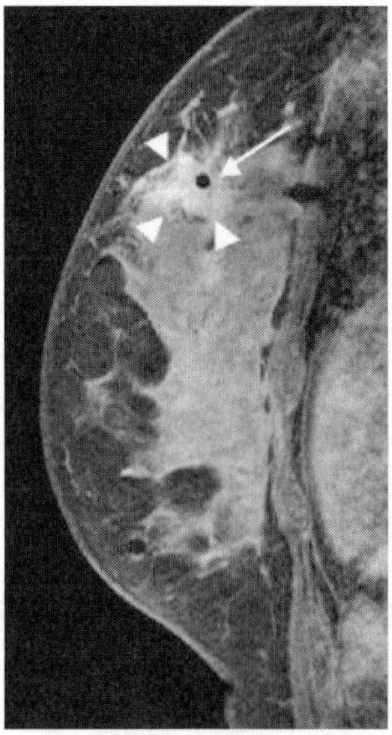

Figure 2.21 Sagittal contrast enhanced fat suppressed gradient echo T1 sequence of the left breast demonstrates suspicious nonmass-like enhancement (NMLE) in the upper outer quadrant (arrow heads). The lesion was not seen on plain film mammography or ultrasound. Therefore, MR image-guided biopsy was indicated. Round hypointense susceptibility artifact (long arrow) represents the biopsy device within the lesion. The biopsy needle was inserted using a lateral approach, perpendicular to this imaging plane. Histology of the lesion revealed invasive ductal breast cancer.

For MR-guided procedures a freehand versus a stereotactic technique may be chosen.

2.3.2 Functional MRI

Functional magnetic resonance imaging (fMRI) has gained tremendous popularity among researchers and clinicians at the end of the twentieth and the beginning of the twenty-first century. The term "functional" has been applied to a range of physiologic parameters interrogated by a variety of MR techniques and capable of being co-registering with high-resolution anatomical images obtained in the same session.

2.3.2.1 MR Angiography, Perfusion Imaging, Cardiac MR

Functional MRI in the more traditional sense also includes classic applications such as MR angiography without the use of IV contrast which at the same time allow a morphologic evaluation of the area of interest. Examples are phase contrast (PC), time-of-flight MR angiography (TOF, Figure 2.20), or functional analysis of blood flow in the heart (Figure 2.22) or of cerebrospinal fluid within cerebral ventricles. In all these techniques blood becomes visible as a hyper- or hypointense signal depending on flow its velocity and direction. A major advantage of these techniques without the use of IV contrast is their capability of quantifying blood flow and relating it to established clinical parameters known from other imaging modalities such as calculating the degree of a vascular stenosis by Doppler ultrasound or assessing the ejection fraction of the left cardiac ventricle by echocardiography.

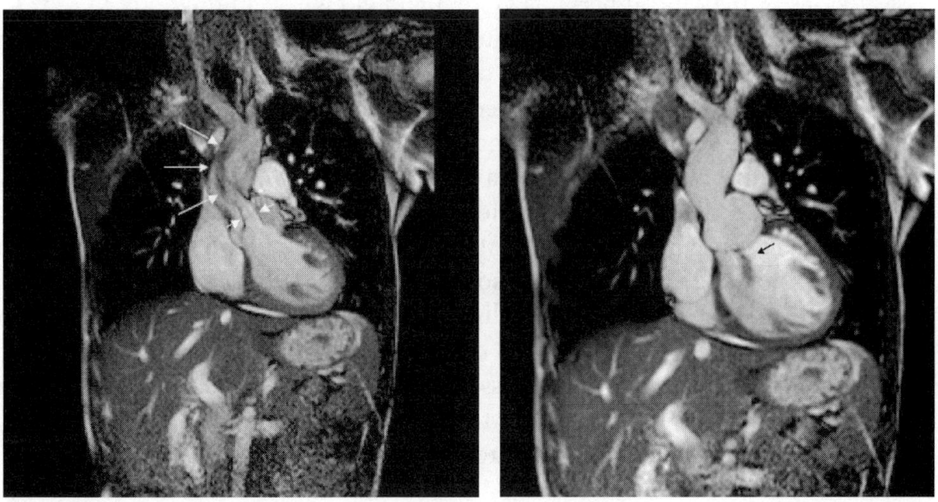

(a) (b)

Figure 2.22 Functional and morphologic evaluation of the heart in a patient with unicuspid aortic valve and resulting aortic regurgitation (technique: coronal balanced steady state free precession cine sequence). (a) Frame taken in systole demonstrates open aortic valve (short arrows) with hypointense abnormal turbulent flow pattern (long arrow). Note that the valve is less open than a normal tricuspid aortic valve would be at this stage. (b) Frame taken in diastole: closed aortic valve and significant jet (arrow) represents aortic regurgitation of 50% as a result of the abnormal valve.

There is increasing use of physiological imaging such as brain MR perfusion which involves the rapid intravenous injection of paramagnetic contrast agents and the calculation of regional signal change over time using repeat imaging every 1 to 2 seconds. By doing a time series analysis on a pixel-by-pixel basis, mapping and quantification of blood flow, blood volume, and transit time may be done over an area of interest.

Clinically brain MR perfusion imaging is used most commonly for strokes, looking for brain regions of abnormally decreased blood flow, or for tumor mapping, looking for areas of abnormally high perfusion. Brain tumors typically show higher metabolic activity than the normal brain and the degree of activity may correlate with the degree of malignancy. Blood flow and blood volume usually correlate with tissue metabolism—most tumors have abnormally high blood flow and this may be used for surgical guidance. In heterogeneously enhancing tumors it can help guide the surgeon to biopsy or resect the most metabolically active and therefore likely the highest grade part of the lesion. Sometimes a relatively slow growing tumor will focally degenerate on follow-up scans into a higher grade cell type. For example, an astrocytoma may degenerate into a glioblastoma multiforma. Also often on anatomic brain MRI it is difficult to distinguish between peritumoral edema and infiltrating tumor. Sometimes MRI perfusion or PET can show this distinction and help the surgeon determine the extent of the resection and better judge the need to resect as much tumor as possible while sparing normal brain function (Figure 2.23).

2.3.2.2 Diffusion Weighted and Tensor Imaging

Diffusion weighted imaging (DWI) has its established role in early stroke detection and to a lesser degree in the distinction between inflammatory and neoplastic lesions of the central nervous system and elsewhere in the body [57, 58]. Diseases that cause breakdown of the integrity of the cellular membrane such as ischemic or inflammatory disorders will cause cytotoxic edema, a swelling of the intracellular compartment. While extracelluar free moving (diffusing) protons, directed by Brownian motion, give a low signal in DWI, protons restricted by intracelluar barriers and macromolecules will cause an increased DWI signal.

The direction of diffusion along axons can be coded by color and major tracts can be inferred by linking similarly directed white matter voxels. Such mapping is commonly called diffusion tensor imaging (DTI) or DT tractography. Its importance lies in the capability to display in three dimensions the nerve fibers of the white matter of the brain based on their intact function (Figure 2.24). DTI can be co-registered with anatomic cross-sectional MRI to visualize the spatial relationship of lesions to major white matter tracts and facilitate surgical planning with the goal of minimizing surgical damage to critical pathways such as the corticospinal tract [59, 60].

2.3.2.3 MR Spectroscopy

Spectroscopy was the first clinical application of MRI decades ago. More recently it has experienced a revival within the field of MR imaging since it has become avail-

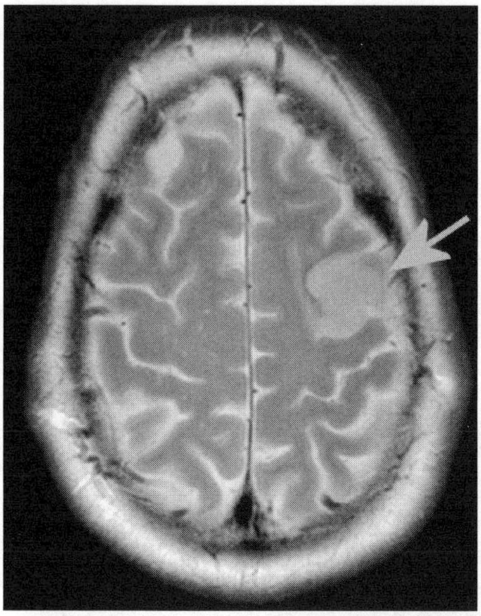

(a)

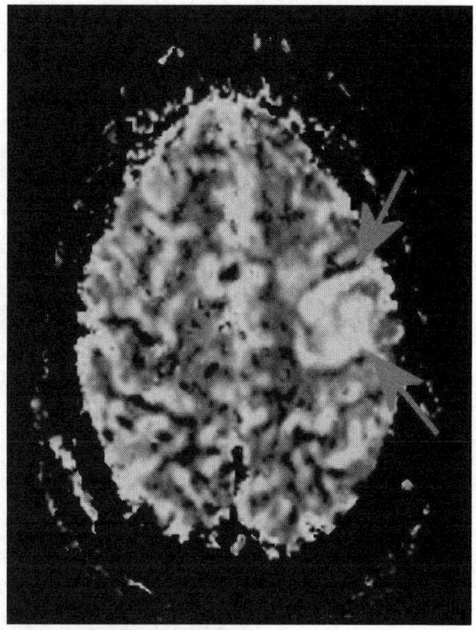

(b)

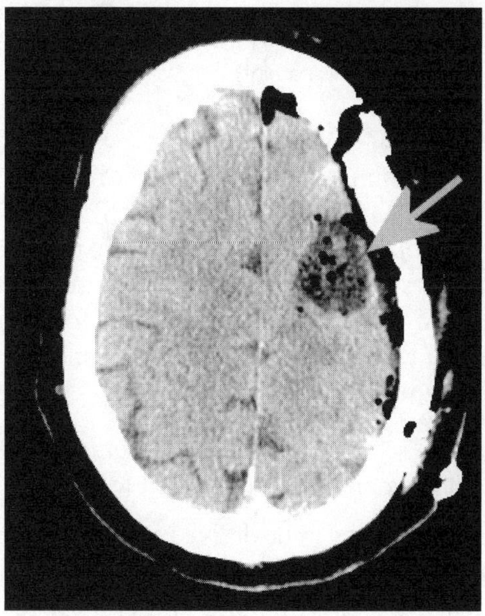

(c)

Figure 2.23 A 62–year-old man with left frontal lesion. (a) Anatomic T2-weighted image shows high signal well-circumscribed lesion in the left frontal lobe near the vertex. Differential diagnosis was multiple sclerosis versus primary brain tumor or metastasis. (b) MR cerebral perfusion scan at 3T using gadolinium bolus power injection during sequential gradient echo T2*-weighted imaging every 2 seconds. This calculated map looks at the negative integral of signal drop out as the contrast passes through each slice which reflects the vascularity of the lesion. In this case, the high vascularity along parts of the lesion indicated this was likely a high grade primary brain tumor. (c) Immediate postoperative CT scan shows appearance after resection using stereotaxic guidance. Pathology revealed glioblastoma multiforma, a high grade tumor.

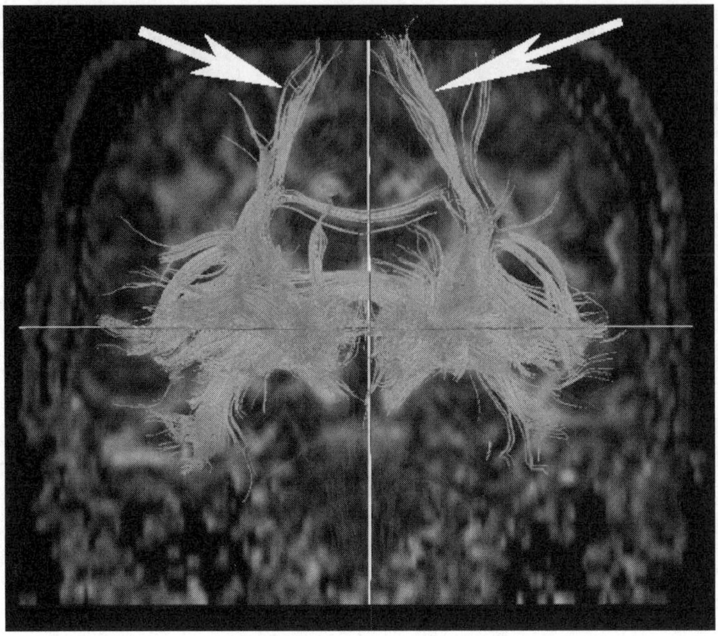

Figure 2.24 Diffusion tensor tractography map in a patient with multiple sclerosis. A critical pathway clinically is the corticospinal tract extending superiorly (arrows) which can be involved in multiple sclerosis (but intact in this patient).

able as a built-in adjunct to morphologic MRI providing useful information about tissue metabolites. MR spectroscopy (MRS) may be able to depict, for example, a higher ratio of choline and creatine to citrate in cancerous tissue than in normal tissue [61]. In tumors of the prostate, brain, or other organs, analysis of these or other substances may aid in the decision process for the correct therapy modality [62] or may facilitate estimation of treatment response earlier than contrast enhanced methods do (Figure 2.25) [63, 64].

2.3.2.4 Blood Oxygen Level Dependent MRI

Another parameter that can be derived from functional MRI is the level of blood oxygenation in a specific area of the body. This technique is called blood-oxygenation level dependent MRI (BOLD) and is a clinical reality in neurosciences [65], but other studies have interrogated its usefulness for detection of parenchymal hypoxemia in other highly vascularized organs as well such as the kidneys, renal grafts, and also in animal experiments in the myocardium [66–68].

Upon activation of a specific area of the brain by repeating motor, sensory, or language tasks, a color map may be calculated displaying the foci showing greater activity during the task versus a rest period. This functional color map may then be registered with the anatomic images. In patients with brain tumors and other lesions undergoing resection, this technique may aid in surgical planning since it demonstrates the location of critical brain centers in relation to the surgical target and may help reduce significant unexpected post-operative neurological deficits. (Figure 2.26).

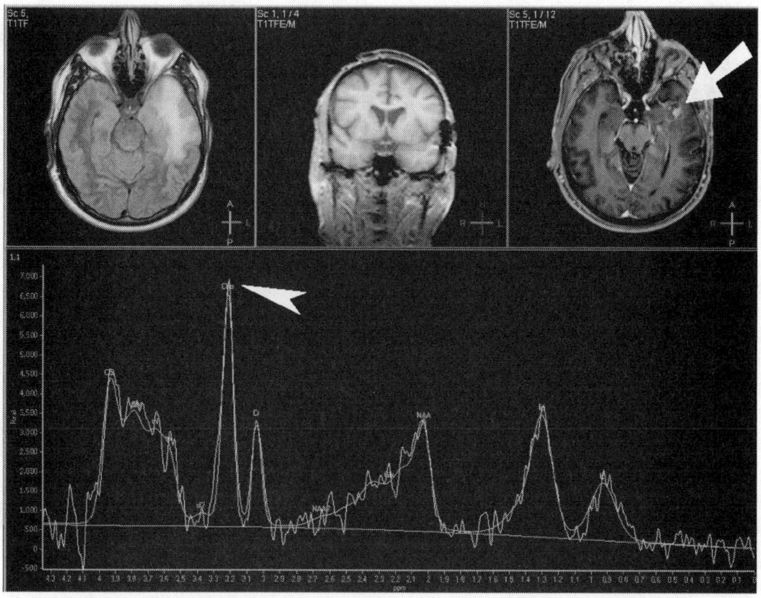

Figure 2.25 Proton single voxel MR spectroscopy using Point RESolved Spectroscopy (PRESS) technique with long TE 144ms. In this patient with mixed anaplastic glioma in the left anterior temporal lobe treated with radiation and chemotherapy, a new focus of enhancement was seen on a 1-year follow-up scan (arrow). This could represent either tumor recurrence or radiation necrosis. Spectroscopy revealed a large choline peak (arrow head) representing high membrane turn over and consistent with tumor recurrence. The patient was therefore treated with gamma knife radiation focused on the region of enhancement.

2.4 Combination of Imaging Modalities

To achieve access to an organ or lesion of interest for a minimally invasive procedure, its anatomic location might preclude a physical approach by one imaging modality alone. In these situations the combination of two established modalities might be helpful to achieve the information needed. Two examples are given, endoscopic retrograde cholangio-pancreatography, which is the physical combination of two very different imaging modes, and fusion imaging, which is the coregistration of two imaging datasets.

2.4.1 Endoscopic Retrograde Cholangio-Pancreatography

Endoscopic retrograde cholangio-pancreatography (ERCP) is the combination of endoscopy and fluoroscopy for the dedicated indication of evaluating the biliary and pancreatic ductal system. It offers immediate opportunity to add a therapeutic procedure such as the incision of the duodenal ampulla (sphincterotomy) or the insertion of a ductal stent in case of a stenosis. The endoscope requires an optical head with side view capabilities to adequately visualize the duodenal ampulla, which in the normal case drain both the common biliary and the main pancreatic duct. Through a working channel and a side hole within the tip of the endoscope, a catheter may be introduced in the ampulla to inject radio-opaque dye into the ductal system. The injection is fluoroscopically monitored and may be documented with spot images and still radiographs (Figure 2.27). Competing diagnostic methods

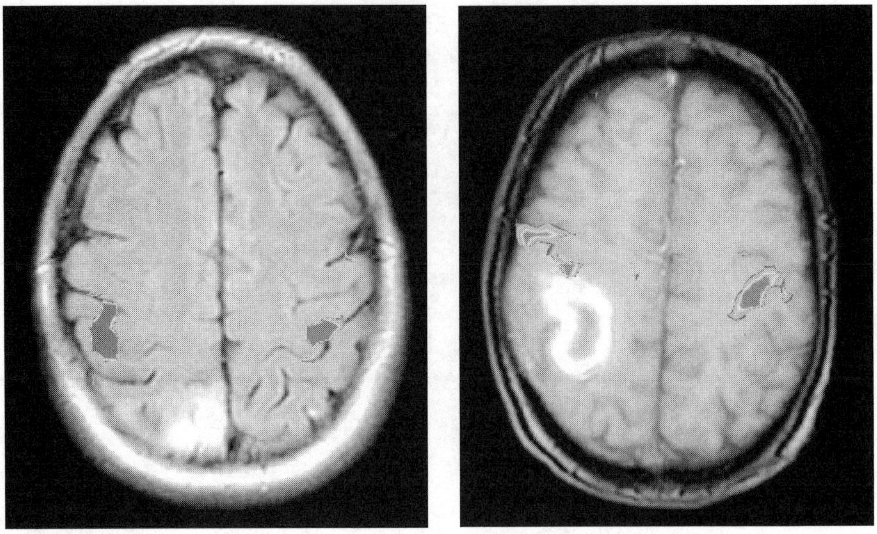

(a) (b)

Figure 2.26 (a) Axial BOLD MRI of a patient with a brain tumor in the right parietal lobe. After a bilateral finger motor task (finger tapping), a color-coded BOLD activation map was calculated demonstrating activity at the expected location of hand sensori-motor cortex along the central sulcus (gray areas bilaterally). The underlying coregistered anatomic FLAIR image demonstrates a high-signal right parietal tumor. Knowing the precise location of the critical hand sensori-motor cortex helps the surgeon to plan a safe tumor resection. (Courtesy of Dr. Kenneth R. Maravilla, University of Washington, Seattle, Washington, Neuroradiology.) (b) Axial BOLD MRI of another patient with a brain tumor in the right parietal lobe. The same functional paradigm as in the patient in (a) was used. Both sensori-motor hand centers are activated. The contrast enhanced T1 weighted coregistered anatomic image demonstrates a peripherally enhancing centrally necrotic metastatic tumor (large white oval ring lesion), which is directly adjcent to the hand motor cortex (small gray areas anterior to enhancing mass) making loss of hand function likely if a complete resection is performed. (Courtesy of Dr. Kenneth R. Maravilla, University of Washington, Seattle, Washington, Neuroradiology.)

such as MR retrograde cholangio-pancreatography (MRCP) offer good diagnostic image quality without the side effects and logistical efforts of the ERCP, but lack the spatial resolution and the option for intervention. However, advantages of MRCP include visualization of the ductal system beyond the occlusion of a duct and cross-sectional image information of the liver, pancreas, and the entire upper abdomen or more organ systems in the same session.

2.4.2 CT Myelography

CT myelography is another method that uses two imaging modalities: it generates CT images of the intrathecal space with iodine contrast in order to outline its anatomic contents or less commonly to show leakage of cerebrospinal fluid.

A needle is inserted under fluoroscopic guidance into the subarachnoid space of the lumbar spine, most commonly at the L2/3 level. A nonionic iodine contrast agent is then injected into the subarachnoid space with correct flow within the cerebral spinal fluid verified with intermittent fluoroscopy. The patient is then transferred to the CT scanner and images of the spinal level of interest are then taken, which are now typically reformatted in sagittal and sometimes coronal planes. Usually performed as a preoperative assessment in patients with severe lower back pain

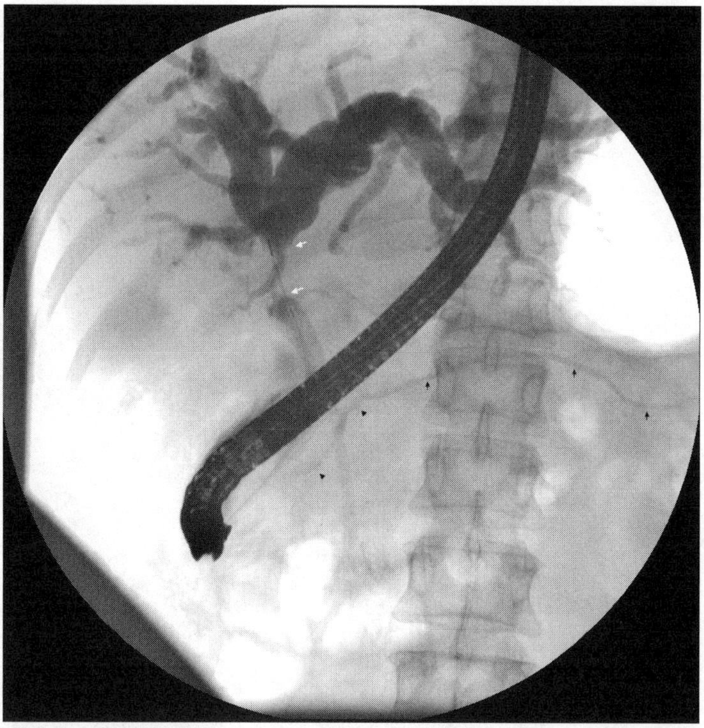

Figure 2.27 Endoscopic retrograde cholangio-pancreatography (ERCP) of a patient with cancer of the bile ducts. A small catheter is advanced through a side opening at the tip of the endoscope into the papilla and further in beyond a high-grade stenosis (the distance between the white arrows) at the bifurcation of the right and left hepatic bile ducts ("Klatskin" tumor). The mass itself is not seen with this method, only the contrast filling defects that are caused by its contour. Note significant dilatation of the intrahepatic bile ducts superior to the stenosis as a sign of bile duct obstruction caused by the mass. Note the normal pancreatic duct (arrow heads), which was contrasted before also through the duodenal ampulla (black arrow heads). Note endoscope projecting between biliary tree and pancreatic duct.

or leg pain and/or weakness, the most common abnormalities seen are intervertrebral disc herniations and bony spurs which may impinge on the contrast-outlined nerve roots. Other less common findings include abnormal clumping of the nerve roots (arachnoiditis), post-operative or traumatic leakage of cerebrospinal fluid, and subtle arachnoid or synovial cysts, which would not be otherwise appreciated using conventional CT with or without intravenous contrast (Figure 2.28).

2.4.3 MR Arthrography

Equivalent to CT myelography, CT arthrography has been used in the past to outline preformed cavities, in this case structures within or adjacent to joints. Nowadays, however, mostly magnetic resonance arthrography (MR arthrogram) is being performed. Direct and indirect arthrographies are distinguished; however, the direct method uses two modalities of imaging: under fluoroscopy guidance a needle is inserted into the joint space and a solution containing an MR contrast agent such as gadolinium is injected. The patient is then transferred to the MR suite and MR images form the joint of interest, mostly the shoulder, are being taken. Mostly traumatic conditions of the glenoid and its cartilages, but also its tendons and

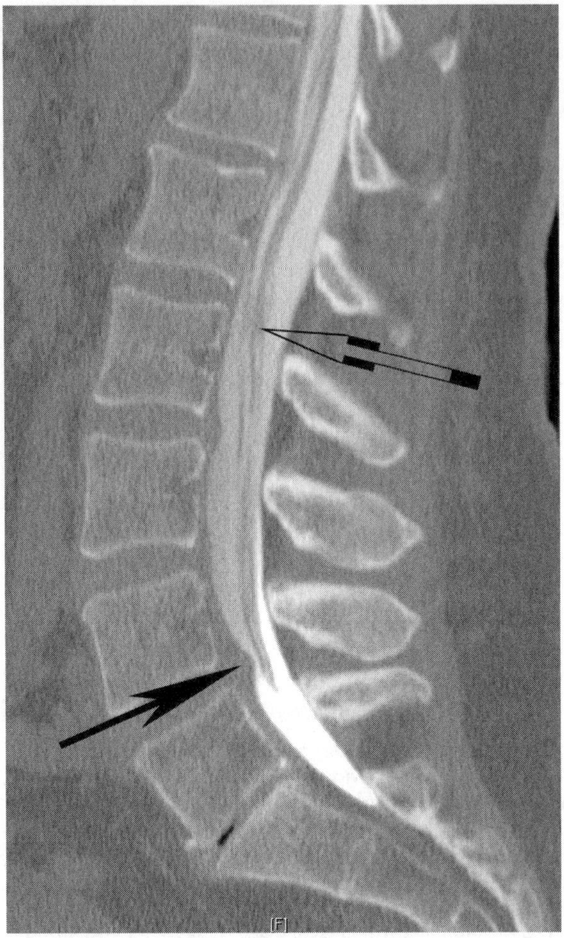

Figure 2.28 Sagittal reconstruction of lumbar CT myelogram following intrathecal injection of iodinated contrast in a patient with lower back pain. The dark arrow shows L4/5 disk herniation indenting the contrast-filled thecal sac. Normal nerve roots (open arrow) are shown forming the cauda equina ("horse's tail") which extend from the spinal cord terminus and exit out the lumbar and sacral foramen. Compression of these nerves can cause pain and weakness.

ligaments, may be better seen when the joint space is distended and contrasted (Figure 2.29).

2.4.4 Fusion Imaging

Modality fusion is the combination of two different imaging modalities with regard to one and the same anatomic area. The intent is to combine anatomic and functional image information.

A clinical reality of fusion imaging is PET-CT. Systems that allow acquisition of image data from both modalities are in use. The CT dataset serves two purposes: it is used for attenuation correction of the PET data and is also used for anatomical coregistration of the PET images. The result is two volume datasets that can be displayed independent and next to each other or in an overlaid and color-coded mode [Figure 2.18(a)].

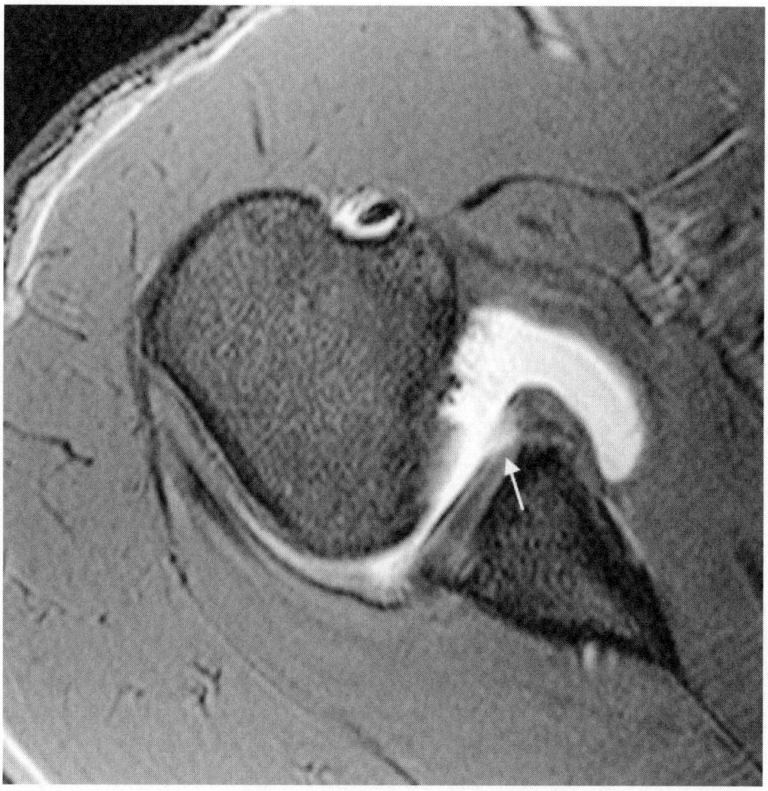

Figure 2.29 Axial proton density MR arthrogram showing glenolabral articular disruption (GLAD) of the cartilage of the right shoulder (arrow). This finding is well seen since the contrast material injected into the joint fills in the cartilaginous gap. (Courtesy Dr. John Hunter, University of Washington Medical Center, Seattle, Washington, Musculoskeletal Radiology, Online Teaching File.)

A relatively new application for fusion imaging is its use for interventional guidance. Datasets from CT or MR exams can be combined with real-time ultrasound to enable access to lesions that are occult to ultrasound alone. These systems usually require a stereotactic approach to coregister the datasets with the interventional device. In these devices previously acquired gapless volume image data sets from CT or MR are transferred into the system [69, 70]. The guidance system then coregisters the volume data either with or without fiducial markers on the patients' skin with the location of the patient in relation to the ultrasound transducer and to the interventional device via receivers such as optical systems. Both the ultrasound transducer and the needle device carry antennas to be registered with the image datasets. Once the system is set up the operator is able to navigate through the CT or MR dataset by moving the transducer over the patients' corresponding body portion. A toggle between the ultrasound and the CT or MR dataset allows seamless superimposed and, if desired, semitransparent display of either imaging modality. In addition, a coregistered biopsy or ablation probe may be inserted and projected as a virtual needle onto the real-time image. As a result of the combined display of the real-time ultrasound image and the overlayed CT or MR image, an interventional device can be positioned into the target even if neither the target nor the needle tip are seen by ultrasound for reasons mentioned in other chapters. Various indications and technical applications have been introduced [1, 69, 70].

Since this kind of virtual navigation system displays image data acquired at a different point in time than the real-time ultrasound does, caution is required when used for lesions targeted in locations that have a close proximity to organs at risk such as stomach and bowel, gallbladder, lungs, and heart. It has to be ascertained that the likelihood for misregistration is minimized to prevent the operator from being misguided. An accuracy of below 2 mm has been reported [69].

Other methods of image fusion combine CT-guided navigational procedures such as radiofrequency ablations of the liver with previously obtained MR datasets [71]. For improved targeting a nonrigid registration system has been developed similar to guidance systems in the brain to minimize misregistration due to brain shift, once the skull has been opened [71, 72].

Other fusion systems have been investigated. Systems combining 99m Tc-MIBI SPECT and MRI fusion for radiation treatment planning of the brain have been recently successfully tested [73]. For brain interventions and surgery, percutaneous and intraoperative guidance through coregistered image datasets of volumetric CT and MR [74] can be provided. Approaches of virtual three-dimensional CT-video fusion for image-guided navigation have been carried out for guiding bronchoscopes to a peritracheal target that was not endoscopically seen [75].

While retrospective registration of PET and MRI has been a routine tool of researchers, its clinical implementation as a prospectively set up whole body fusion system is one of the most promising contributions to the field of fusion imaging. MRI with its excellent soft tissue contrast is mostly used as a morphologic imaging modality. The overwhelming number of three-dimensional MR data sets of the entire body buries the risk of overlooking small, but potentially crucial details such as tumor metastates [76]. PET on the other hand is able to detect subtle oncologic disease before it becomes morphogically distinguishable from its background by other modalities; however, it suffers from its lack of precise anatomic reference frame [76]. Fusion of these two modalities combines the advantages of both, but has a significantly smaller radiation dose than PET-CT does. It also has the potential to be more accurate in the detection and characterization of brain tumors and soft tissue sarcomas than PET-CT [77, 78].

Finally, fusion can be used to enhance the performance of guided procedures by just combining one modality by a previously obtained dataset of its own. One example is CT-guided percutaneous radiofrequency ablation in CT fluoroscopy mode, where low signal-to-noise ratio, absence of contrast, and additional presence of needle in the imaging plane may degrade the image quality to a degree that the target lesion is not seen. In this case solutions have been proposed to link the real-time CT-fluoro image with a previously taken contrast enhanced CT dataset, indicating the position of the probe in the appropriate virtual plane on the preinterventional image set [79]. Other such applications include fusion of preinterventional with real-time MR for guided brain biopsies and surgery, where brain shift would cause misregistration, if the procedure, guided by MR navigation, would not be supported by fusion with real-time MR [72].

With the improving performance of computer hardware and further advanced software developments, virtual navigation utilizing previously recorded datasets and displaying them in a variety of rendition modes, either in two or three dimensions, has become a clinical reality in selected indications and has tremendous potential to contribute to the safety and accuracy of percutaneous or endoscopic minimally invasive or surgical procedures.

Modality fusion is a promising and elegant imaging tool which, when combining morphological and functional or molecular information, has the potential to increase sensitivity and specificity of the detection of diseases and to better monitor treatment responses. As a guidance tool it has the capability to increase accuracy, speed and safety of a procedure.

The success of developments in molecular imaging and other functional imaging modalities may even depend on robust fusion imaging methods that allow the precise co-registration and display of anatomic and nonmorphologic information.

Although this chapter permits only a limited survey of the many varied techniques, diseases, and anatomic structures encompassed by the rapidly growing field of image-guided medical interventions, it can be seen that it has already played an important role advancing the quality and safety of patient care and much more can be expected in the near future.

References

[1] Tang, A. M., et al., "Simultaneous Ultrasound and MRI System for Breast Biopsy: Compatibility Assessment and Demonstration in a Dual Modality Phantom," *IEEE Transactions on Medical Imaging*, Vol. 27, 2008, pp. 247–254.

[2] Molloy, J. A., and S. A. Oldham, "Benchmarking a Novel Ultrasound-CT Fusion System for Respiratory Motion Management in Radiotherapy: Assessment of Spatio-Temporal Characteristics and Comparison to 4DCT," *Med. Phys.*, Vol. 35, 2008, pp. 291–300.

[3] Hoult, D., et al., "The Engineering of an Interventional MRI with a Movable 1.5 Tesla Magnet," *Journal of Magnetic Resonance Imaging*, Vol. 13, 2001, pp. 78–86.

[4] Merkle, E. M., et al. "The Interventional MR Imaging Suite: Magnet Designs and Equipment Requirements," *Magnetic Resonance Imaging Clinics of North America*, Vol. 13, 2005, pp. 401–413.

[5] Fenchel, S., D. Boll, and J. S. Lewin, "Intraoperative MR Imaging," *Magn. Reson. Imaging Clin. N. Am.*, Vol. 11, 2003, pp. 431–447.

[6] Hall, W. A., and C. L. Truwit, "Intraoperative MR-Guided Neurosurgery," *Journal of Magnetic Resonance Imaging*, Vol. 27, 2008, pp. 368–375.

[7] Hushek, S. G., et al., "MR Systems for MRI-Guided Interventions," *Journal of Magnetic Resonance Imaging*, Vol. 27, 2008, pp. 253–266.

[8] Sheafor, D. H., et al., "Abdominal Percutaneous Interventional Procedures: Comparison of CT and US Guidance," *Radiology*, Vol. 207, 1998, pp. 705–710.

[9] Winter, T. C., F. T. Lee, Jr., and J. L. Hinshaw, "Ultrasound-Guided Biopsies in the Abdomen and Pelvis [Review]," *Ultrasound Quarterly*, Vol. 24, 2008, pp. 45–68.

[10] Paulson, E. K., et al., "CT Fluoroscopy-Guided Interventional Procedures: Techniques and Radiation Dose to Radiologists," *Radiology*, Vol. 220, 2001, pp. 161–167.

[11] Weiss, C. N. S., and J. S. Lewin, "MR-Guided Biopsy: A Review of Current Techniques and Applications," *Journal of Magnetic Resonance Imaging*, Vol. 27, 2008, pp. 311–325.

[12] Wilson, S., and P. Burns, "Liver Mass Evaluation with Ultrasound: The Impact of Microbubble Contrast Agents and Pulse Inversion Imaging," *Semin. Liver Dis.*, Vol. 21, 2001, pp. 147–159.

[13] Albrecht, T., et al., "Phase-Inversion Sonography During the Liver-Specific Late Phase of Contrast Enhancement: Improved Detection of Liver Metastases," *Am. J. Roentgenol.*, Vol. 176, 2001, pp. 1191–1198.

[14] Simpson, D. H., C. T. Chin, and P. N. Burns, "Pulse Inversion Doppler: A New Method for Detecting Nonlinear Echoes from Microbubble Contrast Agents," *IEEE Transactions on Ultrasonic Ferroelectric Frequency Control*, Vol. 46, 1999, pp. 372–382.

[15] Quaia, E., "Contrast-Specific Ultrasound Techniques," *La Radiologia Medica*, Vol. 112, 2007, pp. 473–490.

[16] Burns, P. N., S. R. Wilson, and D. H. Simpson, "Pulse Inversion Imaging of Liver Blood Flow: Improved Method for Characterizing Focal Masses with Microbubble Contrast," *Invest. Radiol.*, Vol. 35, 2000.

[17] Albrecht, T., et al., "Stimulated Acoustic Emissions with the Ultrasound Contrast Medium Levovist: A Clinically Useful Contrast Effect with Liver-Specific Properties," *Rofo*, Vol. 172, 2000, pp. 61–67.

[18] Ohlsson, B., et al., "Detection of Hepatic Metastases in Colorectal Cancer: A Prospective Study of Laboratory and Imaging Methods," *Eur. J. Surg.*, Vol. 159, 1993, pp. 275–278.

[19] Leen, E., et al., "Potential Value of Contrast-Enhanced Intraoperative Ultrasonography During Partial Hepatectomy for Metastases: An Essential Investigation Before Resection?" *Ann. Surg.*, Vol. 243, 2006, pp. 236–240.

[20] Romanini, L., et al., "Economic Assessment of Contrast-Enhanced Ultrasonography for Evaluation of Focal Liver Lesions: A Multicentre Italian Experience," *Eur. Radiol.*, Vol. 17, 2007, pp. F99–F106.

[21] http://www.medical.philips.com/main//products/ultrasound/general/iu22/upgrades/vision2008.html#p5.

[22] Blake, G. M., and I. Fogelman, "Technical Principles of Dual Energy X-Ray Absorptiometry," *Seminars in Nuclear Medicine*, Vol. 27, 1997, pp. 210–228.

[23] Park, J. M., et al., "Breast Tomosynthesis: Present Considerations and Future Applications," *Radiographics*, Vol. 27, 2007, pp. S231–S240.

[24] Bachar, G., et al., "Image Quality and Localization Accuracy in C-Arm Tomosynthesis-Guided Head and Neck Surgery," *Medical Physics*, Vol. 34, 2007, pp. 4664–4677.

[25] Eide, K. R., et al., "Initial Observations of Endovascular Aneurysm Repair Using Dyna-CT," *J. Endovasc. Ther.*, Vol. 14, 2007, pp. 50–53.

[26] Flohr, T., et al., "First Performance Evaluation of a Dual-Source CT (DSCT) System," *European Radiology*, Vol. 16, 2006, pp. 256–268.

[27] Achenbach, S., et al., "Contrast-Enhanced Coronary Artery Visualization by Dual-Source Computed Tomography—Initial Experience," *European Journal of Radiology*, Vol. 57, 2006, pp. 331–335.

[28] Wang, G. Y. H., and B. De Man, "An Outlook on X-Ray CT Research and Development," *Med. Phys.*, Vol. 35, 2008, pp. 1051–1064.

[29] Takahashi, N., et al., "Dual-Energy CT Iodine-Subtraction Virtual Unenhanced Technique to Detect Urinary Stones in an Iodine-Filled Collecting System: A Phantom Study," *Am. J. Roentgenol.*, Vol. 190, 2008, pp. 1169–1173.

[30] Boll, D. T., et al., "Coronary Stent Patency: Dual-Energy Multidetector CT Assessment in a Pilot Study with Anthropomorphic Phantom," *Radiology*, Vol. 247, 2008, pp. 687–695.

[31] Schaefer, P. J., et al., "CT Fluoroscopy Guided Biopsy of Small Pulmonary and Upper Abdominal Lesions: Efficacy with a Modified Breathing Technique," *J. Vasc. Interv. Radiol.*, Vol. 18, 2007, pp. 1241–1248.

[32] Rajendran, J. G., et al., "Tumor Hypoxia Imaging with F-18 FMISO PET in Head and Neck Cancer: Value of Pre-Therapy FMISO Uptake in Predicting Survival," *Clin. Can. Res.*, Vol. 12, 2006, pp. 5435–5441.

[33] Rajendran, J. G., and B. Greer, "Expanding Role of Positron Emission Tomography in Cancer of the Uterine Cervix," *J. of Nat. Comp. Can. Network*, Vol. 4, 2006, pp. 463–469.

[34] Rosen, E. L., W. B. Eubank, and D. A. Mankoff, "FDG PET, PET/CT, and Breast Cancer Imaging," *Radiographics*, Vol. 27, 2007, pp. S215–S229.

[35] Vesselle, H., et al., "The Impact of Fluorodeoxyglucose F 18 Positron-Emission Tomography on the Surgical Staging of Non-Small Cell Lung Cancer," *J. Thorac. Cardiovasc. Surg.*, Vol. 124, 2004, pp. 511–519.

[36] Vesselle, H., et al., "In Vivo Validation of 3'deoxy-3'-[(18)F]fluorothymidine ([(18)F]FLT) as a Proliferation Imaging Tracer in Humans: Correlation of [(18)F]FLT Uptake By Positron Emission Tomography with Ki-67 Immunohistochemistry and Flow Cytometry In Human Lung Tumors," *Clin. Cancer Res.*, Vol. 8, 2002, pp. 3315–3323.

[37] Patz, S., et al., "Hyperpolarized 129Xe MRI: A Viable Functional Lung Imaging Modality?" *European Journal of Radiology*, Vol. 64, 2007, pp. 335–344.

[38] Möller, H. E., et al., "MRI of the Lungs Using Hyperpolarized Noble Gases," *Magnetic Resonance in Medicine*, Vol. 47, 2002, pp. 1029–1051.

[39] Kuhl, C., "The Current Status of Breast MR Imaging * Part I. Choice of Technique, Image Interpretation, Diagnostic Accuracy, and Transfer to Clinical Practice," *Radiology*, Vol. 244, 2007, pp. 356–378.

[40] Lu, D. S., S. G. Silverman, and S. S. Raman, "MR-Guided Therapy. Applications in the Abdomen," *Magn. Reson. Imaging Clin. N. Am.*, Vol. 7, 1999, pp. 337–348.

[41] Martin, A. J., et al., "Minimally Invasive Precision Brain Access Using Prospective Stereotaxy and a Trajectory Guide," *Journal of Magnetic Resonance Imaging*, Vol. 27, 2008, pp. 737–743.

[42] Kuhl, C. K., "Current Status of Breast MR Imaging * Part 2. Clinical Applications," *Radiology*, Vol. 244, 2007, pp. 672–691.

[43] Liberman, L., et al., "MRI-Guided 9-Gauge Vacuum-Assisted Breast Biopsy: Initial Clinical Experience," *Am. J. Roentgenol.*, Vol. 185, 2005, pp. 183–193.

[44] Lehman, C. D., et al., "Clinical Experience with MRI-Guided Vacuum-Assisted Breast Biopsy," *Am. J. Roentgenol.*, Vol. 184, 2005, pp. 1782–1787.

[45] Lewin, J. S., et al., "Intraoperative MRI with a Rotating, Tiltable Surgical Table: A Time Use Study and Clinical Results in 122 Patients," *Am. J. Roentgenol.*, Vol. 189, 2007, pp. 1096–1103.

[46] Wacker, F. K., et al., "The Catheter-Driven MRI Scanner: A New Approach to Intravascular Catheter Tracking and Imaging-Parameter Adjustment for Interventional MRI," *Am. J. Roentgenol.*, Vol. 183, 2004, pp. 391–395.

[47] Vogl, T. J., et al., "Malignant Liver Tumors Treated with MR Imaging-Guided Laser-Induced Thermotherapy: Technique and Prospective Results," *Radiology*, Vol. 196, 1995, pp. 257–265.

[48] Stattaus, J. M. S., et al., "MR-Guided Core Biopsy with MR Fluoroscopy Using a Short, Wide-Bore 1.5-Tesla Scanner: Feasibility and Initial Results," *Journal of Magnetic Resonance Imaging*, Vol. 27, 2008, pp. 1181–1187.

[49] Silverman, S. G., et al., "CT Fluoroscopy-Guided Abdominal Interventions: Techniques, Results, and Radiation Exposure," *Radiology*, Vol. 212, 1999, pp. 673–681.

[50] Rofsky, N. M., et al., "MR-Guided Needle Aspiration Biopsies of Hepatic Masses Using a Closed Bore Magnet," *J. Comput. Assist. Tomog.*, Vol. 22, 1998, pp. 633–637.

[51] Sequeiros, R. B., et al., "MR-Guided Interventional Procedures: A Review," *Acta. Radiol.*, Vol. 46, 2005, pp. 576–586.

[52] Smith, K. A., and J. Carrino, "MRI-Guided Interventions of the Musculoskeletal System," *Journal of Magnetic Resonance Imaging*, Vol. 27, 2008, pp. 339–346.

[53] Merkle, E. M., S. G. Nour, and J. S. Lewin, "MR Imaging Follow-Up after Percutaneous Radiofrequency Ablation of Renal Cell Carcinoma: Findings in 18 Patients During First 6 Months," *Radiology*, Vol. 235, 2005, pp. 1065–1071.

[54] Lewin, J. S., S. G. Nour, and J. L. Duerk, "Magnetic Resonance Image-Guided Biopsy and Aspiration," *Top. Magn. Reson. Imaging*, Vol. 11, 2000, pp. 173–183.

[55] Fritz, J., et al., "Real-Time MR Fluoroscopy-Navigated Lumbar Facet Joint Injections: Feasibility and Technical Properties," *European Radiology*, 2008.

[56] Tempany, C., et al., "MR-Guided Prostate Interventions," *Journal of Magnetic Resonance Imaging*, Vol. 27, 2008, pp. 356–367.

[57] Hagmann, P., et al., "Understanding Diffusion MR Imaging Techniques: From Scalar Diffusion-Weighted Imaging to Diffusion Tensor Imaging and Beyond," *Radiographics*, Vol. 26, 2006, pp. S205–S223.

[58] Roberts, T. P., and E. S. Schwartz, "Principles and Implementation of Diffusion-Weighted and Diffusion Tensor Imaging," *Pediatr. Radiol.*, Vol. 37, 2007, pp. 739–748.

[59] Nucifora, P. G. P., et al., "Diffusion-Tensor MR Imaging and Tractography: Exploring Brain Microstructure and Connectivity," *Radiology*, Vol. 245, 2007, pp. 367–384.

[60] Hess, C. P., and P. Mukherjee, "Visualizing White Matter Pathways in the Living Human Brain: Diffusion Tensor Imaging and Beyond," *Neuroimaging Clin. N. Am.*, Vol. 17, 2007, pp. 407–426, vii.

[61] Choi, Y. J., et al., "Functional MR Imaging of Prostate Cancer," *Radiographics*, Vol. 27, 2007, pp. 63–75.

[62] Claus, F. G., H. Hricak, and R. R. Hattery, "Pretreatment Evaluation of Prostate Cancer: Role of MR Imaging and 1H MR Spectroscopy," *Radiographics*, Vol. 24, 2004, pp. S167–S180.

[63] Al-Okaili, R. N., et al., "Advanced MR Imaging Techniques in the Diagnosis of Intraaxial Brain Tumors in Adults," *Radiographics*, Vol. 26, 2006, pp. S173–S189.

[64] Chuang, C. F., et al., "Potential Value of MR Spectroscopic Imaging for the Radiosurgical Management of Patients with Recurrent High-Grade Gliomas," *Technol. Cancer Res. Treat.*, Vol. 6, 2007, pp. 375–382.

[65] Matthews, P. M., and P. Jezzard, "Functional Magnetic Resonance Imaging," *J. Neurol. Neurosurg. Psychiatry*, Vol. 75, 2004, pp. 6–12.

[66] Michaely, H., et al., "Functional Renal Imaging: Nonvascular Renal Disease," *Abdominal Imaging*, Vol. 32, 2007, pp. 1–16.

[67] Sadowski, E. A., et al., "Assessment of Acute Renal Transplant Rejection with Blood Oxygen Level-Dependent MR Imaging: Initial Experience," *Radiology*, Vol. 236, 2005, pp. 911–919.

[68] Wright, K. B., et al., "Assessment of Regional Differences in Myocardial Blood Flow Using T2-Weighted 3D BOLD Imaging," *Magnetic Resonance in Medicine*, Vol. 46, 2001, pp. 573–578.

[69] Banovac, F., et al., "Precision Targeting of Liver Lesions Using a Novel Electromagnetic Navigation Device in Physiologic Phantom and Swine," *Med. Phys.*, Vol. 32, 2005, pp. 2698–2705.

[70] Crocetti, L., et al., "Targeting Liver Lesions for Radiofrequency Ablation: An Experimental Feasibility Study Using a CT-US Fusion Imaging System," *Invest. Radiol.*, Vol. 43, 2008, pp. 33–39.

[71] Archip, N., et al., "Non-Rigid Registration of Pre-Procedural MR Images with Intra-Procedural Unenhanced CT Images For Improved Targeting of Tumors During Liver Radiofrequency Ablations," *Med. Image Comput. Comput. Assist. Interv. Int. Conf.*, Vol. 10, 2007, pp. 969–977.

[72] Archip, N., et al., "Non-Rigid Alignment of Pre-Operative MRI, fMRI, and DT-MRI with Intra-Operative MRI for Enhanced Visualization and Navigation in Image-Guided Neurosurgery," *NeuroImage*, Vol. 35, 2007, pp. 609–624.

[73] Krengli, M., et al., "Delineation of Target Volume for Radiotherapy of High-Grade Gliomas by 99mTc-MIBI SPECT and MRI Fusion," *Strahlentherapie und Onkologie*, Vol. 183, 2007, pp. 689–694.

[74] Mascott, C. R., and L. E. Summers, "Image Fusion of Fluid-Attenuated Inversion Recovery Magnetic Resonance Imaging Sequences for Surgical Image Guidance," *Surgical Neurology*, Vol. 67, 2007, pp. 589–603.

[75] Higgins, W. E., et al.,"3D CT-Video Fusion for Image-Guided Bronchoscopy," *Computerized Medical Imaging and Graphics*, Vol. 32, 2008, pp. 159–173.

[76] Seemann, M., "Whole-Body PET/MRI: The Future in Oncological Imaging," *Technol. Cancer Res. Treat.*, Vol. 4, 2005, pp. 577–582.

[77] Somer, E. J., et al., "PET-MR Image Fusion in Soft Tissue Sarcoma: Accuracy, Reliability and Practicality of Interactive Point-Based and Automated Mutual Information Techniques," *Eur. J. Nucl. Med. Mol. Imaging*, Vol. 30, 2003, pp. 54–62.

[78] Myers, R., "The Application of PET-MR Image Registration in the Brain," *Br. J. Radiol.*, Vol. 75, 2002, pp. 31–35.

[79] Micu, R., et al., "A New Registration/Visualization Paradigm for CT-Fluoroscopy Guided RF Liver Ablation," *Med. Image Comput. Assist. Interv. Int. Conf.*, Vol. 9, 2006, pp. 882–890.

PART II

Interventional Therapy Modalities

CHAPTER 3

Minimally Invasive Endoscopic Surgery and Intraluminal Endoscopy: Videoscopic-Guided Therapy Systems

Allan Haynes and Mika Sinanan

Imperative to conventional open surgical intervention are excellent visualization of the tissues to be affected and free access to permit fine manipulation of these structures. This art was perfected through the twentieth century, with operations devised to alter or remove every organ of the human body to provide relief or cure from disease. Unfortunately, this came at significant cost. When visceral structures deep within the peritoneal or thoracic cavities were involved, generous incisions through the body wall allowing access were necessary, causing a significant physiologic insult to the host organism.

The advent of remote videoscopic imaging in the late twentieth century significantly altered this paradigm of surgical diagnosis and intervention. With accompanying advances in instrumentation and technique, new fields of medicine with videoscopic imaging as the key modality would leap to the forefront, providing near equivalent visualization and manipulation of tissues deep within the body as seen with open techniques, but at much less physiologic cost to the host.

Two distinct disciplines exist that fall into the category of videoscopic-guided therapy: minimally invasive surgery and intraluminal endoscopy. Both rely on similar technology but differ in the way this is applied due to their inherent nature.

Minimally invasive surgery (MIS) involves manipulation of organs and tissues within the abdominal and thoracic cavities, using small incisions in the wall of the human body for introduction of the equipment. The terms laparoscopy and thoracoscopy are often used when discussing MIS involving the abdominal and thoracic cavities, respectively.

Intraluminal endoscopy involves the introduction of equipment through a natural orifice, namely the mouth or the anus, for diagnosis and therapy within the lumen of a hollow viscus (esophagus, stomach, intestine).

This chapter will review the fundamentals underlying the current systems used for videoscopic-guided diagnosis and therapy, some history behind development of the integral components of these systems, how these systems are used practically, and directions of future development for this discipline.

3.1 Minimally Invasive Surgery

Minimally invasive surgery involves performing the equivalent of classic surgical operations through much smaller incisions than what would be needed for conventional surgery. The perceived advantage is that smaller incisions result in improved cosmesis, decreased pain, and most importantly, less overall physiologic insult to the host, allowing quicker healing and recovery.

The essence of MIS lies in the system developed to create an environment allowing visualization and fine manipulation of internal organs through small incisions. The following is a brief description of the system. First, inert gas is introduced into the designated visceral cavity (peritoneal or thoracic cavity), creating a working space. Specially designed access ports called trocars are placed through small incisions made in the abdominal wall to allow access to this space. Through the trocars, visualization of the space is accomplished by use of a videoendoscope, a specialized video camera utilizing a telescopic lens that displays an image on a video monitor. Specially designed instrumentation and devices, discussed in detail later in this chapter, are also introduced through the trocars to manipulate tissues and organs and institute therapy. Figure 3.1 illustrates these basic principles.

3.1.1 Origins of MIS

Defining MIS as a "therapeutic system" is a retrospectively applied perspective. Its early origins lay not in an attempt to design a system for less invasive surgical intervention but to visualize suspected pathology in the peritoneal or thoracic cavity.

The first attempts at laparoscopy date to the early twentieth century. Credit is given to Georg Kelling for performing the first laparoscopy, termed "celioscopy," using a canine in 1901 [1, 2]. Hans Christian Jacobaeus is credited with the first reports of laparo-thoracoscopic techniques in humans, detailed in his 1910 article

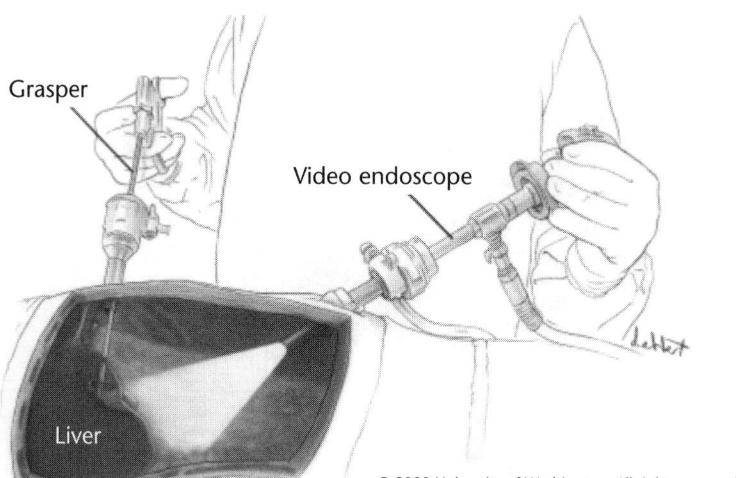

Figure 3.1 Minimally invasive surgery.

"Concerning the Possibility of Applying Cystoscopy in the Examination of the Serous Cavities" [3].

Kelling utilized an instrument developed by Max Nitze in 1872 for retrograde examination of the bladder, the angled cystoscope. Jacobaeus utilized similar instrumentation. It consisted of a hollow metal tube set with lenses and a mirror. This provided transmission of light and thus an image, which was viewed at the proximal end of the scope through an eyepiece. Illumination was provided intracorporeally by an incandescent bulb at the end of the scope. A pneumoperitoneum (injection of air into the peritoneal cavity) was created to provide a working space for viewing via a valved bulb, which allowed introduction of air under pressure into the peritoneal cavity. This rudimentary device was obviously limited in the extent of its applications, but did provide limited visualization of the liver and other peritoneal structures.

For the most part the field lay stagnant over the following decades, being limited to rudimentary diagnostic technique. Some improvements in technique were made, mainly in regard to improving the safety of achieving pneumoperitoneum (injection of air into the peritoneal cavity). In 1924, Richard Zollikofer of Switzerland first recommended carbon dioxide (CO_2) for creation of pneumoperitoneum due to its nonflammable nature and fairly rapid resorption by the peritoneum [1].

Additionally, the introduction of the Veress needle by Janos Veress of Hungary in 1938 greatly decreased the potential for hollow viscus perforation associated with establishment of pneumoperitoneum [1]. The device utilized a spring-loaded blunt tip contained within a cutting core needle. While being pushed through the resistant tissue of the abdominal wall, the force would compress the blunt needle into the core needle, exposing its cutting edge. With entry into the peritoneal cavity, the blunt tip would spring out preventing injury to the contained hollow viscus structures within. His device differed little from the current-day Veress needle shown in Figure 3.2.

It was not until the latter part of the twentieth century that multiple technological advances occurred that would allow the development of the basic system that is used for MIS today. The first of these was the development of the rod lens by Harold Hopkins in 1959. Prior to this, most laparoscopic lenses used a design with multiple lenses along the tubular scope with air interspace. Hopkins discovered that by interspacing glass rods between the lenses in place of air, one could increase light transmission 80 fold and significantly widen the field of vision [4], dramatically improving the quality of the image (Figure 3.3). With the marriage of the lens with recently developed fiber optic technology to provide a high intensity extracorporeal light source, the first high quality laparoscopes would be developed.

The next significant advance was the development of the automatic insufflator by Kurt Semm in 1967 [5]. His device allowed for continuous regulation of pneumoperitoneum to a set pressure and adjustment of the rate of flow of gas into the peritoneal cavity. This provided safe maintenance of a working space within the peritoneal cavity with relative ease and reliability.

The true innovation, which would usher in the era of minimally invasive surgery, was the introduction of the charge-coupled device (CCD) silicon chip image sensor—more commonly referred to as the miniature video camera. While originally adapted to flexible endoluminal endoscopy, it was only a short period of time

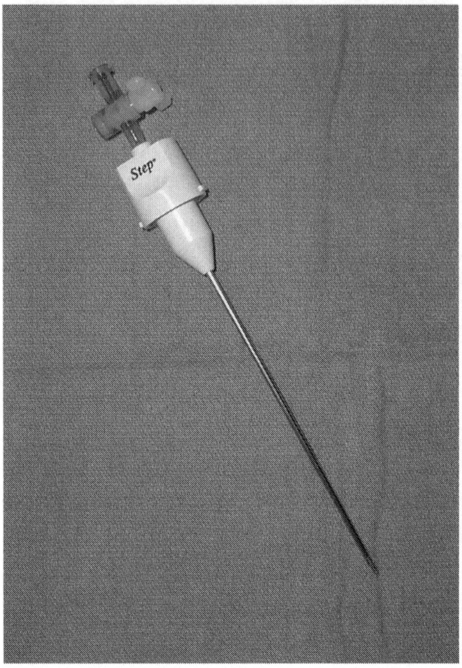

Figure 3.2 Veress needle.

before this was coupled to the Hopkins/Storz telescopic lens to provide a system of functional intracorporeal visualization capable of providing real-time high quality images to a team of individuals, allowing one to coordinate visualization while the other instituted therapy. The pace of advancement after this was exponential. Two years after the introduction of this technology in 1985, the first laparoscopic cholecystectomy would be performed [6]. By 1991, 20,000 surgeons in the United States had received training in the technique of laparoscopic cholecystectomy [6]. Over the following decade, the trend toward minimally invasive surgery would be carried even further, with attempts to adapt virtually every open surgical procedure to its minimally invasive equivalent.

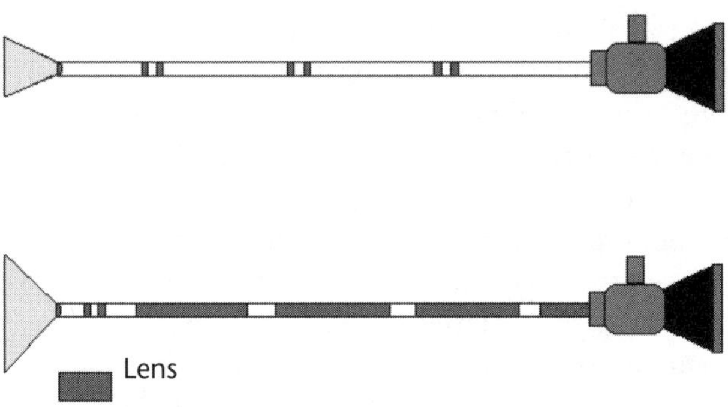

Figure 3.3 Standard air interface lens versus Hopkins rod lens.

3.1.2 MIS—A System for Surgical Therapy

Defining MIS as a "system" is a somewhat novel concept. Most texts providing discussion of MIS in the literature provide a brief history of the discipline and review of the equipment and quickly get into the technical aspects of different operative procedures.

The basic setup of the MIS system has been alluded to earlier in this chapter. However, this brushes the surface in describing a complex system with an array of specialized equipment.

To better characterize MIS as a system, the following section breaks down MIS into integral components and discusses each individually. Each component has specially designed equipment that allows for function of that component of the system.

These components are as follows:

1. Creation of a working space within the designated visceral cavity;
2. Visualization of visceral structures within the working space;
3. Manipulation of visceral structures within this environment to institute therapy.

3.1.2.1 Creation of Working Space

The first objective is to define a well-maintained, easily accessible free space in the designated visceral cavity. As alluded to above, this involves introduction of gas into the visceral cavity and placement of trocars through the body wall to allow access for instruments and the camera. This space in the abdominal cavity is commonly referred to as pneumoperitoneum. The equivalent in the thoracic cavity would be termed pneumothorax, but this is not a commonly used term in this sense.

Creation of a working space in the thoracic cavity is fairly straightforward. In the natural state, the lung entirely fills the thoracic cavity. This state is maintained by positive pressure with inhalation through the airways and negative pressure from the chest wall. Through use of special airway equipment, the lung can be collapsed. The ribs, given their rigid nature, maintain the space. Ambient air enters through the incisions made for port placement.

Creation of this space in the peritoneal cavity is more complex. Unlike the thorax, the abdomen is not rigidly supported. To maintain a space within the abdomen, gas must be introduced and maintained under pressure. In the abdominal cavity, the gas typically used is carbon dioxide. This is due to its relatively benign physiologic nature, and being nonflammable and absorbable into the bloodstream, minimizing the risk of air embolism. The act of introduction of air into the peritoneal cavity is termed insufflation. This is typically accomplished by one of two techniques: the Veress technique or the Hasson technique.

The Veress technique involves placement of a Veress needle, previously described, through the abdominal wall and injection of CO_2 through this needle (Figure 3.4). Once the appropriate pressure is reached, typically 15 mm Hg, the needle is removed. Appropriate trocars are then placed.

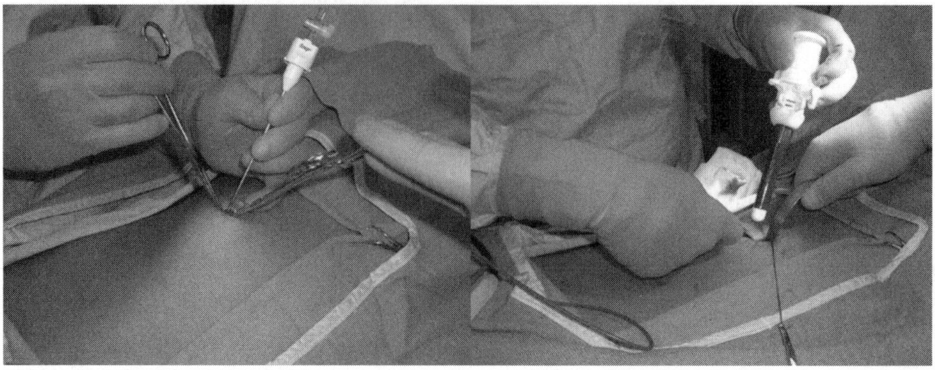

Figure 3.4 Veress and Hasson techniques.

The alternate approach is termed the Hasson technique (Figure 3.4). This involves making a small incision (typically 1 cm) through all layers of the abdominal wall and entering the peritoneal cavity bluntly with the index finger.

The first trocar, a blunt port typically termed a Hasson trocar is introduced through this incision and secured with anchor sutures to the abdominal wall. Insufflation is then achieved through this trocar.

Trocars

Trocars are used to maintain the small incisions through the body wall, facilitating easy access for the videoendoscope and instruments to the working space. As the space for thoracoscopy is naturally maintained, trocars are simple metal sleeves. Those used in the peritoneal cavity are more complex. They are typically designed with diaphragms to maintain the airtight seal necessary to maintain pneumoperitoneum and valves to allow for maintenance insufflation of CO_2.

Some are also designed with balloon valves to maintain better seal at the body wall level. Trocars come in a variety of sizes, with the sleeve typically 5 to 15 mm in diameter. Figure 3.5 illustrates a variety of trocars.

Visiport

When using the Veress technique, insufflation is achieved prior to placement of any ports. Therefore, the first port must be placed blindly, risking injury to peritoneal structures. The Visiport (Figure 3.6) limits this risk by allowing real-time videoscopic visualization through the trocar of tissues being divided as it is placed. A retractable crescent blade at the tip of the device splits tissue in 2-mm increments to allow for advancement of the trocar through tissue in a controlled fashion.

Automatic Insufflator

Throughout a laparoscopic procedure, it is impossible to avoid a small amount of loss of insufflated CO_2, either through escape at the sites of port placement or through slow absorption by the visceral cavity. To maintain a stable pneumoperitoneum, there must be steady, low-level replacement of CO_2 within the peritoneal cavity. However, care must be taken to ensure that pressures to reach a point that would cause physiologic harm. The device that controls this is the automatic insufflator. It allows for adjustable flow of CO_2 by both rate of flow and maximal

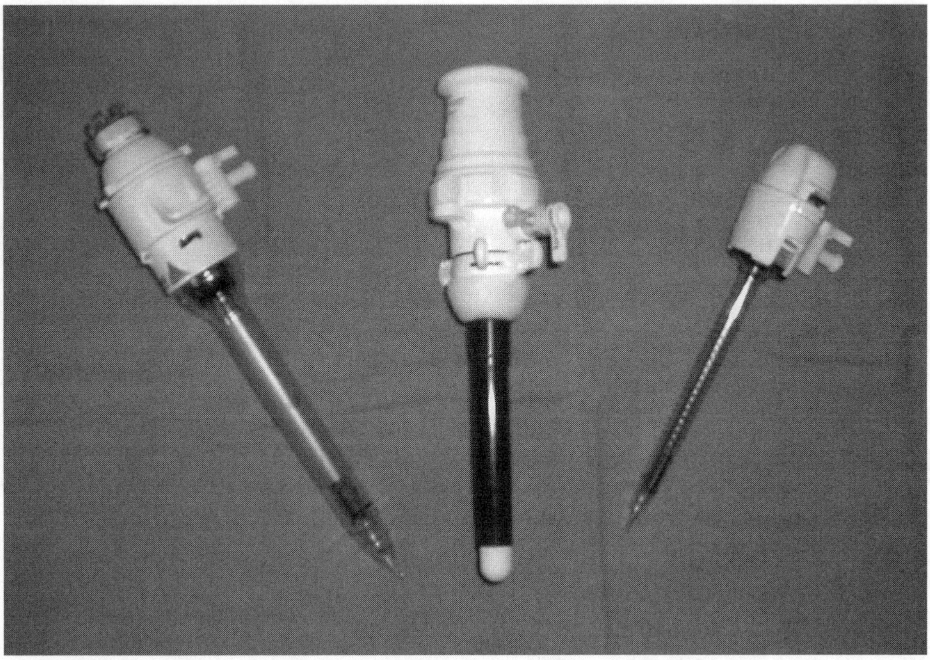

Figure 3.5 Trocars.

pressure, creating a safe, reliable pneumoperitoneum. As discussed previously, this device was invented by Kurt Semm. Figure 3.7 shows a current automatic insufflator. While the ergonomic design has improved over the decades, it is essentially the same device as the original introduced in 1967.

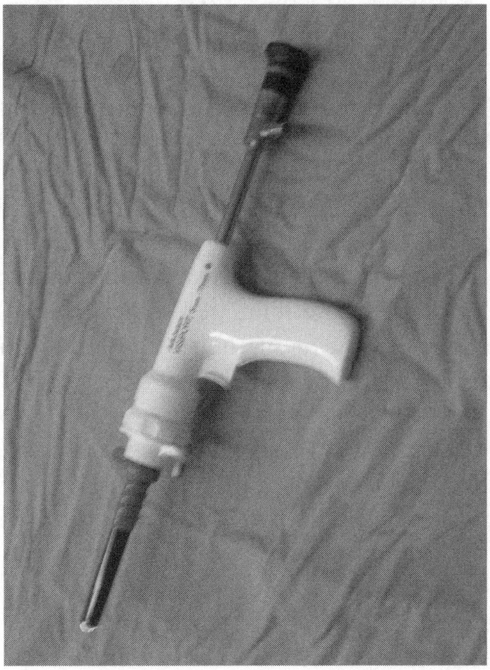

Figure 3.6 Visiport.

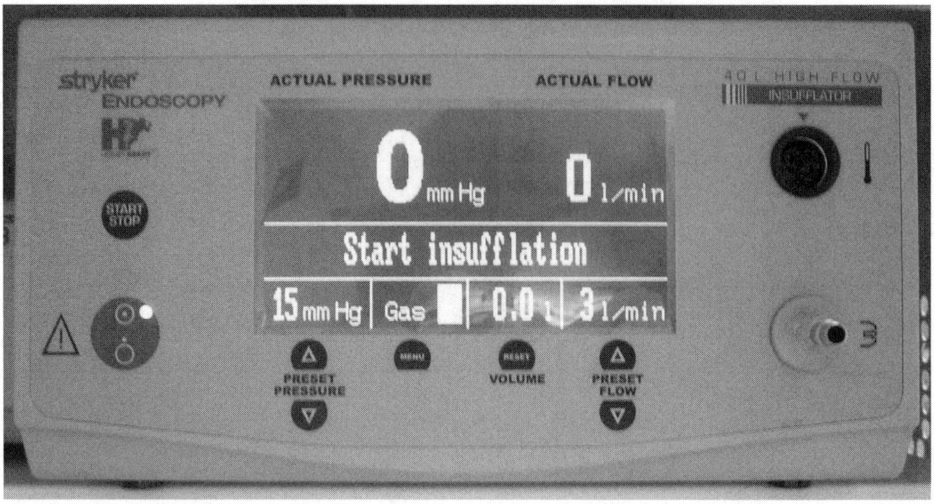

Figure 3.7 The automatic insufflator.

3.1.2.2 Visualization—The Videoendoscope

The videoendoscope allows transmission of light and a visual image respectively into and out of the designated visceral cavity. It is the key innovation that has allowed development of MIS as an alternative to open surgery.

The basic design of the videoendoscope has not changed significantly since its introduction in the 1980s. It consists of three components (Figure 3.8):

1. Hopkins telescopic rod lens;
2. Extracorporeal cold light source;
3. Video camera and associated video monitor.

The design of the rod lens has undergone minimal change since its original development as discussed earlier in the chapter. The telescopic rigid rod structure of the lens is ideally suited for placement through the trocars and allows for controlled telescopic advancement of the distal point of the lens deep into the peritoneal cavity for close-perspective visualization of the viscera. The lenses typically come in 2 diameters, 5 and 10 mm, which correlate with standard trocar diameter. The visual acuity of the 5-mm lens is diminuated somewhat as it allows for passage of less light. The lenses also come in an angled format, which in certain situations, facilitates visualization of visceral structures.

The light source is typically provided by a 250W to 400W high intensity incandescent bulb. Transmission of light from the source to the camera is achieved via a fiber optic cable that connects to the rod lens. Maintaining an extracorporeal light source alleviates difficulty with generation of heat that was associated with early intracorporeal sources.

The video source for the modern surgical endoscope consists of a miniature silicon chip video camera. The palm-size camera is a lightweight, self-contained unit that is hermetically sealed to allow for chemical sterilization so that the scope

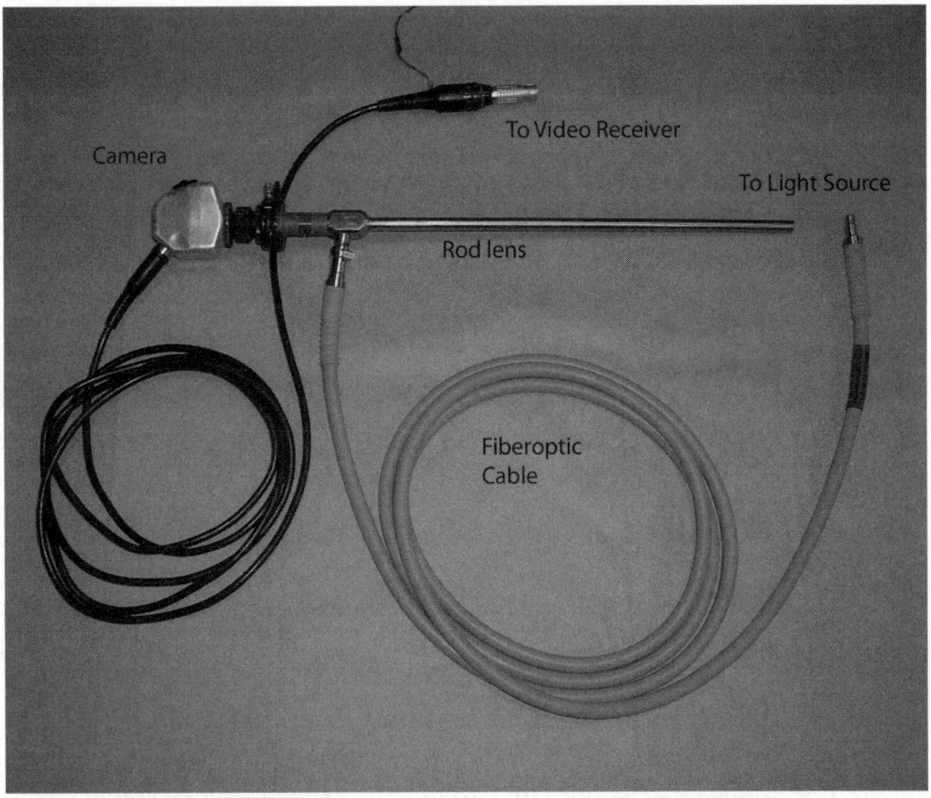

Figure 3.8 The videoendoscope.

can be passed directly onto the operating field. An adaptor clip allows for fixation of the rod lens at its distal end. A cable exits the camera proximally and allows for transmission of a digital image to an associated video monitor.

3.1.2.3 Manipulation of Structures—The Instrumentation of MIS

The two components of the system just described are a means to this end—use of instrumentation to perform an operation, typically involving removal or alteration of a visceral structure, with a result equivalent to classic open surgery.

The "system" aspect of this component is overcoming the limit of performing a complex operation through 5- to 15-mm access points, often at a significant distance from the target structure. This is based on the use of an array of specifically adapted instrumentation.

The basic design of typical MIS instrumentation was established by the time of laparoscopic cholecystectomy and has changed little since that time. This consists of a metal rod, often with ceramic insulation, typically 30 to 40 cm in length. A downsized equivalent of a standard surgical instrument is found at the distal end. The proximal end has a handgrip that is connected to the distal functional end via a lever system that allows control of the instrument. Most also have a component of 360-degree axial rotation to allow for adjustment of the angle of the instrument using the thumb.

Virtually all surgical instrumentation used in open surgery has been adapted in this manner for in the MIS system. This includes not only scissors, graspers, and tissue dissectors as seen in the standard endoscopic surgery instrument set shown in Figure 3.9, but also staplers (Figure 3.10), clip appliers (Figure 3.10), electrocautery, and cholangiography equipment.

Given the difficulty of performing certain tasks with the limited access of the MIS environment, many novel devices unique to this discipline have been developed.

Surgical intervention often requires coordination of irrigation, evacuation of ongoing bleeding, and coagulation of vessels in a rapidly coordinated fashion. Accomplishing this in the MIS environment can be difficult. This has led to the development of devices that combine all three functions in one instrument. The Surgiwand (Figure 3.10) is an example of this type of device.

Retrieval of intact specimens through small incisions can also be challenging. A retrieval system that utilizes a retractable and detachable polyurethane bag, called the Endo-Catch (Figure 3.10), is often utilized for this purpose.

Certain devices have been designed to help overcome the inherent limitations in suturing and knot tying. The Endo-Loop (Figure 3.11) provides the equivalent of a suture ligature. The Endo-Stitch (Figure 3.11) is a suturing device that facilitates intracorporeal suture placement.

3.1.3 Integration of the MIS System: The MIS Operating Suite

The layout of the modern day MIS operating suite is similar to the layout for open surgery, but it must incorporate the additional equipment required for endoscopic surgery. As with open surgery, the patient is appropriately positioned on an operating table in accordance to the planned procedure. The anesthesia team and their equipment are located at the head of the bed. The light source, insufflator, and video camera receiver are typically located on a tower or cart that is placed to the side or the patient. The necessary cables run off the operating field and across the floor to this tower. Monitors are stationed appropriately at the head or foot of the bed as needed for the operating team.

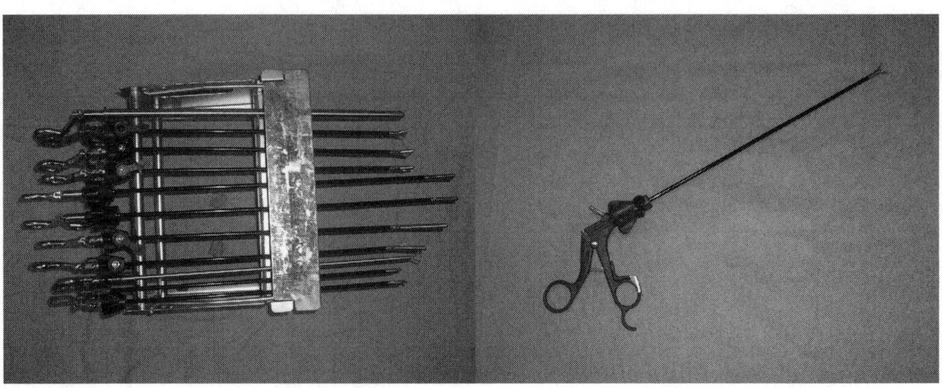

Figure 3.9 Laparoscopic instruments.

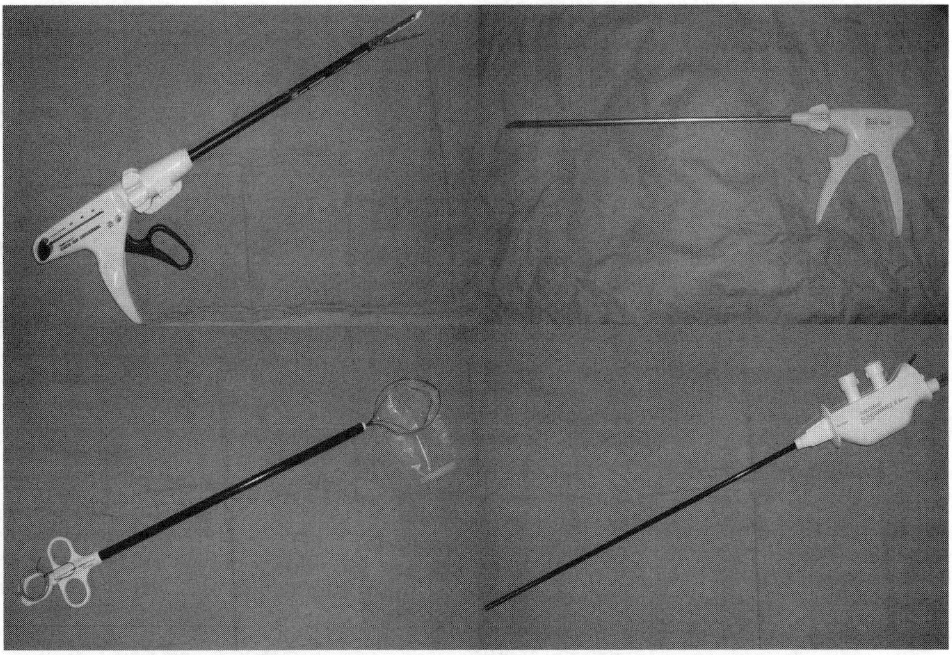

Figure 3.10 Stapler, clipper, Surgiwand, Endo-Catch (from top left clockwise).

The operating surgeon utilizes two instruments, one for tissue manipulation and the other to provide traction. An assistant provides countertraction and runs the video camera. For more complex procedures, a second assistant will run the camera and provide the appropriate image guidance, freeing the first assistant to use instruments in both hands for traction and operative assistance. One of the true complexities of endoscopic surgery lies in coordinating the actions of up to three persons to perform a single complex task.

In recent years, there has been a move toward having specific operating rooms dedicated to laparoscopy. These rooms are laid out to ergonomically maximize access and use of the laparoscopic equipment. A typical suite is shown in Figure 3.12.

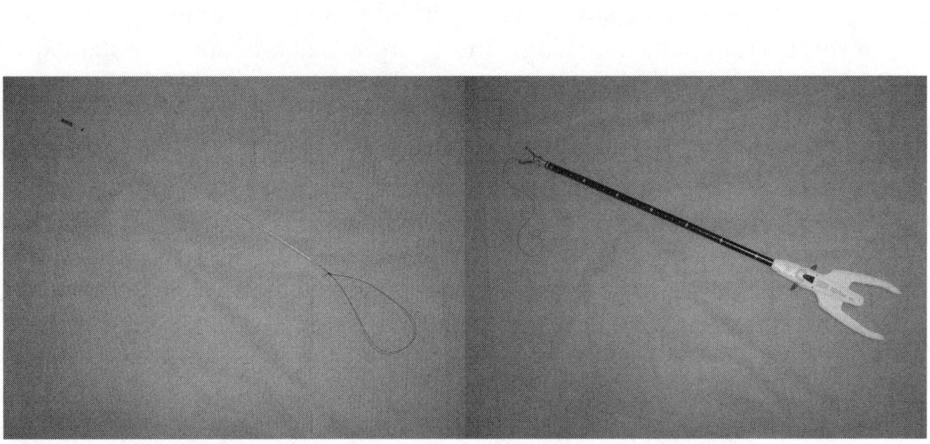

Figure 3.11 Endo-Loop and Endo-Stitch.

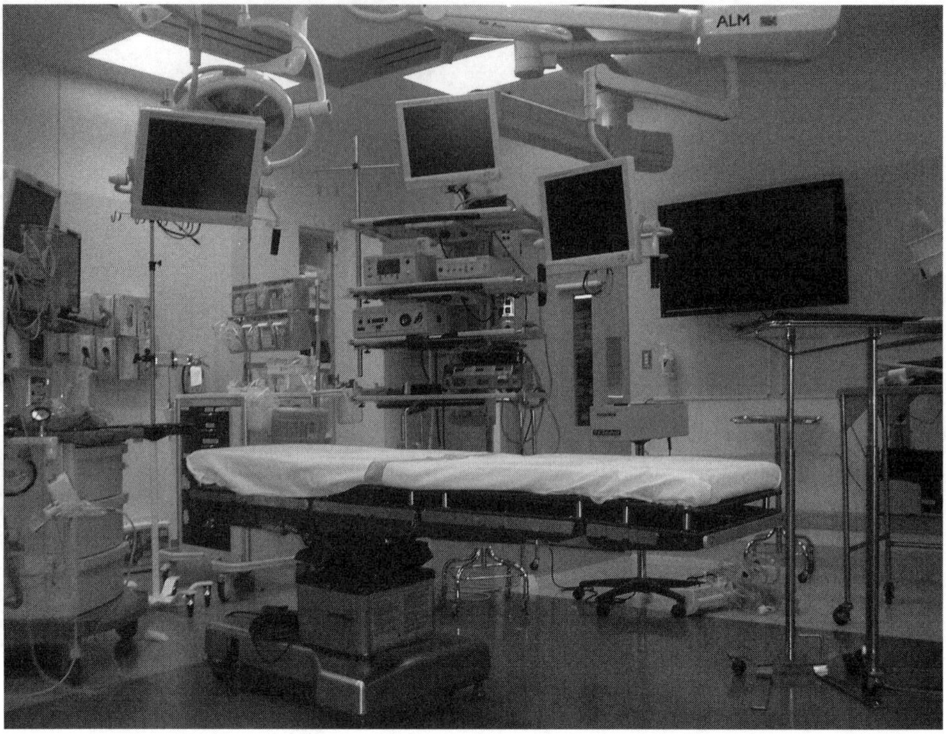

Figure 3.12 The current-day MIS operating suite.

The monitors and equipment are stationed on easily positionable pneumatic booms that facilitate adjustment of the monitors and equipment.

3.1.4 Current-Day MIS: Its Uses and Limitations

The laparoscopic revolution began in the late 1980s with the introduction of laparoscopic cholecystectomy. In lieu of a sizeable subcostal incision and a multiday associated hospital stay and weeks to months of healing and recovery, patients could anticipate a surgery performed through four incisions less that 1 cm in length, less than 24 hours in the hospital, and typically full recovery in a few weeks. This procedure was rapidly adopted by most surgeons and became the standard of care in most industrialized countries by the early 1990s.

Once the benefits of the minimally invasive approach for cholecystectomy became apparent, extensive efforts were made to adapt this technique to other surgical procedures. Some procedures such as gastro-esophageal reflux surgery, splenectomy, adrenalectomy, and hernia repair proved readily adaptable to this modality.

Other procedures, such as colon resection, gastric resection, and pulmonary resection, have more recently been shown to be equivalent operations using the minimally invasive technique.

Even more complex procedures, such as liver resection, pancreatic head resection, and rectal resection, have recently been shown to be feasible using a minimally invasive approach, albeit usually in isolated instances at highly specialized academic centers.

3.2 Intraluminal Flexible Endoscopy

Intraluminal endoscopy is the second major application of videoendoscopy technology. It has become a technical mainstay for diagnostic and therapeutic procedures in many surgical specialties as well as anesthesiology, pulmonary medicine, and gastroenterology. Organ systems for which flexible endoscopic evaluation is routinely carried out are all accessible through natural orifices. These include the upper and lower gastrointestinal tracts (upper endoscopy and sigmoidoscopy or colonoscopy) and the orotracheobronchial system (video laryngoscopy and bronchoscopy). Novel applications of flexible endoscopy have also been described for the nasosinus and genitourinary systems though rigid scopes are still more common due to therapeutic instrumentation requirements and better lighting of a rigid scope.

In its current form, the flexible endoscope is a wonder of technical innovation. Each endoscope includes a halogen light source, flexible fiber optic fibers to carry light to illuminate the target, lenses to carry the image to a tip-mounted CCD chip or back via other coherent fiber optics to an optical viewer, and control systems to change the geometry of the tip so that the endoscope can be steered to a target. Most flexible endoscopies provide an optical view off of the end of the endoscope. Some have been specially modified to provide a side view or to augment visual diagnosis with ultrasound. Therapeutic interventions such as biopsies, injections, cauterization, and delivery of stents or inflatable balloons are facilitated by a user-accessible working port. And of course, this complex instrument must be durable, cleanable, sterilizable, and small enough to match the orifice and lumen of the organ being examined.

3.2.1 Origin of Intraluminal Endoscopy

As previously described, the history of endoscopic development started with rigid scopes using glass lenses. Philipp Bozzini, a German physician and inventor working in the early 1800s developed a rigid but angled scope for evaluating the larynx. Eighty years later, Stoerk (1887) developed an angled esophagoscope. Kelling (1898), also recognized for his enabling work in rigid videoendoscopes for surgery, developed a gastroscope with a partial flexion capability. This was the first endoscope with a maneuverable tip capability, a key enabling feature for current generation endoscopes.

Although the guiding of light by optical refraction was first demonstrated in 1840s, development of glass fibers with a transparent refractive cladding was realized in 1952 by Narinder Singh Kapany. Bundling of fibers to achieve effective image transmission culminated in a flexible fiberoptic gastroscopic design that was patented in 1956 by Hirschowitz, Peters, and Curtiss from the University of Michigan. Intense commercial development by companies in Japan, the United States, and Germany in the ensuing years has created an industry and novel clinical applications dependent on an entire families of endoscopes designed for specialized applications. Indeed, the field continues to evolve with the incorporation of novel illumination techniques (laser or narrow band illumination), combinations of visual and ultrasound imaging, and an array of endoscopically deployable surgical instruments for manipulation of tissue internally.

3.2.2 Diagnostic Flexible Endoscopy

Diagnostic flexible endoscopy is available for evaluation of the nasal passages and sinuses (rhinoscopy), tracheobronchial tree into the lungs (bronchoscopy), joints (arthroscopy), the chest cavity (thoracoscopy), urinary bladder (cystoscopy), colon and rectum (colonoscopy), esophagus, stomach and first part of the small bowel (gastroesophagoscopy), and mid to distal small bowel (enteroscopy).

3.3 Future Directions: Videoendoscopic-Guided Therapy

To be able to offer surgical therapy, one has first to see, and to see with clarity, precision, and accuracy, including accuracy to context and to the three-dimensional relationships that define a safe procedure. The range and severity of disease processes for which an endoscopic option exists continues to expand. Many in the clinical field and industry have predicted that for most surgical procedures, a minimally invasive approach or component, often using videoendoscopic tools to enhance visualization and discrimination of normal from diseased tissue, will become a standard. Goals of this evolution will be to continue offering increased capability, safety, and efficiency thorough smaller and smaller incisions and the option for videocapture as a durable record of the procedure. Videoendoscopic technology will remain a key element of this ongoing revolution in minimally invasive therapy.

References

[1] Modlin, M., M. Kidd, and K. Lye, "From the Lumen to the Laparoscope," *Archives of Surgery*, Vol. 139, 2004, pp. 1110–1126.

[2] Litynski, G. S., and V. Paolucci, "Origin of Laparoscopy: Coincidence or Surgical Interdisciplinary Thought?" *World J. Surg.*, Vol. 22, No. 8, 1998, pp. 899–902.

[3] Litynski, G. S., "Laparoscopy—The Early Attempts: Spotlighting Georg Kelling and Hans Christian Jacobaeus," *JSLS*, Vol. 1, 1997, pp. 83–85.

[4] Morgenstern, L., "Harold Hopkins (1918–1995): Let There Be Light...," *Surgical Innovation*, Vol. 11, No. 4, 2004, pp. 291–292.

[5] Litynski, G. S., "Kurt Semm and an Automatic Insufflator," *JSLS*, Vol. 2, 1998, pp. 197–200.

[6] Jones, D. B., J. S. Wu, and N. J. Soper, *Laparoscopic Surgery: Principles and Procedures*, 2nd ed., New York: Marcel Dekker, 2004.

CHAPTER 4

Image-Guided Radiation Therapy: From Concept to Practice

E. Ishmael Parsai, Michael C. Dobelbower, and Ralph R. Dobelbower

Ionizing radiations have been applied as therapy for cancer and other diseases for more than a century, ever since the discovery of X-rays by Wilhelm Conrad Röntgen in 1895 [1]. The efficacy of radiation therapy depends mainly upon two fundamental principles [2]: the therapeutic ratio and targeting.

4.1 Therapeutic Ratio (TR)

With respect to the treatment of cancer via ionizing radiations,

$$\text{Therapeutic Ratio} \equiv \text{TR} \equiv \frac{\text{Normal Tissue Complication Dose (NTCD)}}{\text{Tumoricidal Dose}} \tag{4.1}$$

Clearly, if TR >> 1.0, then a situation exists wherein the normal tissue complication dose is large compared to the tumoricidal dose; hence, tumor cure without complication can theoretically be achieved. In this context:

$$\text{NTCD} \equiv \text{that dose of radiation necessary to produce side effects in normal tissue} \tag{4.2}$$

and

$$\text{Tumoricidal Dose} \equiv \text{that dose necessary to eradicate the tumor} \tag{4.3}$$

Contrariwise, if tumoricidal dose >> normal tissue complication dose, then TR < 1.0, reflecting a situation in which tumor cure without complication is categorically impossible.

In point of fact, in many clinical scenarios, TR ≈ 1.0. On this account, radiation oncologists use many maneuvers such as fractionation of radiation dose, protraction of dose delivery, radiation sensitizers, radiation protectors and various targeting methods to enhance (increase) the TR toward the objective of tumor cure without complication or untoward side effects of treatment [2].

Another important concept is that adverse effects of radiation treatment come not from irradiation of tumors per se, but from the associated radiation dose to

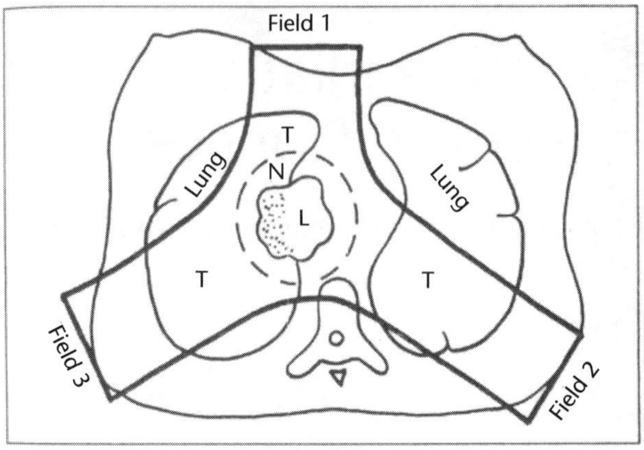

Figure 4.1 Three field radiation treatment plan for a right hilar lesion (L) illustrating the lung tissue as matrix tissue (stippled), normal tissue (N) within the target volume (broken line), and transit tissue (T). (*After:* [2].)

normal tissues. Within the treatment fields applied to any malignant tumor, there exist both malignant and nonmalignant tissues (Figure 4.1). These two categories of tissue behave differently in response to irradiation, and it is this differential response that accounts for the existence of the therapeutic ratio. Furthermore, there appear to be differences between normal cells and malignant cells with respect to the repair of sublethal and potentially lethal radiation injury. Radiation oncologists take advantage of these inherent differences by administering repeated fractions of the radiation dose, allowing sufficient time between dose increments for repair of radiation damage in the normal tissues. Thus, protraction and fractionation of radiation dose can be used to enhance the therapeutic ratio [2].

4.2 Targeting

Of course, the therapeutic ratio can be enhanced by focusing the dose of ionizing radiation upon the diseased tissues. This process of targeting embodies the following two basic principles:

- Put the dose on the disease.
- Spare the normal tissues.

In general, the more effective the targeting is, the greater the enhancement of the therapeutic ratio and the more salutary the effect of radiation treatment. Targeting can be accomplished via a variety of means depending upon the source(s) of the ionizing radiation(s). For example, radioactive pellets, seeds, wires, or needles can be placed into or immediately adjacent to diseased tissues, thereby targeting the area of disease (typically a malignant tumor). Such procedures are referred to as brachytherapy.

More commonly, high-intensity beams of ionizing radiation produced outside the body (e.g., by linear accelerators) are employed to deliver penetrating radiant energy to diseased tissues within the body. Such radiation beams can be cross fired, custom shaped, and modulated in intensity by various means in order to match the radiation dose "cloud" to the physical anatomy of the diseased tissue. During the last decade of the twentieth century and the first decade of the twenty-first century, a radiation treatment delivery technique referred to as the intensity-modulated radiation therapy (IMRT) has gained momentum to the point that it now carries a reputation as the state-of-the-art radiation therapy technology throughout the world. This technology permits the generation of extremely conformal radiation dose distributions (even including concave isodose volumes) that provide conformal coverage of geometrically complex targets as well as avoidance of specific sensitive normal structures.

Image-Guided Radiation Therapy (IGRT)

Various technologies have been used to generate two-dimensional (2D) or three-dimensional (3D) images of patient anatomy to identify the exact location(s) of diseased (commonly cancerous) tissues prior to radiation treatment. In many cases, such image guidance (targeting) is crucial. Targeting is important when radiation treatment fields must be as limited as possible to avoid irradiation of nearby critical normal structures, or when the target of the radiation treatment moves or deforms. Radiation therapy for prostate cancer provides an example: With physiologic filling of the rectum with stool, that organ deforms and the prostate gland actually moves a bit. In such cases, daily image guidance via IGRT (vide infra) is beneficial, especially in the setting of dose escalation. Certain physical characteristics of high energy radiation beams used for treatment render said beams suboptimal with respect to diagnostic radiographic imaging. In other words, radiation beams energetic enough for deep therapy are too energetic to produce good images. Hence, alternative means of imaging are usually necessary for beam targeting. These include:

- Radiography;
- Computerized tomography (CT);
- Magnetic resonance imaging (MRI);
- Positron emission tomography (PET);
- Ultrasonography (US).

4.2.1 Radiography

Conventional radiographic techniques have long been used to facilitate the process of directing beams of therapeutic ionizing radiations toward diseased tissues within the body. The precision of such technology was substantially improved with the development of the radiation therapy simulator. The first such radiation treatment simulation device in the United States was designed and built at the Jefferson Medical College of Philadelphia by Simon Kramer, MD [3]. In the 1960s Dr. Kramer cobbled together some diagnostic radiographic and fluoroscopic equipment in a physical configuration identical to that of his therapy machine, such that the contraption was capable of producing "beam's eye" images as "seen" by the therapy machine. With this device Dr. Kramer was able to simulate radiation therapy fields and plan the actual treatment regimen more accurately and with less radiation exposure to patients than ever before.

4.2.2 Computerized Tomography (CT)

Computerized tomography, which permits imaging the internal anatomy in axial cross-sections, as well as in coronal and sagittal planes, has had a major impact in diagnostic and treatment of malignancies. A very popular modality since the early 1970s, the CT scanner has functioned as the main modality in the planning of the radiotherapy treatment of malignant tumors by providing an exact contour of transverse sections of the body along with a distinct representation of nearby anatomic internal structures. In addition to providing a very powerful diagnostic tool, it provides an opportunity to obtain quantitatively, the "density" of the anatomical structures in the body sections for a very accurate assessment of dose deposition through external radiotherapy. Through treatment planning computers, the isodose curves may be projected on CT slices with inhomogeneity corrections applied, resulting in a realistic prediction of planned treatment. In following up with patients, the successive CT scans will provide physicians with the ability to follow the response of a tumor to treatment, noninvasively. With improved image resolution of CT scanners by at least an order of magnitude in contrast to radiography, the circumstance theoretically provides the possibility to proportionately improve the accuracy of treatment beam targeting. Computerized tomography has proven to provide radiation and medical oncologists with a valuable adjunct in their management of tumor patients. Available techniques such as coregistration of CT data with treatment beam data becomes critically important in such applications; hence, the advent of the CT-based radiation therapy simulator and the CT-based positron emission tomography units, which were technological achievements around the end of the second millennium.

4.2.3 Magnetic Resonance Imaging (MRI)

Radiography and CT both depend upon differential absorption of X-rays by diseased tissues as compared to that by normal tissues. MRI yields images based upon an entirely different tissue characteristic, the relative concentration of hydrogen ions. This has the potential to provide the radiation oncologist with the ability to identify and target diseased tissues in a whole new way. Such potential has yet to be fully exploited.

4.2.4 Positron Emission Tomography (PET)

Positron emission tomography provides a means of identification and localization of abnormally functioning tissues. Coregistration of PET data with treatment beam data also has the potential to provide the radiation oncologist with the ability to identify and target diseased tissues in yet another spectrum of new ways. Such potential has yet to be fully developed.

4.2.5 Ultrasonography (US)

Ultrasonography can provide images of diseased tissues depending upon differential absorption and/or reflection of sonic energy by such tissues as compared to normal tissues. Although US has been employed as an aide to targeting beams of therapeutic ionizing radiation, this application has not been developed to the level of sophistication and utility enjoyed by radiography, CT, PET, and so on.

Present day radiation therapy delivery systems are commonly capable of submillimeter precision with respect to spatial delivery of beams of ionizing radiation. Each of the aforementioned methods of targeting beams of ionizing radiation (radiography, CT, PET, MRI, and US) is heavily dependent upon accurate imaging of diseased and normal tissues. If such imaging cannot be accomplished reliably, technology and techniques for precise delivery of ionizing radiations becomes moot. Likewise, at such levels of precision dose delivery, day-to-day reproducibility of clinical patient immobilization and treatment setup takes on added importance, as does normal physiologic motion of internal body structures. As any hunter will attest, it is always more difficult to hit a moving target than one that is stationary.

The process of IGRT commonly employs a linear accelerator equipped with a kilovoltage (KV) or megavoltage (MV) X-ray imaging device and solid-state X-ray detector. With IGRT, a novel form of scanning, X-ray volume imaging (XVI), is combined with intensity modulated radiation therapy (IMRT). This enables the radiation oncologist to make adjustments based on the position of the target (typically a tumor) as well as that of adjacent critical organs during treatment administration. The first clinical use of this technology took place at The Netherlands Cancer Institute [4] in July 2003, where three cancer patients were treated using the then-new Elekta Synergy system. Figure 4.2 shows an Elekta linear accelerator equipped with a KV imaging arm being used for IGRT.

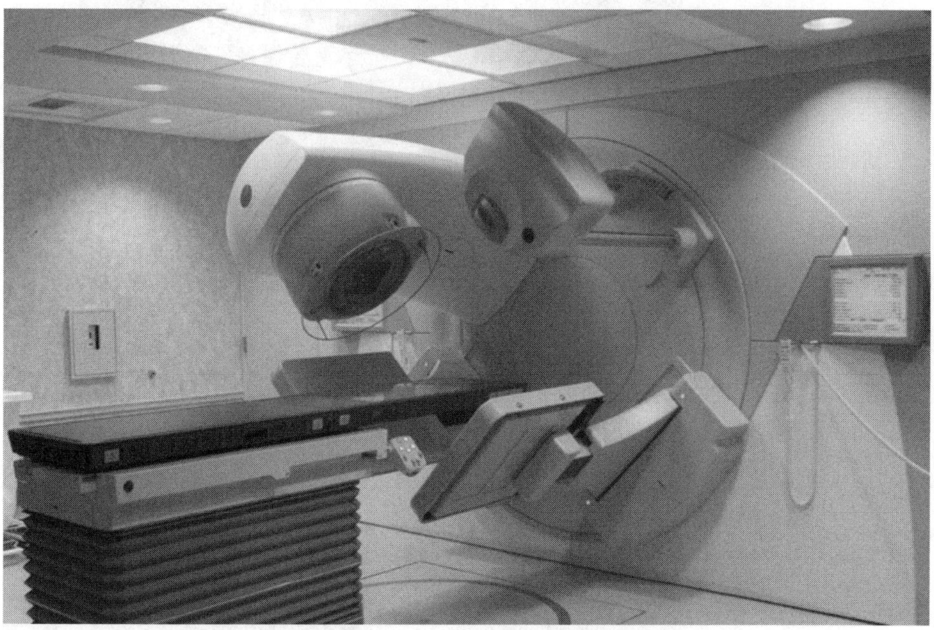

Figure 4.2 Elekta linear accelerator with on-board KV imaging device.

4.3 Methods of Delivering IGRT

To take advantage of existing technology, manufacturers of linear accelerators providing on-board imaging for IGRT combine both IMRT with state-of-the-art 3D X-ray volume imaging technology, an example of which is shown in Figure 4.3.

Aspects of image guidance have long existed. Even with early use of X-ray beams for cancer therapy, the same radiation source could be used for both imaging and treatment. Many devices promoted today as tools specifically dedicated to IGRT have existed for a decade or more, but new attention is focused upon IGRT for several reasons:

- Highly conformal dose distributions delivered by IMRT to complex target volumes are less forgiving with respect to treatment uncertainties.
- Availability of online electronic portal imaging devices (devices that provide images of the treatment beam immediately prior to or even during radiation treatment delivery) has led to improved understanding of treatment uncertainties, and of the need for strategies to further reduce same.
- Development and commercial availability of advanced online imaging technologies, particularly cone-beam CT (CBCT) systems.

In a simplified view of IGRT, an ideal system should have three essential elements:

1. 3D volumetric capabilities for soft tissues (including tumor tissue);
2. Efficient 3D volumetrics acquisition and comparison capabilities for both simulation and administration of treatment;

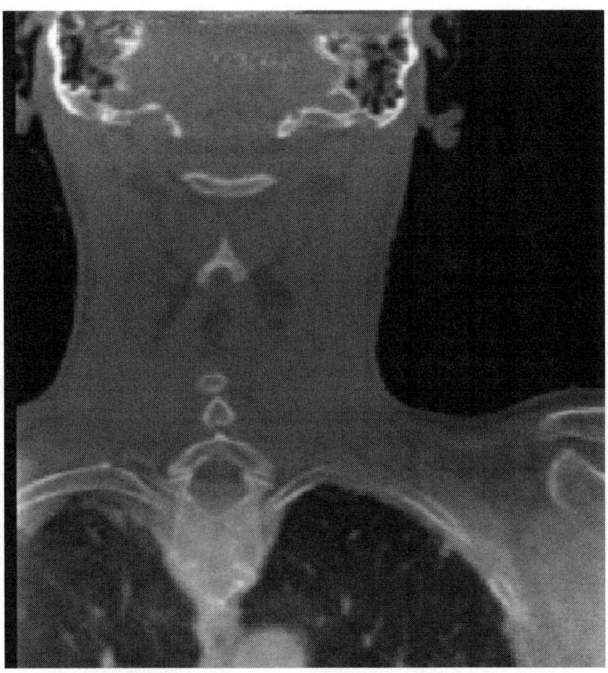

Figure 4.3 The X-ray volume imaging capabilities of Elekta Synergy afford CT-like contrast, thus enabling identification of soft tissue structures such as tumors and organs at risk.

3. Capability for clinically meaningful interventions (precise spatial position adjustments and so forth).

In contrast to this simple definition with well-defined goals, many aspects of IGRT are anything but simple. There is much uncertainty and debate regarding many topics (e.g., 2D versus 3D, kilovoltage versus megavoltage, the use of fiducial markers, and how to minimize the effect of tumor geometry variation during the course of treatment) regarding IGRT.

Conceptually, IGRT can:

- Reduce setup error;
- Account for organ motion;
- Increase accuracy of beam placement;
- Increase precision of radiation dose delivery;
- Lead to reduced treatment toxicity;
- Permit dose escalation;
- Improve treatment outcome.

Such arguments constitute the basis of many research projects, leading to a spate of new literature pertinent to IGRT dose delivery. Investigation of the impact of IGRT upon treatment outcomes will necessitate clinical trials, data from which will take substantial time to collect and analyze. In the short term, we are left with the surrogates of reduction of setup uncertainties and minimization of the effects of organ motion, retreating to the hope that they will translate into improvements regarding radiation treatment outcomes.

4.3.1 Setup Uncertainties

It is generally accepted that there are two types of treatment setup error: systematic and random. Systematic error refers to the difference between the 3D image set (hence, target geometry) acquired at the time of CT simulation, and the target position at the instant of treatment delivery. Random error is the day-to-day spatial deviation from the average target position. Of the two, systematic uncertainty is generally more important because, if uncorrected, it could be propagated throughout the entire course of radiation treatments, and lead to undesirable effects on local disease control [5].

A simplistic method to reduce both systematic and random errors would be to devise a means of intervention to correct the target position based on the 3D images of the tumor and normal tissues acquired at the time of treatment as compared to those acquired at simulation (planning). If that could be accomplished immediately prior to each radiation dose administration based on daily sequential pre-irradiation images, spatial treatment errors could be largely eliminated, but doing so for each of the many treatment sessions (typically 10 to 40 in conventionally fractionated radiotherapy) would be very costly and potentially wasteful. There is general agreement that three to five imaging sessions are usually sufficient for minimization of systematic error [6]. Subsequent periodic (e.g., weekly) imaging checks are routinely performed for continuing quality assurance (QA).

The undesirable dosimetric consequences of random errors are usually less than those of systematic errors. Random errors are generally accounted for in the delineation of the planning target volume (vide infra) [5].

Regardless of the periodicity of the intervention, the simplistic approach outlined above ignores the many complexities inherent in the comparison of 3D volumetrics of tumors and normal tissues as well as the multitude of complexities involved in the implementation of meaningful interventions. Report #62 from the International Commission on Radiation Units and Measurements (ICRU) offers standardized target and uncertainty definitions in addition to dosimetric objectives for specifying geometric constructs and margins as well as means for meaningful interventions [7]. A margin is added around the gross tumor volume (GTV) to take into account potential "subclinical" invasion by tumor. The GTV plus this margin define the clinical target volume (CTV). To ensure that all parts of the CTV receive the prescribed radiation dose, additional margins must be considered to account for geometric variations and uncertainties:

- An internal margin (IM) is added for the variations in position and/or shape and size of the CTV. This defines the internal target volume (ITV).
- A setup margin (SM) is added to take into account all the variations and uncertainties in patient and radiation beam positioning.

The CTV, plus the IM, plus the SM define the planning target volume (PTV) on which the selection of beam size and arrangement is based (Figure 4.4):

$$CTV + IM + SM \equiv PTV \tag{4.4}$$

The reduction of these margins has become a major focus of IGRT objectives because they are associated with toxicity and hence constitute a constraint on dose escalation for tumor control.

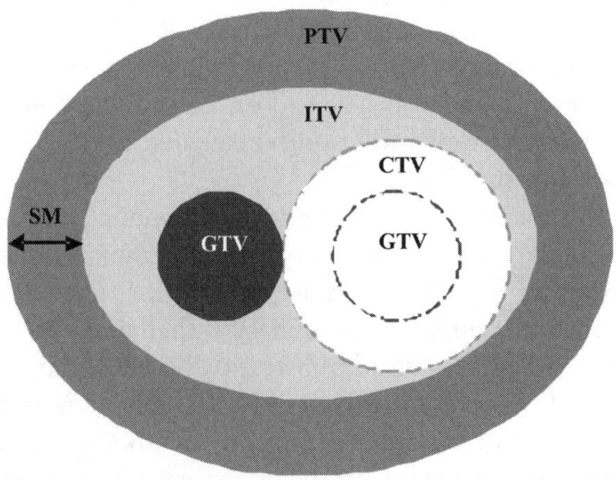

Figure 4.4 Illustrated are gross tumor volume (GTV), clinical target volume (CTV), internal target volume (ITV), and planning target volume (PTV). The entire excursion of GTV and the CTV is contained within the ITV. The PTV can be considered an expansion of the ITV to account for setup margin (SM).

Emphasis on geometric uncertainties in radiation dose delivery has resulted in the development of a variety of imaging and tracking technologies that are now readily available. These highly complex systems integrate tools such as:

- Image generation;
- Image registration to original 3D images;
- Computation of appropriate adjustments;
- Automated spatial corrections.

Modern IGRT systems provide a great deal more information than just what is needed for simple positioning adjustments. Conventional CT scanners are now available in some radiation treatment rooms. With respect to soft tissue image quality, conventional CT seems to be the most satisfactory imaging tool currently available, followed by kilovolt cone beam CT (KVCBCT) and megavolt cone beam CT (MVCBCT).

Target motion and changes in target size and shape compound the complexity of IGRT (e.g., a lung tumor that moves and changes shape with respiration). One aspect of the challenge is maintenance of consistency of tumor geometry throughout the treatment course (i.e., the actual tumor geometry during each treatment should be approximately the same as the reference model built at the time of treatment simulation and used for treatment planning). However, it is not a trivial task to maintain such geometrical consistency because patient geometry, specifically tumor position and shape, can vary from one treatment session to the next and even from moment to moment during any single treatment. Certain current IGRT research projects focus on the issue of how to keep the patient geometry as close as possible to the reference model in the machine coordinate system (vide supra) or how to expeditiously modify the model to accommodate the changing patient/target geometry. Such changes in patient/target geometry originate from a variety of sources, such as:

- Day-to-day variations in patient positioning;
- Patient motion;
- Physiologic organ filling and emptying (e.g., stomach, bladder, etc.);
- Physiologic organ wriggling (e.g., peristalsis, etc.);
- Respiratory motion;
- Cardiac motion.

Figure 4.5 shows time dependent variations of several processes capable of causing changes in target geometry.

4.3.1.1 Interfractional Versus Intrafractional Variations

A course of radiation therapy is generally administered not as a single dose, but as a series of fractional doses delivered at regular intervals that range in frequency from three doses per day to three doses per week. Each dose is referred to as a single "fraction." The most common regimen comprises five fractions weekly, administered as single daily fractions Monday through Friday.

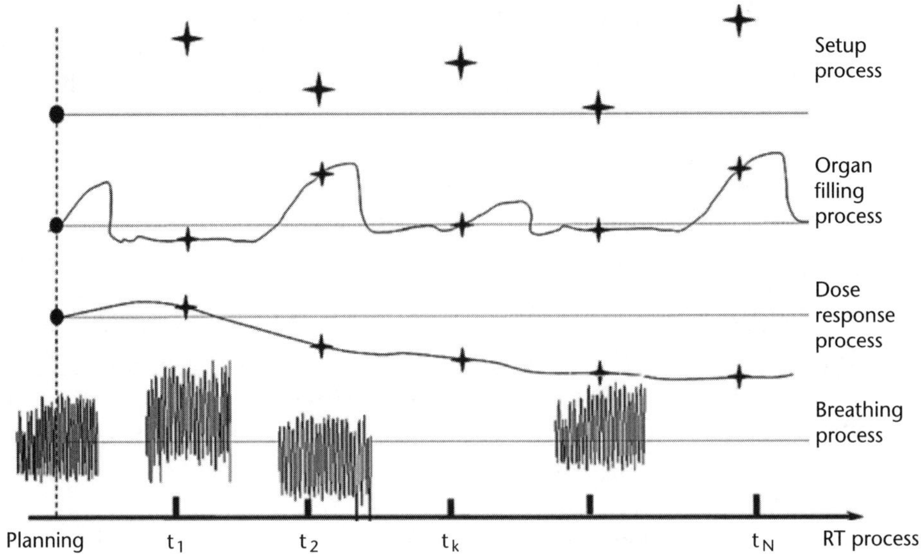

Figure 4.5 Common sources of patient geometry variation during the course of treatment. The horizontal axis represents treatment fractions (t). The vertical axis represents tumor position (in a broad sense, including shape changes). (*From:* [8].)

Variations in patient/target geometry are often described as either "interfractional" or "intrafractional." Interfractional variations occur between one fraction and the next, whereas intrafractional variations occur from moment to moment during administration of a single fraction. Interfractional variation characterizes the deviation of the (average) patient/target geometry during each fractional dose from that of the reference patient/target model established through treatment simulation. Intrafractional variation characterizes instantaneous changes of patient/target geometry, usually caused by internal organ motion. Such uncontrolled movements produce artifacts which degrade the quality of volumetric images.

4.3.1.2 Concerning Uncertainties

Thus far we have discussed a variety of issues concerning the IGRT process and the difficulties in quantifying the clinical benefits therefrom. We recognize the potential of IGRT and believe that such will eventually be realized through carefully designed studies, but that these will take time to complete. As the capabilities of IGRT improve, it will provide the tools to better understand treatment uncertainties and allow re-examination of the concepts of GTV, CTV, and PTV, each of which suffers certain limitations.

We appreciate some uncertainty concerning disease extension beyond that which is visible radiographically, so we surround the GTV with the CTV. To account for organ motion, we encompass the CTV with the ITV, and to account for setup errors, we envelop the ITV with the even larger PTV. Given such practice, it makes little sense to use IGRT to assure that the PTV is within each radiation field, each and every day during a course of conventionally fractionated radiotherapy.

Perhaps, with the passage of time, our understanding of the capabilities of IGRT will mature to a level where we can refine our notions of target volumes to incorporate the concept of an *image guided target volume* (IGTV or PTV_{IG}) as proposed by Ling et al. [9] in 2006. This may be a CTV plus a margin to account for residual setup uncertainty and organ motion when "image guidance" is used during radiation dose delivery. Conceptually the IGTV should be smaller than the corresponding conventional PTV, which could translate into reduced dose to normal tissues immediately adjacent to the target, thus permitting radiation dose escalation and, hopefully, improving local disease control. Viewed in this perspective, IGRT represents a natural progression of the implementation of the basic principles of targeting clinical radiation therapy (Section 4.2).

4.4 Delivery of IGRT

Precision targeting of a tumor volume with external beam radiotherapy requires consideration of positioning uncertainties involved in delivering the intended dose. The CTV consists of the GTV plus a margin to account for subclinical extension of disease plus an additional margin to account for daily setup error and internal organ (or target) movement. Accurate identification of this volume, the PTV, is critical as irradiation of normal tissues contained therein is a major factor contributing to treatment morbidity. Contrariwise, inadequate margins can result in underdosing a portion of the target, thereby leading to treatment failure. More precise targeting of the target volume has resulted in the use of smaller margins, thereby reducing treatment toxicity and/or allowing dose escalation without change in the accompanying toxicity profiles for the organs at risk (OAR).

4.4.1 Adaptive Versus Integrated IGRT Systems

Available image-guidance systems for IGRT can be classified as belonging to one of two main categories: (1) adaptive IGRT and (2) integrated IGRT.

4.4.1.1 Adaptive IGRT Systems

Adaptive IGRT systems (also known as nonintegrated IGRT systems) are those in which the imaging device (commonly a CT scanner) employed for treatment beam guidance is physically located outside the treatment vault [10].

4.4.1.2 Integrated IGRT Systems

Integrated IGRT systems are those in which the imaging device(s) employed for treatment beam guidance is/are actually integrated with the treatment delivery equipment [11–13]. Such imaging equipment may include:

- Kilovoltage (KV) X-ray imaging devices;
- Implanted markers;
- Ultrasound (US) imaging devices;

- Megavoltage (MV) single slice CT (tomotherapy);
- Conventional CT;
- Kilovolt cone beam CT (KVCBCT);
- Megavolt cone beam CT (MVCBCT).

An essential component of any image-guidance system is an image-acquisition device that provides satisfactory soft-tissue contrast and adequate imaging of the target (or target surrogate). The imaging system should be capable of accurate spatial calibration as well as high speed image acquisition and reconstruction. For each treatment session a reference dataset should be available, such as the planning CT images with the GTV contoured. The user should have the ability to define a region of interest so that the target localization software, which provides fast automatic image registration, "knows" the proper part of the image upon which to focus. Of course, the user must be able to use translational, rotational, pitch, yaw, and roll movements to shift the target to the correct position (matching that of the planning CT) before commencing the actual radiation treatment.

4.4.2 Treating Moving Targets

One method to account for target motion [11–21] due to respiration observed at the time of the planning CT scan (simulation) is to add more generous cephalo-caudad margins around the GTV. Thoracic targets (typically lung tumors) are subject to interfraction motion (i.e., changes in position from one treatment session to the next), and intrafraction motion (i.e., changes in position during a single treatment session) (Section 4.1.1). The main contributors to the latter are physiologic respiratory, cardiac and peristaltic organ movements as well as voluntary movements. Figure 4.6 is an example of how much a reference point actually moves during a two second breathing cycle because of respiratory motion.

Methods have been developed for "gating" radiation dose administration based on the 3D locations of fiducial markers implanted in the periphery of lung tumors [13]. Continuous multiview fluoroscopy assures the user that the radiation is being delivered accurately. Schweikard et al. [21] used infrared external markers and implanted radio-opaque markers to periodically reestablish internal/external spatial correlation throughout CyberKnife system irradiation sessions. The BrainLAB Novalis system uses dual X-ray units to track bony landmarks in the treatment region and allow the user to compare these images to digitally reconstructed radiographs (DRRs) based on data collected via simulation. This system is used for stereotactic body radiotherapy (SBRT) using a linear accelerator equipped with a miniature multileaf collimation (mMLC) system, and dual X-ray tubes and detectors for on-board imaging.

Techniques have been developed for respiratory gating based on the positions of external surrogates placed on thorax and/or abdomen [15–17]. Strategies that do not monitor internal anatomy during treatment delivery assume a fixed correlation between the surrogate and the target does not vary during the course of treatment. One method to obviate this issue might be the use of ultra-fast CT scanners in combination with patient breath-holding during scanning. This has proven difficult for many radiotherapy patients, especially for those with compromised pulmonary function.

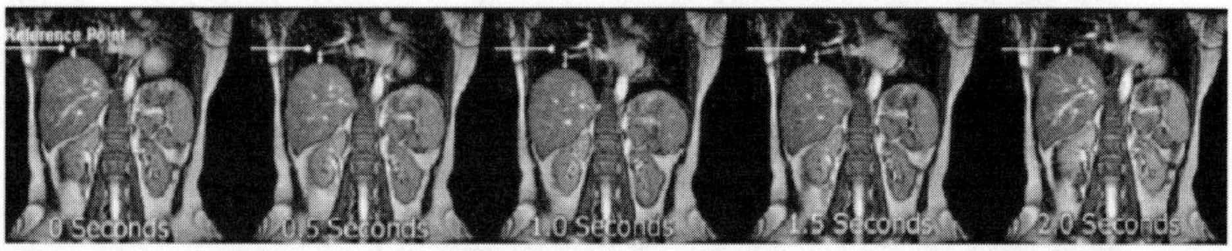

Figure 4.6 Serial CT scans of human chest and abdomen during a 2-second breathing cycle demonstrating actual extent of motion of a reference point due to physiologic respiratory movements. (*From:* [22].)

Another method is to gate the acquisition of CT scan data (i.e., images are only acquired at a particular breathing phase). A more popular technique is respiration-correlated or four-dimensional (4D) CT scanning: At every position of interest along patient's long axis, images are oversampled and each image is tagged with breathing phase information. Following CT scan data acquisition, images are sorted based on corresponding breathing phase signals. Thus, many 3D CT datasets are obtained, each corresponding to a particular breathing phase. Together these constitute a 4D CT dataset that covers the full breathing cycle [18].

4.4.3 Megavolt Cone Beam Computerized Tomography (MVCBCT) System

An MVCBCT system [19] consists of a standard linear accelerator equipped with an amorphous silicon flat panel detector optimized for MV photons. The panel has a flat panel area of approximately 40 × 40 cm (with effective area for imaging of about 25 × 25 cm) with typically 1,024 × 1,024 pixels. The detector is mounted on a retractable support that deploys in less than 10 seconds with a spatial position reproducibility of 1 mm in any direction. The entire imaging system, an illustration of which is presented in Figure 4.7, communicates with the radiation therapy machine control console, the linear accelerator, and a patient database.

The operator has immediate access to applications permitting automatic acquisition of projection images, image reconstruction, CT-to-CBCT image registration, couch position adjustment, and radiation dose delivery. This provides a 3D patient

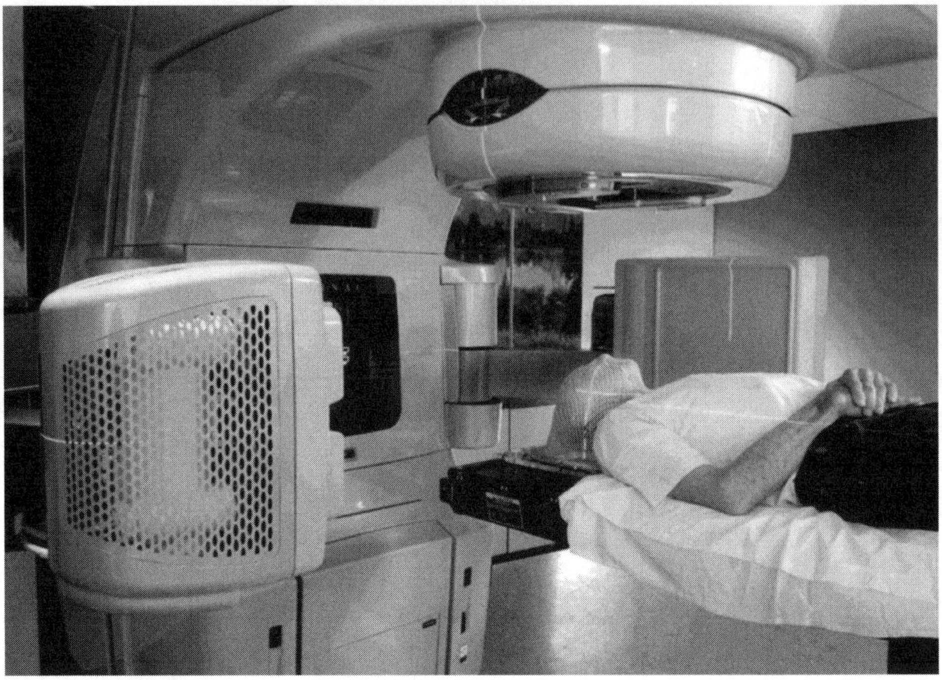

Figure 4.7 A megavoltage cone beam computerized tomography system on board a Varian Linear Accelerator. (*From:* [19].)

anatomy reference volume in the actual treatment position relative to the treatment isocenter just moments prior to dose delivery, which can be tightly aligned to the planning CT images, allowing verification and correction of the patient position, detection of anatomical changes, and dose calculation.

4.4.4 Kilovoltage Cone Beam Computerized Tomography (KVCBCT) System

The KVCBCT system characteristic of most linear accelerators manufactured today enables radiation oncologists to:

- Acquire high-resolution X-ray images to pinpoint disease sites;
- Register such images against reference (planning) images;
- Adjust patient positioning automatically when necessary;
- Accurately deliver radiation treatment;

all within the standard daily treatment time slot.

The KV X-ray source can be used for:

- Volumetric cone-beam CT imaging;
- Fluoroscopy;
- Radiography.

In effect, this technology combines the imaging capabilities of a digital simulator and a CT scanner into the linear accelerator. The ability to employ a treatment-procedure-specific imaging strategy, whether real-time fluoroscopy, radiography, cone-beam CT, or an appropriate combination of all three, has enhanced target localization considerably. Figure 4.8 shows application of localizing fiducial markers that are identified prior to each radiation treatment, permitting the operator, through a process of visual inspection and identification, to identify the region of interest (ROI) for both KV and MV video streams using the electronic portal imaging device (EPID).

A tracking system converts the detected location of the center-of-mass of the fiducial images to the real space coordinates of the reference images and moves the patient into position for radiation dose delivery. The full clinical potential of such systems has yet to be fully exploited. In the future, such systems could conceivably be used to verify treatment position and apply necessary position shifts and rotations to correct for any deviations immediately prior to radiation dose delivery. If target deformation is identified, a corrected treatment plan could be generated just prior to treatment administration. In light of the circumstance that the time required for recontouring and replanning renders such procedure impractical at present, offline treatment analysis may have to be applied for this kind of treatment deviation. The actual dose received by the target could be calculated from the imaging systems onboard the linear accelerator. Regions that receive less or more than the planned dose could be compensated during the remaining treatment fractions through what may become the future of radiation therapy, adaptive four-dimensional treatment planning [24].

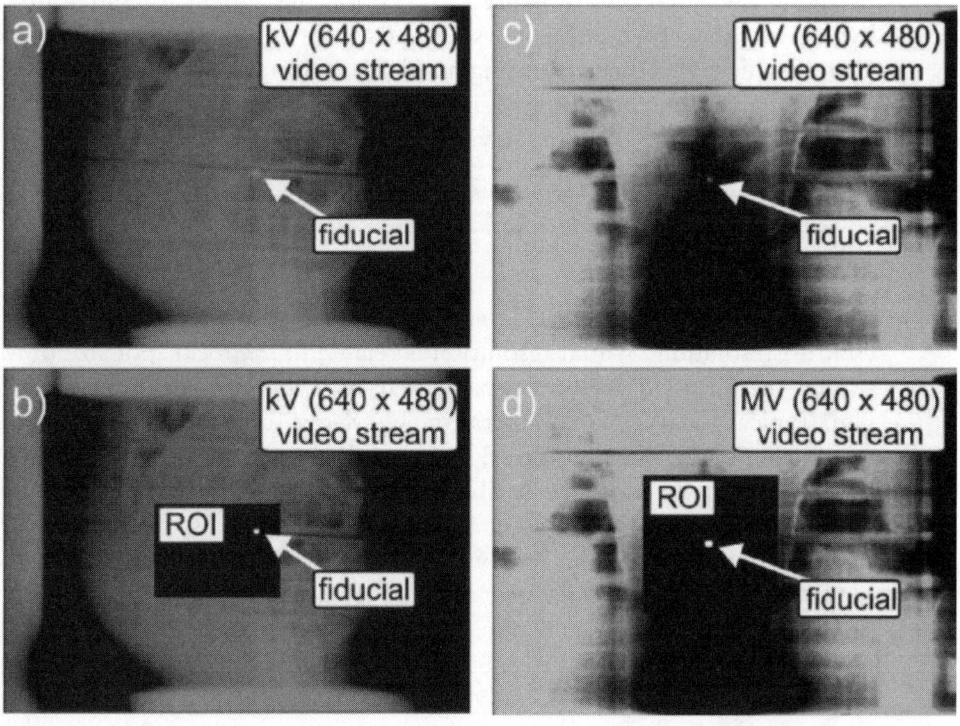

Figure 4.8 Fiducial markers seen on (a, b) kilovolt images and (c, d) megavolt images to localize region of interest (ROI). (*From:* [23].)

4.5 Quality Assurance (QA) for IGRT Systems

The inherent complexities of IGRT systems (Section 4.3.1) require rigorous daily QA assessments to ensure pinpoint accuracy of spatial distribution of radiation dose and stable reproducibility of same. Evaluation of the overall performance of the IGRT system should include checks of [25]:

- Mechanical safety;
- Geometric accuracy (agreement of MV and kV beam isocenters);
- Image quality (resolution and low contrast visibility);
- Image registration capability;
- Position correction accuracy;
- Dose delivery.

4.5.1 Safety Checks

These should match closely the procedures in the acceptance document provided by the manufacturer, including all system interlocks, touch guards, terminate keys, and so on.

4.5.2 Geometric Accuracy

This test verifies coincidence of the isocenters of the kV imaging and the MV treatment system. It is perhaps the most crucial test since the target position identified by the KV imaging system is used to position the patient for radiation dose delivery using the MV treatment system. Lehmann et al. recommended a technique [26] to achieve this objective using an Elekta IGRT system through matching port films taken at different gantry positions. The images are then imported to a system software package to compute deviations from exact coincidence between the two isocenters.

4.5.3 Image Quality

The image quality of an IGRT system is assessed mainly by measuring spatial and contrast resolution. Spatial resolution is related to the focal spot size of the X-ray source, the pixel size of the flat-panel detectors, and the configuration of the system. Typical focal spot diameters for KV X-ray tubes used with IGRT systems range from 0.6 to 1.2 mm [26]. Flat-panel detectors typically have a pixel size of 0.4 mm with a sensitive area of about 20 × 20 cm. Spatial resolution can be quantified by the modulation transfer function (MTF) of the system. Contrast resolution is determined by many factors, such as the initial subject contrast, the X-ray quality, the scattered radiation, and the number of photons used to take the images. Unlike contrast in a film system, the contrast of the digital image is affected mainly by the signal-to-noise ratio [27]. Phantoms with various cylindrical sections (modules), each specially designed for a specific test, are used for these measurements.

4.5.4 Image Registration Accuracy

Most commercial treatment planning systems now use CT imaging as the basis for generation of treatment plans and delineation of tumor volumes. These are supplemented by data from other imaging modalities such as MRI and PET spatially integrated into the CT dataset. With IGRT dose delivery, integrated 4D imaging process (often from multiple modalities) are essential to achieve the required levels of accuracy. This process may be accomplished either manually through matching image datasets by image rotation, translation, and transformation, or as is often the case, automatically through application of some mathematical tool. The user can then visually inspect the matched result.

Even though commercially available image registration packages use complex mathematical tools for improved accuracy (on the order of a few millimeters), their performance is greatly challenged if the image sets are from different modalities. For this reason, combined CT/PET scanners became popular to facilitate fusion of planning CT images with PET images and, to some degree, improve the accuracy thereof. The transformation is made easier by registering the planning CT to the CT from the PET/CT combined scanner first and then setting the resultant transformation as the starting image transformation between the planning CT and PET images.

With image guided IMRT one has the potential to achieve both unparalleled tumor control and sparing of normal tissue. To confidently administer highly conformal radiation to complex three-dimensional volumes, clinicians can track and manage tumor motion in all four dimensions by using *dynamic targeting*, an approach toward image guided motion management that reduces uncertainties in both setup and organ motion. The importance of accuracy in image registration has driven the manufacturers of high energy linear accelerators to produce onboard X-ray Volume Imaging (XVI) to achieve excellent image quality allowing visualization of the tumor and critical soft tissue organs in both 2D and 3D modes. These include 2D planar (static and stereoscopic) imaging, 2D sequence imaging (fluoroscopy), and 3D imaging at treatment time. With all these options available online, the user can reconstruct data sets in any plane with submillimeter resolution in all three dimensions.

4.5.5 Dose Computation and Delivery

The complexities inherent to accurate dose delivery presented by IGRT and adaptive radiotherapy (ART) are significantly different from those of other modes of radiation dose delivery. With four-dimensional radiotherapy or adaptive radiation therapy, one needs to focus effort on per-treatment reproducibility of the time-of-simulation patient geometry by developing an adaptive strategy to accommodate setup errors and anatomic changes. This effort is basically led by various onboard imaging devices such as CBCTs which permit routine updates of the treatment plan as well as modifications applied to the voxel-specific dose prescription from fraction to fraction. To complete this complex task, two classes of algorithms have been discussed in the periodic literature:

- Those adapting to changing geometry (the "manual" approach described by Mohan et al. [28] representing a special example of geometric adaptation);

- Those adapting to geometry and delivered dose (which take into account organ deformations identified immediately prior to radiation dose delivery).

Detailed descriptions of each algorithm lie beyond the purview of this chapter. For related information the reader is referred to [24, 28, 29]. The fact remains that much research needs to be done to develop more sophisticated closed-loop algorithms to search for the best possible ART strategy.

Given the complex interactions among the various sources of error, motion, and the doses delivered to the patient, sophisticated disease-site specific adaptation schemes may be needed. Dose algorithms developed using Monte Carlo (MC) simulations carry the promise of achieving the goals of adaptive IGRT because they can accurately account for details of the fluence delivery (via direct transport of particles through moving MLC segments) as well as patient tissue heterogeneities.

For MC simulation of IMRT, each beam of radiation is divided into many (often 100 or so) beamlets. Through each of these beamlets different amounts of radiation dose are delivered to a given point within the target volume. To achieve this, often a miniature multileaf collimation system (mMLC) made of heavy (high Z) metal is attached to the linear accelerator head. The mMLC modifies the "fluence" of the radiation beam as the head of the linear accelerator rotates around the patient by modulating the beam intensity. For every 5° rotation, the individually controlled beamlets are constantly updated according to the computer prescription. Sensors monitor the accelerator position and keep track of the dose, the beam intensity, and the beam-on time, so that only what has been prescribed is actually delivered. The aim is to achieve a final uniform dose cloud within the target volume by summation of all the radiation doses and to spare (as much as is possible) the surrounding normal structures.

The term "fluence map," then, in simple terms, refers to a planar nonuniform distribution of radiation dose acquired from the sum of all the beamlets within one radiation field.

In radiation treatment of cancer patients, because of the physical shortcomings of accurate delivery per mathematically computed models, we compare deliverable fluence maps (generated by the treatment planning system) to similar measured fluence maps (using the linear accelerator to produce X-rays and some type of detector system), both of which different from a mathematical solution. MC simulation is accepted as the benchmark standard by which other dose computation algorithms are measured.

MC simulation can accurately account for both details of the fluence delivery (via direct transport of particles through moving MLC segments) and patient tissue heterogeneities. In the case of tissue inhomogeneity computations, when compared with algorithms that use, for example, radiologic path-length corrections to account for heterogeneities, MC computations reveal a significant dose difference of nearly 20% in some cases because of failure of the radiologic path-length method to properly account for said heterogeneities. So, "fluence delivery" in the context of this discussion refers to an ideal radiation dose delivery when all parameters of particle transport are considered. Given the current state of development of MC algorithms for radiotherapy treatment planning, however, and the lack of clinical feasibility, the convolution-based dose algorithm seems to be the closest alternative feasible for clinical applications.

4.6 Conclusion

The principle advantage of IMRT lies in sparing the surrounding normal tissues while conforming the high dose volume to the target (commonly a tumor). Since the rapid implementation of IMRT in radiation oncology clinics throughout the world, attention has focused on the need to better account for intrafractional and interfractional spatial uncertainties. This has helped spur development of radiation treatment machines with advanced integrated planar and volumetric imaging capabilities. In addition, advances in both anatomical and functional imaging provided improved capability to define tumor volumes. Such technological advances occurring at a record pace have pushed the frontiers of radiation oncology from IMRT to image guided IMRT, or simply image guided radiation therapy (IGRT). This sophisticated type of targeting is highly dependent upon the radiation oncologist's ability to accurately "see" (or image) the diseased tissue; hence the term, image guided radiation therapy (IGRT).

A future possibility for dose-calculation may be to modify the onboard CBCT (currently used to determine pretreatment patient anatomy for contouring and replanning) for adaptive dose calculation. Ideally, via acquisition of on-treatment CBCT images, the dose can be reconstructed using fluence maps from the treatment plan, which represent the dose to be delivered to the patient since the CBCT is usually acquired before the patient's treatment.

Issues related to Hounsfield units (HUs) and the electron density (or material cross-sections for MC) when CBCT is used could cause imaging artifacts which could affect accurate dose calculations. For CBCT units mounted on linear accelerator gantries, cupping artifacts, ring artifacts, and motion artifacts in three-dimensional and four-dimensional space continue to be problems for dose computation algorithms. Recent research [30] showed that CBCT was adequate for dose calculations for treatments directed to the prostate; however, for treatments directed to the lung, dose differences as large as 5% were observed on the CBCT image set in comparison to the mapped initial planning CT. Motion artifacts not only make it difficult to see the tumor, but they also limit the direct use of CBCT for dose calculation. Long-term solutions are, of course, improvements in scatter correction functions and image quality for CBCT.

References

[1] Röntgen, W. C., "Ueber eine nue Art von Strahlen," *Proc. Würzburg Phisico-Medical Soc.*, December 28, 1895.

[2] Dobelbower, R. R., "Principles and Practical Aspects of Radiation Therapy," in *Handbook of Cancer Chemotherapy*, 4th ed., R. T. Skeel and N. A. Lachant, (eds.), Boston, MA: Little, Brown and Company, 1995, pp. 52–70.

[3] Dobelbower, R. R., "Simon Kramer 1919–2002: Physician, Teacher, Pioneer, Scientist, Leader," *Int. J. Radiat. Oncol. Biol. Phys.*, Vol. 54, No. 3, 2002, pp. 633–634.

[4] Elekta Oncology Systems, *Wavelength Newsletter*, Vol. 8, No. 1, March 2004.

[5] Van Herk, M., "Errors and Margins in Radiation Therapy," *Semin. Radiat. Oncol.*, Vol. 14, 2005, pp. 52–64.

[6] Erridge, S. C., et al., "Portal Imaging to Assess Set-Up Errors, Tumor Motion and Tumor Shrinkage During Conformal Radiotherapy of Non-Small Cell Lung Cancer," *Radiother. Oncol.*, Vol. 66, 2003 pp. 75–85.

[7] International Commission on Radiation Units and Measurements, *Report 62: Prescribing, Recording and Reporting Photon Beams Therapy (Supplement to ICRU Report 50)*, Bethesda, MD, 1999.

[8] Yan, D., et al., "Computed Tomography Guided Management of Interfractional Patient Variation," *Semin. Radiat. Oncol.*, Vol. 15, 2005, pp. 168–179.

[9] Ling, C. C., E. Yorke, and Z. Fuks, "From IMRT to IGRT: Frontierland or Neverland?" *Radiotherapy and Oncology*, Vol. 78, 2006, pp. 119–122.

[10] Yan, D., et al., "An Off-Line Strategy for Constructing a Patient-Specific Planning Target Volume in Adaptive Treatment Process for Prostate Cancer," *Int. J. Radiat. Oncol. Biol. Phys.*, Vol. 48, 2000, pp. 289–302.

[11] Shimizu, S., et al., "Use of an Implanted Marker and Real-Time Tracking of the Marker for the Positioning of Prostate and Bladder Cancers," *Int. J. Radiat. Oncol. Biol. Phys.*, Vol. 48, 2000, pp. 1591–1597.

[12] Court, L., et al., "Evaluation of Mechanical Precision and Alignment Uncertainties for an Integrated CT/LINAC System," *Med. Phys.*, Vol. 30, 2003, pp. 1198–1210.

[13] Jaffray, D. A., et al., "Flat-Panel Cone-Beam Computed Tomography for Image-Guided Radiation Therapy," *Int. J. Radiat. Oncol. Biol. Phys.*, Vol. 53, 2002, pp. 1337–1349.

[14] Shirato, H., et al., "Physical Aspects of a Real Time Tumor Tracking System for Gated Radiotherapy," *Int. J. Radiat. Oncol. Biol. Phys.*, Vol. 48, 2000, pp. 1187–1195.

[15] Vedam, S. S., et al., "Determining Parameters for Respiration-Gated Radiotherapy," *Med. Phys.*, Vol. 28, No. 10, 2001, pp. 2139–2146.

[16] Kubo, H. D., et al., "Breathing Synchronized Radiotherapy Program at the University of California Davis Cancer Center," *Med. Phys.*, Vol. 27, 2000, pp. 346–353.

[17] Ozhasoglu, C., and, M. J. Murphy, "Issues in Respiratory Motion Compensation During External Beam Radiotherapy," *Int. J. Radiat. Oncol. Biol. Phys.*, Vol. 52, 2002, pp. 1389–1399.

[18] Keall, P., "4-Dimensional Computed Tomography Imaging and Treatment Planning," *Semin. Radiat. Oncol.*, Vol. 14, 2004, pp. 81–90.

[19] Pouliot, J., et al., "Low-Dose Megavoltage Cone Beam CT for Radiation Therapy," *Int. J. Radiat. Oncol. Biol. Phys.*, Vol. 61, No. 2, 2005, pp. 238–246.

[20] Keall, P. J., et al., "The Management of Respiratory Motion in Radiation Oncology Report of the AAPM Task Group 76," *Med. Phys.*, Vol. 33, No. 10, 2006, pp. 3874–3900.

[21] Schweikard, A., et al., "Robotic Motion Compensation for Respiratory Movement During Radiosurgery," *J. Computer-Aided Surg.*, Vol. 5, No. 4, 2000, pp. 263–277.

[22] Huntzinger, C., *Image Guided Radiation Therapy*, Palo Alto, CA: Varian Medical Systems, 2004.

[23] Wiersma, M., and L. Xing, "kV + MV Imaging for Real-Time Tracking of Implanted Fiducial Markers," *Med. Phys.*, Vol. 35, No. 4, April 2008.

[24] de la Zerda, A., B. Armbruster, and L. Xing, "Formulating Adaptive Radiation Therapy Planning into Closed-Loop Control Framework," *Phys. Med. Biol.*, Vol. 52, 2007, pp. 4137–4153.

[25] Yoo, S., et al., "A Quality Assurance Program for the On-Board Imager," *Med. Phys.*, Vol. 33, No. 11, 2006, pp. 4431–4447.

[26] Lehmann, J., et al., "Commissioning Experience with Cone-Beam Computed Tomography for Image-Guided Radiation Therapy," *J. App. Clin. Med. Phys.*, Vol. 8, No. 3, 2007, pp. 22–36.

[27] Lee, S.W., et al., "Clinical Assessment and Characterization of a Dual-Tube Kilovoltage X-Ray Localization System in the Radiotherapy Treatment Room," *J. App. Clin. Med. Phys.*, Vol. 9, No. 1, 2008, pp. 1–15.

[28] Mohan, R., et al., "Use of Deformed Intensity Distributions for On-Line Modification of Image-Guided IMRT to Account for Interfractional Anatomic Changes," *Int. J. Radiat. Oncol. Biol. Phys.*, Vol. 61, 2005, pp. 1258–1266.

[29] Mackie, T. R., et al., "Image Guidance for Precise Conformal Radiotherapy," *Int. J. Radiat. Oncol. Biol. Phys.*, Vol. 56, 2003, pp. 89–105.

[30] Yang, Y., et al., "Evaluation of On-Board kV Cone Beam CT (CBCT)-Based Dose Calculation," *Phys. Med. Biol.*, Vol. 52, 2007, pp. 685–706.

CHAPTER 5

Radiofrequency Ablation

Dieter Haemmerich

5.1 Introduction

Radiofrequency (RF) ablation employs electric current in the radiofrequency range (typically ~450 to 500 kHz) to heat biological tissues. While RF heating in the same frequency range has been used for electrosurgical devices since the 1930s, RF ablation saw clinical application more recently in the 1980s and 1990s. The most prevalent applications of RF ablation are for treatment of cardiac arrhythmia and cancer. In this chapter we discuss the biophysics of RF ablation and specific devices for different applications.

5.2 Biophysics of RF Ablation

5.2.1 Physics of RF Heating

During RF ablation, an RF electrode is introduced to the target site under imaging guidance, and the tissue in proximity of the electrode is heated by electric current. In addition to the RF electrode, one or more ground pads (or dispersive electrodes) are required to serve as return path for the electric current; these ground pads are placed either on the patient's back or thighs. Figure 5.1 shows the schematics of an RF ablation system.

While inside the RF generator and cables free electrons carry the electric current, inside tissue there are no free electrons available and ions (Na^+, K^+, Cl^-) serve as charge carriers. The RF current applied via the RF electrode results in ion oscillations in the tissue (Figure 5.2), which in turn cause resistive heating. The amount of heat generated depends on the local current density, which corresponds to the velocity of ion movement. Typically, the highest current densities are observed close to the RF electrode. To quantify the heat generated locally, a parameter called *specific absorption rate* (SAR) is often used, with units of W/kg (i.e., mass related power). To determine the SAR profile of a certain RF electrode, the electric field problem has to be solved, which gives as a result the distribution of electric field strength (E), or current density (J) throughout the tissue. Subsequently we can obtain the SAR profile according to following equation (the local version of Ohm's law) [1]:

$$SAR = \frac{\sigma}{\rho}|E|^2 = \frac{1}{\sigma \cdot \rho}|J|^2 \tag{5.1}$$

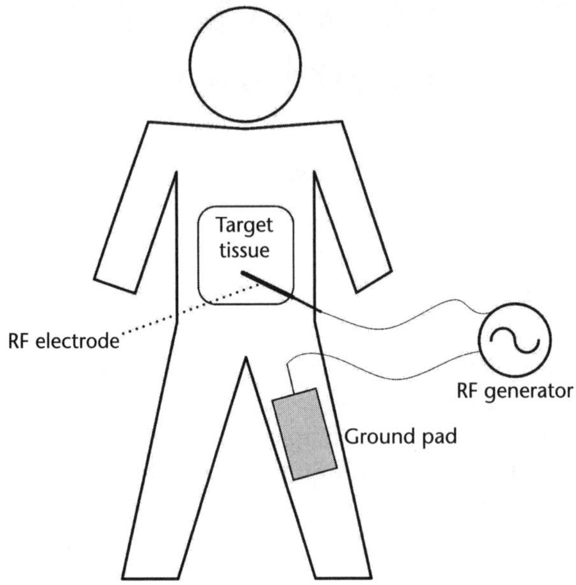

Figure 5.1 RF system schematics. An RF electrode is inserted into the target tissue under imaging guidance. RF energy provided by a generator is applied to the electrode and results in tissue heating around the electrode. A ground pad placed on the patient's thighs or back serves as return path for the RF current.

σ = tissue electrical conductivity
ρ = tissue mass density
E = electric field strength
J = electric current density

Since in general the electric field strength (and accordingly current density) is only sufficiently high to cause considerable direct heating very close to the electrode, thermal conduction contributes considerably towards the tissue temperature profile. The heat transfer problem during RF ablation as well as other ablation

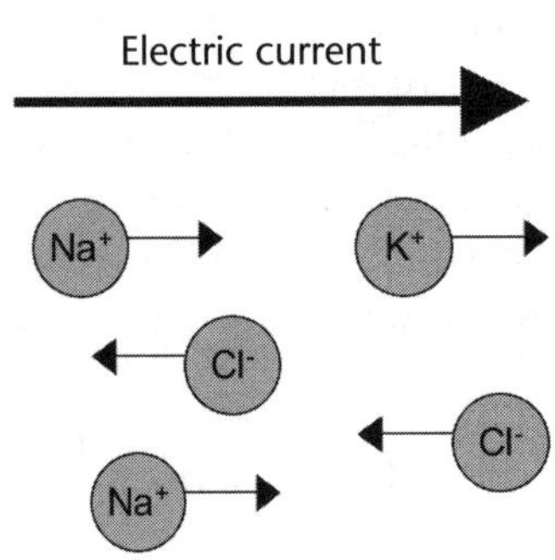

Figure 5.2 Electric current inside tissue is carried by ions. Ion oscillations due to applied RF current results in resistive tissue heating (e.g., for a 500-kHz frequency RF current, the direction of the current changes ~1 million times/sec).

methods can be mathematically described by the following heat transfer equation where T represents tissue temperature [2]:

$$\rho c \frac{\partial T}{\partial t} = \nabla \cdot k \nabla T + Q_{RF} - Q_p \tag{5.2}$$

$$Q_{RF} = SAR \cdot \rho = \sigma \cdot |E|^2 \tag{5.3}$$

Q_{RF} (W/m^3) is the RF energy applied to the tissue around the RF electrode resulting in heating. Blood perfusion carries some heat Q_p (W/m^3) away. Perfusion varies between tissue types, between locations within an organ, and between patients, and may therefore have negligible impact in some cases (e.g., heart) or major impact in other cases (e.g., liver). Once tissue temperature is elevated above body temperature, thermal conduction results in spread of heat through the tissue [first term on right-hand side of (5.2)]. The left-hand side term of (5.2) quantifies the change in tissue temperature depending on specific heat c (J/(kg K)) and mass density ρ (kg/m^3) of the tissue.

Figure 5.3 shows an example of current density profile, and final tissue temperature profile after applying RF energy for 12 minutes to liver tissue in a computer simulation.

The target temperatures during RF ablation are in the range of ~50°C to 110°C (see also Section 5.2.3). Above ~110°C tissue water vaporizes and forms an electrically insulating barrier preventing further RF heating. In addition, vapor formation can result in perforation of the tissue, which may be undesirable, depending on the particular application. Furthermore, a region of carbonized tissue can form

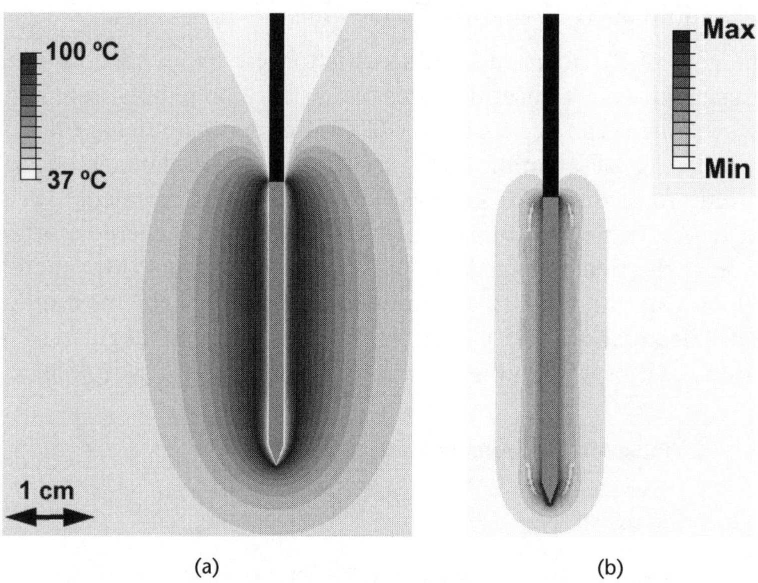

Figure 5.3 Final tissue temperature profile after 12 minutes RF ablation with an internally cooled needle electrode (a), and current density profile (b). The gray electrode region depicts the active RF electrode, and the black needle region is electrically insulated. Current density is high only close to the RF electrode.

at highly elevated temperatures (generally termed "charring"); this carbonization of tissue is irreversible and is electrically insulating as well. Therefore, applied RF power has to be controlled to keep tissue temperature in the target range.

5.2.2 Power Control Algorithms

Initially RF ablation devices applied *constant power* over the treatment period. The power level was chosen by the operator, and there was no feedback control of applied power. This method is still used in electrosurgery units, but is no longer commonly used in RF ablation devices.

Temperature feedback control is often used for ablation devices. One or more thermal sensors (typically thermistors or thermocouples) are located inside the electrode, or at a specified distance from the electrode. Applied power is controlled such that the measured temperature is kept at a specified value. Note however, that when the electrode temperature is measured, this value usually underestimates the maximum tissue temperature (see Figure 5.3).

Impedance feedback control is another commonly used method. Tissue electrical conductivity changes during heating. Initially, tissue becomes electrically more conductive as it is heated due to increases in ion mobility. When tissue vaporization occurs above 100°C, tissue electrical conductivity rapidly drops. These changes in electrical conductivity can be measured via impedance measurements, which give an overall measurement of the electrical connection between RF electrode and ground pad (compare to Figure 5.1). Vapor formation in the tissue can then be detected by those impedance measurements, and applied power controlled accordingly to avoid excessive vapor generation.

5.2.3 Principles of Thermal Tissue Injury

The goal of RF ablation treatments is to destroy a defined tissue region via heat. Tissue injury due to heating is dependent both on temperature and time. Significant tissue damage can occur above ~42°C after many hours; at the target temperatures used during RF ablation (50°C to 100°C), tissue damage occurs in the range of minutes to seconds (see Table 5.1). In general, an exponential relationship is present where, at temperatures above 43°C, with each degree centigrade temperature increase the time required for cell death is cut in half [3]. There are a number of cellular responses due to elevated temperature, but the most prevalent mechanism of cell death above ~45°C is necrosis due to protein coagulation. There are several different terms used in the literature for the zone of tissue destruction. In literature

Table 5.1 Temperature Versus Tissue Effects

Temperature (°C)	*Tissue Effects*
36–38	Normal body temperature
38–42	Fever
> 42	Elevated rates of enzyme activity, cell death possible
45	Protein coagulation and cell death after 1–2 hours
50	Protein coagulation and cell death after 2–3 minutes
60–100	Protein coagulation and cell death instantaneous
> 100	Tissue vaporization, carbonization (charring)

on cardiac RF ablation, "lesion" is generally used. This term was also initially used in tumor ablation literature, but has more recently been replaced by "coagulation zone," "ablation zone," "thermal lesion," or "necrosis zone" to avoid confusion with tumors, which are also frequently called "lesions."

5.3 Cardiac RF Catheter Ablation

5.3.1 Clinical Background

The contraction of the heart is dictated by specific conduction pathways in the heart tissue; these pathways orchestrate the spatial and temporal heart muscle contraction. Abnormalities in these conduction pathways can lead to arrhythmias (i.e., irregular heart beats). For certain cardiac arrhythmias, RF ablation has become the treatment of choice [4], for example, for several types of tachycardias (i.e., the heart is beating too fast, > 150 beats per minute) and for some types of atrial fibrillation (i.e., disorganized, quivering contraction of the atria).

Cardiac RF ablation is performed in a specially equipped laboratory. Typically, x-ray fluoroscopy imaging is employed to guide the procedure while the patient is either anesthetized or under conscious sedation (Figures 5.4 and 5.5). The RF ablation catheter (Figure 5.6) and diagnostic catheters are inserted through veins (typically groin and/or neck) and guided into the heart (see Figure 5.4). The electrophysiologist uses the RF catheter and additional diagnostic catheters that record the electrical activity from different locations inside the heart to determine the mechanism of the arrhythmia and locate the target site of ablation (see Figure 5.5). RF ablation is performed for ~1 minute to destroy the tissue region responsible for the

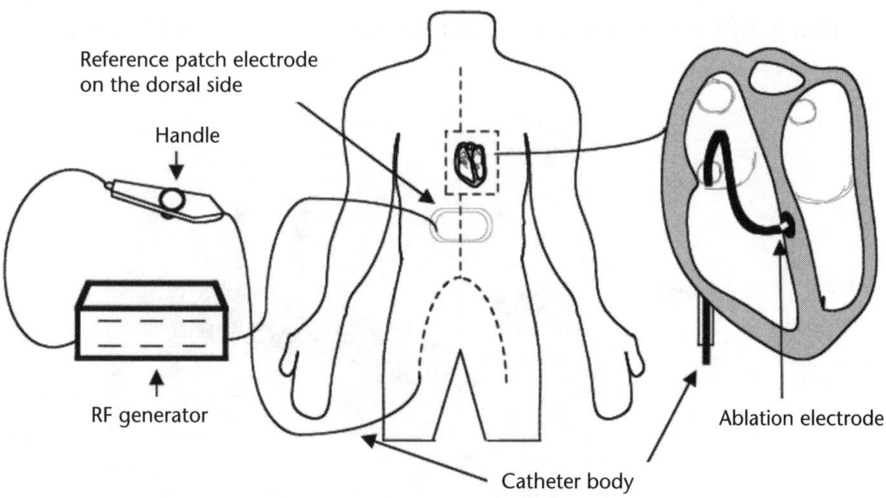

Figure 5.4 Schematics of cardiac RF ablation system. A cardiac RF catheter is inserted through a leg vein, and steered to the target site inside the heart (right figure). A reference patch electrode (i.e., ground pad) is placed on the patient's back. The small black region around the RF electrode at the catheter tip depicts the ablation zone. (*From:* [5]. © 1995 IEEE. Reprinted with permission from Panescu et al.)

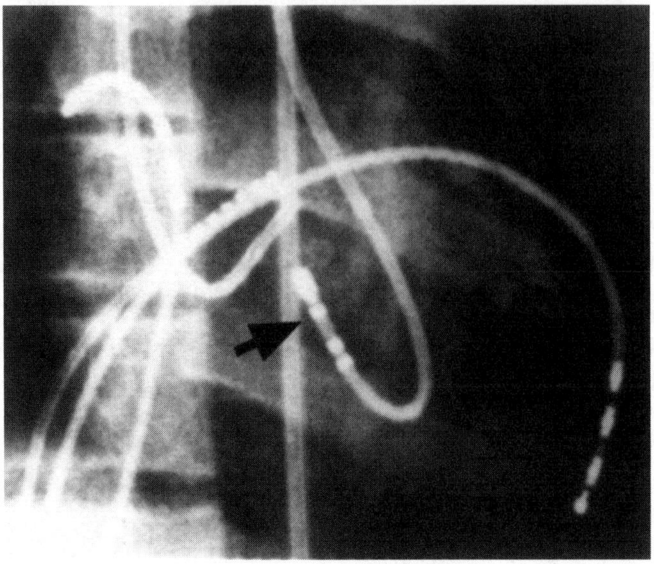

Figure 5.5 X-ray fluoroscopy is typically used to guide cardiac RF ablation procedures. This image taken of a patient's heart shows the RF ablation catheter (arrow), as well as other catheters ("mapping catheters") used to record electrical activity from inside the heart to locate the target site. (Image provided courtesy of Dr. Phil Saul, Medical University of South Carolina.)

arrhythmia, and the patient is discharged typically a few hours after the procedure or may be monitored overnight in the hospital.

5.3.2 Devices

Figure 5.4 shows an overview of an RF ablation procedure, and Figure 5.6 depicts a cardiac RF catheter. Most catheters employ temperature control (see Section 5.2.2) where temperature is measured by a sensor embedded in the electrode

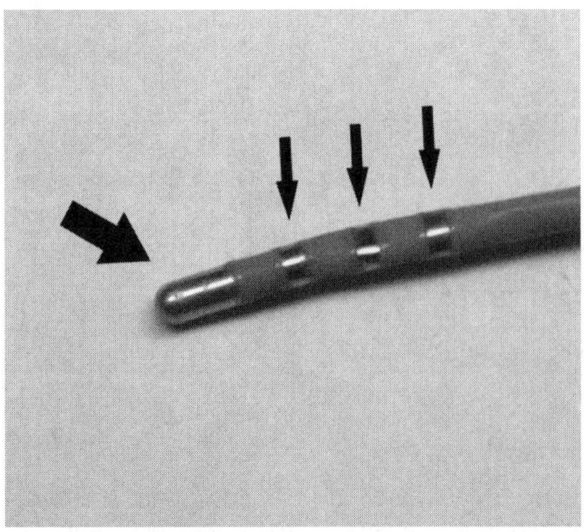

Figure 5.6 Cardiac RF ablation catheter (7F = 2.3-mm diameter). Catheter has an RF electrode (large arrow, 4-mm length) to create the ablation zone, and mapping electrodes (small arrows) to record electrical activity from within the heart.

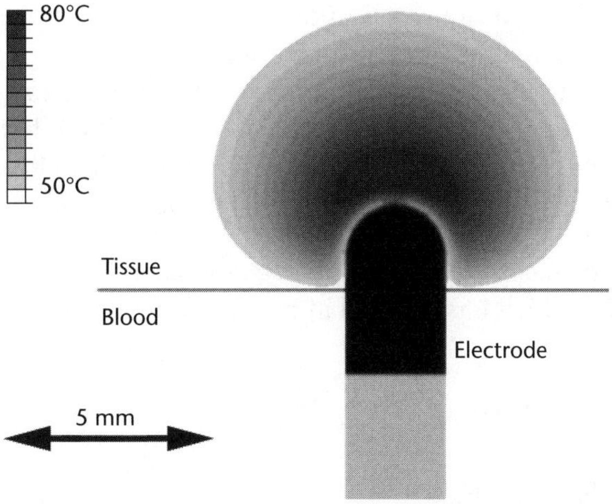

Figure 5.7 The tissue temperature profile in the tissue at the end of a 45-second-long ablation. Since ~50°C is the threshold for cell necrosis, the 50°C isotherm estimates the boundary of cell death.

tip, with target tip temperatures of ~60°C to 80°C and applied power of up to 100W. A single ablation lasts for typically 45 to 60 seconds, and creates a teardrop-shaped ablation zone (Figure 5.7). Note that the location of highest temperature is a few millimeters from the RF electrode, and therefore the measured temperature deviates from the maximum tissue temperature. This issue is of importance since tissue perforations (often called "popping" in the literature due to the sound associated with this event)—which occur at tissue temperature above 100°C—are undesired during cardiac RF ablation. Since actual tissue temperature cannot be accurately measured, ideal treatment parameters (i.e., target tip temperature, time) to maximize ablation zone size while avoiding perforation due to excessive heating are not always known.

Catheters of different sizes are available depending on the desired size of the ablation zone. Newer catheter designs are available that employ internal cooling to create larger ablation zones [6]. For treatment of atrial fibrillation, linear ablation zones are desired. These can be created by dragging a standard catheter or sequentially creating adjacent ablations.

5.3.3 Comparison of Cardiac RF and Cryo-Ablation

More recently, cryo-ablation devices have become clinically available for cardiac applications [7]. These employ cryogenic cooling down to –80°C to create an ice ball in the myocardium, and kill tissue via freezing. The application times are longer compared to RF with typically 4 minutes, and initial devices created smaller lesion sizes compared to RF. However, cryo-ablation has several safety advantages over RF:

- The cryo catheter attaches to the tissue upon freezing preventing any movement from the target site.
- Cryo-ablation is less thrombogenic and the chance of stenosis of coronary vessels is considerably smaller compared to RF.

- RF ablation can result in cardiac perforation due to excessive heating, which is not possible with cryo-ablation.
- The target site can be confirmed by cooling to temperatures where tissue function disappears reversibly (~0°C to 12°C), but resumes after rewarming of the tissue; this is important when ablating close to structures that should not be damaged (e.g., the atrio-ventricular node)

In particular for pediatric patients, the safety advantages of cryo-ablation are attractive [8], which has resulted in increased clinical use in those patient populations.

5.4 RF Tumor Ablation

5.4.1 Clinical Background

RF ablation for the treatment of cancer (i.e., tumor ablation) saw its first clinical application in the early 1990s. An estimated 70,000 tumor ablation procedures were carried out in 2004, with numbers rising an estimated ~20% to 30% annually. Initially, RF ablation was employed for treatment of liver cancer where there was a need for a new treatment modality. Most patients with liver cancer are not candidates for surgery (the standard treatment for liver cancer), for example, due to multiple tumors or tumors located close to large vessels; other available therapies such as chemotherapy and radiation therapy do not work well for liver cancer. Today, RF ablation is the treatment of choice for certain patient populations where surgery is not possible. In addition, it is increasingly used in other organs such as cancer in kidney, lung, bone, and adrenal gland [9, 10].

Tumor ablation can be performed during open surgery or laparoscopy (by a surgeon), or minimally invasive through a small incision in the skin (by an interventional radiologist). The tumor is diagnosed typically by computed tomography (CT) or ultrasound imaging. The same imaging modalities are also usually used to guide the procedure by visualizing the RF applicator and tumor (see Figures 5.8 and 5.9).

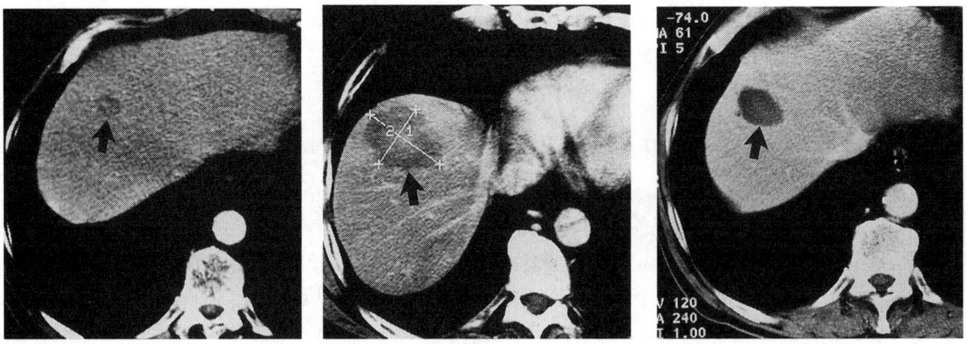

(a) (b) (c)

Figure 5.8 Contrast-enhanced CT is commonly used to identify a tumor (left, arrow). One month after ablation, a follow-up image shows the ablation zone created by two sequential ablations (middle, arrow). The ablation zone is 4.5 × 6.0 cm in diameter (indicated by cursors 1 and 2). A 10-month follow-up image shows the ablation zone decreases in size over time (right, arrow). (Reprinted with permission from Gazelle et al. [11].)

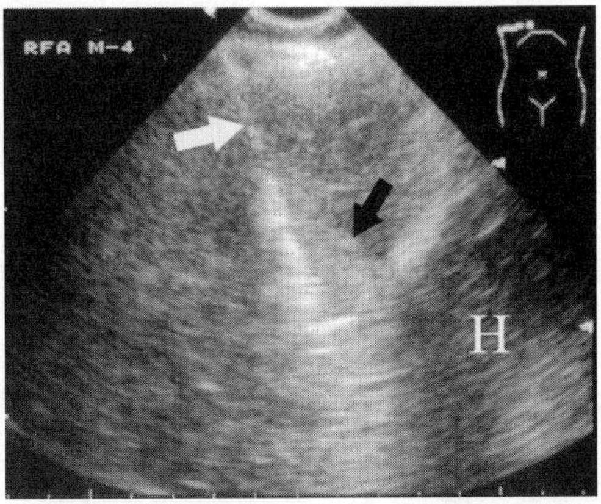

Figure 5.9 Ultrasound image obtained during RF tumor ablation procedure depicts RF electrode (white arrow), and hyperechoic (i.e., white) region around the electrode (black arrow) due to microbubble formation in the heated tissue. (Reprinted with permission from Chen et al. [12].)

The RF electrode is inserted into the tumor (in Figure 5.10 via ultrasound imaging guidance) while the patient is under general anesthesia or conscious sedation. When RF ablation is applied minimally invasive, the patient can typically leave the hospital the same or the next day.

The goal of the tumor ablation procedure is to ablate the tumor including a 1-cm margin of surrounding normal liver tissue. This is because often small islets of cancer cells are surrounding the under imaging visible tumor, and these cells will result in regrowth of the tumor after treatment if they are not ablated. A single ablation can create a necrosis zone of ~3 to 6 cm in diameter within ~12 to 25 minutes,

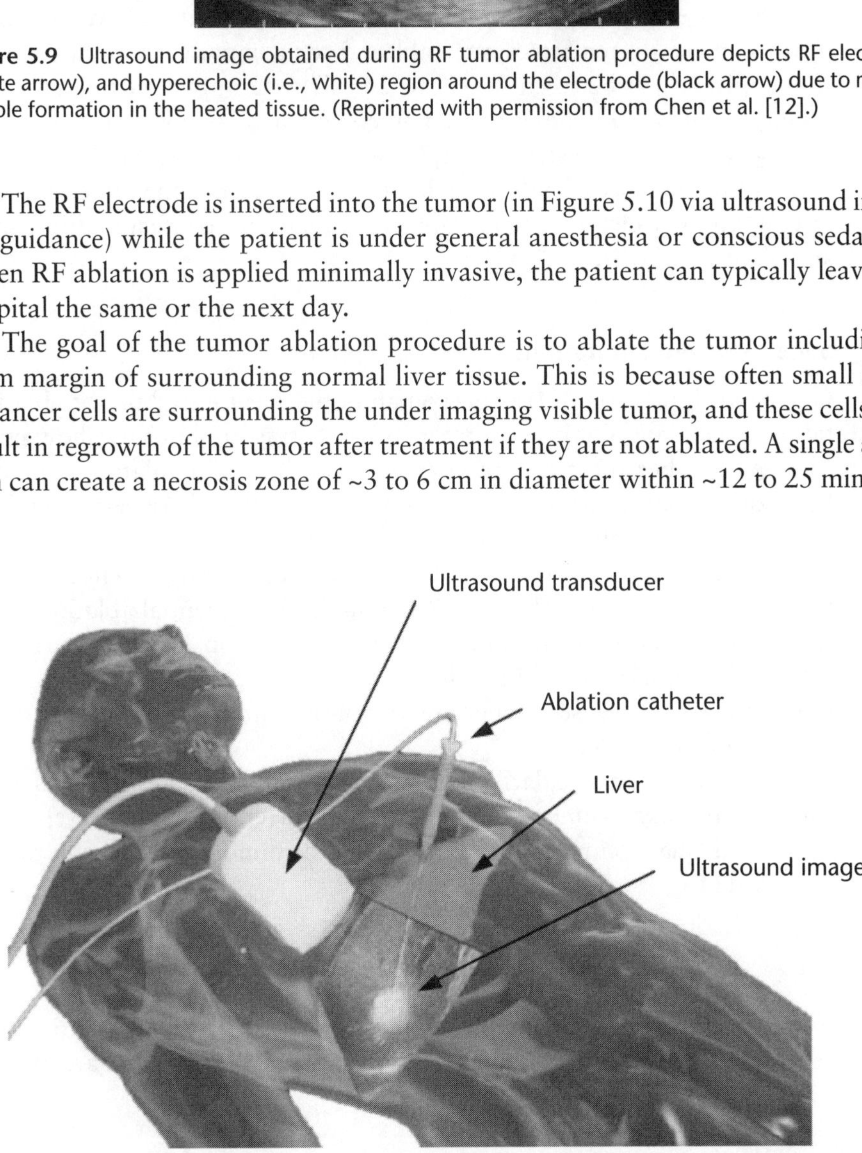

Figure 5.10 Schematics of minimally invasive liver tumor RF ablation procedure. The ablation catheter is inserted through a small incision and steered into the tumor under ultrasound imaging guidance. (Reproduced with permission from Dodd et al. [13].)

depending on the device (see Section 5.4.2). For large tumors multiple overlapping ablations may have to be performed.

5.4.2 Devices

For tumor ablation procedures tissue perforation is not an issue as it is for cardiac procedures. Therefore, higher tissue temperatures up to ~110°C are obtained with the goal of creating a large and reproducible ablation zone. Figure 5.3 shows the tissue temperature profile at the end of an ablation procedure in a computer simulation. The highest temperatures are again close to the electrode, and the necrosis zone encompasses all tissue above ~50°C to 52°C.

There are currently four commercial RF tumor ablation devices available (three of these in the United States; see Table 5.2 for company information). The generators apply power between 200W to 250W, with application times of ~12 to 25 minutes. Figure 5.11 shows two commercially available RF electrodes.

All RF ablation systems except one (Switching controller, Valleylab, Boulder, Colorado) allow use of only a single electrode at a time; the switching controller allows up to three electrodes to create larger ablations, or treat multiple small tumors simultaneously [14].

5.4.3 Current Limitations

One major limitation of RF ablation and other heat-based tumor ablation modalities is inadequate interprocedural imaging. Ultrasound images show microbubbles (Figure 5.9), but these do not correlate well with the ablation zone dimensions. Ultrasound contrast agents show coagulated regions where perfusion is absent, but these are not available yet in the United States.

The size of the ablation zone of current devices is still often not adequate to treat large tumors in a single ablation. When multiple sequential ablations are required, the procedure becomes technically complex since no information is available on extent of prior ablations; this is likely one of the reasons resulting in increased tumor recurrence rates seen when treating large tumors (> 3 cm) due to incomplete ablation of the tumor.

Large vessels, particularly in organs with high blood perfusion such as the liver, act as heat sinks. Tumor regions located adjacent to large vessels often do not achieve adequate temperatures; the chances of tumor recurrence in those cases are increased [15].

5.4.4 Comparison of Tumor RF, Microwave, and Cryo-Ablation

While RF ablation is worldwide the most widely used tumor ablation method, microwave ablation and cryo-ablation are also clinically used and are briefly reviewed below.

Cryo-Ablation

Cryo tumor ablation has been in clinical use much longer than heat-based modalities, with the earliest applications in the 1960s. Cryo-ablation systems employ

Table 5.2 RF Ablation Device Manufacturers

Application	*Company*	*Device Name*
Cardiac	Biosense-Webster (Diamond Bar, CA) www.biosensewebster.com Tel. 800-729-9010	Stockert 70
	Boston Scientific (Natick, MA) www.bsci.com Tel. 888-272-1001	Cobra Chilli EPT-1000XP
	Cardima (Fremont, CA) www.cardima.com Tel. 800-354-0102	Revelation
	Medtronic (Minneapolis, MN) www.medtronic.com Tel. 763-514-4000	Atakr
	St. Jude Medical (St. Paul, MN) www.sjm.com Tel. 800-328-9634	Livewire
Tumor	Boston Scientific (Natick, MA) www.bsci.com Tel. 888-272-1001	RF 3000
	Celon (Teltow, Germany) www.celon.com Tel. +49-3328-3519-0	CelonSurgical
	AngioDynamics (Queensbury, NY) www.angiodynamics.com Tel. 800-772-6446	Model 1500X
	Valleylab (Boulder, CO) www.valleylab.com Tel. 800-255-8522	Cool-Tip
Endometrial	Cytyc (Marlborough, MA) www.cytyc.com Tel. 800-442-9892	Novasure
Endovascular	VNUS Medical Technologies (San Jose, CA) www.vnus.com Tel. 888-797-8346	ClosurePlus
Cornea	Refractec (Irvine, CA) www.refractec.com Tel. 800-752-9544	Viewpoint CK NearVision CK
Enlarged Prostate	Medtronic (Minneapolis, MN) www.medtronic.com Tel. 800-328-2518	Prostiva RF

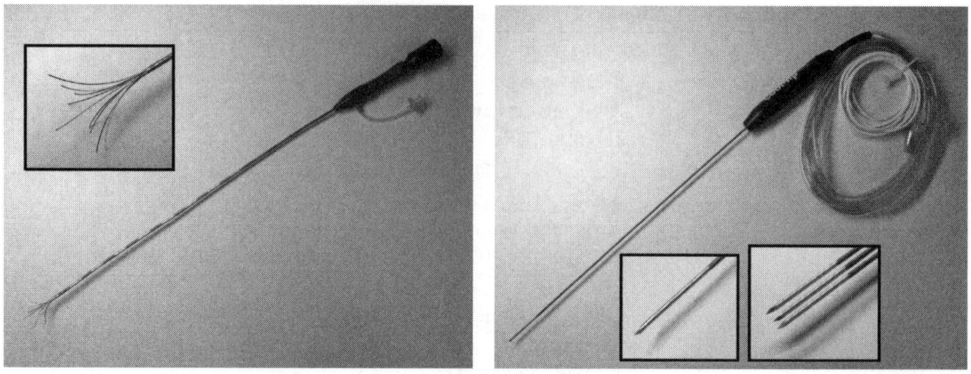

(a) (b)

Figure 5.11 Commercial RF electrodes for tumor ablation. (a) Multiprong electrode, with magnified electrode tip shown in insert. The prongs are extended once the catheter is placed in the tumor. (b) Cooled needle electrode, available as single or three-needle cluster (see magnified inserts). Active electrode at the tip is 3 cm (single) or 2.5 cm long (cluster), and is internally cooled by circulating water.

cryogenic cooling mediated by either argon or nitrogen to obtain probe temperatures down to –160°C. So far, cryo-ablation has been mainly used during open surgery, since the comparably large probe sizes made application during minimally invasive procedures not viable. Recently, smaller probes have become commercially available that are suited for minimally invasive treatment. The major advantage of cryo-ablation over heat-based methods is that the ice ball is clearly visible under imaging, in particular with ultrasound imaging. It should be noted however that the ice ball does not exactly correspond to the boundary of the necrosis zone, but typically extends several millimeters beyond. Cryo-ablation also allows the use of multiple cryo probes to create large ice balls.

Microwave Ablation

Microwave (MW) ablation has been clinically used in Asia for several years for treatment of small tumors with generic MW antennas. Only recently have commercial devices been announced, and these will likely be available in the near future. The possible advantages over RF ablation include shorter treatment times due to higher possible tissue temperatures, as MW propagation is not limited by tissue vaporization or charred tissue. MW ablation also seems less affected by perfusion mediated cooling in initial studies. Furthermore, multiple MW antennas can be used simultaneously for treatment of large tumors.

5.5 Other Applications of RF Ablation

5.5.1 Endometrial Ablation

Thermal ablation has become an accepted treatment modality for women with uterine bleeding that do not respond to standard treatments such as drugs and scraping of the endometrium (i.e., lining of the uterus). During treatment, the whole endometrium is ablated within typically 3 to 10 minutes [16]. While most devices use heated aqueous solutions to ablate the tissue, there is also an RF-based device available (Novasure, Cytyc, Marlborough, Massachusetts) that employs mesh electrodes with power applied between two meshes in bipolar fashion. RF energy is applied for 1.5 to 2 minutes, and power is controlled by tissue impedance.

5.5.2 Endovascular Ablation

Endovascular ablation is a treatment modality for varicose veins (i.e., visible, dilated and twisted veins near the skin surface). Varicose veins most often affect legs and thighs, where insufficiencies in the venous valves result in blood pooling and vein enlargement. Treatment options aim to close the affected veins and include surgical stripping, injection of a drug that results in vein swelling and closure, and ablation.

During ablation, a catheter is introduced into the vein; subsequently, the vessel wall is heated resulting in collagen shrinkage above ~60°C, and closure of the vein. Laser- and RF-based endovascular ablation devices are commercially available. The RF device (ClosurePlus, VNUS Medical, San Jose, California) employs a catheter equipped with multiple electrodes arranged in a Christmas tree like configuration. The electrodes are extended inside the vein and are in direct contact with the endovascular surface. Temperature sensors located at the electrode's tips are employed for temperature feedback control of the applied power, with target temperatures of ~85°C.

5.5.3 Corneal Ablation

Many vision disorders are the result of shape imperfections of the cornea. Treatments aim to correct the shape and include surgical methods where part of the cornea is removed and ablative methods where part of the cornea is heated resulting in shrinkage.

While laser ablation is the more commonly used ablative method, an RF-based device has also been available for several years now. RF pulses of ~1W power are applied for a few seconds to a very thin electrode (90-μm diameter and 450-μm long) to produce the intended heating and shrinkage effects [17].

5.5.4 Other Applications

In addition to the applications above, RF ablation is investigated for other applications such as prostate cancer, brain tumors, Parkinson's disease, and chronic pain (i.e., ablation of the nerve fibers responsible). For treatment of enlarged prostates (benign prostate hyperplasia, or BPH) a commercial device is available (Prostiva RF, Medtronic, Minneapolis, Minnesota).

References

[1] Haemmerich, D., "Tissue Ablation," in *Wiley Encyclopedia of Medical Devices and Instrumentation, Volume* 6, 2nd ed., J. G. Webster, (ed.), New York: John Wiley & Sons, 2006, pp. 362–379.

[2] Diller, K. R., J. W. Valvano, and J. A. Pearce, "Bioheat Transfer," in *CRC Handbook of Thermal Engineering, Volume 4*, F. Kreith, (ed.), Boca Raton, FL: CRC Press, 2000, pp. 114–215.

[3] Dewhirst, M. W., et al., "Basic Principles of Thermal Dosimetry and Thermal Thresholds for Tissue Damage from Hyperthermia," *Int. J. Hyperthermia*, Vol. 19, May-June 2003, pp. 267–294.

[4] Wilber, D. J., D. L. Packer, and W. G. Stevenson, *Catheter Ablation of Cardiac Arrhythmias: Basic Concepts and Clinical Applications*, Malden, MA: Blackwell Publishing, 2007.

[5] Panescu, D., et al., "Three-Dimensional Finite Element Analysis of Current Density and Temperature Distributions During Radio-Frequency Ablation," *IEEE Transactions on Biomedical Engineering*, Vol. 42, September, 1995, pp. 879–890.

[6] McGreevy, K. S., et al., "Comparison of a Saline Irrigated Cooled-Tip Catheter to Large Electrode Catheters with Single and Multiple Temperature Sensors for Creation of Large Radiofrequency Lesions," *J. Interv. Card. Electrophysiol.*, Vol. 14, December 2005, pp. 139–145.

[7] Skanes, A. C., et al., "Cryoablation: Potentials and Pitfalls," *J. Cardiovasc. Electrophysiol.*, Vol. 15, October 2004, pp. S28–S34.

[8] Miyazaki, A., et al., "Cryo-Ablation for Septal Tachycardia Substrates in Pediatric Patients: Mid-Term Results," *J. Am. Coll. Cardiol.*, Vol. 45, February 15, 2005, pp. 581–588.

[9] Gillams, A. R., "The Use of Radiofrequency in Cancer," *British Journal of Cancer*, Vol. 92, May 23, 2005, pp. 1825–1829.

[10] van Sonnenberg, E., *Tumor Ablation*, 1st ed., New York: Springer, 2005.

[11] Gazelle, G. S., et al., "Tumor Ablation with Radio-Frequency Energy," *Radiology*, Vol. 217, 12/2000 2000, pp. 633–646.

[12] Chen, M. H., et al., "Large Liver Tumors: Protocol for Radiofrequency Ablation and Its Clinical Application in 110 Patients—Mathematic Model, Overlapping Mode, and Electrode Placement Process," *Radiology*, Vol. 232, July 2004, pp. 260–271.

[13] Dodd, G. D., et al., "Minimally Invasive Treatment of Malignant Hepatic Tumors: At the Threshold of a Major Breakthrough," *Radiographics*, Vol. 20, January-February 2000, pp. 9–27.

[14] Laeseke, P. F., et al., "Multiple-Electrode Radiofrequency Ablation of Hepatic Malignancies: Initial Clinical Experience," *AJR Am. J. Roentgenol.*, Vol. 188, June 2007, pp. 1485–1494.

[15] Lu, D. S., et al., "Influence of Large Peritumoral Vessels on Outcome of Radiofrequency Ablation of Liver Tumors," *J. Vasc. Interv. Radiol.*, Vol. 14, October 2003, pp. 1267–1274.

[16] Cooper, J., and R. J. Gimpelson, "Summary of Safety and Effectiveness Data from FDA: A Valuable Source of Information on the Performance of Global Endometrial Ablation Devices," *J. Reprod. Med.*, Vol. 49, April 2004, pp. 267–273.

[17] Berjano, E. J., J. L. Alio, and J. Saiz, "Modeling for Radio-Frequency Conductive Keratoplasty: Implications for the Maximum Temperature Reached in the Cornea," *Physiol. Meas.*, Vol. 26, June 2005, pp. 157–172.

CHAPTER 6

Microwave Ablation

Christos S. Georgiades and Jean-Francois Geschwind

6.1 Introduction

Image-guided therapies encompass a variety of relatively new interventions that avail themselves either as a replacement to more invasive surgical procedures or as altogether new treatment options in cases where there was none. Image-guided interventionalists, usually interventional radiologists, "marry" their imaging expertise with skills in using minimally invasive probes to treat disease deep within the human body. One of these, percutaneous ablation, has emerged as a very attractive alternative for the treatment of certain cancers as well as other amenable conditions such as certain types of chronic pain. Ablation refers to the "killing" of a well-defined, targeted volume of tissue by chemical or thermal means, which, however, cannot distinguish between normal and diseased tissue, therefore some form of image guidance is required. Ablation methods currently in clinical use are summarized in Figure 6.1. The term "percutaneous" refers to another attribute these procedures have in common: they are all guided by an imaging modality, be it ultrasound (US), computed tomography (CT), magnetic resonance imaging (MRI) or fluoroscopy (Fluoro) through the skin thus avoiding the need for an incision. Ablative methods are generally divided into chemical and thermal ones with distinct applications and objectives. Chemical ablative methods use a substance to effect the death of the targeted tissue that comes in contact with it. Common chemicals currently in clinical use include acetic acid, ethanol, and certain anticancer compounds. Thermal methods of ablation utilize hyper- (burning) or hypothermia (freezing or cryo-ablation) to kill tissue. Of the four methods used to ablate tissue by causing hyperthermia [radiofrequency ablation (RFA), microwave ablation (MA), high frequency ultrasound (HIFU), and laser coagulation (LC)], this chapter is devoted to microwave ablation.

6.2 Physics and Physiology of Microwave Ablation

The microwave spectrum is arbitrarily defined as the portion of the electromagnetic spectrum whose frequency range is bounded by 300 MHz and 300 GHz; or whose wavelength is between 1 mm and 1m (Figure 6.2). Currently available microwave ablation generators operate between 900 MHz and 2.45 GHz [1–4]. The antenna (i.e., microwave probe) acts as the source of microwave radiation. As the rapidly alternating electromagnetic field is applied in tissue (adjacent to the tip of the probe), the available dipoles (i.e., water) begin to vibrate as they try to align with this

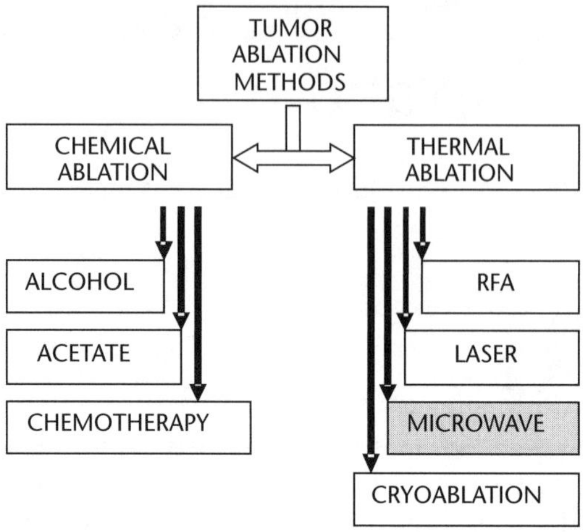

Figure 6.1 Tumor ablation can be affected by a variety of methods, which are divided into chemical or thermal methods. The vast majority of ablations performed in the United States are based on thermal means, most commonly radiofrequency. Laser ablation is more popular in Europe, whereas cryo-ablation is becoming increasingly popular in the United States, especially for kidney tumors and bone lesions. Alcohol, acetate, and chemotherapy ablations are increasingly unpopular as they require multiple sessions to achieve the efficacy of a single session thermal ablation.

alternating field. This effect is noticeable up to 2 cm away from the microwave source [2]. Dielectric hysteresis—that is, the lag of vibrational response by the dipoles to the actual alternating field—results in the conversion of part of the energy in the form of heat [5]. This energy is deposited within the 2-cm ablation zone (distance from the probe or antenna) and does not rely on tissue thermal conductivity [6] for efficient energy transfer. Energy is transferred farther than 2 cm as frictional

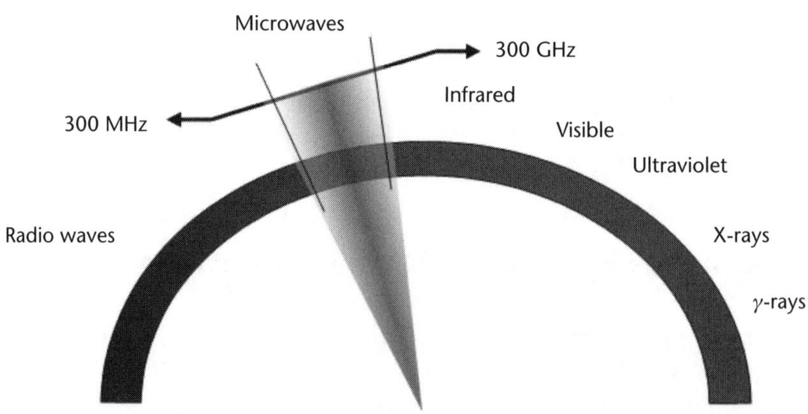

Figure 6.2 The microwave spectrum is the part of the electromagnetic spectrum (EM) with wavelengths shorter than 1m and longer than 1 mm, or frequencies between 300 MHz and 300 GHz. EM radiation is composed of a magnetic and an electric field oscillating synchronized at orthogonal angles to each other. The interaction between the EM radiation and tissue depends on the frequency of oscillation. For example, high frequency radiations (γ-rays or X-rays) result in ionization, ultraviolet rays cause superficial skin burns, and radio- or microwaves result in deeper energy deposition (ablations). The degree of damage depends on the energy deposited by the radiation and is related to the amplitude of the EM wave.

losses couple molecules beyond this zone [3]. This is dependent on tissue thermal conductivity and therefore desiccation or charring of the tissue will limit further energy deposition beyond the 2-cm boundary. Herein lies the major advantage of microwave ablation versus radiofrequency ablation. RFA has a very short direct ablation range (2 mm), while the rest of the ablation zone depends on tissue thermal conductivity. It is therefore more vulnerable to tissue desiccation [6], which causes tissue to lose its thermal/electrical conductivity and effectively thwarts further expansion of the ablation zone (Figure 6.3). The effect of tissue desiccation (charring) around the probe is showcased in Figure 6.4. In reality, the microwave spectrum is part of the radiofrequency spectrum, with the former occupying the higher frequency ranges of the latter (ultra-, super-, and extremely-high frequency).

Thermal ablative methods (i.e., microwave) cause coagulative tissue necrosis by increasing the temperature of the tissue around the probe and maintaining it at adequately high levels for a long enough time. Both temperature and duration are critical factors in effecting a large and effective ablation zone. Figure 6.5 shows the duration of ablation required to cause tissue death at certain temperatures.

6.3 Current Microwave Ablation Technology

The microwave ablation system is composed of a power generator and the antenna (or probe, which is connected to the generator). Contrary to RFA, no grounding pads are necessary. Currently, the only system approved for human use in the United States is the Vivant Medical (Mountain View, California), which has

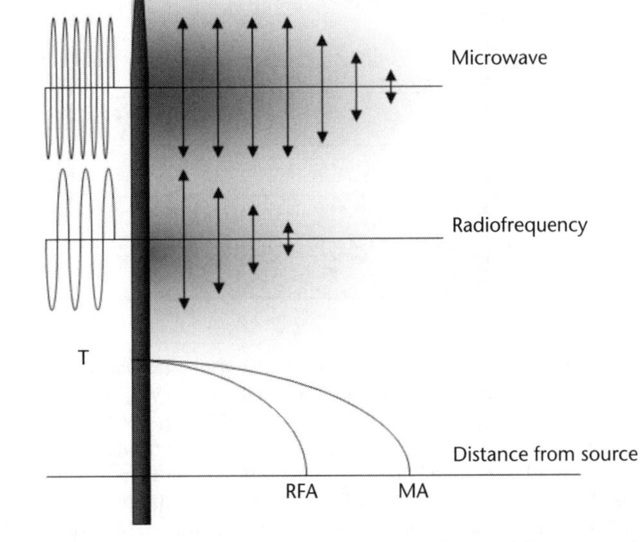

Figure 6.3 Comparison between RFA and microwave coagulation. Microwaves have a higher frequency of vibration and directly excite water molecules farther away from the source (probe) than radiowaves. This results in a larger ablation zone and less dependence on tissue thermal conductivity for effective ablation.

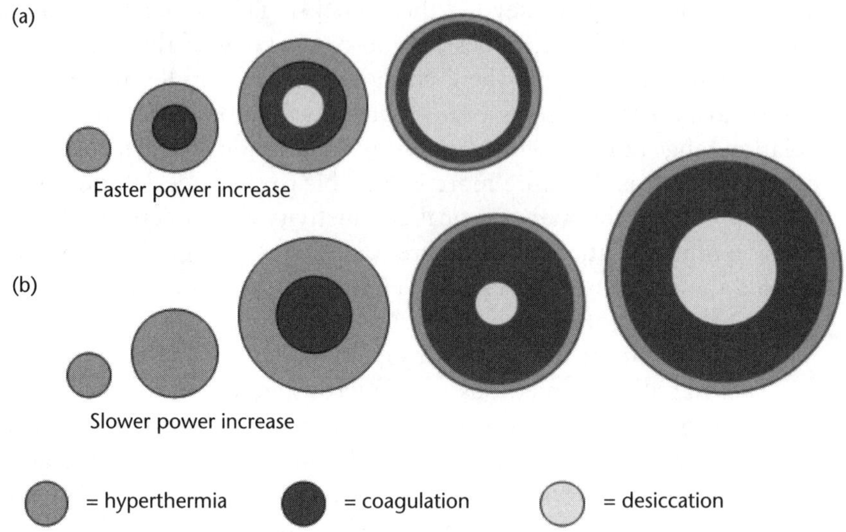

Figure 6.4 A "thought experiment" comparing the eventual ablation zone between (a) a faster power increase and (b) a slower power increase ablation. Early during the ablation the tissue around the probe is heated, however the temperature is not high enough to cause coagulation. As more power is deposited the temperature gradually increases reaching levels that result in tissue death. Tissue death around the probe with the faster power increase ensues earlier. With further energy deposition, tissue temperature increases further, desiccating the tissue. Again, desiccation of the tissue around the probe occurs earlier in the experiment with faster power increase (a). The desiccated tissue is a poor conductor of heat and therefore it limits further extension of the ablation zone. On the other hand in the case of slower power increase, tissues farther away from the probe are heated effectively as the lack of desiccation allows prolonged energy deposition and farther heat conduction.

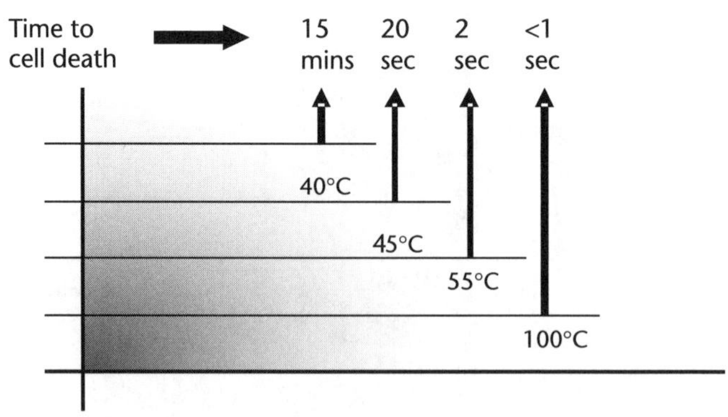

Figure 6.5 Response of mammalian tissue to hyperthermia. Maintaining human cells in vitro at 40°C for at least 15 minutes results in cell death. However, inhomogeneities in the thermal map during ablation mean that some cells within the ablation zone will be heated to less than that and ablation will be ineffective. At 45°C tissue death ensues within 20 seconds, whereas at 50°C to 60°C within 2 seconds. At 100°C cell death is instantaneous. However, this is not ideal as water boiling will result in gas formation which severely limits further heat deposition and conduction as well as visualization of the lesion under certain imaging modalities (i.e., ultrasound). The ideal ablation results in a slow, gradual and uniform tissue temperature increase to at least 60°C. Once this is achieved, further energy deposition and temperature increase to 100°C will not limit the ablation zone and therefore can be performed. However, a fast temperature increase to 100°C within minutes will almost certainly result in inadequate ablation.

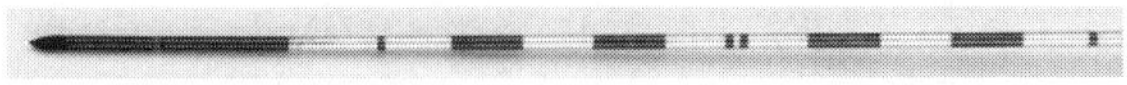

Figure 6.6 The Vivant Medical microwave ablation probe has a 14-gauge (4.4 mm) diameter shaft. Under ideal circumstances it can result in a maximum effective ablation of 5.5 cm (long axis) by 2.5 cm (short axis). (Image courtesy of Dr. Damian Dupuy, Brown Medical School.)

recently been acquired by Vally Lab (Colorado). Though the technology is relatively simple and other systems do exist outside the United States, because this ablation technique is newer and safety and efficacy data lag those of others, U.S. Food and Drug Administration (FDA) approval also lags. The generator produces a power output of up to 60W at frequencies between 900 MHz and 2.45 GHz. The antenna is a 14g single tipped probe [2] (Figures 6.6 and 6.7). The ablation zone depends on power, target organ, and duration of ablation. For example, an oval ablation zone was observed in the liver with a long axis of 5.5 cm, whereas the same settings resulted in a 4-cm-long axis ablation zone in the lung (45W for 10 minutes) [2]. For larger lesions one can use more than one probe inserted in parallel (cluster) to ensure complete coverage of the target lesion. The same study confirmed another advantage of microwave ablation versus RFA; that is, it is less susceptible to heat sink. Heat sink refers to inadequate ablation as a result of tumor cooling by the

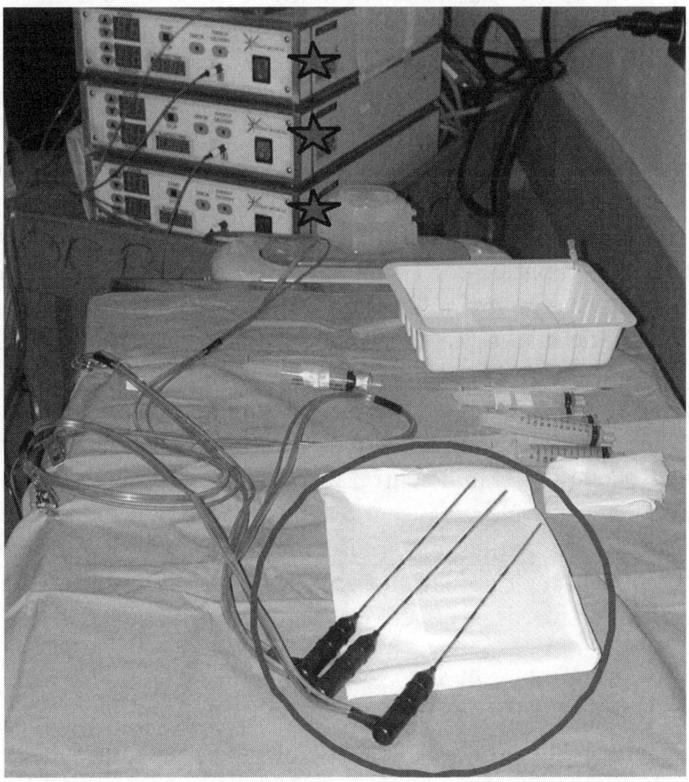

Figure 6.7 Equipment setup for the Vivant Medical microwave ablation system. The power generators are shown stacked in the background. One can use as many probes as desired in order to effectively ablate the entire tumor. (Image courtesy of Dr. Damian Dupuy, Brown Medical School.)

flowing blood in a nearby vessel. Because RFA depends on tissue thermal conductivity for adequate ablation, tumors near vessels larger than 3 mm may not be ablated completely. Another system (not available in the United States) is the Microtaze (Alfresa, Osaka, Japan) 2.45-GHz microwave generator. It uses a 1.6-mm diameter, 25-cm-long, brass probe coated with silver/gold that is MR compatible. In vivo studies have documented oval necrosis of 3 × 2 cm at 60W for 60 seconds [1]. However, studies support using more than one probe if the lesion size is greater than 2 cm because of the uncertainty of the probe location [7]. Alternatively, circular probes that have a larger ablation zone can be used [8]. In soft tissue, 63% of the energy is deposited within a radius of 8 mm from the probe, whereas 95% of the energy is deposited at 12 mm [9]. This means that the effective direct ablation radius is up to 2.5 mm with additional ablation, dependent on temperature conduction. Because microwave ablation technology is newer than RFA, long-term studies are limited as is the availability of ablation systems. However, the advantages described above are likely to push microwave technology more into clinical use.

6.4 Clinical Applications

6.4.1 Liver Cancer

Hepatocellular carcinoma (HCC) is the most common solid (nonskin) malignancy in the world mainly due to hepatitis C (in the West) and hepatitis B (in the East). The vast majority of patients is unresectable at presentation (75% to 85%) and is left only with nonsurgical options. Chemotherapy has traditionally been ineffective in treating HCC. Even with the recent approval of Sorafenib, the most effective systemic chemotherapy drug for HCC thus far, survival is only improved by approximately 12 weeks [10]. Therefore ablative techniques are quite important palliative treatment options. In addition, studies have shown that ablation of liver HCC 3 cm or less results in similar survival rates compared to surgery. The efficacy of microwave ablation for HCC has been established; however, large, prospective comparison studies are lacking [11, 12].

Metastatic disease to the liver (i.e., colon cancer, breast cancer) presents a unique clinical challenge. Studies have shown that in the case of colon and breast cancer resection of a limited number of metastases may improve survival. However, repeat liver resections may not be possible in cases of limited liver function reserve or when the lesion is in a central location. Percutaneous ablation for such lesions is especially attractive because it results in much less collateral liver injury, is much less invasive, the patient has a faster recovery period, and may be repeated more often. The efficacy of ablation depends on lesion size and location, not on tumor type, and therefore is as effective as for HCC (Figure 6.8).

6.4.2 Lung Cancer

Lung cancer is the number-one cause of cancer mortality in the United States with about 220,000 new cases per year in 2006. More than 90% of cancer patients are current or ex-smokers, and emphysema complicates the course of treatment. For many patients with advanced emphysema, surgery or anesthesia is not an option,

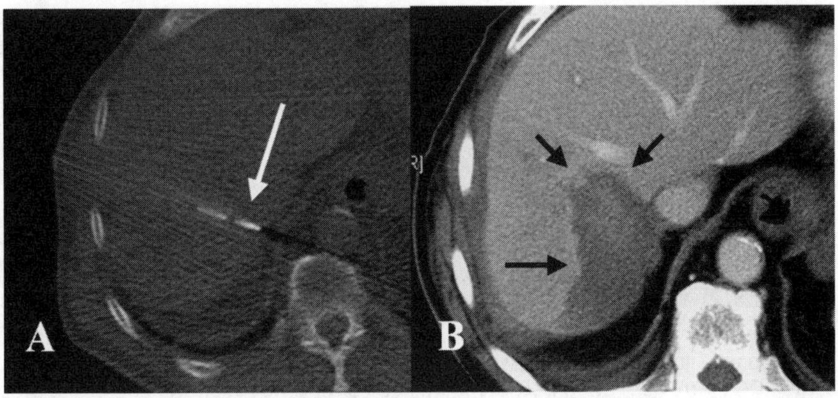

Figure 6.8 CT-guided, percutaneous microwave ablation for colon cancer metastasis to the liver. Intraprocedure CT image (A) shows the microwave probe with its tip (arrow) in segment 7 of the liver. The tumor is not visible because of the lack of intravenous contrast administration. Axial, contrast enhanced CT image immediately post ablation (B) shows the extent of the ablation zone (arrows) demarcated by the lack of contrast enhancement. (Image courtesy of Dr. Damian Dupuy, Brown Medical School.)

and thus minimally invasive treatments are especially important. Percutaneous ablation of lesions 4 cm or less (Figure 6.9) has been shown to be quite effective, though again prospective randomized trials have not yet been published. Microwave ablation is reportedly less painful than RFA. This is a significant advantage for lung cancer patients, many of whom cannot tolerate general anesthesia.

6.4.3 Kidney Cancer

Renal cell cancer (RCCa) has dramatically increased in incidence during the past decade. This is mainly due to the liberal use of CT, which allows for the detection

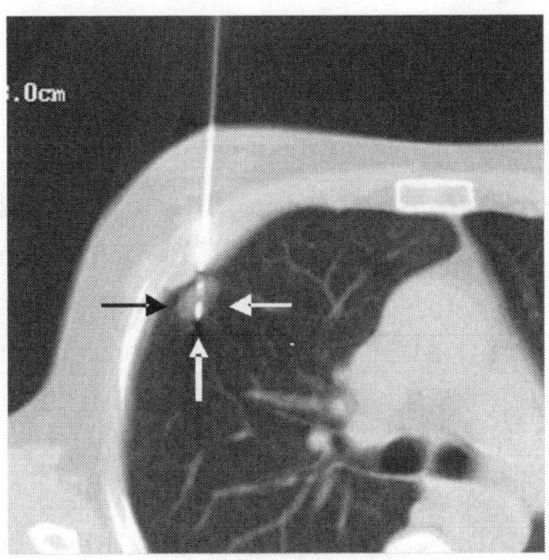

Figure 6.9 CT-guided, percutaneous microwave ablation for primary nonsmall cell lung cancer. The 1.5-cm lesion is outlined by arrows and surrounds the tip of the microwave ablation probe. Such minimally invasive procedures allow the treatment of tumors on an outpatient basis and are shorter, safer, and less expensive than traditional surgery. (Image courtesy of Dr. Damian Dupuy, Brown Medical School.)

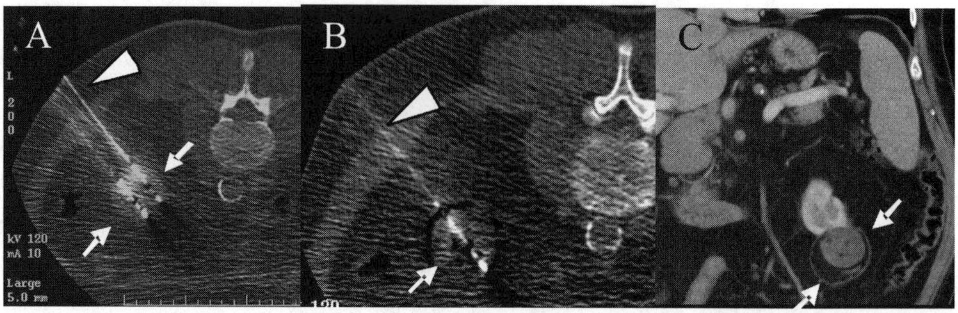

Figure 6.10 CT-guided, percutaneous microwave ablation for renal cell carcinoma (RCCa). Intraprocedure CT image (A) shows two probes (arrowhead) placed in parallel with their active tips within the RCCa (arrows). Intraprocedure image at a later time (B) shows one of the probes (arrowhead) in the tumor and a thin rim of gas surrounding the tumor (arrow) indicative of high temperature achieved. Coronal reconstructed, contrast enhanced CT image 2 years after ablation (C) shows the lesion as a nonvascularized (dead) region surrounded by the ablation rim (arrows) representing the extent of the ablation. (Image courtesy of Dr. Damian Dupuy, Brown Medical School.)

of asymptomatic renal masses. Because most of these masses are detected incidentally (while the patient is being worked up for something else), they are small and amenable to percutaneous treatment. Percutaneous treatments such as microwave ablation, RFA, and cryo-ablation are becoming very popular treatment options for these patients. They obviate the need for surgery, have a faster recovery rate and fewer complications, and are less expensive. Additionally they offer an alternative to patients who because of comorbid conditions are not surgical candidates. One of the risks associated with kidney ablations is hemorrhage, as the kidney is a very vascular organ. Cryo-ablation, though painless, has a higher risk for hemorrhage compared to RFA or microwave ablation because the latter two coagulate any damaged vessels. Microwave ablation is better tolerated than RFA and requires less frequent use of general anesthesia (Figure 6.10). It may therefore become a better alternative than RFA for treating RCCa.

6.5 Discussion

Image-guided, percutaneous tumor ablation is becoming an increasingly popular treatment option for cancer patients. Of all the ablation modalities, heat ablation is by far the most commonly used one. Owing to longer experience and older technology, radiofrequency ablation use is more widespread than microwave ablation. However, recent reports have indicated certain advantages for microwave ablation over RFA. They include a larger ablation zone, less susceptibility to heat sink effect, less pain, and faster ablation. If these advantages are born out in further clinical studies, microwave ablation will likely become a very important solid tumor treatment modality. In designing future ablation techniques one has to consider certain variables. First, the probe design must be such that it is easy to use (thin to limit injury and rigid for better guidance). It must also be visible under the imaging methods used for guidance. Equally important, probes should be compatible with magnetic resonance (MR) imaging guidance. Ultrasound guidance is more versatile than the others (CT or MR). The operator controls both the ultrasound probe and the microwave ablation probe. This provides real-time, continuous imaging feedback to the operator who can adjust either or both of the probes to approach the tumor in a safe and effective way. On the other hand, ultrasound suffers from lower image resolution and tissue characterization compared to CT and MR. In addition, once the ablation starts and microtubules form as a result of temperature increase, ultrasound loses its ability to penetrate beyond these microtubules resulting in loss of detail along the distant part of the ablation zone. CT guidance has better tissue discrimination and resolution; however, because of radiation concerns, continuous imaging is not feasible. Therefore the operator obtains one cross-sectional image at regular intervals and adjusts the ablation probe accordingly. MR offers both advantages (i.e., it provides effective and continuous image guidance without exposing personnel to ionizing radiation). However, both the probe and the power supply cable must be designed in such a way as to allow operation in a high magnetic field environment, which is not currently feasible.

Other design ideas that can be very useful for physicians performing image-guided percutaneous ablations include coupling the probe to the imaging modality, providing real-time tissue temperature maps and designing robotic probe guidance. What is certain is that thermal ablations of solid tumors will continue to expand in scope and frequency of use, and that ablation technology needs to catch up with associated imaging modalities and clinical requirements.

References

[1] Kurumi, Y., et al., "MR-Guided Microwave Ablation for Malignancies," *Int. J. Clin. Oncol.*, Vol. 12, 2007, pp. 85–93.

[2] Simon, C. J., D. E. Dupuy, and W. W. Mayo-Smith, "Microwave Ablation: Principles and Application," *RadioGraphics*, Vol. 25, 2005, pp. S69–S83.

[3] Nikfarjam, M., V. Muralidharan, and C. Christophi, "Mechanisms of Focal Heat Destruction of Liver Tumors," *Journal of Surgical Research*, Vol. 127, 2005, pp. 208–223.

[4] Simon, C. J., et al., "Intraoperative Triple Antenna Hepatic Microwave Ablation," *AJR*, Vol. 187, 2006, pp. W333–W340.

[5] Mantero, S., et al. "Hyperthermia in the Treatment of Cholangiocarcinoma: Development and Testing of an Endobiliary Microwave Device," *Cardiovasc. Intervent. Radiol.*, Vol. 26, No. 4, 2003, pp. 379–385.

[6] Meredith, K., et al., "Microwave Ablation of Hepatic Tumors Using Dual-Loop Probes: Results of a Phase I Clinical Trial," *J. Gastrointest. Surg.*, Vol. 9, 2005, pp. 1354–1360.

[7] Izzo, F., "New Approaches to the Treatment of Hepatic Malignancies Other Thermal Ablation Techniques: Microwave and Interstitial Laser Ablation of Liver Tumors," *Annals of Surgical Oncology*, Vol. 10, No. 5, 2003, pp. 491–497.

[8] Yu, N. C., et al., "Hepatocellular Carcinoma: Microwave Ablation with Multiple Straight and Loop Antenna Clusters—Pilot Comparison with Pathologic Findings," *Radiology*, Vol. 239, No. 1, 2003, pp. 269–275.

[9] Tabushe, K., "Basic Knowledge of a Microwave Tissue Coagulator and Its Clinical Applications," *J. Hep. Bil. Pancr. Surg.*, Vol. 5, 1998, pp. 165–172.

[10] Llovet, J. M., et al., "For the SHARP Investigators Study Group Journal of Clinical Oncology. Sorafenib Improves Survival in Advanced Hepatocellular Carcinoma (HCC): Results

of a Phase III Randomized Placebo-Controlled Trial (SHARP Trial)," *ASCO Annual Meeting Proceedings, Part I*, Vol. 25, No. 18S (June 20 Supplement), 2007.

[11] Shibata, T., et al., "Small Hepatocellular Carcinoma: Comparison of Radiofrequency Ablation and Percutaneous Microwave Coagulation Therapy," *Radiology*, Vol. 223, 2002, pp. 331–337.

[12] Lu, M. D., et al., "Hepatocellular Carcinoma: US-Guided Percutaneous Microwave Coagulation Therapy," *Radiology*, Vol. 221, 2001, pp. 167–172.

CHAPTER 7

Lasers and Photodynamic Therapy (PDT) in Imaging and Therapy

Keyvan Moghissi and Mark Stringer

Lasers and their use in surgery, photodynamic therapy, and photodiagnosis are relatively recent advances, despite the fact that the underlying principles of each have been under investigation for almost a century. Clinical exploitation of these practices was initiated in the 1960s but only gathered real momentum some 10 years later following the introduction of reliable, commercially available laser technology [1–4]. Parallel clinical and research efforts have subsequently resulted in a wide range of applications, described extensively in a substantial number of publications across diverse areas of science and medicine. The greatest impact of laser surgery and photodynamic therapy (PDT) has been, and continues to be, in oncology. In this chapter we review laser surgery, PDT, and photodiagnosis within the general theme of image-guided therapy. In this context, it is important to note that the term "laser surgery" is used throughout the chapter to describe a procedure in which lasers are used in interventions with therapeutic intention. The term is employed because controlled laser radiation can incise, excise, ablate, eradicate, and repair, all of which are attributes of "surgery/surgical intervention."

The chapter is divided into two major parts, describing lasers and photodynamic processes, respectively. Each part is subdivided in order to cover principles, methods, and major indications in the context of imaging and therapy. The description of PDT also encompasses the principles of photodiagnosis based specifically upon fluorescence imaging, which includes both autofluorescence (AF) detection and drug-enhanced fluorescence (photodynamic) diagnosis.

7.1 Lasers

7.1.1 Definitions

The term LASER is an acronym for light amplification by stimulated emission of radiation. This is a description of the physical process whereby a specific type of light energy is produced, though the term is now more generally applied to the device itself. Although a multiplicity of different lasers have been developed that can operate across a broad range of the electromagnetic spectrum, it is only those emitting radiation in the ultraviolet, visible, and infrared spectral regions that have found direct clinical applications. Therefore, laser light is not expected to cause genetic modification which might induce malignancy.

A laser consists of a material with suitable optical properties (the gain medium) that is located within a highly reflective optical resonant cavity. The gain medium, which may be in gaseous, liquid, or solid form depending upon the type of laser, is supplied with energy, most often from an electrical or an optical source. This is a process known as pumping. By pumping at an appropriate rate, a large fraction of the atoms or molecules that make up the gain medium are temporally promoted into energetic states. One way that equilibrium can be restored to this type of system is in the release of energy by *spontaneous* emission. This occurs in all directions, but since the optical resonant cavity (in its simplest arrangement) consists of two mirrors aligned longitudinally on either side of the gain medium, it is only the light traveling along this axis that is reflected back into the medium to release energy as *stimulated* emission. What follows is a cascade process where the stimulated emission continues to be reflected back and forth, each time passing through the gain medium, thereby becoming amplified. One of the two mirrors that form the resonant cavity (the output coupler) is partially transparent, allowing the laser beam to propagate beyond the confines of the cavity.

7.1.2 The Characteristics of Laser Light

The gain medium, method and rate of pumping, and design of resonant cavity, all have an influence upon the precise properties of the resultant laser beam. Also, many lasers contain additional elements that affect properties such as the wavelength and the shape of the beam. There are, however, three fundamental characteristics that define how a laser beam differs from other light sources:

1. The beam is *monochromatic*, which denotes that the laser emission comprises a single output wavelength.
2. The output is *collimated* so that the radiation propagates in a narrowly confined beam, with a low divergence.
3. The laser radiation is *coherent*, which defines a close phase relationship between all components of the emitted beam.

Some types of gain medium are able to sustain continuous laser emission. These provide a continuous wave (CW) output, with the output power controllable by means of variation of the pumping power. However, many types of laser can only emit radiation in the form of pulses. Depending upon laser type, these pulses may have a duration ranging from milliseconds (10^{-3}s) to femtoseconds (10^{-15}s). One of the results of generating a laser pulse with even only moderate energy content is that the *peak* power of the pulse can be very high. Indeed, ultra-fast pulses are associated with enormous peak powers, far beyond what can be achieved with any other type of light source. Also, when it is considered that the beam can be focused to a very small spot size (diameters of microns are routine), the associated power density is such as to have significant effects upon the interaction with the target material.

7.1.3 The Laser-Tissue Interaction

The interaction between an incident laser beam and human tissue is very complex and depends not just on the laser parameters but also upon the tissue type, its degree of blood perfusion (and blood oxygenation), as well as the nature of tissue abnormality. The consequences of the interaction may be separated into those that are therapeutic and those that are diagnostic. The former may be defined in terms of the changes which occur in structure and composition of tissue, whereas the latter generally involve no permanent effect upon the tissue but induces an optical response that can be used as a signature of disease. It is important to note that tissue comprises a complex mixture of heterogeneously distributed cellular-related molecules as well as structured ground substance. The two mechanisms which ultimately determine the effects of laser-tissue interaction are absorption and scattering, the latter including surface reflection. Both properties play important roles in determining the type and severity of tissue manifestations and structural injuries (lesions).

The light absorption of a particular tissue depends upon the relative concentrations of different molecules, each with a characteristic absorption spectrum. For example, although water is transparent across the visible range, it is highly absorbing in sections of the ultraviolet and infrared bands. Therefore, for laser wavelengths in these regions, penetration is limited to depths of significantly less than 1 mm. Reduced absorption in the visible and near-infrared wavelengths allows deeper light penetration into tissue, with an interaction depth up to several millimeters. However, the presence of blood has a major effect upon the penetration of blue and green wavelengths, as a consequence of the strong absorption properties of hemoglobin. Similarly the concentration of melanin in skin dictates penetration across the entire visible spectrum. Scattering is most commonly an elastic interaction, in which only the direction of light propagation is changed. The spatial distribution and intensity of scattered light depends upon the size and shape of the scattering particles. Multiple scattering events each impose a change of direction and the light distribution is rapidly diffused, with a loss of laser coherence. Even for laser wavelengths where absorption in tissue is low, scattering is effective in limiting the depth of light penetration, and in defining the radial distribution of the optical energy at the tissue surface. Therefore the chemical composition and physical (and hence optical) properties of each component of tissue influence the anatomical and physiopathological manifestations when exposed to specific laser radiation.

Both absorption and scattering play important roles in determining the type and severity of tissue manifestations and structural injuries (lesions). The laser wavelength determines the radial distribution of the optical energy at the tissue surface and the depth of light penetration. Ultraviolet and far-infrared wavelengths are unable to penetrate tissue effectively, limiting the interaction to depths of less than 1 mm. On the other hand, radiation in the visible and near-infrared range penetrates better into tissue, due to reduced absorption, with an interaction depth of several millimeters in the near-infrared (IR).

Besides the wavelength, a number of other factors related to the laser light are operational in determining the tissue response, the most important of which are:

- Power, expressed in units of watts (W). This may be the average power, which is the energy delivered every second, or the peak power, which is the energy in an individual pulse divided by the pulse duration ($E/\delta t$).
- Irradiance (fluence-rate, or power density), expressed in terms of W/cm^{-2}.
- Radiant exposure (fluence, or energy-density), expressed as $Joules/cm^2$.

When performing laser surgery in clinical practice, an understanding of the specific laser/tissue interaction, combined with the knowledge of anatomo-physiological consequences of such an interaction, is essential. However, the number of variables involved, including different types of tissues and their associated optical properties, often prevents a full theoretical analysis, and empirical evidence is often the basis of progress.

7.1.4 Types of Lasers

Lasers are named after the material that forms the gain medium. Many solid crystalline materials, semiconductors, liquids, gases, as well as electrons in a vacuum, have been employed to provide laser output over a wide wavelength range from X-rays to the far infrared band. Although many types of laser emit at only one wavelength (NdYAG = 1,064 nm, Ruby = 694 nm) or in a discrete set of lines (Argon ion = 6 lines from 457.9 nm to 514.5 nm, CuVapour = 511, 578 nm), dye lasers employ the broad fluorescence emission band from an organic dye compound to allow tunability over a range defined by the specific dye. Also, in addition to the availability of the fundamental output wavelength, efficient nonlinear electro-optical techniques such as frequency-doubling and tripling extend the range of coherent output to shorter wavelengths. Considering the range of output parameters available, current laser technology offers a variety of capabilities. Only relatively few lasers, however, have ever reached the corridors of clinics and even fewer have passed the threshold of an operating theater to become a routinely adopted clinical tool because of lack of knowledge of their usefulness in connection with indications and absence of trials in clinical settings. The lasers used in clinical practice generally fall into two groups, as described next.

7.1.4.1 Thermal Lasers

This group comprises devices which radiate in specific sections of the visible spectrum (generally at wavelengths shorter than 600 nm) and in the infrared. Examples include:

- Pulsed dye laser: operating around 590 nm, used for the treatment of port-wine stains;
- Carbon dioxide (CO_2) laser: wavelength 10,600 nm;
- Neodymium Yttrium Aluminium Garnet (NdYAG) laser: wavelength 1,060 nm.

The latter two examples have been extensively used in laser surgery. In addition, a number of semiconductor diode lasers, which operate within the range of near infrared wavelengths, have more recently been introduced for clinical work. These offer turn-key operation (with no complex setup, alignment, and calibration procedures involved) in a compact package that is specifically designed for clinical use. Infrared medical systems usually include a low-power red aiming laser beam allowing precise delivery of the (invisible) therapeutic laser beam.

7.1.4.2 Nonthermal Lasers

In this group the interaction between laser light and tissue is not generally mediated through the generation of heat but via changes in cell metabolism and tissue composition. An example is the use of lasers that emit light in the red part of the spectrum that are effective at inducing the photophysical and photochemical processes that form the basis of PDT.

7.1.5 Anatomo-Pathological Features of the Laser-Tissue Interaction (Tissue Injuries)

For infrared lasers the light-tissue interaction is expressed macroscopically as thermal injuries of different severity depending on the radiant exposure and the optical properties of target tissue. The least macroscopic manifestation is "shrinkage" of the tissue due to evaporation of the water component of cells and interstitial ground substance. Under high radiant exposure, water evaporation leads to serious injury and cell death when charring takes place. At a yet higher level of exposure, complete evaporation of tissue ensues. The latter event results in loss of tissue equivalent to surgical incision and/or ablation as a visible (macroscopic) effect. (See Figure 7.1.)

Microscopically, changes from the focal point of the laser beam outwards are: complete loss of tissue substance, complete coagulation necrosis (death of cells by the thermal energy), and various degrees of severely injured and dying cells and then normal cellular structure. In the case of CO_2 lasers these changes are superficial and limited in extent, whereas for NdYAG lasers the changes are deep and more extensive.

Ex vivo experiments on animal tissue/organs as well as in vivo studies on human tissue/organs at operation have permitted the establishment of correlation between

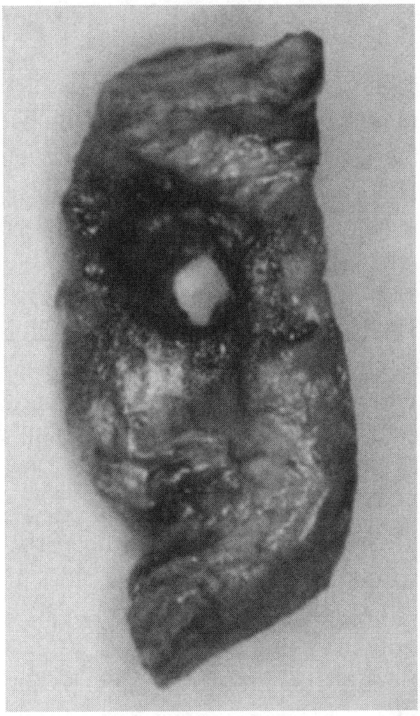

Figure 7.1 Pulmonary tissue (ex vivo) exposed to NdYAG laser radiation (radiant exposure 50 to 60 j/cm^2). Note: complete evaporation of the parenchyma at the center of the impact with charring around.

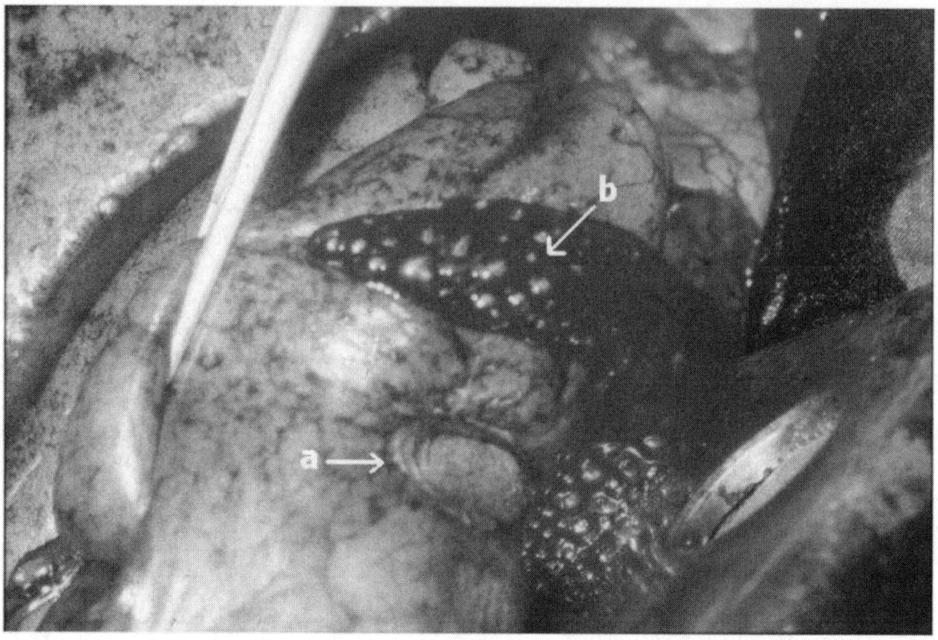

Figure 7.2 This shows ventilating lung at operation. (a) A short incision made by noncontact mode of NdYAG laser. There is no bleeding or any air leak from pulmonary alveoli. (b) A similar incision made by surgical electro-diathermy shows both bleeding as well as a considerable air leak.

radiant exposure and effect in terms of total evaporation, charring, and other pathological effects [5, 6].

In lung tissue (parenchyma), with its very high vasculature, the following observations were made: a high power setting of > 50W with the beam in noncontact mode, delivered at a distance of 0.7 to 2 cm, caused evaporation of tissue and an incision of 2- to 5-mm depth with little or no bleeding or air leak (Figure 7.2). In comparison, an incision made with electro-diathermy operating in coagulation and cutting mode resulted in bleeding and considerable air leak [5].

Ex vivo experiments in which the normal part of a lung excised for cancer and irradiated with NdYAG laser beam of > 50W for 20 seconds showed complete evaporation at the focal center of the beam, which presented as a funnel-shaped crater. (See Figure 7.1.) The surrounding wall of the crater showed charring (burned tissue). On microscopic examination five zones could be identified [Figure 7.3(a–c)]:

1. Normal unaffected lung tissue.
2. A zone of incomplete coagulative necrosis. In this zone there was oedema and distortion of tissue structures.
3. A zone of complete coagulative necrosis.
4. Charring zone.
5. A zone of central evaporation. There was no trace of tissue; all vascular and broncho-alveolar structures had disappeared. The horizontal extent and depth of the crater were proportionate to the power density and radiant exposure.

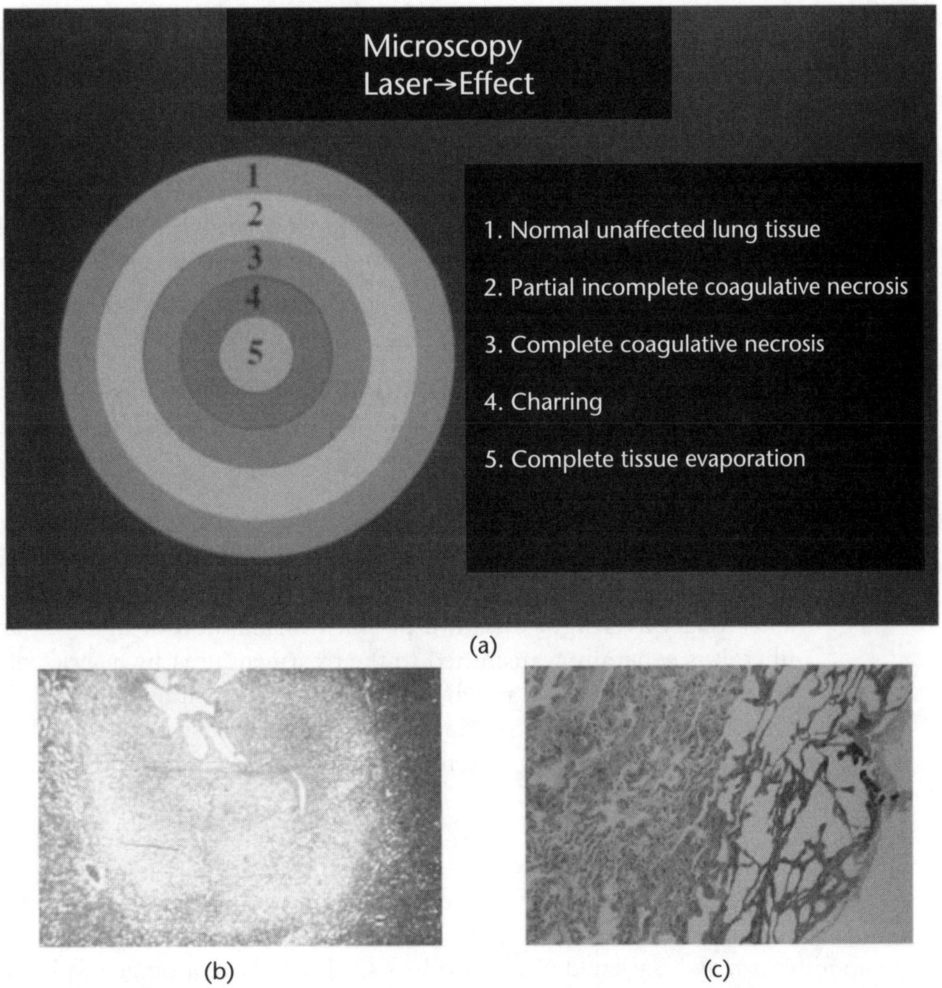

Figure 7.3 (a) Irradiation of lung tissue by high power NdYAG laser showing five zones from the center of impact outwards. (b) At the center there is total evaporation of the tissue surrounded by charring and coagulative necrosis. (c) More externally there is a zone of partial coagulative necrosis followed by normal parenchyma. The extent of total evaporation and partial necrosis relates to the fluence and proximity of the emitting laser fiber to the target.

The thickness of the wall showing dead or seriously injured tissue varied from 2 to 5 cm from the center of the beam focus.

In general, the changes observed in pulmonary tissue can be replicated in other normal and abnormal tissue and may be taken as the basic principles of laser surgery using thermal lasers.

7.1.6 Laser Surgery with Thermal Lasers: What Are the Advantages over Conventional Surgical Methods?

Some of the prominent advantages of the use of thermal lasers for surgical operations are:

- Precision of surgery, when it is important to avoid collateral damage to surrounding normal structure.

- Nontouch technique. This avoids transmission of infective organisms.
- Provision of minimal access (minimally invasive) operations. This is due to the possibility of endoscopic surgical operation.
- Laser incision/ablation is attended by less bleeding than conventional type of surgery due to the hemostatic effect of laser energy.
- Sealing of lymphatic channel (contraction of the lymphatic vessel wall). This is relevant to cancer surgery in particular since the lymphatic channels are the preferred way of propagation of neoplastic (epithelial) cells/carcinoma.

7.1.6.1 The CO_2 Laser

This is a molecular gas laser emitting at 10,600 nm. The beam is usually coupled with a low power red laser aiming beam. In this way the principal beam can be accurately directed to the target.

Important characteristics of this laser are:

- Water displays a large absorption coefficient at the laser output wavelength.
- Many standard clinical units allow a power output of 25W to 40W.
- This long wavelength does not permit transmission of light via an optical fiber. It is generally transmitted to the treatment area by a series of mirrors, contained within tubes and articulated joints. This limits the use of the CO_2 laser in deep body cavities since most of the body systems must be accessed by endoscopic equipment which cannot accommodate this form of beam transmission equipment.

Clinical Indications of the CO_2 Laser

The CO_2 laser is used in a variety of skin conditions and lesions in the more accessible body areas. For example, in dermatology, many tumors and other skin conditions may be ablated or excised by CO_2 laser. Also, a range of plastic surgery and skin resurfacing procedures can be undertaken. Other indications include treatment of mucosal lesions in the mouth and laryngo-pharynx, anal and vulvar intraepithelial neoplasia.

7.1.6.2 The NdYAG Laser

The wavelength of this laser (1,064 nm) lies in the near-infrared part of the spectrum. The standard NdYAG laser is a crystalline material (Yttrium Aluminium Garnet) doped with neodymium ions. Clinical systems are available which can produce 100W or more. The beam can be transmitted through optical fibers to remote sites and through the small biopsy channel of endoscopic equipment. The NdYAG laser thus is an important and invaluable surgical tool.

For the past 25 years, the NdYAG laser has been used in a variety of conditions, either alone [6–12], or in association with other treatment modalities [13–19]. In most clinical settings advantage is taken of one or all the effects of the laser in relation to a given tissue. These are:

- Incision;
- Hemostasis;

- Sealing of small (1-mm diameter) blood vessels or lymphatics;
- Sealing of terminal broncho-alveolar divisions in lung.

Much of the clinical work using the NdYAG laser has involved its endoscopic application, in which the laser has been used to evaporate/eradicate malignant obstructive tumors within the airway or upper/lower gastrointestinal tract [6, 8, 10, 11]. However, the use of this laser in association with conventional surgery has also been reported [6, 16–20].

The most impressive result of the NdYAG laser has been, and continues to be, in connection with its use in relief of malignant bronchial or esophageal obstruction caused by lung and esophageal cancer, respectively. In these, the laser is used either alone or in a multimodal therapy setting [8, 9, 13].

Between 50% and 60% of lung cancer cases are bronchogenic, meaning that the tumor initiates within the bronchial wall and grows in all directions, especially within the bronchial lumen. This would cause increasing obstruction and accompanying symptoms, particularly dyspnoea.

Diagnosis and staging in lung cancer is made using clinical imaging and endoscopic techniques [21, 22].

The indications for the NdYAG laser are in:

1. *Advanced stage disease with major endoluminal bronchial malignant obstruction.* In such conditions there is a collapse of the lung corresponding to the localization of the obstructed bronchial division. This would cause corresponding ventilatory deficiency. The relief of such an obstruction with the use of NdYAG laser is carried out bronchoscopically, under vision, using an appropriate light dose. It is important to focus the red aiming beam on to the tumor and then proceed to lasing the tumor using a high power setting [> 50W] for 4 to 5 seconds; this will cause evaporation of the tumor. [See Figure 7.4(a).] If any bleeding occurs, a lower power setting (15W to 20W) is used to coagulate the blood and achieve homeostasis. The operation is continued until clearance of the lumen is completed. Within 1 to 2 hours of the procedure, the results of the laser application will become evident:

- Subjectively with improved breathing and objectively by increase in ventilatory parameters;
- Radiologically, with expansion of previously collapsed lobe/segments of the lung [Figure 7.4(b, c)];
- Endoscopically, by opening of previously blocked lumen.

2. *Local excision of peripheral lung tumor.* In such cases it is necessary to identify the nature and the topography of the lesion. To this end a variety of imaging and endoscopic techniques are employed. Some of these lesions are within the substance of the lung peripherally, near the inner chest wall and beyond the segmental bronchi. They are, therefore, not amenable either to bronchoscopic visualization sampling or interventional bronchoscopy therapeutic procedures. Some are sampled by CT-guided needle biopsy. A few might be visualized by thoracoscopic examination and biopsy under vision,

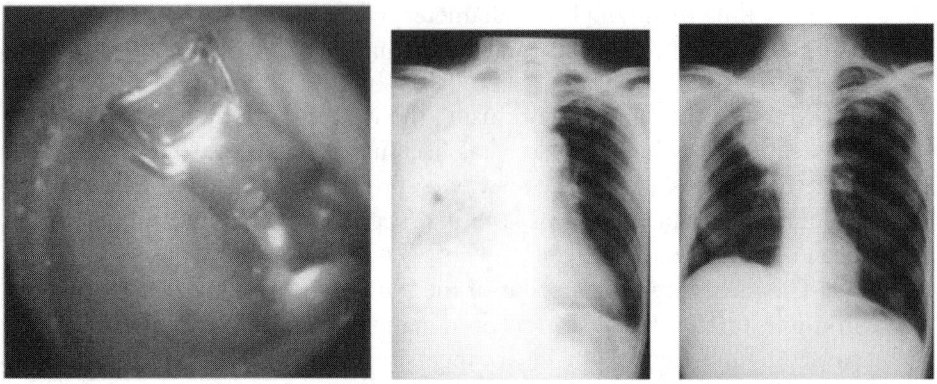

(a) (b) (c)

Figure 7.4 (a) Beam of the laser (NdYAG) coupled with helium-neon laser guiding light focusing at the tumor in the main stem bronchus. (b) Almost complete collapse of the right lung in consequence of the above bronchial obstruction. (c) Following laser treatment a good reexpansion of the previously collapsed lung.

and a small number might have to have standard operation of thoracotomy to access the lesion and carry out biopsy or excision biopsy.

The excision of such a tumor involves exposure of the tumor using conventional methods of surgery. The lesion is then excised employing thermal properties of the laser. This is, in fact, local excision, which permits a parenchyma saving operation to be undertaken. The principle of the procedure was first described in 1980; since then many hundreds of patients have benefited from the method [19].

Fiber Optic Delivery Fibers

Light emitted by many lasers in the visible and near-infrared range of wavelength can be transmitted through flexible optical fibers which have a glass core (diameter 6 to 250 micrometers) which is surrounded by reflecting glass or plastic cladding (10 to 150 micrometers thick). These have greatly expanded the range of indications of lasers. The optical fibers transmit light efficiently with very little loss through the cladding. Both the diameter and type of optical fibers used for delivering the emitted light from the laser to the patient vary according to the wavelength of the laser and whether there is a necessity of a cooling system at the delivery site. This is particularly relevant to infrared lasers (wavelength 1,064 nm) when they have to be used in their noncontact mode, which needs a cooling system (diameter fiber 0.7 mm). Those in which the application is by contact mode—for example, D60 (manufactured by Diomed Ltd., United Kingdom) with its wavelength within the near-infrared wavelength in the region of 900 nm—use a fiber with a diameter of 600 μm.

The optical fiber used in connection with the laser application in photodynamic therapy, exemplified by the D630—wavelength 630 nm (Diomed Ltd., United Kingdom)—has a larger diameter of 1.7 mm.

Applicators

In laser surgery, the delivery of light to the target tissue or organ needs an appropriate *applicator* which accommodates the light delivery device of the laser system.

The applicator should be compatible with the requirement of the anatomical site and adaptable to the needs of the operation and the operator. As such, the design of the applicator for the ultimate destination of the light to the anatomical site should have input by the user/practitioner.

Thoracoscopic Laser Surgery

With the emergence of video-assisted thoracoscopic surgery, thermal lasers (both CO_2 and NdYAG) have been used in pleural and pulmonary peripheral (subpleural) lesions. The method consists of:

- The use of standard minimally invasive thoracoscopic surgical instrumentation (akin to laparoscopic surgery) which provides access to visual examination of the thoracic cavity projected on to a monitor and recorded via a video system. This is referred to as video assisted thoracoscopic surgery (VATS).
- Identification of the lesion over the surface of the lung or within the thoracic (pleural) cavity.
- Introduction of the laser fiber through the biopsy channel of the device followed by laser radiation of the lesion visualized on the monitor.

Video-thoracoscopic laser surgery has been used in cases of emphysematous bullae and pneumothorax. In the former the bulla shrinks when radiated by a thermal laser. In the latter a small air leak from a periphery of the lung can be sealed and laser abrasion of the parietal pleural can be accomplished to promote pleurodesis, which is the object of the operation [17, 20].

7.2 The Photodynamic Processes

7.2.1 Photodiagnosis/Fluorescence Imaging

7.2.1.1 Introduction

Cyto/histology is the gold standard of pathological diagnosis, and clinicians rely on a number of methods to localize and sample (biopsy) a lesion such as a tumor for histo-pathological examination. Localization is also important in treatment using *interventional procedures*. Clinicians deploy a variety of methods in localization of a lesion including visualization and the use of imaging techniques such as radiology (in its broad sense to encompass computed tomography and positron emission tomography scan). The advent of fiber optics and, in particular, the development of fiber optic endoscopy for the past 40 to 50 years has expanded the field of visual examination to include inspection of remote areas within the interior of hollow organs and body cavities and has greatly assisted localization and sampling of suspected abnormalities. Furthermore, endoscopic techniques have allowed the emergence of a whole range of new methods: minimal access/minimally invasive laparoscopic surgery, thoracoscopic and video assisted thoracoscopic surgery, and interventional endoscopy, which are now routinely practiced in every clinic throughout the world.

In the case of cancer, the detection/diagnosis of the lesion at its early stage of development is of crucial importance since treatment at this stage is generally attended by long-term complete response and cure of the disease [23, 24]. It is well known, however, that detection of early stage (superficial) cancer using standard imaging techniques and/or endoscopic devices with the use of white light is difficult and often unrewarding in the presence of occult cancers. This is because of the low discriminative power of these techniques to distinguish between normal and slightly abnormal tissue. In contrast, spectroscopic and fluorescence imaging provides a better visual expression of early lesions (voir infra under Sections 7.2.1.2 through 7.2.1.4).

7.2.1.2 Principle

Fluorescence refers to the reemission of optical radiation, following the absorption of light energy. In molecular systems, the fluorescence consists of an emission band at lower energies (longer wavelengths) than that of the excitation wavelength (the absorbed light). The difference in tissue optical properties is related to the differences in both tissue architecture and chemical compositions. In the UV and visible part of the spectrum the tissue optical properties are largely dominated by endogenous chromophores (light absorbing components) each with their specific chemical composition. Some chromophores are nonfluorescent and solely absorb light (e.g., hemoglobin). Others absorb and emit light with a characteristic fluorescence emission band. In practical terms abnormal tissue displays fluorescence output that is modified compared to that of normal tissue. Although this may often not be directly visually perceptible, image processing methods can define different coloring between normal and abnormal (neoplastic) tissue. Interest in the application of fluorescence techniques goes back to 1924 and the observation of Policard who reported that porphyrins, accumulated in tumor tissue, displayed fluorescent emission when exposed to Wood's light [25]. In the 1940s and 1950s efforts were focused on administration of fluorescent markers to assist in cancer detection. In 1960 Lipson and colleagues reported that hematoporphyrin derivative (HPD) was capable of localizing in malignant tumors and that the exposure of such tumors to an appropriate light could assist in their detection [26, 27]. Interestingly, the same authors also treated a case of breast cancer using HPD for photosensitization and subsequent exposure to filtered light from a Xenon arc-lamp, resulting in objective evidence of response [28]. In the 1970s through to the early 1980s most investigators and clinicians were focused on the introduction to clinical practice of diagnostic fluorescence imaging based on photosensitization of the target followed by the exposure of the presensitized tissue to the light (usually laser) of an appropriate wavelength; the principle derived from this is introduced by Lipson et al. [28–31].

In 1991 Hung and colleagues reported the use of autofluorescence methods in normal and malignant bronchial lesions [32]. Later, Lam and colleagues were involved in the development and clinical use of the first generation of "Xillix" Laser Induced Fluorescence Endoscopy (LIFE) for bronchoscopic fluorescence imaging [33]. The method has proved effective for localization of early neoplastic lesions. Currently, there are two methods of fluorescence imaging in clinical practice, as described next.

7.2.1.3 Autofluorescence Technique

This method uses the principle outlined above, based on displaying differential fluorescence emission between normal and abnormal diseased tissue, on exposure to a blue light. Autofluorescence has found its greatest use in conjunction with bronchoscopy (visual examination of the tracheo-bronchial tree). Also, the method is now being investigated in the upper and lower gastro-intestinal tract for detection of mucosal abnormalities.

Autofluorescence bronchoscopy (AFB) has become a routine method of investigation. In many countries it is carried out by the respiratory physician and surgeon, together with its counterpart white light bronchoscopy (WLB). Its major indications are:

- Localization/detection of pre- and early neoplastic lesions of central type (endobronchial) lung cancer. Its sensitivity in detecting/localizing intraepithelial mucosal neoplasia is four to five times greater than WLB [33]. (See Figure 7.5.)
- Guidance to sampling. AFB is particularly useful in occult (central) lung cancer when the cytology of sputum may show malignant cells but radiology of the chest (CT scan) and even WLB appear completely normal.
- Detection of multifocal lesions.
- Delineation of the extent of the lesion, which assists the surgeon to carry out complete surgical resection, minimizing the rate of neoplastic infiltration of at the margin of the resection.
- Guidance to interventional procedures in early stage cancer. This is particularly relevant to treatment of early lung cancer with PDT (see Section 2.2).
- Monitoring efficacy of interventional bronchoscopy method.

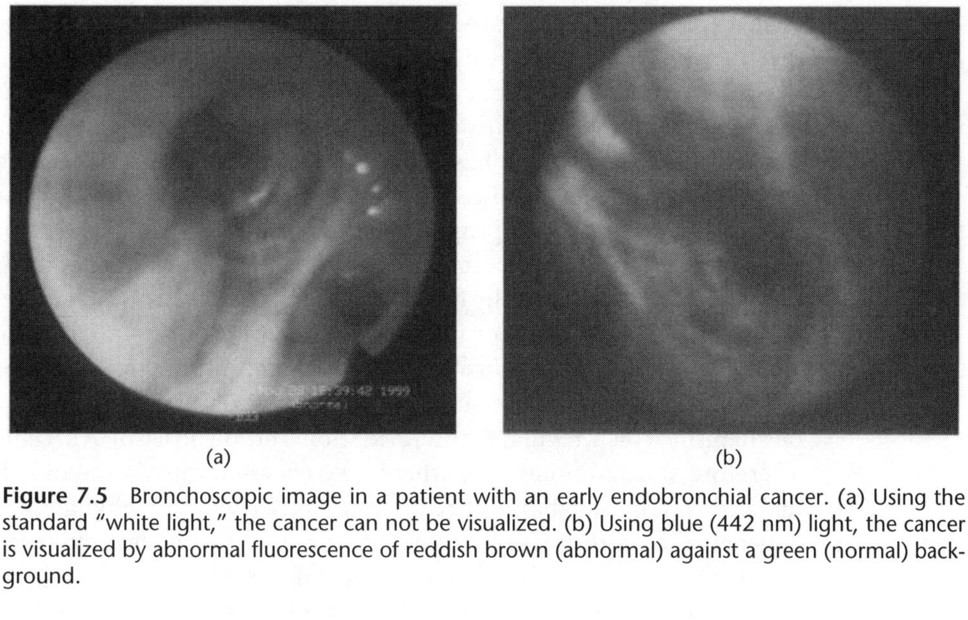

(a) (b)

Figure 7.5 Bronchoscopic image in a patient with an early endobronchial cancer. (a) Using the standard "white light," the cancer can not be visualized. (b) Using blue (442 nm) light, the cancer is visualized by abnormal fluorescence of reddish brown (abnormal) against a green (normal) background.

- Bronchoscopic post-operative surveillance of patients who had resectional surgery for lung cancer to diagnose tumor recurrence at its early stage or to detect metachronous/synchronous lesions.

7.2.1.4 Drug Induced Fluorescence Imaging (DIF)

This method is based on selective presensitization of malignant tissue followed by appropriate illumination. Essentially, this involves loading tissue with a fluorescent marker in such a way that only the clinical target contains a sufficient quantity of marker, so that it may be identified by absorption of light and reemission at longer wavelengths. The concept of drug induced tumor detection was conceived over 50 years ago and its progressive development has been continued by a number of researchers, clinicians, and scientists [25–31, 34]. In bronchogenic cancer the method was initially investigated and practiced for detection and guided bronchoscopic PDT of early stage lung cancer by a number of authors in Europe, the United States and Japan with the use of systemic photosensitizer [29–31, 35]. Later, topical sensitization was introduced using 5-aminoluvulinic acid to generate the fluorescence image [35, 36].

In comparison with autofluorescence, induced fluorescence can exhibit a stronger contrast and, therefore, could have a higher sensitivity with less false-positive results (i.e., discrepancy between positive fluorescence and negative cyto/histology for malignancies). However, the method is dependant on prephotosensitization, and hence localization of the drug in the target tissue. This, in practice, presents with a number of practical problems, the most important of which are:

- The difficulty of presensitization of some tissues such as bronchial mucosa other than by systemic administration of the drug;
- Systemic presensitization leads to prolonged residual photosensitization of normal tissue (particularly skin) after the drug is administered intravenously. Whilst patients will accept the inconvenience of restrictions for therapy, neither they nor medical ethical principles permit the use of a systemic photosensitizer for diagnosis alone. It follows that, currently, presensitization for DIF can be undertaken with the use of drugs, which could be administered topically. The drug which has been in use in recent years is the "pro-drug" 5-Aminoluvulinic acid (ALA) and its derivatives. This, like its predecessor HPD, has a double edged property of presensitizing for DIF and also presensitization for PDT [35–37]. It is relevant to note that ALA is not itself a photosensitizer but is a naturally occurring (endogenous) chemical synthesized in the cell, which is a precursor to the formation of proto-porphyrin IX (PpIX), which, in turn, is the precursor of heme, an important constituent of hemoglobin. In a normal stable situation there exists a feedback on the control mechanism which regulates the formation and disposal of ALA and PpIX. Therefore, in conditions where there is no excess accumulation of heme, normal cells retain the ability of regulating PpIX level. In malignant cells there appears to be a decrease in enzymatic activity of the enzyme ferrochelate which participates in the regulation of PpIX level. This would account for excess PpIX in the tumor and the fluorescence when exposed to light.

At the present time ALA-DIF is used clinically in a number of circumstances, but still as clinical research trials:

1. Skin, delineating the boundary of the superficial skin lesions [38];
2. Bladder for detection of superficial bladder tumors [35–37];
3. Brain tumors as guided therapy method [39].

The practical application of DIF involves presensitization using ALA or one of its derivatives [methyl/hexyl ALA]. This is administered topically and after a period of time allowing capture (absorption), to carry out illumination using specific light to exhibit fluorescence. The light used to induce ALA fluorescence is usually at the short wavelength boundary of the visible spectrum (~405 nm).

7.2.2 Photodynamic Therapy

7.2.2.1 Definition and Mechanisms

PDT is a treatment method with three components; a chemical photosensitizer (the drug), a light of an appropriate wavelength, and oxygen. The original principle of PDT was observed in the laboratory of Raab in the early 1900s [40, 41]. In the 1960s the idea was investigated for possible cancer treatment by Lipson and colleagues [28]. It was Dougherty and colleagues, however, who initiated experimental and clinical trials [3, 41–43]. In the presence of oxygen the interaction between the drug and light promotes the release of singlet oxygen and other cytotoxic agents which brings about tissue destruction. The mechanisms involved in PDT include both cellular and vascular components. At the cellular level energy transfer from the activated photosensitizer to molecular oxygen results in the generation of singlet oxygen as well as radicals which have a cytotoxic effect. These affect the cell membrane, mitochondria, and other subcellular structures. Vascular components relate to ischemic effects, resulting from shutdown of host vasculature and neoangiogenesis. The overall result is cell and tissue necrosis.

In clinical practice PDT has been used largely for the treatment of localized cancer and is performed as a two-step procedure. First, the chemical photosensitizer is administered to the patient, either topically or systemically. Such a photosensitizer should have the ability to localize preferentially (but not exclusively) into the cancer (lesion) compared with normal tissue. After an interval of hours or days (depending on the drug used) the presensitized lesion is exposed to light of a specific wavelength. The presence of molecular oxygen, which is available in the living tissue, is, by definition, essential to induce the photodynamic effect.

Clinical PDT originated in the 1960s when Lipson, Blades, and Gray reported the use of hematoporphyrin derivative to treat a patient with breast cancer [28]. In the 1980s a number of investigators began clinical trials in a variety of common cancers notably of the lung, esophagus, skin, and head and neck [4, 44–50]. Worldwide there are now several thousands of patients who have received PDT for cancer. There are also a number of photosensitizers available, several of which have been licensed by the regulatory bodies in the United States, Europe, Japan, and many other countries [51]. Porfimer Sodium (Photofrin Axcan Pharma Inc., Canada) is the most extensively used photosensitizer with approved indications for lung and esophageal cancer. This is used systemically by intravenous administration followed 24 to 72 hours later by illumination with 630-nm laser light. Of the topical photosensitizers 5-Amino-Levulinic acid (pro-drug) is currently the most extensively used photosensitizer in dermatology [52]. At the present time, more compact light sources, using both laser and nonlaser technology, have been developed that make this type of treatment more accessible [53].

7.2.2.2 Special Characteristics of PDT

As a treatment method PDT has many special characteristics, which make its use for cancer treatment attractive.

- It is a target guided and lesion orientated therapy. In fact, surgery apart, PDT is one of the most effective methods of treatment to focus on a lesion with little or no significant collateral injury to normal tissue. This characteristic is derived from:
  - The relative affinity of the photosensitizing drug to concentrate predominantly in the tumor compared with normal tissue (i.e., selective presensitization of the target);
  - Selective absorption of light by the presensitized tissue;
  - The process of illumination involves the delivery of light in such a manner as to provide controlled illumination by the operator of the presensitized target tissue.
- PDT is a minimal invasive procedure. It is usually carried out without the need to resort to conventional surgical technique. In most cases, the illumination is carried out endoscopically.
- PDT is a repeatable method of treatment. This is important since in cases of local recurrence and metachronous cancer it permits preservation of normal tissue.

From the anatomo-pathological perspective PDT produces cell death of the diseased (cancer) tissues and preserves the normal tissue. Total eradication macroscopically and microscopically is interpreted as complete response (CR). Partial response (PR) refers to total or at least 50% of disappearance of the lesion macroscopically but persistence of the tumor on microscopic examination. No response defines continuous growth.

7.2.2.3 Practical Aspects of PDT: Indications and Techniques

PDT is essentially a local treatment method, the application of which requires identification, localization (topography), and the size of the target lesion. The major indication of PDT is in oncology, and selection of patients is based on the standard protocol of workup for cancer to evaluate tumor burden and staging. It is then important to consider which of the treatment options (alone or in combination) would be most suitable for the case. Current consensus on the role of PDT in oncology is that it has a place alone or in conjunction with any or all of the three "standard" cancer therapy methods, which are surgery, radiotherapy, and chemotherapy.

Indications

The indications of PDT in the majority of the common cancers (e.g., lung, esophagus, skin, and head and neck) depend on the stage of the tumor at presentation, with the caveat that PDT is basically a local treatment method.

Two major types of cases qualify for the treatment:

- Locally advanced cancers with bulk, which cause symptoms. PDT in such cases is used for symptom relief and to improve function "locally" as well as to ameliorate performance status generally. In such a case the primary goal is provision of a better quality of life for as long as possible. [See Figure 7.6(a–c).]
- Early stage cancer in which PDT is used for patients who are not eligible for surgical treatment. The principal goal is to achieve survival benefit and long-term CR amounting to cure of the disease. (See Figure 7.7.)

It is important to note that surgical resection is the first choice option for a patient with an early cancer. However, the patient becomes ineligible for surgical option:

- When the operation is not technically feasible;
- If the general condition and the function status are deemed inadequate for the proposed operation;

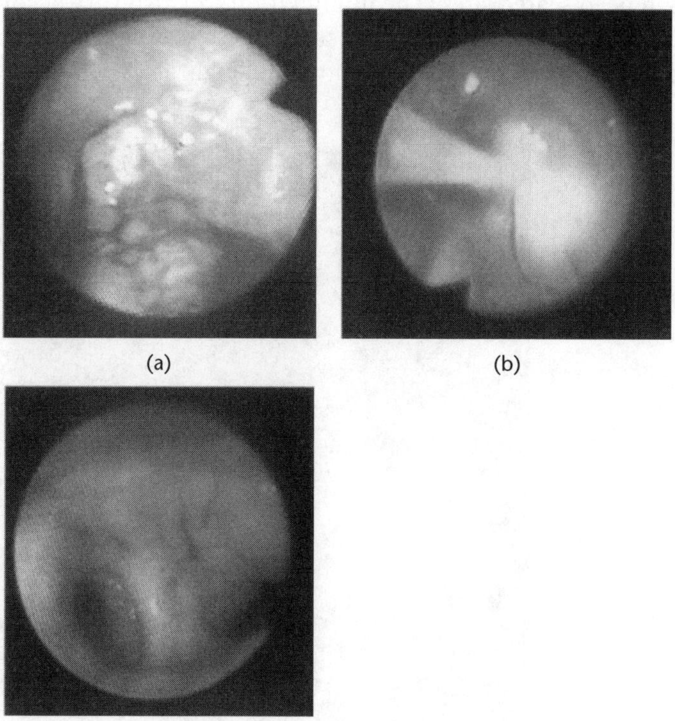

(a) (b) (c)

Figure 7.6 (a) Bronchoscopic view of the left upper lobe bronchus of the lung with a complete blockage by a tumor. (b) Bronchoscopic view of the interstitial illumination (diffuser within the tumor mass). (c) Bronchoscopic view of the same bronchus 1 month following bronchoscopic PDT with Photofrin, showing no evidence of any endoluminal tumor.

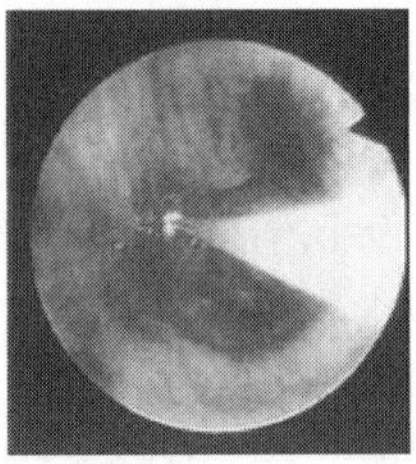

Figure 7.7 This shows endoscopic illumination of an early stage esophageal cancer using the laser optical fiber, which in this case is passed through the biopsy channel of the instrument for the delivery of the laser light.

- When the quality of survival is predicted to be compromised by surgical resection;
- When the patient does not consent to surgery.

PDT Techniques

In locally advanced cases systemic presensitization, with intravenous injection of the drug, is usually required. Illumination is carried out interstitially (intra-tumor), using an appropriate wavelength laser and a suitable fiber optic applicator.

In an early stage type of cancer the presensitization may be performed by topical administration of the drug when the lesion is superficial and involves exposed part of the body such as the skin, mouth, and external genitalia and by systemic route in deep-seated sites. The illumination can also vary according to the practical feasibility of application. In cases such as skin tumors illumination with light emitting diode (LED) array devices is possible (Figure 7.8). In the case of internal organs

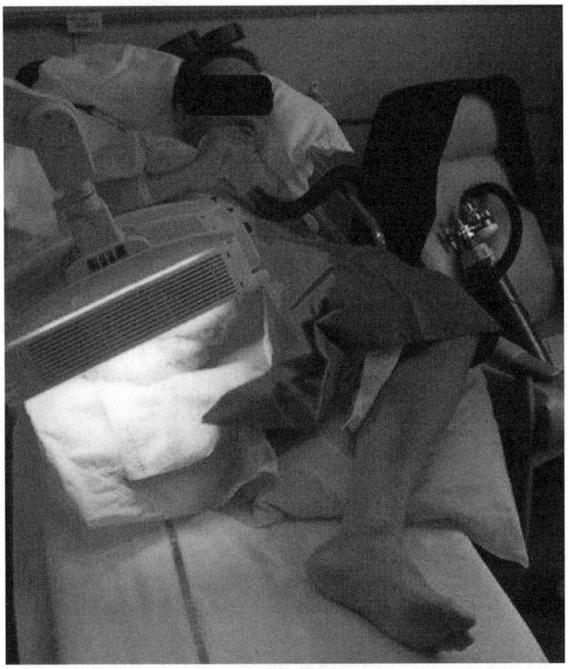

Figure 7.8 Illumination of the skin using LED array. In this case ALA was used for topical photosensitization.

with either advanced or early stage tumor, illumination of the presensitized tissue (tumor) requires laser light and fiber optic delivery systems in order to illuminate the target tissue.

7.2.2.4 Illustration of PDT in Practice

Illustration of Topical—ALA (Amino-Levulinic Acid) PDT

Typical indication for such an application is a flat-type basal cell carcinoma of the skin. The sequence of steps in the procedure is as follows:

- Information to patient and informed consent.
- Diagnosis and delineation of the extent of the lesion. For the latter a fluorescence technique may be used.
- Topical administration of the drug. This is done by applying ALA cream or gel to the lesion, which is kept in position and in darkness via an occlusive dressing for ≥ 4 hours.
- Illumination. This is carried out using either a laser light delivering 100 Jcm^{-2} of the lesion or an LED array designed to deliver an equivalent light dose.
- The patient is discharged 30 to 60 minutes after illumination. Response to treatment is evaluated 3 to 4 weeks and then 3 months later. As a rule such superficial lesions heal completely without scarring after small ulceration following treatment and the long-term result is excellent in 82% of cases showing no recurrence after 1-year follow-up [52].

Illustration of Case of Systemic Photosensitization and Laser Light Illumination

A typical example of this concerns an endo-bronchial lung cancer using Photofrin (Porfimer sodium) as the drug of choice. Photofrin is currently the drug that has a license for lung cancer application from a number of authorities in the world. The sequence of steps in the procedure is as follows:

- Diagnosis/workup including localization and delineation of the lesion using white light and autofluorescence bronchoscopy.
- Information to patient and consent.
- Systemic presensitization using intravenous Photofrin (2 mg/kg/body weight).
- Latent period. This is the time between administration of the drug to illumination, which is 24 to 72 hours.
- Illumination. This is carried out bronchoscopically using 630-nm laser light. The delivery fiber of the light is inserted into the biopsy channel of bronchoscope and illumination is carried out with the cylindrical diffuser end of the optical fiber. In locally advanced cases the diffuser is placed within the tumor, thus providing interstitial therapy [Figure 7.6(b)]. In some cases, such as the one illustrated in Figure 7.9, the lesion was an early cancer and could not be defined with white light instrumentation. Therefore, the illumination was carried out guided by autofluorescence vision (imaging) (Figure 7.9).

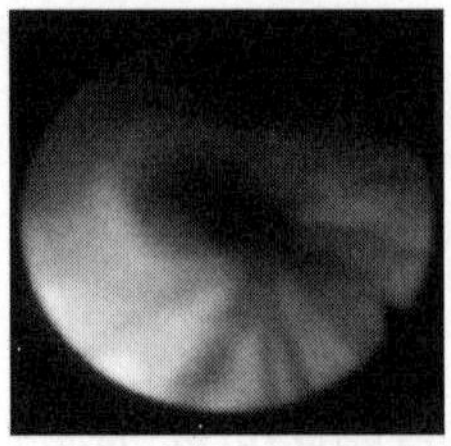

Figure 7.9 This illustrates illumination assisted by fluorescence bronchoscopy to delineate and target the cancer which was not visible by standard white light.

7.3 Conclusion

In this chapter we have given an outline of what lasers are, how the laser light interacts with tissue, and what ensues from such an interaction. The injury sustained by the tissue as a result of its exposure to a laser beam depends on the type of tissue and its structure, and the characteristics of laser emission, in terms of continuous or pulsed output, wavelength, and power.

Notwithstanding the great variety of available lasers offering a wide range of output characteristics, from the clinical usage point of view we have broadly classified them into thermal and nonthermal lasers, depending upon their principal mode of action upon the tissue. In clinical practice thermal lasers are essentially used as surgical tools for incision, excision, or ablation with the advantage of coagulation and sealing of the small capillary vessels. The nonthermal lasers affect the metabolism of the tissue and are used principally for photodiagnosis and photodynamic therapy.

In the context of imaging and therapy, using nonthermal type of lasers is more relevant in that:

- They can be used for fluorescence imaging, either by inducing autofluorescence, or in conjunction with a chemical photosensitizer (to enhance the fluorescence effect) as in drug induced fluorescence.
- They can be employed for photodynamic therapy, where the target tissue is presensitized by a chemical photosensitizer whose absorption band matches the wavelength of the laser light. The generation of highly reactive singlet oxygen results in the destruction of the target tissue, by necrosis. Currently the technique is applied to a variety of conditions but most commonly in cases of localized cancer.

In both types of lasers the use of custom-made light delivery systems, often incorporating flexible optical fibers, permits controlled application of the laser light to lesions in body cavities and/or tubular organs.

In the future, the development of new sensitizers, with more specific tumor localizing properties, would permit better imaging of the tumor and more precise use of photodynamic therapy. This would amount to precision surgery without the need for the use of conventional surgical methods and within the minimal access/minimal invasive setting.

References

[1] Goldman, L., J. M. Ingleman, and D. F. Richfield, "Impact of the Laser on Nevi and Melanomas," *Arch. Dermat.*, Vol. 90, 1964, pp. 71–75.

[2] Minton, J. P., N. C. Andrews, and J. E. Jesseph, "Pulsed Laser Energy in the Management of Multiple Pulmonary Metastases," *J. Thorac. Cardiovasc. Surg.*, Vol. 54, 1967, pp. 707–713.

[3] Dougherty, T. J., et al., "Photoradiation for the Treatment of Malignant Tumours," *Cancer Res.*, Vol. 38, 1978, pp. 2628–2635.

[4] Hayata, Y., et al., "Haematoporphyrin Derivative and Laser Photoradiation in the Treatment of Lung Cancer," *Chest*, Vol. 81, 1982, pp. 264–277.

[5] Moghissi, K., M. Dench, and E. Neville, "Effects of the Non-Contact Mode of YAG Laser on Pulmonary Tissues and Its Comparison with Electro Diathermy. An Anatomo-Pathological Study," *Lasers in Medical Science*, Vol. 4, 1989, pp. 17–23.

[6] Moghissi, K., and K. Dixon, "Neodymium Yttrium Aluminium Garnet Laser for Excision of Pulmonary Nodule: An Institutional Review," *Laser Med. Sci.*, 2008.

[7] Dumon, J. F., et al., "Treatment of Tracheo-Bronchial Lesions by Laser Photo-Resection," *Chest*, Vol. 81, 1982, pp. 278–284.

[8] Personne, C., et al., "Indications and Technique for Endoscopic Laser Resection in Bronchology: A Critical Analysis Based upon 2284 Resections," *J. Thorac. Cardiovasc. Surg.*, Vol. 91, 1986; pp. 710–715.

[9] Moghissi, K., and K. Dixon, "Bronchoscopic NdYAG Laser Treatment in Lung Cancer 30 Years On: An Institutional Review," *Laser Med. Sci.*, Vol. 21, 2006; pp. 186–191.

[10] Kiefhaber, P., G. Nath, and K. Mortiz, "Endoscopic Control of Massive Gastro-Intestinal Haemorrhage by Irradiation High Power Neodymium YAG Laser," *Prog. Surg.*, Vol. 15, 1977, pp. 140–155.

[11] Krasner, N., et al., "Palliative Laser Therapy for Malignant Dysphagia," *Gut.*, Vol. 28, 1987, pp. 792–798.

[12] Hainz, H., et al., "Prostate Laser Operation: The Cheapest Therapy 872 Cases," *Acta. Urol. Biol.*, Vol. 66, 1998, pp. 3–5.

[13] Renwick, P., V. Whitton, and K. Moghissi, "Combined Endoscopic Laser Therapy and Brachytherapy for Palliation of Oesophageal Carcinoma: A Pilot Study," *Gut.*, Vol. 33, 1992, pp. 435–438.

[14] Chung, P. S., et al., "Anticancer Effect of Combined Intratumour Cisplatin Injection and Interstitial KTP Laser Therapy on Xenografted Squamous Cell Carcinoma," *J. Clin. Laser Med. Surg.*, Vol. 21, 2003, pp. 23–27.

[15] Christiansen, H., et al., "Long Term Follow Up After Transoral Laser Microsurgery and Adjuvant Radiotherapy for Advanced Recurrent Squamous Cell Carcinoma of the Head and Neck," *Int. J. Radiat. Oncol. Biol. Phys.*, Vol. 65, 2006, pp. 1067–1074.

[16] Moghissi, K., "Local Excision of Pulmonary Nodular (Coin) Lesions with Non-Contact Yttrium Aluminium Garnet Laser," *J. Thorac. Cardiovasc. Surg.*, Vol. 97, 1989, pp. 147–151.

[17] Sharpe, D. A. C., D. Dixon, and K. Moghissi, "Thoracoscopic Use of Laser in Intractable Pneumothorax," *Eur. J. Cardiothorac. Surg.*, Vol. 8, 1994, pp. 34–36.

[18] Rolle, A., et al., "Is Surgery For Multiple Lung Metastases Reasonable? A Total of 328 Consecutive Patients with Multiple Laser Metastatectomies with a New 1318 nm NdYAG Laser," *J. Thorac. Cardiovasc, Surg.*, Vol. 131, 2006, pp. 1236–1242.

[19] Moghissi, K., M. Dench, and P. Goebells, "Experience in Non-Contact NdYAG Laser in Pulmonary Surgery," *Eur. J. Cardiothorac. Surg.*, Vol. 2, 1988, pp. 87–94.

[20] Wakabayashi, A., M. Brenner, and R. A. Kayaleh, "Thoracoscopic Carbon Dioxide Laser Treatment of Bullous Emphysema," *Lancet*, Vol. 337, 1991, pp. 881–883.

[21] Moghissi, K., and J. A. C. Thorpe, "Clinical Manifestations and Diagnostic Methods," in *Moghissi's Essentials of Thoracic & Cardiac Surgery*, 2nd ed., K. Moghissi, J. A. C. Thorpe, and F. Ciulli, (eds.), Amsterdam: Elsevier, 2003, pp. 13–29.

[22] Moghissi, K., "Bronchopulmonary neoplasms," in *Moghissi's Essentials of Thoracic & Cardiac Surgery*, 2nd ed., K. Moghissi, J. A. C. Thorpe, and F. Ciulli, (eds.), Amsterdam: Elsevier, 2003, pp. 119–135.

[23] Kato, H., "Photodynamic Therapy for Lung Cancer: A Review of 19 Years Experience," *J. Photochem. Photobiol. B*, Vol. 42, 1998, pp. 96–99.

[24] Moghissi, K., et al., "Photodynamic Therapy in Early Central Lung Cancer: A Treatment Option for Patients Ineligible for Surgical Resection," *Thorax*, Vol. 62, 2007, pp. 391–395.

[25] Policard, A., "Etudes sure les aspects affects par des tumours experimental examinées á la luminiere de Woods," *C. R. Soc. Biol.*, Vol. 91, 1924, pp. 1423–1425.

[26] Lipson, R. L., and E. J. Blades, "The Photodynamic Properties of a Particular Haematoporphyrin Derivative," *Arch. Dermatol.*, Vol. 82, 1960, pp. 508–516.

[27] Lipson, R. L., E. J. Blades, and A. M. Olsen, "The Use of a Derivative of Haematoporphyrin in Tumour Detection," *J. Nat. Cancer. Inst.*, Vol. 26, 1961, pp. 1–10.

[28] Lipson, R. L., E. J. Blades, and M. J. Gray, "Haematoporphyrin Derivative for Detection and Management of Cancer," *Cancer*, Vol. 20, 1967, pp. 2255–2257.

[29] Profio, A. E., D. R. Doiron, and E. G. King, "Laser Fluorescence Bronchoscopy for Localisation of Occult Lung Tumours," *Med. Phys.*, Vol. 6, 1979, pp. 523–525.

[30] Cortese, D. A., et al., "Clinical Application of a New Endoscopic Technique for Detection of Insitu Bronchial Carcinoma," *Mayo Clin. Proc.*, Vol. 54, 1979, pp. 635–642.

[31] Hyata, Y., et al., "Fluorescence Fibreoptic Bronchoscopy in Diagnosis of Early Stage Lung Cancer," *Rec. Res. Cancer Res.*, Vol. 82, 1982, pp. 124–130.

[32] Hung, J., et al., "Autofluorescence of Normal and Malignant Bronchial Tissue," *Laser Surg. Med.*, Vol. 11, 1991, pp. 99–105.

[33] Lam, S., et al., "Localisation of Bronchial Intraepithelial Neoplastic Lesions by Fluorescence Bronchoscopy," *Chest*, Vol. 113, 1998, pp. 696–702.

[34] Kelly, J. F., and J. F. Snell, "Haematoporphyrin Derivative: A Possible Aid in the Diagnosis and Therapy of Carcinoma of the Bladder," *J. Urol.*, Vol. 115, 1976, pp. 150–151.

[35] Kennedy, J. C., R. H. Pottier, and D. C. Pross, "Photodynamic Therapy with Endogenous Protoporhyrin IX: Basic Principles and Present Clinical Experience," *J. Photochem. Photobiol. B*, Vol. 1, 1990, pp. 143–148.

[36] Kreigmair, M., et al., "Fluorescence Photodetection of Neoplastic Urothelial Lesions Following Installation of 5-Aminoleuvululinic Acid," *Urology*, Vol. 44, 1994, pp. 836–841.

[37] Jichlinski, P., et al., "Clinical Evaluation of a Method for Detecting Superficial Surgical Transitional Cell Carcinoma of the Bladder by Light Induced Fluorescence of Protoporhyrin IX Following the Topical Application of 5-Aminoleuvulinic Acid: Preliminary Results," *Laser Surg. Med.*, Vol. 20, 1997, pp. 402–408.

[38] Orenstein, A., G. Kostenich, and Z. Malik, "The Kinetics of Protoporhyrin Fluorescence During ALA-PDT in Human Malignant Skin Tumour," *Cancer Lett.*, Vol. 120, 1997, pp. 229–234.

[39] Eljamel, S., "Brain Photodiagnosis (PD), Fluorescence Guided Resection (FGR) and Photodynamic Therapy (PDT) Past, Present and Future," *Photodiagnosis and Photodynamic Therapy*, Vol. 5, 2008, pp. 29–35.

[40] Raab, O., "On the Effect of Fluorescence Substances on Influsoria Z," *Biol.*, Vol. 39, 1900, pp. 524–526.

[41] Kessel, D., "Photodynamic Therapy from the Beginning," *Photodiagnosis and Photodynamic Therapy*, Vol. 1, 2004, pp. 3–7.

[42] Dougherty, T. J., et al., "Photoradiation Therapy Cure of Animal Tumour with Haematoporphyrin and Light," *J. Natl. Cancer Inst.*, Vol. 55, 1975, pp. 115–121.

[43] Dougherty, T, J., "Photodynamic Therapy of Malignant Tumours," *Crit. Rev. Oncol. Hematol.*, Vol. 2, 1984, pp. 83–116.

[44] Balchum, O. J., D. R. Doiron, and G. C. Huth, "Photodynamic Therapy of Endobronchial Lung Cancer Employing the Photodynamic Action of the Haematoporphyrin Derivative," *Lasers Surg. Med.*, Vol. 14, 1984, pp. 13–30.

[45] McCaughan, J. S., Jr., "Photoradiation of Malignant Tumours Presensitised with Haematoporphyrin Derivative," *Prog. Clin. Biol. Res.*, Vol. 170, 1984, pp. 805–827.

[46] Schuller, D. E., J. S. McCaughan, Jr., and R. P. Rock, "Photodynamic Therapy in Head and Neck Cancer," *Arch. Otolaryngol.*, Vol. 111, 1985, pp. 351–355.

[47] McCaughan, J. S., Jr., T. E. Williams, Jr., and B. H. Bethel, "Palliation of Esophageal Malignancy with Photodynamic Therapy," *Ann. Thorac. Surg.*, Vol. 40, 1985, pp. 113–120.

[48] Goldman, L., R. O. Gregory, and M. La Plant, "Preliminary Investigative Studies with PDT in Dermatologic and Plastic Surgery," *Lasers Surg. Med.*, Vol. 5, 1985, pp. 453–456.

[49] Moghissi, K., and K. Dixon, "Is Bronchoscopic Photodynamic Therapy a Therapeutic Option in Lung Cancer?" *Eur. Resp. J.*, Vol. 22, 2003, pp. 535–541.

[50] Keller, G. S., D. R. Doiron, and G. U. Fischer, "Photodynamic Therapy in Otolargyngology, Head and Neck Surgery," *Arch. Otolaryngol.*, Vol. 111, 1985, pp. 758–761.

[51] Allison, R., et al., "Photosensitisers in Clinical PDT," *Photodiagnosis and Photodynamic Therapy*, Vol. 1, 2004, pp. 27–42.

[52] Clark, C., et al., "Topical 5-Aminolaevulinic Acid Photodynamic Therapy for Cutaneous Lesions; Outcome and Comparison of Light Sources," *Photodermatol. Photoimmunol.*, Vol. 19, 2003, pp. 134–141.

[53] Mang, T. S., "Lasers and Light Sources for Photodynamic Therapy: Past, Present and Future," *Photodiagnosis and Photodynamic Therapy*, Vol. 1, 2004, pp. 43–48.

Selected Bibliography

Allison, R. R., et al., "A Clinical Review of PDT for Cutaneous Malignancies," *Photodiagnosis and Photodynamic Therapy*, Vol. 3, 2006, pp. 214–226.

Juzeniene, A., and J. Moan, "The History of PDT in Norway: Part I: Identification of Basic Mechanisms of General PDT," and "Part II: Recent Advances in General PDT and ALA-PDT," *Photodiagnosis and Photodynamic Therapy*, Vol. 4, 2007, pp. 3–11 and pp. 80–87.

Mang, T., et al., "Autofluorescence and Photofrin-Induced Fluorescence Imaging and Spectroscopy in an Animal Modal of Oral Cancer," *Photodiagnosis and Photodynamic Therapy*, Vol. 3, 2006, pp. 168–176.

Martin, N. E., and S. M. Hahn, "Interstitial Photodynamic Therapy for Prostate Cancer: A Developing Modality," *Photodiagnosis and Photodynamic Therapy*, Vol. 1, 2004, pp. 123–136.

Mitra, A., and G. I. Stables, "Topical Photodynamic Therapy for Non-Cancerous Skin Conditions," *Photodiagnosis and Photodynamic Therapy*, Vol. 3, 2006, pp. 116–127.

Moghissi, K., and K. Dixon, "Update on the Current Indications, Practice and Results of Photodynamic Therapy in Early Central Lung Cancer (ECLC)," *Photodiagnosis and Photodynamic Therapy*, Vol. 5, 2008, pp. 10–18.

Morton, C. A., "How to Optimise Topical Photodynamic Therapy in Dermatology," *Photodiagnosis and Photodynamic Therapy*, Vol. 3, 2006, pp. 112–115.

Schleyer, V., and R. M. Szeimies, "ALA/MAL-PDT," in *Dermatology in Photodynamic Therapy with ALA: A Clinical Handbook*, R. Pottier et al., (eds.), The Royal Society of Chemistry, India: Macmillan, 2006.

Tardivo, J. P., et al., "Methylene Blue in Photodynamic Therapy: From Basic Mechanisms to Clinical Applications," *Photodiagnosis and Photodynamic Therapy*, Vol. 2, 2005, pp. 175–191.

Zeng, H., A. McWilliams, and S. Lam, "Optical Spectroscopy and Imaging for Early Lung Cancer Detection: A Review," *Photodiagnosis and Photodynamic Therapy*, Vol. 1, 2004, pp. 111–122.

CHAPTER 8

Image-Guided Cryotherapy: An Emphasis on Liver Tumors

David F. Schaeffer and Charles H. Scudamore

Cryosurgery (in situ freezing) is the destruction of a tumor by means of ice crystal formation. The procedure involves the placement of a vacuum insulated cryoprobe into the center of the tumor under visual or ultrasonography guidance. The frozen tumor is then left in situ to be reabsorbed.

Cryotherapy in the setting of primary and secondary malignant liver tumors has been reported to be an effective procedure as compared to best supportive care and has been shown to produce an overall survival of 46% to 89% in patients followed up for at least 20 months. It is of particular value in cases where surgical resection is difficult due to the proximity of vessels, extensive infiltration of tumor, or cirrhosis. As such, cryotherapy has been advocated as an alternative or adjuvant to tumor resection. Cryotherapy has typically been performed using open surgery guided by ultrasonography; however, recent studies have reported the use of minimally invasive access for liver tumor cryoablation and magnetic resonance imaging (MRI) for intraprocedural monitoring.

This chapter discusses image-guided cryotherapeutic ablation of tumors, with a focus on primary and secondary liver tumors, as well as an in-depth view on cryobiology, surgical and radiological technique, advantages and disadvantages of this procedure, and therapeutic consequences.

8.1 Introduction

Percutaneous cryotherapy is a nonvascular interventional procedure and is one of several included in the category of image-guided thermal tumor ablation. Other procedures in this category are heat-based treatments, including radiofrequency ablation (RFA), microwave ablation (MWA), laser ablation (LA), and high-intensity focused ultrasound (HIFU), which are aimed at depositing energy interstitially to coagulate tissue. Cryotherapy is intended to destroy cells by freezing the tissue well below zero degrees centigrade (°C), inducing cell death.

The local freezing of tumor has a documented history in the medical field as an accepted clinical application, either in an open setting, laparoscopically, or percutaneously. The following paragraphs are aimed at highlighting cryotherapy as a locally ablative treatment option for patients with nonresectable liver tumors, either of primary or secondary origin.

Both primary and secondary liver tumors are a common medical problem. Primary liver tumors in the form of hepatocellular carcinoma (HCC) are increasing in incidence globally due to the prevalence of hepatitis B (HBV) and hepatitis C (HCV) infection, both of which are major causes of cirrhosis and subsequent development of HCC [1]. HCC is a very rapidly progressing disease with a poor prognosis [2]. Furthermore, secondary liver tumors are frequently encountered as metastatic disease of colorectal carcinoma (CRC), where two-thirds of patients have liver metastasis by the time of their death [3, 4]. These are detected synchronously with the primary tumor in 25% of patients and metachronously in a further 40% [5]. For CRC hepatic metastasis, survival is determined by the number and extent of metastases, but only 5% to 10% of these are surgically resectable [5]. Median survival with CRC liver metastases is 4.5 to 15 months.

While surgical resection is well established as the gold standard in primary and secondary liver tumors, only a minority of patients, 10% to 20%, are candidates for surgical resection due to limited hepatic reserve and tumor modality [6]. The 5-year survival rate after resection is 25% to 35% [2].

Percutaneous local ablative therapies (PLAT) have emerged as definitive therapies for small HCCs (< 3 cm) [7]. The basic principle is to apply these techniques in patients with a limited number of intrahepatic deposits that are not totally resectable due to their location in the liver. Tumor ablation can be used alone, as a PLAT procedure, or in association with surgical liver resection.

8.2 Cryobiology

Freezing and thawing tissue results in necrosis. It is important to note, however, that cryotherapy applies a direct damage, injury to the individual cells at the time of the therapy, as well as an indirect damage to the tissue as a whole by impairing the microvasculature [8]. The ability of cryotherapy to eradicate tumor tissue is dependent on the exposure of the entire tumor to the lethal freezing process, which differs from the principles of radiation, which is dependent on the nuclear characteristics of individual cells. Cellular survival during cryoablation not only depends on the freezing and thawing rates but, most importantly, upon the lowest temperature reached and the hold time at subzero degrees centigrade [9]. Depending on the cryogen and the size of the cryo-applicator, the tip of each applicator can reach temperatures as low as –196°C. At such temperatures the tumor tissue surrounding the probe is frozen. During the cryoablative process, ice initially forms outside the cell, increasing the extracellular concentration. The freezing rates are high enough to impair cellular function only within a few millimeters of the cryoprobe [10]. The lipid membranes initially block ice crystal formation from building upon inside the cells, leading to an osmotic imbalance. Thus, the resulting direct cellular injury is two-fold: (1) intracellular ice formation, and (2) solution effects—the macroscopic appearance is that of a spherical or elliptical volume of frozen tissue, referred to as an *iceball* (see Figure 8.1).

Despite the fact that intracellular ice formation is usually a lethal event associated with irreversible membrane damage, it is not known if cell death is a cause or a result of this ice formation [11–14]. The majority of the iceball experiences lower

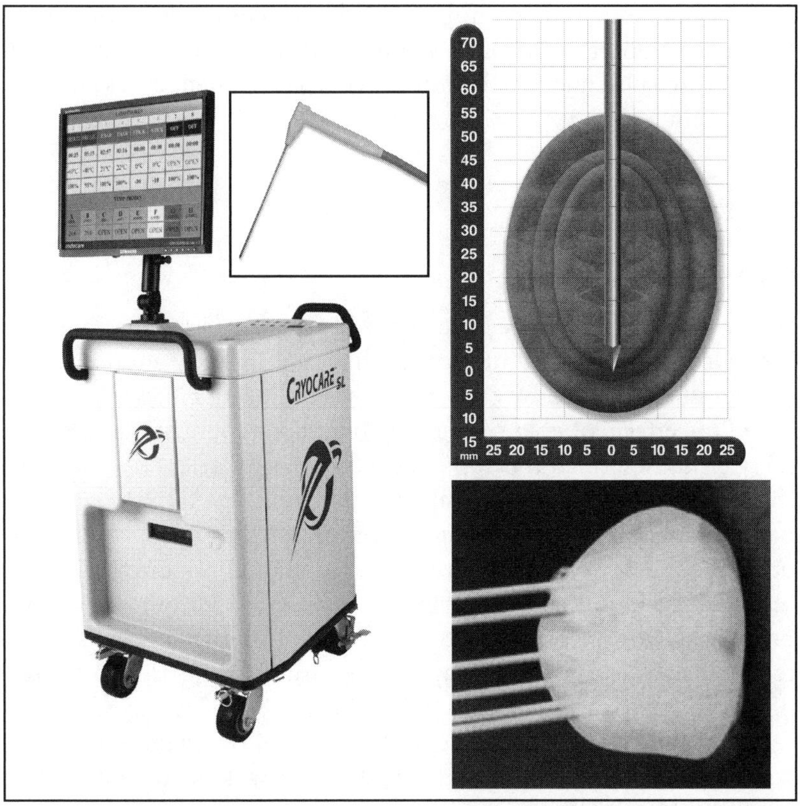

Figure 8.1 A typical cryotherapy generator used in interventional radiology and surgery alike. The inset shows one of the cryoprobes used for the ablation of primary or secondary liver tumors. On the right-hand side a graphic depiction of the "iceball" formation is given. (Images courtesy of Endocare, Inc.)

freezing rates that lead to cellular dehydration resulting from the osmotic imbalance [10]. This process has been referred to as *solution effect*. While several hypotheses exist, no consensus has been found to its physical basis. One hypothesis speculates that the solute concentration alone is responsible for the damage [15], while others conclude that shrinkage beyond a critical minimum volume leads to irreversible membrane damage [16, 17]. A third hypothesis focuses on the principle that proteins with salt bridges within the cytoplasm move into solution due to exposure to high salt concentration [18]. This would lead to a decrease in the intracellular salt concentration causing salt to move through the cation channels into the cytoplasm. Upon thawing, the proteins will reform their salt bridges and release salt due to the dilution of the cytoplasm with water influx.

Another important aspect in cryoablative therapy is the timeline. Direct injury does not destroy all cells. In the hours and days following the initial assault, indirect damage occurs. A main contributing factor is the damage of endothelial cells surrounding the tumor leading to ischemia and thus enhancing the destructive process within the iceball. Several studies have postulated that this secondary mechanism might be the leading cause of cell death within cryosurgery [19, 20]. Furthermore, recent studies have suggested that apoptotic pathways are induced during cryotherapy [20, 21].

Animal models of cryoablation-induced multisystem injury have shown activation of the transcription factor complex nuclear factor κB (NF-κB) in lung and liver tissue, with subsequent elevation of NF-κB dependent cytokines, such as TNFα and interleukin-6 [22].

8.3 Cryotherapy

8.3.1 Historical Aspects

Injury due to cold has been recognized from earliest times and the corresponding references can be found in both civilian and military sources. The prevention and cure of illness caused by cold were known during Hippocratic times. Hippocrates noted the effects of cold on the inhabitants of countries with cold climates. In AD 25, Celsius described the appearance of the skin after cold injury and noted that if the injury was severe, dry gangrene appeared. In AD 70 Galen described the loss of sensation which accompanies injury in his discourse, "Pain as a means of diagnosis." The Carthaginian mercenaries in Hannibal's army which crossed the Alps in 218 B.C. found that smearing their bodies with oil was an effective means of preventing frost-bite, similar to the forces of Alexander the Great, who found protection using sesame juice. Napoleon's surgeon-general, von Larrey, made detailed observations of the effects of cold on his patients. He described erythema and blistering of the skin after freezing and also noted that gangrene was not an inevitable consequence of freezing if exposure was not prolonged, and furthermore described uneventful healing.

Cryosurgery, the operative destruction of pathological tissue by cold, was first used when suitable refrigerants became available in the nineteenth century. In 1851 Dr. James Arnott was the first to make use of the therapeutic effects of low temperatures in the destruction of tumors [23]. The use of carbon dioxide snow and liquid air in the treatment of naevi and other skin lesions [24, 25] was followed by the use of other refrigerants, especially liquid nitrogen. Other therapeutic uses of low temperatures in surgery continued to be developed, such as hypothermia, especially in early heart surgery [26].

This longstanding application of cryotherapy has led to its use in different specialties, ranging from dermatology, urology, gynecology, and cardiology to hepatobiliary surgery.

8.3.2 Imaging Modalities for Percutaneous Cryotherapy

Open cryosurgery has been employed by surgeons for many years for the focal destruction of abdominal tumors. The pioneer work here was performed in the liver. With the advances of thinner cryo-applicators, the possibility of percutaneous cryotherapy became apparent, but also required a suitable imaging modality for monitoring the iceball formation. While ultrasound (US) was initially used to apply percutaneous cryotherapy due to the high echogenicity of the iceball [27, 28], which allowed good visualization, the focus has switched in recent years to using MRI. Quite rapidly it became apparent that magnetic resonance imaging (MRI) provides a good visualization of frozen tissue due to the sharp contrast between frozen and

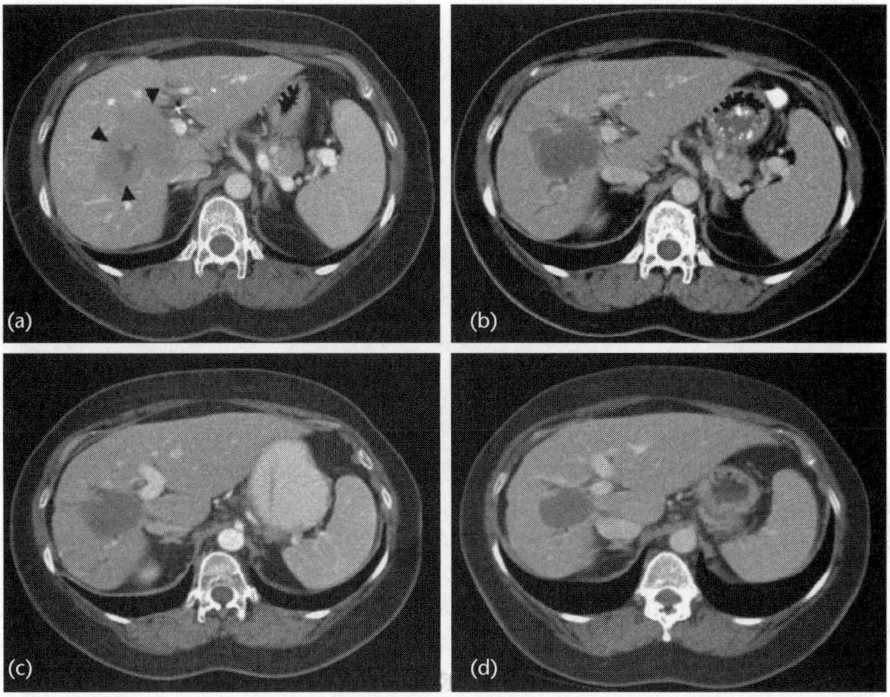

Figure 8.2 Serial CT images of a 6- to 7-cm hepatic mass near the inferior vena cava (a) precryotherapy and at (b) 3-month, (c) 7-month, and (d) 12-month post-initial cryoablative treatment. Note the presence of the typical iceball and its recession in diameter over time. (Images courtesy of Peter Littrup, MD.)

unfrozen regions. Ice can also be viewed with CT but the contrast between frozen and unfrozen tissue is not as good as with MRI [28, 29] (see Figure 8.2). Table 8.1 compares imaging modalities used in cryotherapy.

8.3.3 MRI-Guided Cryotherapy

The late 1980s and early 1990s brought the first experimental data on using MRI for freezing tissue. These early trials demonstrated that frozen tissues were readily visualized under MRI in an especially sharp contrast to unfrozen regions, drawing attention to the potential for MRI to guide cryotherapy clinically [30, 31]. The sharp contrast was already evident in images acquired with a gradient echo pulse sequence in a 0.1T scanner as well as with T1-weighted (T1w) rapid acquisition

Table 8.1 Imaging Modalities Used in Cryotherapy

US	Ultrasound provides high contrast of ice compared to soft tissue and thus leads to good visualization of the iceball.
CT	Ice presents only a moderate contrast on CT images. Soft tissue and especially fat lacks a good contrast of the ice formation, whereas it is completely absent within bone. The low density area created by the iceball may mimic an abscess or infarct region.
MRI	Magnetic resonance images give a high contrast of ice within soft tissue, as well as within bone.

relaxation-enhanced imaging at 1.5T. Since ice is a very solid structure, it has ultrashort T1 and T2 relaxation times, which result in a signal void under nearly all MRI pulse sequences. The above mentioned signal void of frozen tissue presents with a high contrast-to-noise ratio (CNR) related to unfrozen tissue. This results in a sharply marginated iceball that can be viewed in 3D (see Figure 8.3). The entire volume of frozen tissue can be viewed, unlike under US, where the iceball is partially hidden due to acoustic shadowing. The high percentage of water in frozen tissue thus exhibits a very low signal during the actual cryotherapeutic procedure. Besides demonstrating the possibility of visualizing the ice formation with the help of MRI, these early experiments proved that MR images could be acquired with scan times that were short enough to monitor the dynamic processes of freezing and thawing. In 2001 this was subsequently reported in normal porcine kidney in vivo [32]. Ice can also be viewed with the help of CT images, but one has to be aware that the contrast between frozen and unfrozen tissue is not as good as with MR images [33, 34].

The two most important intraprocedural aspects in cryoablative therapy in general are covering the target completely by the iceball and avoiding damage to surrounding structures. MRI is best suited for this aspect, as it provides the ability to monitor the freezing process in 3D over a suitable timescale. The outcome results described in the remainder of this chapter show that these procedures are technically feasible and can be performed safely with good clinical results in select patients in a range of organ systems.

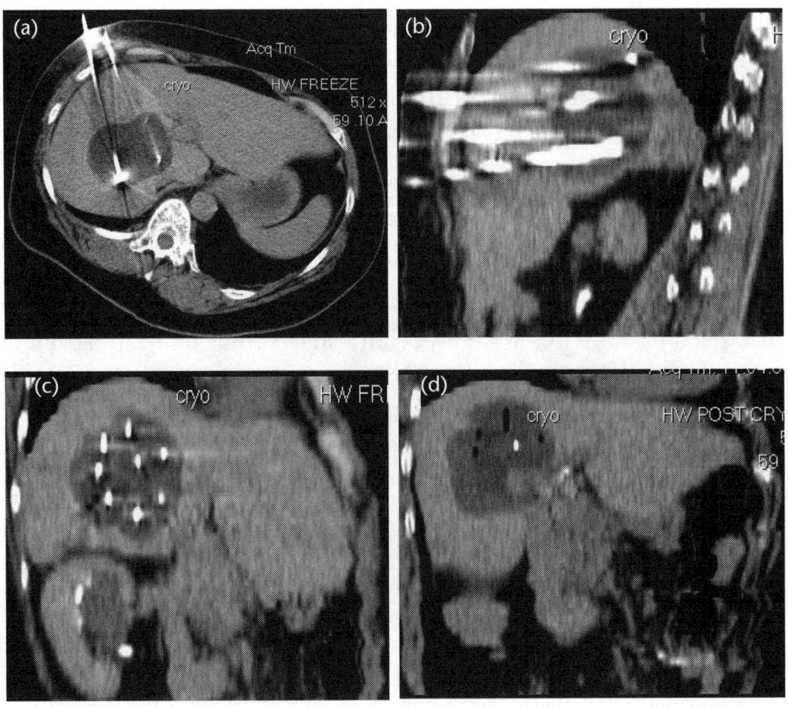

Figure 8.3 Procedural serial CT image of percutaneous cryotherapy of a 7-cm hepatic mass (a) and cranial MRI images demonstrating the placement of the cryoprobes (b–d). This figure is also highlighting the difference between CT and MRI imaging. (Images courtesy of Peter Littrup, MD.)

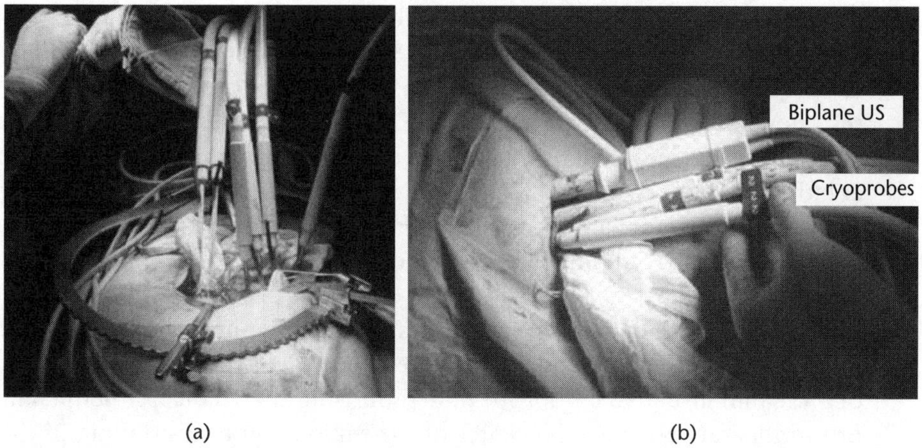

Figure 8.4 (a) Application of cryoablative therapy during open laparotomy. (b) Due to the extensive diameter of the hepatic tumor, several cryoprobes are used at the same time in conjunction with an ultrasound probe. (Images Courtesy of Peter Littrup, MD.)

8.4 Clinical Applications of Cryotherapy

8.4.1 Liver

Traditionally, cryotherapy requires laparotomy to place the needles and deliver therapy [35] (see Figures 8.4 and 8.5). This approach has been reported to encounter a treatment-related mortality rate of 2% [36]. Percutaneous ethanol injection

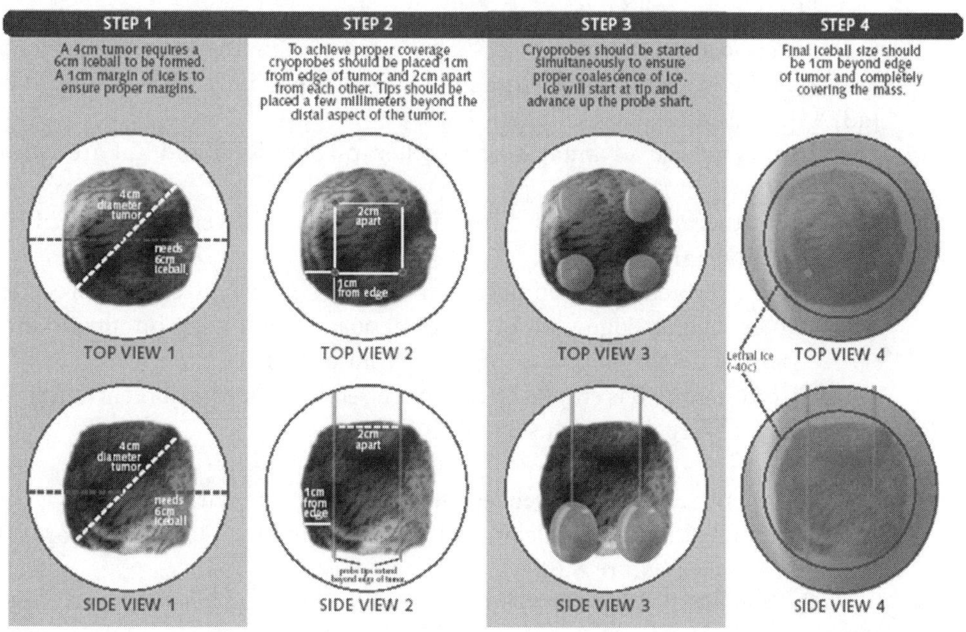

Figure 8.5 During the cryoablative therapy it is important to ensure that an adequate diameter around the tumor is achieved with the application of the cryoprobes. (Images Courtesy of Endocare, Inc.)

(PEI) has been shown to be effective for small HCCs, but is not as effective for CRC metastases [37]. Livraghi et al. [38, 39] demonstrated very elegantly that the technique has an equivalent survival to surgery with a 3-year survival of 79% for resection and 71% for PEI.

Radiofrequency ablation (RFA) is becoming a widely used technique for the ablation of primary or secondary liver tumors. Alternating electric currents in the range of radiofrequency waves (460 kHz) are applied from a generator, agitating ions in tissue surrounding a RFA probe. This causes localized heating and subsequent thermal necrosis.

The principle of cryosurgery is destruction of tumor by means of ice crystal formation [40] and consequential solute effects. This occurs through the placement of a vacuum insulated cryoprobe under ultrasound guidance, either percutaneously or intraoperatively, into the center of the tumor. Upon positioning of the probe it is anchored into place by rapidly lowering the probe temperature up to –195°C. Freezing is produced by a variety of methods; the most convenient of which seems to be to force nitrous oxide (N_2O) through a flow restrictor near the tip of the cryoprobe. The gas expansion causes the absorption of large amounts of heat through the Joule–Thomson effect. This is not the only method available; some systems rely on the expansion of other gases (e.g., argon) or force cryological coolants (e.g., liquid nitrogen) through the probe. The intent in all cases is to destroy tissue by bringing it to very low temperatures.

Freezing is started by circulating liquid nitrogen at –196°C through the cryoprobe, with one to three cycles of 15 minutes each applied. Lethal temperatures in the tissue of below –20°C are achieved. The probe is then withdrawn and the track filled with gel foam [41]. The effect of the iceball is monitored intraoperatively via ultrasound. The anterior margin of the frozen perimeter is seen as an area of increased echogenicity. MRI can clearly identify the iceball as it expands as a sharply marginated tear drop or ellipsoid shaped area of signal void on all sequences [42]. However, the frozen periphery does not correlate precisely with the necrotic margin [43, 44].

The therapeutic advantages of cryotherapy over RFA and PEI are as follows:

1. Cryotherapy can be used near large vessels with very little risk of thrombosis, contrary to RFA.
2. The interface of frozen/unfrozen liver can be visualized intraprocedurally as an echogenic edge with posterior acoustic shadowing on ultrasound or as a sharply demarcated area of signal void on MRI.
3. Cryotherapy has shown to be more effective in terms of recurrence rates than RFA in large tumors (> 3 cm) [39].

Post-operatively, the treated lesion can be followed with CT or MRI, showing a low density area on CT, mimicking an infarct or abscess [45] or as an area of signal void on MRI (see Figure 8.6).

Like any locally ablative therapy within the liver, cryotherapy also carries risks. Those include hemorrhage, pleural effusion, abscess formation, biliary strictures or perforation, small vessel ischemia, platelet consumption, and splitting of the liver capsule.

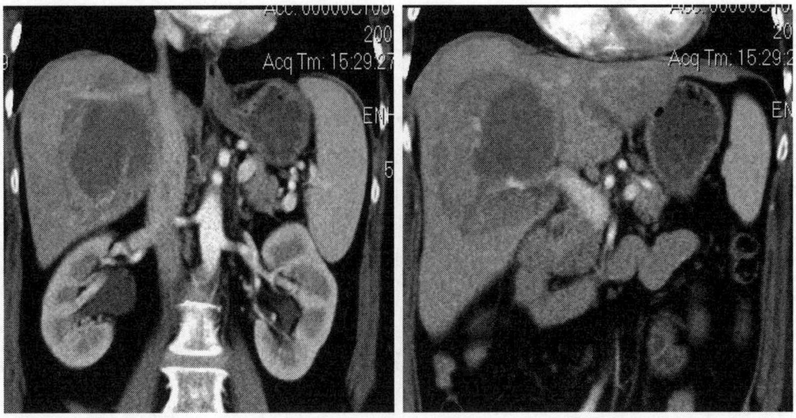

Figure 8.6 Cranial MRI images of hepatic mass treated in Figure 8.3 at day 2 postprocedure. Note the typical iceball. (Images courtesy of Peter Littrup, MD.)

Another complication is the so-called cryoshock phenomenon [46]. Multisystem injury and subsequent systemic inflammation response syndrome (SIRS) is a recognized complication of large-volume cryoablation, due to an overexpression of inflammatory mediators, predominantly produced by macrophages.

In this context one has to take a report by Chapman et al. [47] into consideration, which showed that hepatic cryoablation, but not radiofrequency ablation, induces NF-κB activation in the nonablated liver and lung, and is associated with acute lung injury. The authors made mention that this observation on a molecular level was correlating with the clinical observation of increased incidence of multisystem organ injury, including adult respiratory distress syndrome (ARDS). This report has led to a reevaluation of cryotherapy within the liver and more and more centers are thus relaying on RFA. However, cryoablative therapy does still have its place in hepatobiliary surgery in certain settings. With the advent of percutaneous cryoablative techniques the advantages of a very cost-effective method have become apparent. The highly visible ice increases the ability to protect adjacent structures and allows for a treatment alternative for patients with tumors near painful sites (i.e., diaphragm, chest wall).

Several studies have looked at the outcome of intraoperative US-guided cryotherapy in both primary and secondary liver tumors. In a retrospective review of 18 patients with unresectable CRC metastases treated with intraoperative cryosurgery, Onik et al. [41] could demonstrate a complete remission in 22% and a mean survival time of 21.4 months. In a metanalysis of cryosurgery in primary and secondary liver lesions completed by Lee et al. [48], the authors found an overall survival of 46% to 89% in patients with a minimum follow-up time of 20 months.

The authors stratified the lesions most suitable for cryoablative therapy into the following categories:

1. Less than four lesions in multiple lobes;
2. Lesions near the portal vein, which may preclude conventional surgical resection;
3. Patients with a limited hepatic reserve, who could not undergo resection.

Another paper published results of MR-guided percutaneous cryoablation of 15 hepatic tumors, 14 metastasis, one haemangioma, in 12 patients [42]. The authors could demonstrate that MR-guided therapy, performed in an open 0.5 T magnet, was both feasible and safe, resulting in no major complications. Post-procedural Gadolinium enhanced MRI at 24 hours demonstrated 75% or more necrosis of the lesions in 8 of 12 patients [42]. In a study including 308 patients, Bilchik et al. [45] compared cryosurgery with RFA alone and cryosurgery combined with RFA in unresectable primary and secondary liver tumors. The morbidity of the procedure was decreased in the group, which combined cryosurgery with RFA, as compared with cryosurgery alone. Recurrence rates for small tumors (< 3 cm) were similar for cryosurgery and RFA. However, RFA was less suitable for large tumors (> 3 cm) with a local recurrence rate of 38% for RFA treated patients compared with 17% for cryosurgery treated patients [45].

A common approach in primary and secondary liver is the laparoscopic staging of the tumor followed by in situ ablation within the liver [45, 49, 50]. In a Phase I study of percutaneous cryotherapy for colorectal liver metastasis, Huang et al. [51] demonstrated that percutaneous cryotherapy is not only feasible, but might lead to an added survival benefit, especially if performed in conjunction with a chemotherapeutic regiment.

8.4.2 Kidney

Nephron sparing surgery presents a challenge to the surgeon. Multiple renal tumors are not rare and can be difficult to resect without complication. Renal tumors up to 3 cm in diameter can be destroyed in situ by cryotherapy. In 2005 Silverman et al. [52] reported on initial experience in treating 26 kidney tumors in 23 patients with MRI-guided cryotherapy. Of 26 tumors, 24 (92%) had no evidence of disease at a mean follow-up of 14 months. These initial results were supported by Kodama et al. [53], who treated a patient with five bilateral tumors, two of which were treated in one session and three in another.

In summary, one can conclude that success depends on tumor location and size. Complete ablation was achieved in exophytic tumors, located away from the central sinus, with diameters up to 5 cm, while it was harder to achieve in centrally placed tumors adjacent to the renal sinus. Initial concerns that adjacent bowel or pleura would prevent a percutaneous approach have been lessened by the use of 5% dextrose instilled around the tumor to displace adjacent structures that could be injured.

8.4.3 Gynecological Applications in Uterine Fibroids and Breast Cancer

Several reports have been published describing the application of percutaneous cryotherapy in the advent of uterine leiomyomata [54, 55]. Overall, these reports concluded that percutaneous image-guided cryotherapy was a feasible procedure that was well suited for the task and effective at relieving symptoms caused by uterine fibroids.

In 2004 Morin et al. [56] reported the treatment of 25 patients with breast carcinoma with a "treat-and-resect" protocol to demonstrate the feasibility of MRI-guided cryotherapy in the breast. Surgical excision was undertaken 4 weeks following cryotherapy, which led to total ablation of 13 of the 25 tumors treated. This stands in contrast to a recent report by Pusztaszeri et al. [57], who reported good technical coverage of the tumors, but variable response to the therapy. Two patients (20%) had a complete response and others had various degrees of residual disease seen on pathology, raising the possibility that ductal carcinoma in situ may be more resistant to cryotherapy. Cryotherapy may have a future as a therapeutic option within the gynecological field to treat uterine leiomyoma, but more studies are needed to assess the feasibility for treating breast cancer by cryotherapy.

8.4.4 Prostate

Transcutaneous and percutaneous ablation techniques have gained popularity as a minimally invasive treatment option for primary and recurrent prostate cancer [58, 59]. Only one randomized controlled trial is available for cryoablation within prostatic tissue. In general, the median follow-up time is short and the definition of the available biochemical progression-free survival varies highly among studies. No data have been reported on cancer-specific or overall mortality. Ellis et al. [60] reported the main study for 12 months about cryotherapy as primary treatment for localized prostate cancer. A total of 416 consecutive patients were treated with a mean follow-up of 20 months. The 4-year biochemical disease-free survival was 79.6%, incontinence was observed in 4% at 6 months, and 41% of patients recovered potency at 12 months. Erectile dysfunction remains an issue after cryoablation and is the reason why some authors have proposed to treat only the lobe with a positive core biopsy. Bahn et al. [61] reported a series of 31 patients with unilateral tumor identified by color Doppler ultrasonography and confirmed by targeted and systematic biopsy. With a mean follow-up of 70 months, biochemical disease-free status was maintained by 92.8% of patients and a 96.0% negative-biopsy rate was observed. Potency was maintained by 48.1% of patients and another 40.7% were potent with oral pharmaceutical assistance.

One randomized trial compared cryotherapy versus radiotherapy for patients with clinically locally advanced prostate cancer. Six months of hormonal therapy with LHRH agonist was administered starting 3 months before the date of cryosurgery or the first radiotherapy session. Sixty-four patients were included with a mean follow-up time of 37 months. The 4-year biochemical recurrence-free survival rate for radiotherapy and cryotherapy groups were calculated at 47% and 13%, respectively ($P = 0.027$), indicating that the results of cryotherapy are significantly less favorable than those for radiotherapy. Incontinence was observed in 7% of patients treated by cryotherapy [62].

This conclusion supports a previous retrospective study [63] on 21 high-risk prostate cancer patients treated by percutaneous prostate cryoablation. With a median follow-up of 41 months, the PSA failure rate was 52.9% at 24 months.

8.5 Current Status, Limitations, and Future Aspects

Surgical excision remains the definitive standard treatment of focal tumors. However, ablation provides an option for nonsurgical candidates, or those in whom surgery or chemotherapy has failed, or where indications include pain palliation or quality of life issues, preferably within the context of multidisciplinary meeting and consensus.

Despite reasonably good results with the application of cryotherapy in different organ systems, there are still limitations to this application. One major limitation is our lack of understanding the complete effects of cryotherapy on tissue. A recent publication [64] demonstrated quite nicely that the freezing process itself has different temperature profiles in different organ systems. This highlights the different capacities of tissue to conduct thermal energy and may lead to organ specific "freezing" protocols or organ specific probe developments.

Image-guided ablation is well established in many different organ systems including the liver. The current status of percutaneous cryotherapy shows that it may be performed safely and with good clinical results. Technical advances in the radiological field with high-resolution CT scanners and an MRI environment that allow interventional procedures, will definitely lead to more and more interventional procedures, and cryotherapy is well positioned to play a major role in many organ systems.

References

[1] Grasso, A., et al., "Radiofrequency Ablation in the Treatment of Hepatocellular Carcinoma—A Clinical Viewpoint," *J. Hepatol.*, Vol. 33, No. 4, 2000, pp. 667–672.

[2] Kulik, L. M., "Advancements in Hepatocellular Carcinoma," *Curr. Opin. Gastroenterol.*, Vol. 23, No. 3, 2007, pp. 268–274.

[3] Greenway, B., "Hepatic Metastases from Colorectal Cancer: Resection or Not," *Br. J. Surg.*, Vol. 75, No. 6, 1988, pp. 513–519.

[4] Finlay, I. G., et al., "Resection with Cryotherapy of Colorectal Hepatic Metastases Has the Same Survival as Hepatic Resection Alone," *Eur. J. Surg. Oncol.*, Vol. 26, No. 3, 2000, pp. 199–202.

[5] Weaver, M. L., D. Atkinson, and R. Zemel, "Hepatic Cryosurgery in Treating Colorectal Metastases," *Cancer*, Vol. 76, No. 2, 1995, pp. 210–214.

[6] Taura, K., et al., "Implication of Frequent Local Ablation Therapy for Intrahepatic Recurrence in Prolonged Survival of Patients with Hepatocellular Carcinoma Undergoing Hepatic Resection: An Analysis of 610 Patients over 16 Years Old," *Ann. Surg.*, Vol. 244, No. 2, 2006, pp. 265–273.

[7] Lencioni, R. A., et al., "Small Hepatocellular Carcinoma in Cirrhosis: Randomized Comparison of Radio-Frequency Thermal Ablation Versus Percutaneous Ethanol Injection," *Radiology*, 2003, Vol. 228, No. 1, pp. 235–240.

[8] Hoffmann, N. E., and J. C. Bischof, "The Cryobiology of Cryosurgical Injury," *Urology*, Vol. 60, No. 2, Suppl. 1, 2002, pp. 40–49.

[9] Smith, D. J., et al., "A Parametric Study of Freezing Injury in AT-1 Rat Prostate Tumor Cells," *Cryobiology*, Vol. 39, No. 1, 1999, pp. 13–28.

[10] Bischof, J. C., et al., "Cryosurgery of Dunning AT-1 Rat Prostate Tumor: Thermal, Biophysical, and Viability Response at the Cellular and Tissue Level," *Cryobiology*, Vol. 34, No. 1, 1997, pp. 42–69.

[11] Muldrew, K. and L. E. McGann, "The Osmotic Rupture Hypothesis of Intracellular Freezing Injury," *Biophys. J.*, Vol. 66, No. 2, Pt. 1, 1994, pp. 532–541.

[12] Toner, M., E. G. Cravalho, and M. Karel, "Cellular Response of Mouse Oocytes to Freezing Stress: Prediction of Intracellular Ice Formation," *J. Biomech. Eng.*, Vol. 115, No. 2, 1993, pp. 169–174.

[13] Toner, M., E. G. Cravalho, and D. R. Armant, "Water Transport and Estimated Transmembrane Potential During Freezing of Mouse Oocytes," *J. Membr. Biol.*, Vol. 115, No. 3, 1990, pp. 261–272.

[14] Hubel, A., et al., "Intracellular Ice Formation During the Freezing of Hepatocytes Cultured in a Double Collagen Gel," *Biotechnol. Prog.*, Vol. 7, No. 6, 1991, pp. 554–559.

[15] Lovelock, J. E., "The Haemolysis of Human Red Blood-Cells by Freezing and Thawing," *Biochim. Biophys. Acta.*, Vol. 10, No. 3, 1953, pp. 414–426.

[16] Meryman, H. T., "Modified Model for the Mechanism of Freezing Injury in Erythrocytes," *Nature*, Vol. 218, No. 5139, 1968, pp. 333–336.

[17] Meryman, H. T., "Osmotic Stress as a Mechanism of Freezing Injury," *Cryobiology*, Vol. 8, No. 5, 1971, pp. 489–500.

[18] Muldrew, K., et al., "Kinetics of Osmotic Water Movement from Rabbit Patellar Tendon and Medial Collateral Ligament Fibroblasts," *Cryo Letters*, Vol. 22, No. 5, 2001, pp. 329–336.

[19] Gage, A.A. and J. Baust, "Mechanisms of Tissue Injury in Cryosurgery," *Cryobiology*, Vol. 37, No. 3, 1998, pp. 171–186.

[20] Baust, J. M., B. Van, and J. G. Baust, "Cell Viability Improves Following Inhibition of Cryopreservation-Induced Apoptosis," *Vitro Cell Dev. Biol. Anim.*, Vol. 36, No. 4, 2000, pp. 262–270.

[21] Clarke, D. M., et al., "Chemo-Cryo Combination Therapy: An Adjunctive Model for the Treatment of Prostate Cancer," *Cryobiology*, Vol. 42, No. 4, 2001, pp. 274–285.

[22] Blackwell, T. S., et al., "Acute Lung Injury After Hepatic Cryoablation: Correlation with NF-Kappa B Activation and Cytokine Production," *Surgery*, Vol. 126, No. 3, 1999, pp. 518–526.

[23] Arnott, J., *On the Treatment of Cancer by the Regulated Application of an Anaesthetic Temperature*, London: J. Churchill, 1851, p. 32.

[24] White, A., "Liquid Air, Its Application in Medicine and Surgery," *Medical Records*, Vol. 56, 1899, pp. 109–112.

[25] Pusey, W., "The Use of Carbon Dioxide Snow in the Treatment of Naevi and Other Lesions of the Skin," *JAMA*, Vol. 49, 1907, pp. 1354–1356.

[26] Bigelow, W. G., W. K. Lindsay, and W. F. Greenwood, "Hypothermia; Its Possible Role in Cardiac Surgery: An Investigation of Factors Governing Survival in Dogs at Low Body Temperatures," *Ann. Surg.*, Vol. 132, No. 5, 1950, pp. 849–866.

[27] Onik, G., et al., "Ultrasonic Characteristics of Frozen Liver," *Cryobiology*, Vol. 21, No. 3, 1984, pp. 321–328.

[28] Cohen, J. K., "Cryosurgery of the Prostate: Techniques and Indications," *Rev. Urol.*, Vol. 6, Suppl. 4, 2004, pp. S20–S26.

[29] Schuder, G., et al., "Preliminary Experience with Percutaneous Cryotherapy of Liver Tumors," *Br. J. Surg.*, Vol. 85, No. 9, 1998, pp. 1210–1211.

[30] Isoda, H., "Sequential MRI and CT Monitoring in Cryosurgery—An Experimental Study in Rats," *Nippon Igaku Hoshasen Gakkai Zasshi*, Vol. 49, No. 12, 1989, pp. 1499–508.

[31] Matsumoto, R., et al., "MR Monitoring During Cryotherapy in the Liver: Predictability of Histologic Outcome," *J. Magn. Reson. Imaging*, Vol. 3, No. 5, 1993, pp. 770–776.

[32] Shingleton, W. B., et al., "Percutaneous Cryoablation of Porcine Kidneys with Magnetic Resonance Imaging Monitoring," *J. Urol.*, Vol. 166, No. 1, 2001, pp. 289–291.

[33] Tacke, J., et al., "Imaging of Interstitial Cryotherapy—An In Vitro Comparison of Ultrasound, Computed Tomography, and Magnetic Resonance Imaging," *Cryobiology*, Vol. 38, No. 3, 1999, pp. 250–259.

[34] Sandison, G. A., et al., "X-Ray CT Monitoring of Iceball Growth and Thermal Distribution During Cryosurgery," *Phys. Med. Biol.*, Vol. 43, No. 11, 1998, pp. 3309–3324.

[35] Vogl, T. J., et al., "Liver Metastases: Interventional Therapeutic Techniques and Results, State of the Art," *Eur. Radiol.*, Vol. 9, No. 4, 1999, pp. 675–684.

[36] Sarantou, T., A. Bilchik, and K. P. Ramming, "Complications of Hepatic Cryosurgery," *Semin. Surg. Oncol.*, Vol. 14, No. 2, 1998, pp. 156–162.

[37] Amin, Z., S. G. Bown, and W. R. Lees, "Local Treatment of Colorectal Liver Metastases: A Comparison of Interstitial Laser Photocoagulation (ILP) and Percutaneous Alcohol Injection (PAI)," *Clin. Radiol.*, Vol. 48, No. 3, 1993, pp. 166–171.

[38] Livraghi, T., et al., "Percutaneous Ethanol Injection in The Treatment of Hepatocellular Carcinoma in Cirrhosis. A Study on 207 Patients," *Cancer*, Vol. 69, No. 4, 1992, pp. 925–929.

[39] Livraghi, T., et al., "No Treatment, Resection and Ethanol Injection in Hepatocellular Carcinoma: A Retrospective Analysis of Survival in 391 Patients with Cirrhosis," Italian Cooperative HCC Study Group, *J. Hepatol.*, Vol. 22, No. 5, 1995, pp. 522–526.

[40] Gage, A. A., "History of Cryosurgery," *Semin. Surg. Oncol.*, Vol. 14, No. 2, 1998, pp. 99–109.

[41] Onik, G., et al., "Ultrasound–Guided Hepatic Cryosurgery in the Treatment of Metastatic Colon Carcinoma. Preliminary Results," *Cancer*, Vol. 67, No. 4, 1991, pp. 901–907.

[42] Silverman, S. G., et al., "MR Imaging-Guided Percutaneous Cryotherapy of Liver Tumors: Initial Experience," *Radiology*, 2000, Vol. 217, No. 3, pp. 657–664.

[43] Lee, F. T., Jr., et al., "Hepatic Cryosurgery with Intraoperative US Guidance," *Radiology*, Vol. 202, No. 3, 1997, pp. 624–632.

[44] Brewer, W. H., et al., "Intraoperative Monitoring and Postoperative Imaging of Hepatic Cryosurgery," *Semin. Surg. Oncol.*, Vol. 14, No. 2, 1998, pp. 129–155.

[45] Bilchik, A. J., et al., "Cryosurgical Ablation and Radiofrequency Ablation for Unresectable Hepatic Malignant Neoplasms: A Proposed Algorithm," *Arch. Surg.*, Vol. 135, No. 6, 2000, pp. 657–662; discussion pp. 662–664.

[46] Seifert, J. K. and D. L. Morris, "World Survey on the Complications of Hepatic and Prostate Cryotherapy," *World J. Surg.*, Vol. 23, No. 2, 1999, pp. 109–113; discussion pp. 113–114.

[47] Chapman, W. C., et al., "Hepatic Cryoablation, But Not Radiofrequency Ablation, Results in Lung Inflammation," *Ann. Surg.*, Vol. 231, No. 5, 2000, pp. 752–761.

[48] Goldberg, S. N., et al., "Tissue Ablation with Radiofrequency: Effect of Probe Size, Gauge, Duration, and Temperature on Lesion Volume," *Acad. Radiol.*, Vol. 2, No. 5, 1995, pp. 399–404.

[49] Pearson, A. S., et al., "Intraoperative Radiofrequency Ablation or Cryoablation for Hepatic Malignancies," *Am. J. Surg.*, Vol. 178, No. 6, 1999, pp. 592–599.

[50] Wallace, J. R., et al., "Ablation of Liver Metastasis: Is Preoperative Imaging Sufficiently Accurate?" *J. Gastrointest. Surg.*, Vol. 5, No. 1, 2001, pp. 98–107.

[51] Huang, A., et al., "Phase I Study of Percutaneous Cryotherapy for Colorectal Liver Metastasis," *Br. J. Surg.*, 2002, Vol. 89, No. 3, pp. 303–310.

[52] Silverman, S. G., et al., "Renal Tumors: MR Imaging-Guided Percutaneous Cryotherapy—Initial Experience in 23 Patients," *Radiology*, Vol. 236, No. 2, 2005, pp. 716–724.

[53] Kodama, Y., et al., "MR-Guided Percutaneous Cryoablation for Bilateral Multiple Renal Cell Carcinomas," *Radiat. Med.*, Vol. 23, No. 4, 2005, pp. 303–307.

[54] Sewell, P. E., et al., "Real-Time I-MR-Imaging—Guided Cryoablation of Uterine Fibroids," *J. Vasc. Interv. Radiol.*, Vol. 12, No. 7, 2001, pp. 891–893.

[55] Cowan, B. D., et al., "Interventional Magnetic Resonance Imaging Cryotherapy of Uterine Fibroid Tumors: Preliminary Observation," *Am. J. Obstet. Gynecol.*, Vol. 186, No. 6, 2002, pp. 1183–1187.

[56] Morin, J., et al., "Magnetic Resonance-Guided Percutaneous Cryosurgery of Breast Carcinoma: Technique and Early Clinical Results," *Can. J. Surg.*, Vol. 47, No. 5, 2004, pp. 347–351.

[57] Pusztaszeri, M., et al., "Histopathological Study of Breast Cancer and Normal Breast Tissue After Magnetic Resonance-Guided Cryotherapy Ablation," *Cryobiology*, Vol. 55, No. 1, 2007, pp. 44–51.

[58] Chin, J. L., D. Lim, and M. Abdelhady, "Review of Primary and Salvage Cryoablation for Prostate Cancer," *Cancer Control*, Vol. 14, No. 3, 2007, pp. 231–237.

[59] Marberger, M., "Energy-Based Ablative Therapy of Prostate Cancer: High-Intensity Focused Ultrasound and Cryoablation," *Curr. Opin. Urol.*, Vol. 17, No. 3, 2007, pp. 194–199.

[60] Ellis, D. S., T. B. Manny, Jr., and J. C. Rewcastle, "Cryoablation as Primary Treatment for Localized Prostate Cancer Followed by Penile Rehabilitation," *Urology*, Vol. 69, No. 2, 2007, pp. 306–310.

[61] Bahn, D. K., et al., "Focal Prostate Cryoablation: Initial Results Show Cancer Control and Potency Preservation," *J. Endourol.*, Vol. 20, No. 9, 2006, pp. 688–692.

[62] Chin, J. L., et al., "Randomized Trial Comparing Cryoablation and External Beam Radiotherapy for T2C-T3B Prostate Cancer," *Prostate Cancer Prostatic Dis.*, Vol. 11, No. 1, 2008, pp. 40–45.

[63] El Hayek, O. R., et al., "Percutaneous Prostate Cryoablation as Treatment for High-Risk Prostate Cancer," *Clinics*, Vol. 62, No. 2, 2007, pp. 109–112.

[64] Permpongkosol, S., et al., "Thermal Maps Around Two Adjacent Cryoprobes Creating Overlapping Ablations in Porcine Liver, Lung, and Kidney," *J. Vasc. Interv. Radiol.*, Vol. 18, No. 2, 2007, pp. 283–287.

CHAPTER 9

Gamma Knife Radiosurgery

Arjun Sahgal, Lijun Ma, May Tsao, and David Larson

The Gamma Knife is a precise minimally invasive radiation delivery system designed specifically for intracranial stereotactic radiosurgery. Like other image-guided radiotherapy systems, the goal of the Gamma Knife is to deliver a high dose of radiation to the target area while sparing adjacent normal brain tissue. Since the procedure requires a large dose of radiation delivered in a single treatment session, the design principles of the Gamma Knife system are significantly different from other radiotherapy devices. The distinctive features of the Gamma Knife include: (1) rigid skull fixation, (2) use of a large number of focal beams, (3) short source-to-focal distance, and (4) serial repositioning of the patient to achieve conformal dose distributions. In 2006, the latest Gamma Knife system, the Perfexion, was released and it represents a major innovation. This will be the focus of this review.

Radiosurgery refers to radiation therapy delivered in a single fraction, of a high biologically effective dose, to a small intracranial target (typically up to 3 to 5 cm) whose precise position and configuration is known in three dimensions. With the advent of new technologies such as MRI and CT image-guidance [1], stereoscopic X-ray imaging [2, 3], and robotic linear accelerators [4, 5], this approach has been extrapolated to the radiosurgical treatment of tumors beyond the brain using non-Gamma Knife technologies. Stereotactic body radiotherapy/radiosurgery is currently under investigation in many sites including the spine and lung [5–8]. This chapter will focus on intracranial radiosurgery with the Gamma Knife, a radiosurgery device designed specifically for treating brain indications. Gamma Knife technology has been in practice for at least 30 years with well-described tumor control and toxicity rates [9, 10]. The latest Gamma Knife unit, the Perfexion, was introduced in 2006 and will be discussed in detail.

9.1 History of the Gamma Knife Development

The Gamma Knife was initially designed to focus therapeutic radiation emitted from Colbalt-60 (^{60}Co) sources to create ablative focused lesions in the brain. This technology is based on the vision of Dr. Lars Leksell who invented the first stereotactic radiosurgery unit [11]. It is important to note that stereotactic refers to "spatial fixation," and this is achieved with the Gamma Knife using a stereotactic head frame. This invasive frame provides rigid immobilization of the head and localization of the target within a three-dimensional rectilinear coordinate system associated with the frame (x, y, and z axes).

Previous Gamma Knife Models

1968 Model S	1986 Model U	1987 Model B	1999 Model C	2004 Model 4C
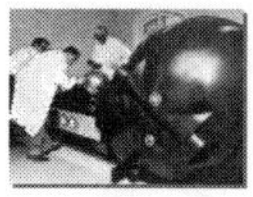	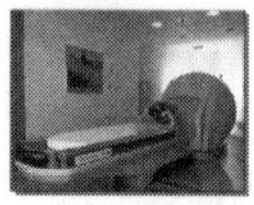	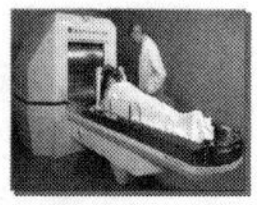	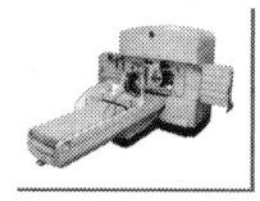	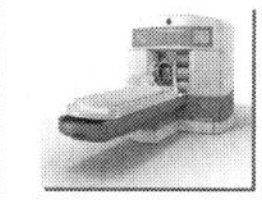
2 delivered	*27 delivered*	*127 delivered*	*152 delivered*	*49 delivered*
Sheffield, Buenos Aires	Decreased body dose Computer dose planning	New collimator design 1998 further decrease in body dose	Semi-robotic patient positioning Improved dose conformity	Still in production Improved software Merge/fusion capability

Figure 9.1 A pictorial of pre-2006 Gamma Knife units.

The Gamma Knife (manufactured by Elekta AB) consists of up to 201 ^{60}Co sources directed radially inward through beam-defining collimators to a common point of intersection (an *isocenter*). Each source emits gamma rays of an average energy of 1.25 MeV. With scores of intersecting beams centered on the target, the radiobiologic effective dose at the isocenter is very large and drops off rapidly within a few millimeters. Therefore, much of the brain receives a low and clinically insignificant dose. The dose rate at the isocenter is ~300 cGy/min. The distinctive features of Gamma Knife technology include: (1) rigid target fixation, (2) use of a large number of focal beams, (3) short source-to-focal distance, and (4) serial repositioning of the patient's head to achieve a conformal dose distribution.

Several Gamma Knife models based on this basic design premise have been produced over the years as illustrated in Figure 9.1. Key components of most pre-Perfexion models consist of 201 cobalt sources, 40-cm source-to-focal point distance, a movable couch, four collimator "helmets" consisting of 201 source collimator apertures that allow for beams of 4-, 8-, 14-, or 18-mm diameter (each helmet is designed to accommodate one beam diameter only), collimator plugs to block individual beam apertures, a console control unit, patient positioning and monitoring devices, and a computerized treatment planning system.

Linear accelerator (LINAC) based radiosurgery has also been used extensively and was developed in the 1980s. This approach requires a conventional LINAC modified with a tertiary circular collimator, or a micro-multileaf collimator (miMLC), and couch stabilizer system [12–15] (Figure 9.2). LINAC radiosurgery systems are designed to deliver noncoplanar converging beam arcs or dynamic rotation beams (with simultaneous gantry and couch rotation) at the isocenter. These systems are still in use in many centers around the world. There is yet to be any evidence that these systems provide inferior clinical outcomes or worse toxicities as compared to the Gamma Knife, though creation of complex isodose distributions to conform to nonspherical shapes is more challenging and limited as compared to the Gamma Knife.

As the Gamma Knife design evolved, the Gamma Knife Models B and C were the first to incorporate an automatic couch driving mechanism and a semi-

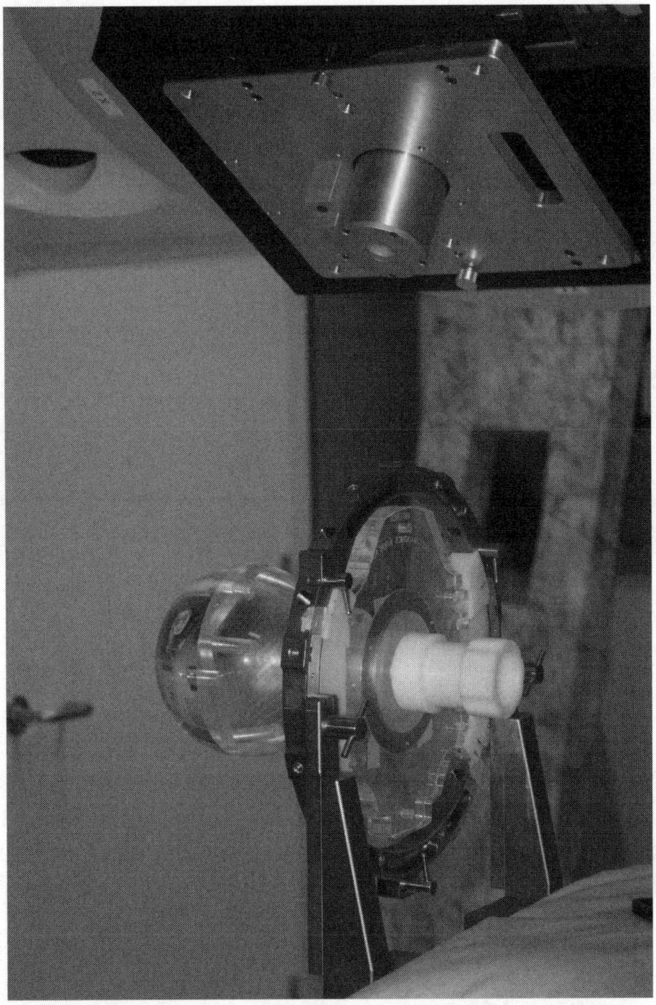

Figure 9.2 In-house stereotactic Lucy 3D QA Phantom (Standard Imaging, Inc.) developed at the Sunnybrook Odette Cancer Center. It is pictured mounted here with the Radionics BRW Head-Ring. The stereotactic cone assembly is in place in the accessory tray holder in the gantry above. (Figure provided by Dr. David Beachy, Sunnybrook Odette Cancer Center, University of Toronto, Toronto, Canada.)

automatic patient positioning assembly. For example, the Gamma Knife Model B and C patient positioning device consists of the Leksell G-frame [16] locked into an automatic positioning system (APS). The APS represented a major step forward in reducing treatment time as the patient no longer had to be manually shifted to every required isocenter position. The APS device uses three sets of micro stepping motors to position the stereotactic frame along three major orthogonal axes (x, y, and z axes) relative to the center of the helmet (the head position is automatically adjusted). The positional accuracy of the APS system is specified to be less than 0.2 mm, which is improved over the 0.5 mm accuracy of the manual setup assembly using trunnions and metal bars attached to the stereotactic frame. For treatment delivery, the couch moves the patient into the radiation unit and then docks the helmet with the center of the radiation unit to deliver the dose at isocenter. Once

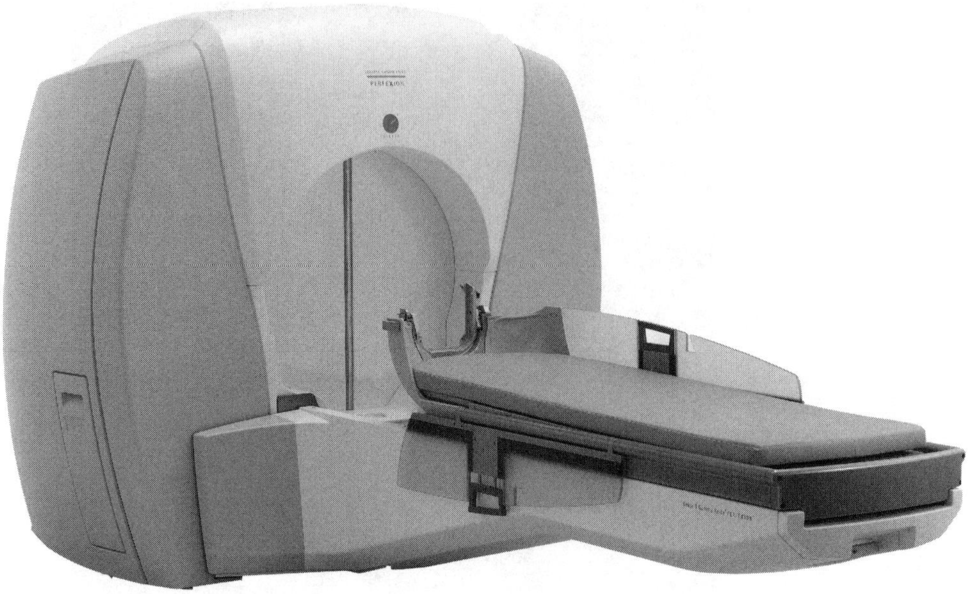

Figure 9.3 The Perfexion unit. (Figure provided by Elekta AB.)

finished, the couch retracts, and another set of the coordinates are positioned either manually or via the APS device for the additional delivery.

The newest generation of Gamma Knife systems, the Perfexion (Figure 9.3), was introduced in 2006 and represents a major design innovation, setting this unit apart fundamentally from prior models. The first units installed worldwide were in Marseille, France, London, England, and Fremont, California.

9.2 Mechanical Design of the Perfexion

A summary of the new design specifications is provided in Table 9.1, and will be briefly discussed. The unit now contains 192 ^{60}Co sources (instead of 201 ^{60}Co sources of prior models) arranged in a cone section configuration. This new cone-based design (as opposed to the prior hemispherical arrangement with helmets) with independently moving sectors of collimators results in varying source-to-isocenter distance (37.3 to 43.3 cm). Figure 9.4 illustrates a comparison of the previous hemispherical fixed collimator design to that of the Perfexion. The majority of the sources are closer to the isocenter than the prior design, resulting in a slightly greater dose rate for a given source activity.

The collimator system is based on a 12-cm-thick tungsten (apparently the world's largest machined piece of tungsten) collimator array, and during fabrication multiple rings of collimating holes are drilled directly into the one tungsten piece collimator creating three beam sizes of 16, 8, and 4 mm in diameter at the isocenter. There are thus 192 16-mm diameter collimators, 192 8-mm diameter collimators, and 192 4-mm diameter collimators. Just beyond the tungsten collimator assembly are eight sliding source sectors, each of which contains 24 sources. Figure 9.5 is an illustration representing the design relative to a patient's head.

Table 9.1 Summary of Current Design Specifications for the Perfexion

192 cobalt-60 sources
Single tungsten collimator with eight individual sectors of 4-, 8-, and 16-mm beam aperture size
Greater treatment range: 160 mm in the x and y dimension and 260 mm in the z dimension
The patient is automatically positioned to required isocenter positions without being shifted into a defocus position
Motorized couch for patient shifts to required isocenter positions (no APS system) with accuracy of <0.05 mm [42]
No collimator helmets
Greater ease of frame placement with a simple docking mechanism
Shielding doors move horizontally as opposed to vertically
Mechanical accuracy >0.5 mm over entire range [42]
LGP PFX treatment planning system:
No multiple matrices required
Dynamic shaping function allows easy blocking of OAR
Significantly lower extra-cranial doses as compared to prior Gamma Knife models

This unique independently moving sector design allows great flexibility in the number and diameter of beams intersecting at the isocenters. Furthermore, individual sectors can be blocked in order to conform the isodose distribution at the target (a Gamma Knife isodose distribution refers to a three-dimensional dose distribution in which the maximum dose within the designated target receives about twice the dose received by the edge of the target; this 50% isodose level conforms tightly around the target while minimizing the volume of normal brain tissue exposed to lower isodoses). All sector positions are adjusted with servo-controlled motors located in the sector drive unit. The introduction of the moving source design represents a paradigm shift in the Gamma Knife radiation transport system, as in all previous Gamma Knife models the sources are all encapsulated and fixed in space. Manual collimator helmet changes are no longer required, and intermediate

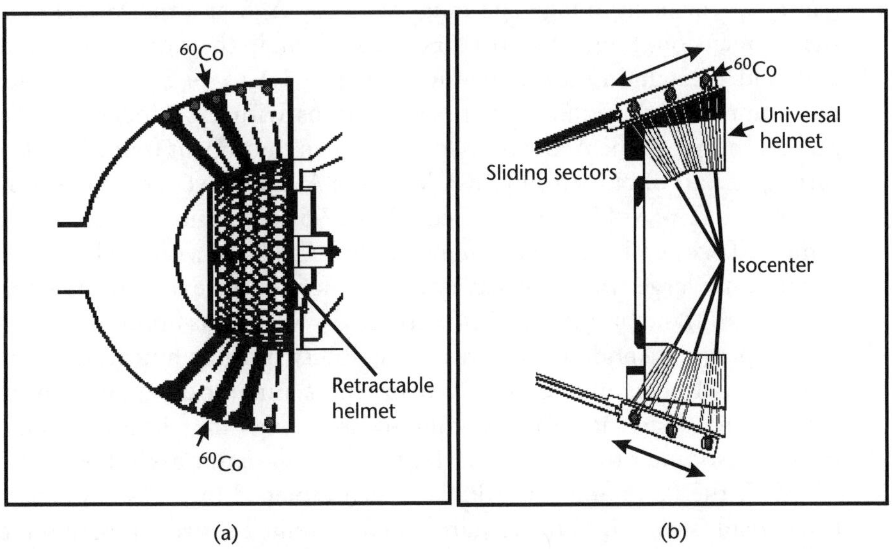

Figure 9.4 Illustration of design differences in beam transport and collimation process of (a) prior Gamma Knife models versus (b) the latest Perfexion system. (Figure provided by Elekta AB.)

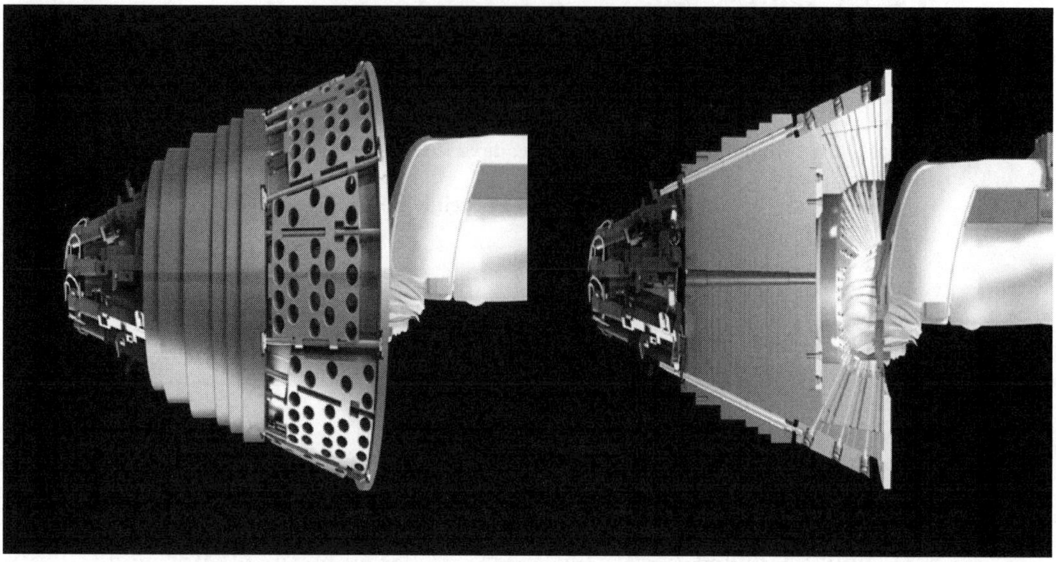

Figure 9.5 A schema of the conical collimator system with a cross-section illustrated on the left and the complete collimator in place on the right and both relative to a patient's head.

collimator sizes can be created within any sector by serially superimposing different collimator sizes with different relative weights (i.e., the beam-on time). Plugs are no longer required for beam shaping, as the blocking feature of individual sectors obviates the need of this time consuming process. Figure 9.6 illustrates a distribution outlining the 40% isodose to which 15 Gy was prescribed to, using the Perfexion, for this meningioma. The shot menu indicated for shot #3 the complexity of the collimation used where sectors of 4, 8, and 16 mm are used in addition to sector blocking (B).

For very lateral tumors, or for multiple tumors far apart within the brain, the APS system of the Gamma Knife Model C/4C required manual rather than automatic patient positioning. The range with the APS and the Model C is 8.2 cm in the x dimension (range, 5.9 to 14.1 cm), 12.0 cm in the y dimension (range, 4 to 16 cm), and 15.3 cm in the z dimension (range, –1.1 to 14.2 cm). Therefore, manual positioning is still required in these situations with the Model C/4C, and this requires removal of the APS unit following which the patient frame is locked manually through a pair of bars (trunnions). With the APS removed, the range now increases in the x (10 cm, 5–15) and y (15 cm, 2.5–17.5) dimension to accommodate lateral tumors. This step is time-consuming and not required with the Perfexion due to its significantly larger radiation cavity (which defines the extent of treatable target location within the brain). The Perfexion cavity volume is approximately three times that of previous models. The greater flexibility in the x and y range of ~16 cm (x range, 2 to 18 cm; and y range, 1 to 19 cm) is a major design improvement. In the z direction (along the patient's cranio-caudad axis) the physical distance is 26 cm from the isocenter to the inner surface of the collimator assembly.

With the Perfexion, the APS has been replaced by a system in which the entire patient is shifted to the required predetermined coordinates, and the treatment couch now serves as the patient positioning system (PPS). The stereotactic frame is anchored directly onto the couch top. For treatment delivery, the source sectors are

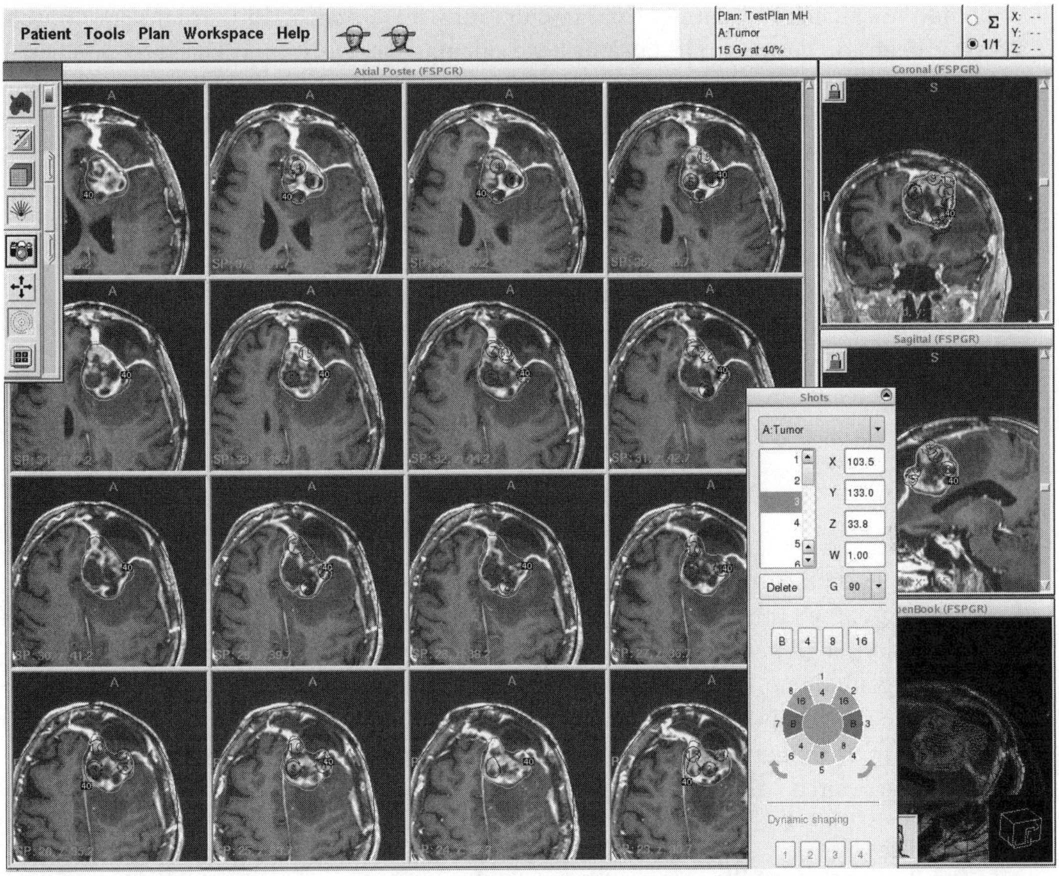

Figure 9.6 Shot menu from the LGP PFX treatment planning system indicating the various combinations of collimator selections for each of the eight sectors and ability to block sectors. (Figure provided by Dr. Mostafa Heydarian, Princess Margaret Hospital, University of Toronto, Toronto, Canada.)

initially in the off-position. Once the treatment couch has moved the patient to the specified coordinates, the source sectors slide into the designated collimation hole location (e.g., 16 mm, 8 mm, 4 mm, or off) within 3 seconds, and the dose is delivered to the patient. Once completed, the source sectors slide into the next position if a different beam configuration is required, and the couch repositions the patient to a new set of coordinates. The entire sequence repeats itself until the treatment finishes. Manual patient positioning is still required for head angulation, and the gamma angles available are 70, 90, and 110 degrees.

9.3 Treatment Planning

9.3.1 Principles

The Gamma Knife treatment planning process involves acquiring 3D imaging studies (CT, MR, or Digital Subtraction Angiography) of the brain, registering the 3D imaging studies with the patient frame coordinates, positioning single or multiple isocenters of different beams to create optimal 3D dose distributions, and exporting the calculated treatment parameters into the Gamma Knife treatment console for beam-on delivery. The current dose calculation algorithm is based on geometric ray-tracing plus empirical data of off-axis dose profiles of each collimator. The final dose distribution is typically normalized to the maximum dose inside the target volume.

Two parameters are commonly used to quantify the quality of the treatment plan. The first parameter is the maximum dose over prescription dose ratio (MDPD), which is defined as the ratio of maximum dose value over the prescription isodose value (e.g., if 50% of the maximum dose is used for the prescription isodose line, then the MDPD = 2). MDPD measures the dose uniformity inside the target. A large value of MDPD indicates a high degree of dose inhomogeneity.

The second parameter is conformity index (CI), which is defined as follows:

$$CI(p) = \frac{V_p}{V_t} \times \frac{V_{pt}}{V_t}$$

where V_p is the volume of the prescription isodose line, V_t is the target volume, and V_{pt} is the target volume that lies inside the selected isodose line. Based on this definition, a CI value of 1.0 means the prescription isodose line perfectly matches the target volume. One of the major goals of Gamma Knife treatment planning is to achieve the best possible CI for a given prescription isodose line. A typical CI value of 1.0 to 2.0 is generally considered acceptable for a Gamma Knife treatment plan and the desired value varies depending on the disease treated.

9.3.2 Treatment Planning with the Perfexion

The new treatment planning system, the Leksell GammaPlan PFX (LGP PFX), is a major advance. No longer are multiple matrices required in the planning of multiple tumors, and each target has its own prescribed dose. Within each of the eight sectors, individual collimator sizes can be selected to allow for shaping of the isodose distribution according to the target volume (Figure 9.6). This is a major advance leading to treatment planning of complex three-dimensional shapes with ease. Dose shaping around organs at risk (OAR) was previously based on a collimator plug patterns requiring manual placement into the collimator helmet, a now obsolete procedure. The Perfexion "dynamic shaping" function has made blocking of an OAR a much simpler process as the computer software designs the optimal beam use around what the operator defines as a OAR. The process of shaping a dose distribution around an OAR is now less time-consuming due to the sector blocking design, as opposed to manually plugging the collimator helmet to create the blocking pattern required.

9.4 Clinical Data

Initial Gamma Knife technology was conceptualized for the treatment of intractable cancer pain, craniopharyngioma, and pituitary adenoma. Today, a spectrum of malignant or benign tumors and functional disorders are treatable with radiosurgery and are comprehensively highlighted in Tables 9.2 to 9.4. Common indications will be discussed below in some detail.

9.4.1 Principles of Radiosurgery Dose Selection and Prediction of Outcome

Several factors influence the dose to prescribe and the outcome following radiosurgery. Fundamentally, the tumor volume/dimension is the most important factor in determining the dose to prescribe as one must balance the goal of tumor control against normal tissue toxicity [9]. Generally, the larger the tumor volume, the lower the dose prescribed. The Kjellberg risk prediction curve [17, 18] describes the risk of radionecrosis as a function of target volume and radiosurgical dose. Although the data on which this plot was derived is limited, the plot may help guide radiosurgical prescriptions in situations where clinical data is sparse and optimal dose is unknown.

Examples of other factors to consider can be categorized under patient, tumor, and treatment factors. An example of a *patient factor* to consider in predicting outcome is the patient's underlying medical condition. Consider the case of an acoustic neuroma in a neurofibromatosis type 2 patient. This population may have lower tumor control rates with radiosurgery as compared to patients with sporadic acoustics [19]. Factors relating to the patient's functional status should also be considered for patients treated for metastatic brain disease. There is considerable controversy as to the clinical benefit of radiosurgery alone or in conjunction with whole brain radiotherapy (WBRT) as a radiosurgical boost for elderly patients, and/or patients with poor performance status, and/or uncontrolled extracranial disease [20–22]. *Tumor factors* can influence the goals of radiosurgery treatment and the dose to prescribe. For example, in benign diseases such as acoustic neuromas, the aim of radiosurgery is to halt further growth of the tumor as opposed to a complete tumor radiographic response, and we prescribe a much lower dose than we would for metastatic disease [23]. *Treatment factors* such as prior embolization in patients with arteriovenous malformations (AVM) should be considered as there has been an association with a lower chance of complete obliteration following radiosurgery [24]. Common doses to prescribe for different tumor types and medical conditions are summarized in Tables 9.2 to 9.4.

Table 9.2 Typical Doses and Outcomes for Selected Benign Tumors

Indication	*Typical Doses (to periphery of target)**	*Results*
Acoustic neuroma	12–14 Gy	Tumor control: 87%–100% Facial nerve toxicity: 2% Trigeminal nerve toxicity: 5% Hearing preservation: 33%
Meningioma	12–14 Gy	Tumor control: ~90%
Arteriovenous malformation	15–25 Gy	Complete obliteration: ~70% Permanent neurologic complication: ~4%
Pituitary adenoma (nonfunctional)	14–16 Gy	Tumor control: 93%–100%
Pituitary adenoma (functional)	20–25 Gy	Hormone normalization: 80%

*Prescription doses may vary due to individual patient factors, target volume/characteristics, and doses to nearby critical structures.

Table 9.3 Typical Doses and Outcomes for Selected Malignant Tumors

Indication	*Typical Doses (to periphery of target)**	*Results*
Brain metastases	< 20 mm: 24 Gy 21–30 mm: 18 Gy 31–40 mm: 15 Gy	Overall brain control: 47%–92% (with whole brain radiotherapy) Overall brain control: 24% (with radiosurgery alone)
Recurrent glial tumors	< 20 mm: 24 Gy 21–30 mm: 18 Gy 31–40 mm: 15 Gy	Survivals variable. Small patient numbers reported
Chordoma/chondrosarcoma	12–20 Gy	Small patient numbers reported

*Prescription doses may vary due to individual patient factors, target volume/characteristics, and doses to nearby critical structures.

9.4.2 Benign Tumors

9.4.2.1 Acoustic Neuroma

Patients selected for radiosurgery have small acoustics which are generally less than 3 cm in diameter at the largest. A dose of 12 to 14 Gy to the periphery of an acoustic neuroma is associated with similar local control rates as compared to higher doses but with a much improved side-effect profile [23, 25–28]. Mature data have been reported by the Pittsburgh group who report on 216 patients treated with a marginal dose of 12 to 13 Gy and a median follow-up of 5.7 years [28]. They report a 10-year resection-free control rate of 98% [28]. For those with serviceable hearing, 44% maintained the same level of hearing and a 100% and 95% rate on unchanged facial nerve and trigeminal nerve function, respectively [28]. Whether fractionated stereotactic radiotherapy results in better hearing preservation rates is a matter of current debate [29].

9.4.2.2 Meningioma

Radiosurgery is used for selected patients with benign meningioma either as initial management or after previous treatment such as surgery or external fractionated radiation therapy. The optimal dose in the treatment of benign meningioma is unclear. There is a suggestion, however, that marginal doses at/or exceeding 15 Gy may not be associated with improved local control [30, 31]. Long-term data on 36 cranial base meningiomas with a mean follow-up of 103 months (10 to 133 months), and a median marginal dose of 17 Gy, reported a 94% tumor control rate (33% reduced in size) [32].

Table 9.4 Typical Doses and Outcomes for Selected Functional Disorders

Indication	*Doses (to Dmax)*	*Results*
Trigeminal neuralgia	70–80 Gy	60% complete pain relief (with or without medications) 2 years: 4% dysesthesias
Tremor	130 Gy at Dmax using 4 mm collimator	2 years: 87% clinically "good" results with no significant morbidity
Epilepsy	20–24 Gy marginal dose to medial temporal lobe	Ongoing analysis

9.4.2.3 Arteriovenous Malformations

Radiosurgery is an important tool in the treatment for AVM and in particular for deep AVM where surgery poses significant risk [33]. Other modalities used alone or in combination with radiosurgery include surgical resection and embolization. Optimal doses for AVMs are not clear. However, a dose response relationship, with higher doses resulting in a higher chance of complete obliteration, has been reported [34]. This is balanced by the risk of side-effects when using higher doses. As such, doses are often selected based on the volume of the nidus target, and based on the location of the nidus in terms of proximity to critical surrounding structures. A large experience of 400 AVMs treated by the University of Tokyo Hospital Group, with a median follow-up of 65 months and a median marginal dose of 20 Gy, reported obliteration rates of 82% at 5 years [35].

9.4.2.4 Pituitary Adenoma: Nonfunctional

Stereotactic radiosurgery can be used for the management of progressive or recurrent small, well-defined, pituitary adenomas. However, patients with tumors exhibiting significant suprasellar extent may not be good candidates for radiosurgery as the dose to the optic chiasm would be prohibitive. In these cases, surgical resection, fractionated stereotactic radiation therapy, or conformal external beam radiotherapy may be preferred.

In balancing tumor control with risk of pituitary hormone insufficiency, a dose of 14 to 16 Gy is typically used. The dose to tumor may be further lowered in order to keep the chiasm dose to safe levels (generally less than 8 to 10 Gy). Mature data has been recently reported by the Mayo Clinic, on 62 treated patients with a median follow-up of 64 months and a median marginal dose of 16 Gy. They report 95% tumor growth control at 7 years and 60% of the tumors had reduced in size. The actuarial risk of developing new anterior pituitary deficits at 5 years was 32% [36].

9.4.2.5 Pituitary Adenoma: Functional

For functional pituitary adenomas, the goals of treatment include hormone normalization and tumor control. In patients with acromegaly or pituitary prolactinomas, the Pittsburg Group reported that a maximum marginal tumor dose of at least 20 Gy (while respecting optic chiasm radiation tolerance) was associated in biochemical remission in approximately 80% of patients [37]. In 12 patients with growing ACTH producing pituitary adenomas (after bilateral adenalectomy), the use of radiosurgery was associated with 86% tumor growth control [37]. Twenty percent of patients may experience new anterior pituitary deficits. Other reported complications include temporal lobe necrosis, asymptomatic internal carotid artery stenosis, and unilateral blindness [37].

9.4.3 Malignant Tumors

9.4.3.1 Brain Metastases

Patients who were eligible for radiosurgery are typically those with small brain metastases and good performance status. Radiosurgery as a boost after whole brain radiotherapy results in improved local brain control as compared to whole brain radiotherapy alone based on a landmark Radiation Therapy Oncology Group (RTOG) randomized trial comparing WBRT versus WBRT plus a radiosurgery boost for patients with one to three brain metastases [20]. Despite the improvement in local control, this did not translate into an improvement in overall survival. A Japanese randomized trial comparing radiosurgery alone versus radiosurgery and whole brain radiotherapy for patients with one to four brain metastases reported no significant difference in overall survival between the two arms. However, overall brain control was significantly better upon the addition of whole brain radiotherapy [21].

Toxicity with combined WBRT and radiosurgery has been reported to be minimal. The RTOG 95-08 trial [20] reported that 6% of patients treated developed grades 3 and 4 late toxicities, while the Japanese reported a 5% risk of radionecrosis and leukoencephalopathy of the 65 patients treated with WBRT and radiosurgery. With radiosurgery alone, as studied in the Japanese randomized trial [21], of 67 patients treated only one patient developed radiation necrosis and one patient had a radiologic diagnosis of leukoencephalopathy. Whether radiosurgery alone is better in terms of quality of life and neurocognitive outcomes as compared to a combined approach remains uncertain. A recent randomized study comparing prophylactic WBRT to no WBRT for extensive stage small cell lung cancer patients reported significantly greater rates of fatigue, loss of appetite, nausea and vomiting, leg weakness, and a trend (nonsignificant difference, $p=0.07$) towards poorer cognitive function with WBRT [38].

Only one Phase 1 dose escalation study has been conducted for radiosurgery in patients with brain tumors less than 4 cm [9, 39]. These patients had prior external beam radiotherapy and the maximum tolerated dose for tumors less than 20 mm in size, between 21 to 30 mm in size, and 31 to 40 mm in size were 24, 18, and 15 Gy, respectively. In the less than 20 mm cohort the maximum tolerated dose was not reached at 24 Gy due to reluctance among the investigators for further dose escalation. These doses form the basis of radiosurgery dose prescriptions.

9.4.3.2 Glial Tumors

The use of a radiosurgery boost with external beam radiotherapy was examined by the RTOG trial 93-05, which randomized glioblastoma patients to external beam radiotherapy alone versus external beam radiotherapy and radiosurgery boost [40]. Both arms also included the use of BCNU chemotherapy. No difference in overall survival was observed with a median survival of 13.6 months in the external beam radiotherapy arm and 13.5 months in the radiosurgery boost arm. In general, radiosurgery boost as up-front treatment for glial tumors remains investigational.

For selected recurrent small glial tumors after previous standard external beam radiation therapy, radiosurgery may be offered. No randomized prospective trials have evaluated this therapeutic option for this indication (glial tumors at relapse). It remains unclear whether there is a survival benefit using radiosurgery as salvage as compared to competing strategies such as chemotherapy, debulking surgery, or best supportive care.

9.4.4 Functional Disorders

9.4.4.1 Trigeminal Neuralgia

Patients with typical trigeminal neuralgia may be offered radiosurgery for pain relief. The typical dose for this condition is 70 to 80 Gy prescribed to the maximum dose (Dmax or 100% isodose line) using a single 4-mm collimator [41]. Increasing the radiosurgical dose (70 Gy compared to 90 Gy), or the number of shots (1 or 2), has not produced an improvement in pain outcomes. The higher doses were associated with a significant increase in the rate of sensory complications [41].

Complete pain relief on or off pain-relieving medication occurs in approximately 75% of patients, but less than 60% maintain this outcome at 2 years [41]. Dysaesthesias affecting quality of life has been reported in 4% of patients treated with 70 Gy to Dmax.

9.5 Conclusion

Currently, a shift in paradigm exists with the development of the Perfexion Gamma Knife system [42]. This machine now allows: (1) the elimination of detachable helmets for beam collimation, (2) an expanded maneuvering space of the patient head, (3) increased delivery speed, and (4) improved flexibility of combining different beams of varying sizes from multiple directions. These developments will allow more isocenters to be used and therefore the capacity for more complex tightly shaped isodose dose distributions. The efficiency of the system will also likely increase the capacity for patient treatments at centers using this technology. The indications for radiosurgery continue to be an active area of research; however, radiosurgery is a standard of care for several indications.

References

[1] Chang, E. L., et al., "Phase I/II Study of Stereotactic Body Radiotherapy for Spinal Metastasis and Its Pattern of Failure," *J. Neurosurg. Spine*, Vol. 7, 2007, pp. 151–160.

[2] Ryu, S., et al., "Patterns of Failure After Single-Dose Radiosurgery for Spinal Metastasis," *J. Neurosurg.*, Vol. 101, Suppl. 3, 2004, pp. 402–405.

[3] Yin, F. F., et al., "A Technique of Intensity-Modulated Radiosurgery (IMRS) for Spinal Tumors," *Med. Phys.*, Vol. 29, 2002, pp. 2815–2822.

[4] Yu, C., et al., "An Anthropomorphic Phantom Study of the Accuracy of Cyberknife Spinal Radiosurgery," *Neurosurgery*, Vol. 55, 2004, pp. 1138–1149.

[5] Sahgal, A., et al., "Proximity of Spinous/Paraspinous Radiosurgery Metastatic Targets to the Spinal Cord Versus Risk of Local Failure," *Int. J. Radiat. Oncol. Biol. Phys.*, Vol. 69, 2007, p. S243.

[6] Sahgal, A., D. A. Larson, and E. L. Chang, "Stereotactic Body Radiosurgery for Spinal Metastases: A Critical Review," *Int. J. Radiat. Oncol. Biol. Phys.*, Vol. 71, 2008, pp. 652–665.

[7] Sahgal, A., et al., "Image-Guided Robotic Stereotactic Body Radiotherapy for Benign Spinal Tumors: The University of California San Francisco Preliminary Experience," *Technol. Cancer Res. Treat.*, Vol. 6, 2007, pp. 595–604.

[8] Timmerman, R. D., et al., "Stereotactic Body Radiation Therapy in Multiple Organ Sites," *J. Clin. Oncol.*, Vol. 25, 2007, pp. 947–952.

[9] Shaw, E., et al., "Single Dose Radiosurgical Treatment of Recurrent Previously Irradiated Primary Brain Tumors and Brain Metastases: Final Report of RTOG Protocol 90-05," *Int. J. Radiat. Oncol. Biol. Phys.*, Vol. 47, 2000, pp. 291–298.

[10] Kased, N., et al., "Gamma Knife Radiosurgery for Brainstem Metastases: The UCSF Experience," *J. Neurooncol.*, 2007.

[11] Leksell, L., "The Stereotaxic Method and Radiosurgery of the Brain," *Acta Chir. Scand.*, Vol. 102, 1951, pp. 316–319.

[12] Bourland, J. D., and K. P. McCollough, "Static Field Conformal Stereotactic Radiosurgery: Physical Techniques," *Int. J. Radiat. Oncol. Biol. Phys.*, Vol. 28, 1994, pp. 471–479.

[13] Lutz, W., K. R. Winston, and N. Maleki, "A System for Stereotactic Radiosurgery with a Linear Accelerator," *Int. J. Radiat. Oncol. Biol. Phys.*, Vol. 14, 1988, pp. 373–381.

[14] Podgorsak, E. B., et al., "Dynamic Stereotactic Radiosurgery," *Int. J. Radiat. Oncol. Biol. Phys.*, Vol. 14, 1988, pp. 115–126.

[15] Leavitt, D. D., et al., "Intensity-Modulated Radiosurgery/Radiotherapy Using a Micromultileaf Collimator," *Med. Dosim.*, Vol. 26, 2001, pp. 143–150.

[16] Leksell, L., et al., "A New Fixation Device for the Leksell Stereotaxic System. Technical Note," *J. Neurosurg.*, Vol. 66, 1987, pp. 626–629.

[17] Kjellberg, R. N., et al., "Bragg-Peak Proton-Beam Therapy for Arteriovenous Malformations of the Brain," *N. Engl. J. Med.*, Vol. 309, 1983, pp. 269–274.

[18] Kjellberg, R. N., et al., "Proton-Beam Therapy in Acromegaly," *N. Engl. J. Med.*, Vol. 278, 1968, pp. 689–695.

[19] Mathieu, D., et al., "Stereotactic Radiosurgery for Vestibular Schwannomas in Patients with Neurofibromatosis Type 2: An Analysis of Tumor Control, Complications, and Hearing Preservation Rates," *Neurosurgery*, Vol. 60, 2007, pp. 460–468.

[20] Andrews, D. W., et al., "Whole Brain Radiation Therapy with or Without Stereotactic Radiosurgery Boost for Patients with One to Three Brain Metastases: Phase III Results of the RTOG 9508 Randomised Trial," *Lancet*, Vol. 363, 2004, pp. 1665–1672.

[21] Aoyama, H., et al., "Stereotactic Radiosurgery Plus Whole-Brain Radiation Therapy vs. Stereotactic Radiosurgery Alone for Treatment of Brain Metastases: A Randomized Controlled Trial," *JAMA*, Vol. 295, 2006, pp. 2483–2491.

[22] Mehta, M. P., et al., "The American Society for Therapeutic Radiology and Oncology (ASTRO) Evidence-Based Review of the Role of Radiosurgery for Brain Metastases," *Int. J. Radiat. Oncol. Biol. Phys.*, Vol. 63, 2005, pp. 37–46.

[23] Flickinger, J. C., D. Kondziolka, and L. D. Lunsford, "Dose and Diameter Relationships for Facial, Trigeminal, and Acoustic Neuropathies Following Acoustic Neuroma Radiosurgery," *Radiother. Oncol.*, Vol. 41, 1996, pp. 215–219.

[24] Andrade-Souza, Y. M., et al., "Embolization Before Radiosurgery Reduces the Obliteration Rate of Arteriovenous Malformations," *Neurosurgery*, Vol. 60, 2007, pp. 443–451.

[25] Weil, R. S., et al., "Optimal Dose of Stereotactic Radiosurgery for Acoustic Neuromas: A Systematic Review," *Br. J. Neurosurg.*, Vol. 20, 2006, pp. 195–202.

[26] Flickinger, J. C., et al., "Acoustic Neuroma Radiosurgery with Marginal Tumor Doses of 12 to 13 Gy," *Int. J. Radiat. Oncol. Biol. Phys.*, Vol. 60, 2004, pp. 225–230.

[27] Andrews, D. W., et al., "Stereotactic Radiosurgery and Fractionated Stereotactic Radiotherapy for the Treatment of Acoustic Schwannomas: Comparative Observations of 125 Patients Treated at One Institution," *Int. J. Radiat. Oncol. Biol. Phys.*, Vol. 50, 2001, pp. 1265–1278.

[28] Chopra, R., et al., "Long-Term Follow-Up of Acoustic Schwannoma Radiosurgery with Marginal Tumor Doses of 12 to 13 Gy," *Int. J. Radiat. Oncol. Biol. Phys.*, Vol. 68, 2007, pp. 845–851.

[29] Szumacher, E., et al., "Fractionated Stereotactic Radiotherapy for the Treatment of Vestibular Schwannomas: Combined Experience of the Toronto-Sunnybrook Regional Cancer

Centre and the Princess Margaret Hospital," *Int. J. Radiat. Oncol. Biol. Phys.*, Vol. 53, 2002, pp. 987–991.

[30] Kondziolka, D., J. C. Flickinger, and B. Perez, "Judicious Resection and/or Radiosurgery for Parasagittal Meningiomas: Outcomes from a Multicenter Review," Gamma Knife Meningioma Study Group, *Neurosurgery*, Vol. 43, 1998, pp. 405–413.

[31] Flickinger, J. C., et al., "Gamma Knife Radiosurgery of Imaging-Diagnosed Intracranial Meningioma," *Int. J. Radiat. Oncol. Biol. Phys.*, Vol. 56, 2003, pp. 801–806.

[32] Zachenhofer, I., et al., "Gamma-Knife Radiosurgery for Cranial Base Meningiomas: Experience of Tumor Control, Clinical Course, and Morbidity in a Follow-Up of More Than 8 Years," *Neurosurgery*, Vol. 58, 2006, pp. 28–36.

[33] Andrade-Souza, Y. M., et al., "Radiosurgery for Basal Ganglia, Internal Capsule, and Thalamus Arteriovenous Malformation: Clinical Outcome," *Neurosurgery*, Vol. 56, 2005, pp. 56–63.

[34] Karlsson, B., I. Lax, and M. Soderman, "Can the Probability for Obliteration After Radiosurgery for Arteriovenous Malformations Be Accurately Predicted?" *Int. J. Radiat. Oncol. Biol. Phys.*, Vol. 43, 1999, pp. 313–319.

[35] Shin, M., et al., "Analysis of Nidus Obliteration Rates After Gamma Knife Surgery for Arteriovenous Malformations Based on Long-Term Follow-Up Data: The University of Tokyo Experience," *J. Neurosurg.*, Vol. 101, 2004, pp. 18–24.

[36] Pollock, B. E., et al., "Gamma Knife Radiosurgery for Patients with Nonfunctioning Pituitary Adenomas: Results from a 15-Year Experience," *Int. J. Radiat. Oncol. Biol. Phys.*, Vol. 70, 2008, pp. 1325–1329.

[37] Szeifert, G., et al., "Radiosurgery and Pathological Fundamentals," *Prog. Neurol. Surg. Ed. Basel: Karger*, Vol. 20, 2007.

[38] Slotman, B., et al., "Prophylactic Cranial Irradiation in Extensive Small-Cell Lung Cancer," *N. Engl. J. Med.*, Vol. 357, 2007, pp. 664–672.

[39] Buatti, J. M., et al., "RTOG 90-05: The Real Conclusion," *Int. J. Radiat. Oncol. Biol. Phys.*, Vol. 47, 2000, pp. 269–271.

[40] Souhami, L., et al., "Randomized Comparison of Stereotactic Radiosurgery Followed by Conventional Radiotherapy with Carmustine to Conventional Radiotherapy with Carmustine for Patients with Glioblastoma Multiforme: Report of Radiation Therapy Oncology Group 93-05 Protocol," *Int. J. Radiat. Oncol. Biol. Phys.*, Vol. 60, 2004, pp. 853–860.

[41] Lopez, B. C., P. J. Hamlyn, and J. M. Zakrzewska, "Stereotactic Radiosurgery for Primary Trigeminal Neuralgia: State of the Evidence and Recommendations for Future Reports," *J. Neurol. Neurosurg. Psychiatry*, Vol. 75, 2004, pp. 1019–1024.

[42] Lindquist, C., and I. Paddick, "The Leksell Gamma Knife Perfexion and Comparisons with Its Predecessors," *Neurosurgery*, Vol. 61, 2007, pp. 130–140.

CHAPTER 10

Ultrasound Mediated Drug and Gene Delivery

Victor Frenkel

Therapeutic ultrasound is best known for its ability to thermally ablate tissue, which has been shown to be effective for the treatment of tumors and uterine fibroids. Nondestructive exposures, however, may be used for enhancing drug and gene delivery, where the mechanisms for doing so are predominantly nonthermal. Presently, low intensity, nonfocused beams are being used in physical therapy for enhancing local transdermal delivery of therapeutically beneficial agents. However, there is a multitude of preclinical examples in the literature demonstrating how focused ultrasound beams can be used to generate increases in the permeability of deeper tissues for enhancing the delivery of conventional agents, as well as for deploying and activating drugs and genes using specially tailored vehicles and formulations. In this chapter, the development of these applications will be described and an emphasis will be placed on the relevant ultrasound mechanisms involved. By using image guidance to deliver the ultrasound energy safely and efficiently for these applications, therapeutic ultrasound holds much promise to further the treatment of cancer and other diseases.

10.1 Introduction

Precisely half a century has passed since the first therapeutic ultrasound application was demonstrated. Using a simple multielement device to concentrate the ultrasound energy, William Fry and his colleagues showed that they could produce precise focal lesions within the central nervous system of animals. Although craniotomies were required for the procedures, the results demonstrated the potential of therapeutic ultrasound and heralded a new era in biomedical research and development [1]. Not long afterward the procedure showed its suitability for human treatment when used to selectively ablate regions of the basal ganglia in patients with Parkinson's disease [2]. Today, a variety of tissues are being treated by this process, including uterine fibroids and tumors of different types such as those in the breast and prostate [3]. The devices used to deliver the energy deep into the body rely on sophisticated image guidance systems based diagnostic ultrasound and magnetic resonance imaging (MRI), allowing for delineation of the tissue to be targeted, and therefore accurate and safe treatment planning. Furthermore, these imaging modalities also enable validation that proper treatment has been carried out by monitoring for tissue boiling (looking for high echogenicity of the tissues) as with ultrasound, or employing

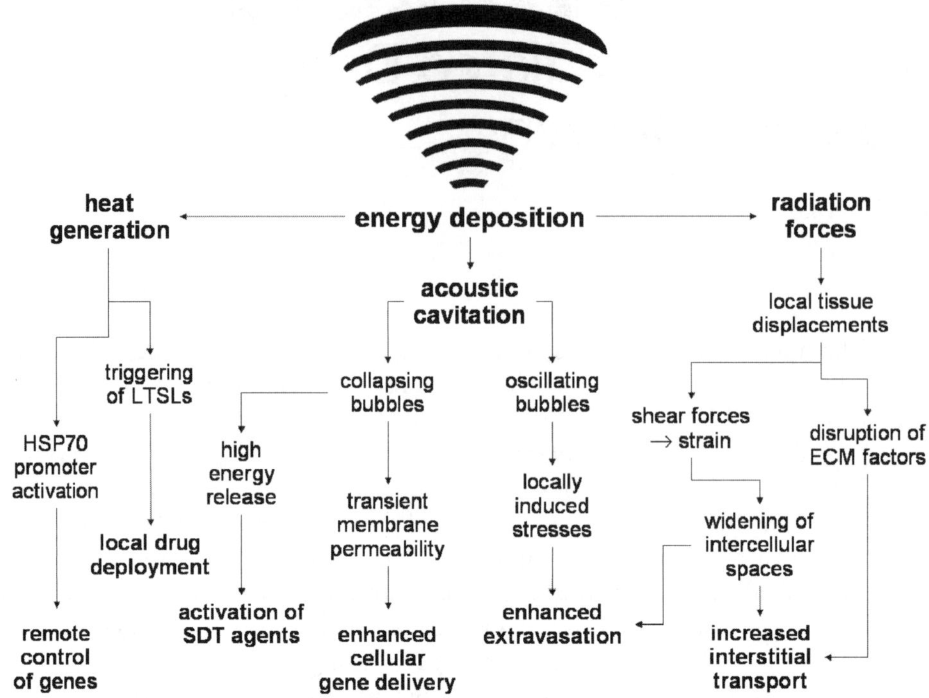

Figure 10.1 A schematic representation showing how energy deposited by focused ultrasound exposures can, through various mechanisms, enhance the delivery or activity of drugs and genes. ECM: extracellular matrix; HSP: heat shock protein; LTSLs: low temperature sensitive liposomes; SDT: sonodynamic therapy.

thermal mapping capabilities as with MRI to validate that the correct thermal dose (TD) has been delivered. Some MR guided systems can actually employ feedback loops to automatically compensate for tissue inhomogeneities and in that way enable real-time correction of exposure duration to provide the correct TD.

Whereas ablation requires relatively high rates of energy to be deposited in order to irreversibly destroy tissue, today a variety of therapeutic ultrasound applications are being developed using relatively lower rates of energy deposition. These employ pulsed exposures that lower the temporal-averaged intensity and therefore limit the rate of energy deposition. As a consequence temperature elevations can be lowered below the cytotoxic level and mechanisms more mechanical in nature will prevail for ultrasound/tissue interactions that are typically nondestructive. The majority of these applications involve improving the delivery of drugs and genes to targeted tissues, or activating these agents using a variety of novel carriers or formulations (see Figure 10.1). In this chapter, these applications will be reviewed and described in context of the ultrasound mechanisms that make them possible.

10.2 Ultrasound Mechanisms for Enhancing Drug and Gene Delivery

10.2.1 Heat Generation

The generation of heat is the best-known mechanism of ultrasound for producing bioeffects, and clearly the best understood. Heat generation occurs from the absorption of energy, where the volumetric rate of heating is directly proportional to the specific absorption coefficient of the tissue being treated, as well as the frequency and intensity of the ultrasound wave, and inversely proportional to the specific heat of that particular tissue, as well as its density [4]. The amount of heat that will be generated, and the temperature elevation that will ultimately occur, is dependant on the tissue's own heat diffusion coefficient and convective heat loss from the vasculature, where heating itself can increase perfusion. At tissue interfaces, discontinuities in impedance will generate even greater heat [5], and also if acoustic cavitation is occurring, where bubbles will increase the absorption of acoustic energy [6]. In certain circumstances, where changes in the tissue occur due to heating itself (e.g., coagulation for ablative exposures), or if there is boiling and/or nonlinear propagation of the acoustic wave, the process of heating can become even more complex, and consequently even more difficult to predict [7].

10.2.2 Acoustic Cavitation

Acoustic cavitation is considered the most important of all the nonthermal ultrasound mechanisms in regards to its potential for producing effects in biological tissues, especially those that enhance drug delivery. Cavitation has been broadly defined as the growth, oscillation, and collapse of small stabilized gas bubbles in a fluid medium in response to the varying pressure field of a sound wave [8]. Cavitating bubbles in an ultrasound field grow by the process of rectified diffusion, where the net amount of gas diffusing into a bubble during its expansion is greater than that diffusing out during contraction. This type of activity can be divided into two distinct types: (1) stable (i.e., noninertial) cavitation bubbles persist for a relatively large number of acoustic cycles, where the bubble radius will vary about an equilibrium value, determined by the driving frequency; and (2) transient (i.e., inertial) cavitation bubbles will grow faster, expanding two to three times their resonant size, oscillating unstably, and finally collapsing in a single compression half-cycle [9]. It has been proposed that damage to biological tissues can potentially occur from the activity of stable cavitation bubbles [10]. However, it is generally accepted that the main mechanism for creating structural changes in intact cells is inertial cavitation, where these changes include nondestructive increases in membrane permeability [11] and also irreversible damage [12].

The most important factors that have been identified to affect acoustic cavitation are the number and availability of small stabilized gas bubbles (cavitation nuclei) [8, 11]. An increase in cavitation activity will occur with an increase in the number of nuclei available [13], being ubiquitous in nondegassed water and other liquids, but scarce in animal tissues [8]. The available physical space for bubbles to form and grow is another important factor that will determine whether cavitation will occur or not. As a result of these factors, it is difficult to induce cavitation within cells and the extracellular matrix [14]. Conversely, the vasculature possesses both cavitation nuclei and the required dimensions to enable cavitation to occur when the ultrasound pressure fields is high enough. Indeed, it is the peak rarefractional pressure of the ultrasound exposure that controls the onset of cavitation [13].

A variety of phenomena can occur when a cavitating bubble collapses in an open medium. Large increases in localized temperature occur at the point of collapse, which can cause thermal dissociation of water molecules and the consequent formation of hydroxyl molecules [9]. The types of "sonochemical" effects that may result from the formation of free radicals include damage to DNA (in aqueous solution), inactivation of proteins and enzymes, and peroxidation of lipids (including those in the cell membrane) [12].

By far the most pronounced effects of inertial cavitation will occur when a bubble collapses near a rigid boundary, while surrounded by body of fluid that is relatively large in comparison to the bubble diameter [13]. Compared to a bubble collapsing in an open medium (as described above), the boundary will impose constraints in fluid flow causing the bubble to collapse asymmetrically. The far side of the bubble will impact and penetrate the bubble surface closest to the boundary, generating what has been called a wall-direct re-entrant [15], where pressures can be as high as 10^9 Pa and jet velocities greater than 100 m s^{-1} [16]. Jet formation has been captured using high speed photography, as well as the manner by which these may compress and crack tissue surfaces [17], and render them pitted and damaged [17, 18]. For a comprehensive review on acoustic cavitation, see Kimmel [13].

10.2.3 Acoustic Radiation Forces

When providing ultrasound exposures at relatively high amplitudes, phenomena associated with nonlinear acoustics will typically occur. Under such conditions a transfer of momentum may result from the ultrasound wave to the medium, generating a unidirectional force in the direction of the propagating wave; also known as a radiation force. These forces are proportional to the rate of energy being applied and the absorption coefficient of the medium, while inversely proportional to the speed of sound of the ultrasound wave in the medium [4]. If large enough, radiation forces are capable of causing local displacements of tissue in the region of the focal zone of the HIFU beam, where the degree of displacement is primarily determined by the elastic (Young's) modulus of the tissue [19]. Radiation forces can produce motion in a fluid medium in the form of a steady flow (also known as acoustic streaming) [4]. The velocity of the stream will be proportional to the ultrasound intensity, the surface area of the transducer, and the attenuation coefficient of the medium, and inversely proportional to the medium's bulk viscosity and speed of sound [20]. Acoustic streaming has been shown to reduce heating from exposures to ultrasound, by increasing convective heat loss [21], and also increasing mass transport of nanoparticles for improved transdermal delivery [22, 23].

10.3 Applications

10.3.1 Sonophoresis

Although enhancing transdermal delivery with ultrasound (i.e., sonophoresis) does not require image guidance, this procedure does deserve mention; especially since it is presently the only one being used in the clinic for ultrasound mediated delivery. Investigations on using ultrasound to enhance drug delivery through the skin have been ongoing for more than half a century. The advantage of such a technique is achieving needle-free drug delivery, where low intensity exposures are given using nonfocused plane-wave transducers applied directly to the body [24]. The most important transport barrier for delivering drugs transdermally is the outer-most layer of the skin, the stratum corneum (SC) [25]. Studies into the mechanisms of this technique have indicated that acoustic cavitation acts to disrupt the lipid bilayers of the SC to create channels for improved transport through it. In addition to local applications of sonophoresis, such as the delivery of anti-inflammatory agents [24] and analgesics [26], that are already being used in the clinic, preclinical investigations have shown enhanced delivery of various large molecules such as insulin [27] and vaccines [28]. Kost et al. [29] have also demonstrated how the permeability enhancing effects of these exposures on the skin can be used to extract analytes from the skin and consequently monitor glucose noninvasively. Similar exposures have also been employed to enhance transport across the cornea of various molecules, where increased permeability of the cornea's stroma appears to occur from minor, and reversible, structural alterations created in the epithelium. This type of direct ocular drug delivery is presently being developed to treat diseases such as glaucoma [30–32]. Controlled exposures at an epithelial-fluid interface have also been shown to produce controlled levels of tissue erosion, where the rate limiting factor for its progression was found to be the diffusion rate of cavitation nuclei from the fluid through the disrupted tissue [18]. Exposures of this type were found to enhance the tissue's permeability to the inward flux of nanoparticles, and may potentially be used for the relatively new field of ultrasound mediated delivery in moist epithelial tissues [22]. For an in-depth review on sonophoresis, see Mitragotri and Kost [33].

10.3.2 Blood Brain Barrier Disruption

Advances in multimodality imaging, along with multielement array transducers, have enabled the development of prototype devices for accurately and safely carrying out high intensity focused ultrasound (HIFU) exposures directly through the intact skull [34]. In addition to using these exposures for ablating tissue [35], they can also be used for disrupting the blood brain barrier (BBB) with [36] and without [37] the addition of contrast agents (UCAs). UCAs are typically protein or lipid based microbubbles (on the order of a few microns in diameter) that contain air or gas, providing high echogenicity, and generally used for ultrasound imaging of the vasculature. Administering UCAs to the vasculature, which serve as cavitation nuclei, enable more predictable activity of acoustic cavitation and lowers the intensity threshold for its onset [37]. Although not precisely known, the mechanism by which this procedure enhances delivery is thought to be related to the stabile oscillation of cavitating bubbles, which generate mechanical stress in the blood vessel walls to increase their permeability, while causing little or no damage to the brain tissue itself. This process is reversible, and could potentially enable the delivery of other therapeutic agents to the brain (e.g., thrombolytic agents, and also new compounds to treat chronic brain diseases) that are not normally able to passively penetrate in to it. The standard image guidance modality for these types of exposures is with MRI [34], where the procedure has been shown to effectively facilitate the delivery of MR contrast agents [38], antibodies [39], and liposomal doxorubicin [40]. For a more comprehensive review on BBB disruption, see Hynynen [41].

10.3.3 Thrombolysis

Ultrasound has been used to enhance thrombolysis, both on its own and with the addition of thrombolytic agents [42]. Clot dissolution may be carried out using invasive strategies such as catheter-delivered transducer devices [43], or using noninvasive devices such as transcutaneous Doppler transducers [44]. Regarding the use of ultrasound to enhance the efficacy of thrombolytic agents, a number of in vitro studies have been carried out to elucidate the mechanisms by which this improved activity is achieved. The consensus of these studies is that nonthermal mechanisms are primarily, if not exclusively, involved; especially acoustic cavitation. Studies in fibrin gels, and later in clots, have demonstrated how ultrasound can induce reversible fiber disaggregation [45], improve fluid flow [46], and consequently enhance the penetration of tissue plasminogen activator (tPA) [47]. Furthermore, in vivo studies using UCAs showed that addition of these bubbles could improve ultrasound mediated thrombolysis, both with [48, 49] and without [50] thrombolytic agents. Novel strategies using ultrasound for thrombolysis continue to be developed, such as loading tPA into echogenic liposomes, where the agent is then released locally within clots with an ultrasound exposure [51].

In the studies mentioned above, relatively low rates of ultrasound energy deposition were being used. More recently, pulsed-HIFU exposures have demonstrated the ability to noninvasively enhance tPA mediated thrombolysis. In vitro studies have shown how pretreatment of clots with these exposures make the clots more permeable to enable improved binding and penetration of tPA [52]. By producing these effects, improved rates of thrombolysis were found compared to using only tPA, where the results were corroborated by higher D-dimer levels with HIFU and tPA, compared to tPA alone [53]. Follow-up studies in rabbits, using a novel clot model in the marginal ear vein, demonstrated that significantly improved thrombolytic rates using the same exposures could be reproduced in vivo. Preliminary histological analysis showed the exposures to be safe, where no deleterious effects occurred in the endothelium of the treated vessels, or in the surrounding tissue [54]. See Pfaffenberger et al. [42] for an in-depth review of ultrasound mediated thrombolysis.

10.3.4 Gene Delivery

Sonoporation

Inertial cavitation (i.e., collapsing bubbles) can be employed to transiently enhance the permeability of individual cells for improving the delivery of genes and drugs. This process has been coined sonoporation, since it uses sound energy, instead of electrical energy (for electroporation), to produce pores to enhance the permeability of cellular membranes. The fact that pores can be created in cell membranes in a nonlethal manner is not surprising since the fatty acids in the membranes tend to associate with one another and exclude water [55]. Fechheimer et al. [56] first demonstrated the process of sonoporation by exposing a cell suspension of live slime mold amoebae in the presence of dextrans labeled with fluorescein, which, because of their size, were normally impermeable to the cells. As a result of the ultrasound exposures, the fluorophore was taken up in approximately 40% of the cells. Soon afterwards, this process was then shown to also be suitable for use in mammalian cells for delivering DNA [57], and consequently opened up an entire new field of endeavor for using ultrasound to enhance gene delivery.

The mechanisms behind sonoporation have only recently been described with the assistance of suitable technological advances. Ohl et al. [58] used high speed photography to demonstrate the formation of wall-direct re-entrant jets, due to asymmetrical bubble collapse (as described above), that are associated with delivery of molecules to individual cells. Image capture at frame rates higher than the ultrasonic frequency enabled visualizing the direct correlation between cell deformation and consequent alterations in cell membrane permeability [59]. Other techniques have also been developed to shed light on this process. For example, Deng et al. [60] measured increases in transmembrane current in Xenopus oocytes, which indirectly proved the formation of pores, whose presence would cause a decrease in membrane resistance. Many studies (especially those in vitro) have reported how sonoporation can be made more efficient by the addition of UCAs, where these stabilized microbubbles serve as cavitation nucleation agents [59]. Adding UCAs is especially crucial for in vivo applications for improving transfection, where a dearth of cavitation nucleation sites limits this process.

Cardiovascular System

In the majority of preclinical studies, the technique of choice for enhancing gene delivery is to infuse naked DNA into an isolated vessel, followed by local ultrasound exposures of various modalities (e.g., focused, nonfocused, and intraluminal). Naked DNA is the simplest nonviral gene delivery system, being easy and inexpensive to produce [61], and possessing low toxicity and immunogenicity [62]. It is, however, considered to be unsuitable for systemic administration because of the presence of serum nucleases [63], and on its own it produces overall lower levels of expression compared to viral vectors or nonviral, liposomal vectors.

The advantage of this kind of a procedure is that transfection is restricted to a specific target tissue or organ, which is essential, for example, when using suicide genes that do not possess any targeting factors such as tissue specific promoters. Another advantage is that less DNA and UCAs (if being used) will be required and that these agents will be concentrated for increasing transfection efficiency. Combining ultrasound exposures with plasmid DNA and UCAs to enhance local gene transfection in an isolated blood vessel was demonstrated by Hashiya et al. [64], where a catheter-based ultrasound device was used in a rat carotid artery. In a second study, noninvasive pulsed-HIFU exposures were used in combination with plasmid DNA infused into isolated segments of the carotid artery of rabbits. Compared to minimal levels of gene expression detected when just administering the DNA alone, exposures significantly enhanced expression, and were further enhanced when UCAs were added, indicating sonoporation as an active mechanism for transfection. The addition of UCAs also lowered the intensity threshold for inducing damage in the treated vessels, which occurred in the form of visible hemorrhages in the vessel walls [65]. By far, the greatest interest for the use of sonoporation is in gene therapy applications for treating ailments of the cardiovascular system. In one study, for example, this procedure was used to enhance delivery of E2F decoy oligodeoxynucleotides, resulting in improved inhibition of intimal hyperplasia following balloon injury in a carotid artery model in rats [64]. Another potential application is for the delivery of genes for increasing vascularization of the heart muscle in order to ameliorate congestive heart failure [66].

Although sonoporation is a reversible process, and therefore nondestructive, cavitation activity (especially inertial cavitation) is extremely nonuniform and hard to control, where some of the cells that are exposed will ultimately undergo irreversible damage that leads to cell death [18]. Substantial increases in tissue temperature can also occur as a result of the cavitation during ultrasound exposures [6, 67], and temperature elevations capable of harming cells may also occur from viscous dissipation in the coating of UCAs [68]. For a comprehensive review on using sonoporation for gene delivery, see Miller [69].

Other Tissues/Organs

Using pulsed-HIFU to enhance delivery and consequent therapeutic effects of locally administered DNA has also been shown in other tissue models. Schratzberger et al. [70] injected the gene for beta-galactosidase directly into ischemic hind limbs of rabbits and found expression levels to increase when administrations were followed by pulsed-HIFU exposures. Increased levels of expression were also observed when exposures were given prior to injections; however, these were lower than when exposures followed the administrations. An improvement in neovascularization was then achieved when the reporter gene was substituted with that for vascular endothelial growth factor (VEGF). In a second study, DNA for human factor IX (for the treatment of hemophilia B) was injected directly into the liver of mice and then followed by pulsed-HIFU exposures. Significant increases in gene expression occurred using this procedure in comparison to injection alone. Further increases were found with the addition of UCAs. Increased levels of expression were correlated with higher peak negative pressure of the exposures, but not as well with longer pulse duration. Above a pressure threshold, damage was observed in the liver; however, this was transient and was found to be reversed in a matter of days [71].

Solid Tumors

For most advanced cancers the treatment of choice is chemotherapy, even though it is rarely curative, especially for solid tumors [72]. Although the large variety of anticancer agents are effective for killing tumor cells in monolayers, grown in culture, in vivo they are unable to reach all cells that are able to regenerate the tumors [73]. Decades of meticulous study of the microenvironment of solid tumors has enabled the identification of a number of factors responsible for nonuniform and insufficient levels of anti-cancer agents being delivered. These are mainly the result of abnormalities in both the vasculature and the extracellular matrix, leading to deficiencies in transvascular and interstitial transport, respectively [74], which ultimately affects the bioavailability and consequent efficacy of chemotherapeutic agents [75]. In order to overcome these barriers for uniform and adequate drug delivery, considerable effort has gone in to modifying the tumor microenvironment. For example, McKee et al. [76] recently showed that the co-injecting of collagenase with an oncolytic virus in human melanoma xenografts in mice improved interstitial distribution of the virus and consequently enhanced growth inhibition of the tumors compared to the virus on its own. Increasing infusion pressures of local administration of viral vectors may also improve distribution for obtaining similar results [74]. Other physical techniques, such as hyperthermia, have been shown to increase extravasation of liposomes by apparently modulating organization of the endothelium [77]. In this and the next section a variety of strategies will be described on using therapeutic ultrasound exposures for improving the delivery of genes to solid tumors in order to improve the treatment of cancer.

Intratumoral infusion of DNA is one of the possible administration strategies for cancer gene therapy, and at present, the most commonly used method when using viral vectors in clinical trials [78]. The majority of preclinical studies performed to date for cancer gene therapy have also involved direct injections or slow (automated) infusions into the targeted tumors. There are several advantages of using intratumoral infusions over systemic delivery. One is circumvention of the transvascular barrier; especially important for large vectors such as viruses. Furthermore, interstitial transport may be enhanced through generation of a transient pressure gradient that may increase convection, as well as induce tissue deformation, leading to increased connectedness and pore size in the interstitium. And since distribution of vectors is restricted to the tumors, toxicity of normal tissue is minimized or even eliminated [74]. Recent studies, however, have demonstrated that infusions can enhance convective transport into the leaky tumor microvasculature and consequently increase the dissemination of viral vectors [78].

A number of preclinical studies have demonstrated how pulsed-HIFU exposures may be used to increase the therapeutic efficacy of cancer gene therapy procedures involving direct administrations. In one study, Quijano et al. [79] worked with tumor necrosis factor alpha (TNFα), which is a multifunctional cytokine capable of producing cytotoxic effects against cancer epithelial cells, as well as indirect effects in tumor associated vasculature [80]. Single intratumoral injections of TNFα, following pulsed-HIFU exposures, improved growth inhibition of a murine squamous cell carcinoma tumor model in comparison to injections alone. Gross morphology and histology showed that tumors receiving the combination treatment had a larger region of necrosis surrounding the needle track compared to injections alone, which is consistent with the therapeutic effects that were observed. In a follow-up study, combination treatment of the exposures and injections of fluorescent nanospheres showed better penetration of the fluorophores than injections alone [81]. A subsequent study used the same combination procedure with a more clinically relevant agent and corresponding tumor model. Here, slow infusions of an attenuated adenovirus expressing tumor necrosis factor–related apoptosis-inducing ligand (TRAIL) were used. TRAIL is known to induce apoptosis in cancer cells, while being nontoxic in most normal host cells. The tumor model was a human esophageal carcinoma, and the vector possessed a tissue-specific promoter to the cell line, meaning that the TRAIL would only be expressed in the tumor cells. The experimental procedure involved infusions of the vector preceded by pulsed-HIFU exposures. This combination treatment was found to produce better growth inhibition of the tumors compared to the infusions on their own [82].

Some studies have used a reversed strategy in which pulsed-HIFU exposures followed local administration of DNA in to tumors. Miller and Song [83] injected naked DNA that encoded for the reporter gene, luciferase, together with UCAs in a murine renal carcinoma tumor model, after which they gave their exposures. This combination treatment produced higher levels of gene expression compared to without the exposures or without the UCAs, as well as significantly lower growth rates of the tumors. Increasing both pulse duration and peak rarefractional pressure amplitude (the most important exposure parameter affecting cavitation activity) caused further decreases in tumor growth rates; however, no decreases in expression of the reporter gene were observed. The decrease in gene expression was apparently due to a reduction in the overall number of viable cells, and not lower transfection efficiency. Huber and Pfisterer [61] injected plasmid DNA encoding for beta-galactosidase into Dunning prostate tumors in rats, and then gave pulsed-HIFU exposures. In their study, where UCAs were not used, significant increases in the expression of the reporter gene were found compared to injections alone.

In the studies described above, where direct injections into tumor were used, it is assumed that increases in gene expression were due to the mechanism of sonoporation when exposures followed administration of the DNA. Even when UCAs were not used, introducing a needle in the tissue, along with fluid, will provide cavitation nuclei, as well as the physical space for bubble activity. However, when the exposures are given prior to administrations, sonoporation can be ruled out because of the long lag time (on the scale of minutes) between exposures and administrations. Mechanistic investigations into these exposures, where relatively high intensities are used and low duty cycles, have shown that the thermal dose generated is not sufficient for enhancing delivery [84]. Furthermore, acoustic cavitation does occur; however, it is sporadic and typically confined to vascular rich regions such as the outer surface of the tumors and the overlying skin [85]. These observations are supported by histological analysis, which shows red blood cell extravasation to occasionally occur but not whole-scale destruction of parenchymal cells. As previously mentioned, drug delivery applications based on acoustic cavitation usually require the addition of UCAs to keep results reproducible. The relative dearth of cavitation nuclei in the interstitium, as well as lack of physical space for bubble growth [14] would further preclude cavitation as a contributing mechanism.

Frenkel et al. [53] have proposed the generation of radiation forces, and the displacements they produce, as the most likely nonthermal, noncavitational mechanism for enhancing delivery when pulsed-HIFU exposures are given. Displacements are nonuniform within the focal zone, and further disparities in displacement will occur at the boundary of the focal zone and the adjacent region of tissue just outside of it [19]. Shear forces can potentially be created between any two adjacent regions of tissue experiencing nonuniform displacement, where the consequent strain is expected to work first on the relatively weaker structural elements in the tissue such as junctions between individual cells (e.g., desmosomes between parenchymal cells). The key to this proposed mechanism is the magnitude of the displacements, being typically on the order of tens of microns [53, 86]. Investigations are still ongoing to determine whether or not this mechanism is a valid one.

10.3.5 Remote Activation/Deployment of Drugs and Genes

So far, a variety of ways have been discussed on how ultrasound can be used to either create changes in the tissues for enhancing drug delivery (at a cellular or whole tissue level). This last section will discuss more recent developments of using ultrasound for improving the efficacy of drug treatment, where energy is directly absorbed by the agents for their activation or through locally induced chemical reactions. Some novel applications will also be discussed involving deployment or manipulation of drug carriers using thermal and nonthermal.

Heat Sensitive Liposomes

One of the ways that has been found to improve delivery of drugs is to encapsulate them in liposomes. Liposomes will preferentially accumulate in solid tumors due to a combination of a leaky vasculature and a lack of functional lymphatics, and also decrease the volume of distribution, which ultimately lowers systemic toxicity [87]. Enhanced tumor drug accumulation can be augmented by incorporating lipid-conjugated polyethylene glycol (PEG) into the liposome membrane. The result of doing so will further lower the liposomes volume of distribution and prolong clearance time, due to the protective barrier provided by the PEG against interactions with plasma proteins and the reticuloendothelial system (RES) [88]. Liposomes are typically stable in the range of physiological temperatures, however they can be designed to undergo a phase transition when heated, which renders them more permeable and consequently releases their payload [89]. By combining these thermosensitive liposomes (TSLs) with an external heat source, such as microwaves [90] or infrared lasers [91], a certain degree of targeting can be achieved where the TSLs will release their payload where the local tissue temperatures are elevated [89]. The delivery of various types of anticancer agents, including cisplatin [92], methotrexate [93], and doxorubicin [94], have been improved when these agents were encapsulated in TSLs in combination with a local source of hyperthermia.

To date, a number of preclinical studies have been reported where HIFU exposures, as a source of hyperthermia, were combined with TSLs. In one of these, an MR contrast agent (gadolinium) was loaded into the TSLs where the triggering temperature of the liposomes was set to thermal ablation levels (i.e., approximately 57°C). Using an MR guided HIFU system and imaging for T1-weighted signal intensity enhancement, the study demonstrated that indeed temperature elevations were achieved for ablating the targeted tissue [95].

In contrast, for drug delivery purposes, TSLs that trigger in the nondestructive hyperthermia range of 39°C to 41°C are more commonly used [94]. These low temperature sensitive liposomes, or LTSLs, were used by Dromi et al. [96] with pulsed-HIFU exposures that typically generate temperature elevations of only 4°C to 5°C [97]. When combining the exposures with the LTSLs, significantly enhanced delivery of doxorubin was found in murine breast cancer tumor xenografts, compared to a commercial nonthermosensitive liposome (i.e., Doxil). This enhanced local drug delivery was subsequently shown to improve growth inhibition of the treated tumors. This type of drug/device combination was subsequently found to be improved using a split-focus HIFU transducer, where increases in the spatial rates of drug deployment were obtained [98].

Remote Control of Gene Expression

One of the requirements for safe and effective gene therapy treatments is both spatial and temporal control of transgene expression. Up until now, some procedures have been discussed for improving spatial targeting of gene delivery; however, these did not include mechanisms for temporal control. Transgene expression can be controlled temporally using promoters that respond to external chemical factors such as antibiotics [99, 100] or small molecules [101]. An obvious drawback to such a system is that transgene expression will also occur in regions where genes were unintentionally delivered through inaccurate targeting [102]. Even when using intratumoral infusions, too high of an infusion pressure may lead to systemic leakage from the injection site [78].

Nondestructive HIFU exposures have been shown to cause significant upregulation of a variety of genes including glucose regulated proteins (GRP), stress proteins (SP), and heat shock proteins (HSP) [103]. In eukaryotic cells, HSP transcription is robustly initiated within minutes of exposures to elevated temperatures above those for maximum growth. To date, a number of preclinical studies have been carried out using HSP promoters to control in vivo transgene expression [102]. While various types of HSPs have been identified to respond well to heat, HSP70 has demonstrated best overall response, being the first to be repressed in the absence of stimulus [104].

HSP promoters have been used with HIFU exposures for temporally controlling gene expression. Liu et al. [105] generated relatively high temperatures (60°C) for short durations (5 seconds) in tumors cells transfected with a bioluminescent reporter gene to significantly enhance gene expression. The majority of studies using HIFU exposures for remote control of gene expression, however, seem to employ lower temperature elevations with longer exposures. This alternative regimen has been used in tumors [106], in the liver [107], and in the prostate [108]. These latter studies employed MRI guided HIFU devices, which not only allowed for accurate targeting of the exposures, but incorporated real-time, automated, feedback control of the required temperature elevation, which is capable of compensating for perfusion and tissue inhomogeneity—two factors known to effect heat generation. For a comprehensive review on using HIFU exposures with HSP promoters for temporal and spatial control of therapeutic genes, see Moonen [109].

Mechanically Activated Drug Carriers

The ability to chemically engineer a wide range of materials and drugs has created a new field of unlimited possibilities for using ultrasound to remotely deploy therapeutically relevant agents. Studies have shown, for example, how biodegradable polymers implanted in rodent skin may be degraded in a controlled fashion by topical ultrasound exposures for releasing drugs incorporated within them. Factors for controlling the release include the polymeric matrix, the molecular weight of the incorporated drug, as well as the various ultrasound exposure parameters [110]. Preclinical studies have also demonstrated how targeted drug release can be achieved using systemically administered carriers, where extracorporeal ultrasound induces reversible changes in those carriers to deploy the agents. Examples of this type of carrier include polymeric micelles [111] and liposomes [112]. Similar to using TSLs (described above), the benefit gained by this type of strategy is through an increase in local drug delivery to a targeted region for enhancing efficacy, while concomitantly minimizing systemic exposure to the drug and the subsequent side effects associated with its use. Compared to using TSLs, however, acoustic cavitation has been identified as the ultrasound mechanism for causing release of these agents from these different carriers.

Sonodynamic Therapy

Among the novel ways that ultrasound exposures can be used is a technique known as sonodynamic therapy (SDT). As one would expect, the name is derived from photodynamic therapy (PDT), which is a more established technique using light to activate anti-tumor agents [113]. The first compounds evaluated in SDT studies were those typically used in PDT. One of the earlier studies demonstrating proof of concept for SDT found synergistic effects when combining ultrasound exposures with the agents in regard to improving growth inhibition of targeted tumors [114]. Whereas the mechanisms involved in SDT are complex, it is generally accepted that they are mediated by acoustic cavitation, where activation of the anti-tumor agents is by the generation of radicals that are capable of initiating chain peroxidation of lipids in cellular membranes [115]. Limited penetration of light through tissue restricts PDT treatments to relatively small tumors on or under the skin, or with endoscopes or fiber optic catheters for reaching the lining of some internal organs [113]. Since focused ultrasound exposures can noninvasively treat regions deep in the body, it therefore has a major advantage over PDT [115]. For a comprehensive review on SDT, see Rosenthal et al. [115].

Additional Manipulation of Drug Carriers

Various biological phenomena have been documented that directly result from the creation of acoustic radiation forces. Mihran et al. [116] demonstrated, using single pulses at short duration and low energy, that the forces generated could modify the excitability of myelinated sciatic nerves in frogs in vitro. In in vivo experiments in the heart of frogs, radiation forces were also found to reduce aortic pressure and induce premature ventricular contractions [117]. These forces were also found to interrupt the flow in blood vessels in the eyes of rabbits [118]. Radiation forces are also being investigated in regard to their employment for drug delivery applications. They have demonstrated the ability to modulate the position and velocity of flow of UCAs in the vasculature, where redistribution of the agents was found for distances of even centimeters from the luminal space towards the walls of the vessels, at velocities exceeding 0.5 m/s [119]. A number of unique drug delivery strategies are presently being tested based on this novel use of radiation forces, including the facilitation of receptor-ligand mediated adhesion of drug carrying nanoparticles [120] and the deflection of drug carriers towards a vessel's wall prior to fragmentation for enhancing local deposition of the agent [121]. In the latter application, energy being released from the fragmentation of the carrier is thought to also potentially create effects in the vessel wall for enhanced local delivery [122]. Furthermore, the unique interaction of ultrasound with UCAs is being employed to create drug carriers that reversibly transform from stealth agents (that evade the immune system for increased circulation) to ones with increased adhesion for improved binding [123]. See Ferrara et al. [122] for a comprehensive review on how these types of interactions can be used for potential drug and gene delivery applications.

10.4 Conclusion

Looking back to the first pioneering studies carried out on the use of ultrasound in biological tissues, one can chart a remarkable advance in the understanding of how ultrasound energy interacts with the tissues, which has enabled a rich variety of applications to be proposed and developed. Hand in hand with this understanding have been the advances in the technology of applying this energy and guiding and monitoring it. This includes more simple systems that employ diagnostic ultrasound [124], and the newest and most sophisticated ones that use MRI for both treatment planning, and real-time MR thermometry to validate that a sufficient thermal dose was delivered, as well as for ensuring that only the targeted tissues were affected [38]. While ultrasound and MRI are presently being used in clinical devices employing focused ultrasound, computed tomography (CT) [125] and optical 3D tracking [126] have also been evaluated and have shown potential for guiding these exposures.

Although still mostly in preclinical development, the largest range of applications for therapeutic ultrasound is presently for enhancing the delivery of an ever increasing assortment of therapeutic agents, which themselves possess a variety of formulations and functions. These applications will hopefully be in the clinic in the near future to help improve the treatment of a host of different diseases including cancer, cardiovascular diseases, and chronic brain diseases.

Acknowledgments

The author would like to thank Ms. Hilary A. Hancock for thoughtful comments in the revision of this chapter. This research was funded in part by the NIH intramural research program.

References

[1] Fry, W. J., "Intense Ultrasound in Investigations of the Central Nervous System," *Adv. Biol. Med. Phys.*, Vol. 6, 1958, pp. 281–348.

[2] Fry, F. J., H. W. Ades, and W. J. Fry, "Production of Reversible Changes in the Central Nervous System by Ultrasound," *Science*, Vol. 127, No. 3289, 1958, pp. 83–84.

[3] Kennedy, J. E., "High-Intensity Focused Ultrasound in the Treatment of Solid Tumors," *Nat Rev Cancer*, Vol. 5, 2005, pp. 321–327.

[4] Nyborg, W. L., "Mechanisms for Bioeffects of Ultrasound Relevant to Therapeutic Applications," in *Emerging Therapeutic Ultrasound*. J. Wu and W. L. Nyborg, (eds.), New York: World Scientific Publishing Co., 2006.

[5] Haken, B. A., L. A. Frizzell, and E. L. Carstensen, "Effect of Mode Conversion on Ultrasonic Heating at Tissue Interfaces," *J Ultrasound Med.*, Vol. 11, No. 8, 1992, pp. 393–405.

[6] Sokka, S. D., R. King, and K. Hynynen, "MRI-Guided Gas Bubble Enhanced Ultrasound Heating in In Vivo Rabbit Thigh," *Phys. Med. Biol.*, Vol. 48, No. 2, 2003, pp. 223–241.

[7] Khokhlova, V. A., et al., "Effects of Nonlinear Propagation, Cavitation, and Boiling in Lesion Formation by High Intensity Focused Ultrasound in a Gel Phantom," *J. Acoust. Soc. Am.*, Vol. 119, No. 3, 2006, pp. 1834–1848.

[8] Barnett, S. B., et al., "Current Status of Research on Biophysical Effects of Ultrasound," *Ultrasound Med. Biol.*, Vol. 20, No. 3, 1994, pp. 205–208.

[9] Suslick, K. S., "Homogenous Sonochemistry," in *Ultrasound: Its Chemical, Physical and Biological Effects*, K. S. Suslick, (ed.), New York: VCH Publishers, Inc., 1988.

[10] Lewin, P. A., and L. Bjorno, "Acoustically Induced Shear Stresses in the Vicinity of Microbubbles in Tissue," *J. Acoust. Soc. Am.*, Vol. 1, No. 3, 1982, pp. 728–734.

[11] Bommannan, D., et al., "Sonophoresis: II. Examination of the Mechanism(s) of Ultrasound Enhanced Transdermal Drug Delivery," *Pharm. Res.*, Vol. 9, No. 8, 1992, pp. 1043–1047.

[12] Riesz, P., and T. Kondo, "Free Radical Formation Induced by Ultrasound and Its Biological Implications," *Free Radic. Biol. Med.*, Vol. 13, 1992, pp. 247–270.

[13] Kimmel, E., "Cavitation Bioeffects," *Crit. Rev. Biomed. Eng.*, Vol. 34, No. 2, 2006, pp. 105–161.

[14] Simonin, J. P., "On the Mechanisms of In Vitro and In Vivo Phonophoresis," *J. Control Release*, Vol. 33, 1995, pp. 125–141.

[15] Zhang, S., J. H. Duncan, and G. L. Chamine, "The Final Stage of Collapse of a Cavitation Bubble Near a Rigid Wall," *J. Fluid. Mech.*, Vol. 257, 1993, pp. 147–181.

[16] Dear, J. P., J. E. Field, and A. J. Walton, "Gas Compression and Jet Formation in Cavities Collapsed by a Shock Wave," *Nature*, Vol. 377, 1988, pp. 505–508.

[17] Kodama, T., and K. Takayama, "Dynamic Behavior of Bubbles During Extracorporeal Shock-Wave Lithotripsy," *Ultrasound Med. Biol.*, Vol. 24, No. 5, 1998, pp. 723–728.

[18] Frenkel, V., E. Kimmel, and Y. Iger, "Ultrasound-Induced Cavitation Damage to External Epithelia of Fish Skin," *Ultrasound Med. Biol.*, Vol. 25, No. 8, 1999, pp. 1295–1303.

[19] Lizzi, F. L., et al., "Radiation-Force Technique to Monitor Lesions During Ultrasonic Therapy," *Ultrasound Med. Biol.*, Vol. 29, No. 11, 2003, pp. 1593–1605.

[20] Dymling, S. O., et al., "A New Ultrasonic Method for Fluid Property Measurements," *Ultrasound Med. Biol.*, Vol. 17, No. 5, 1991, pp. 497–500.

[21] Wu, J., A. J. Winkler, and T. P. O'Neill, "Effect of Acoustic Streaming on Ultrasonic Heating," *Ultrasound Med. Biol.*, Vol. 20, No. 2, 1994, pp. 195–201.

[22] Frenkel, V., E. Kimmel, and Y. Iger, "Ultrasound-Facilitated Transport of Silver Chloride (AgCl) Particles in Fish Skin," *J. Control Release*, Vol. 68, 2000, pp. 251–261.

[23] Frenkel V., et al., "Preliminary Investigations of Ultrasound Induced Acoustic Streaming Using Particle Image Velocimetry," *Ultrasonics*, Vol. 39, No. 3, 2001, pp. 153–156.

[24] Mitragotri S. "Healing Sound: The Use of Ultrasound in Drug Delivery and Other Therapeutic Applications," *Nat. Rev. Drug Discov.*, Vol. 4, No. 3, 2005, pp. 255–260.

[25] Lavon, I., et al., "Bubble Growth Within the Skin by Rectified Diffusion Might Play a Significant Role in Sonophoresis," *J. Control Release*, Vol. 12, No. 117, Pt. 2, 2007, pp. 246–255.

[26] Katz, N. P., et al., "Rapid Onset of Cutaneous Anesthesia with EMLA Cream After Pretreatment with a New Ultrasound-Emitting Device," *Anesth. Analg.*, Vol. 98, No. 2, 2004, pp. 371–376.

[27] Kost, J., "Ultrasound-Assisted Insulin Delivery and Noninvasive Glucose Sensing," *Diabetes Technol. Ther.*, Vol. 4, No. 4, 2002, pp. 489–497.

[28] Tezel, A., et al., "Low-Frequency Ultrasound as a Transcutaneous Immunization Adjuvant," *Vaccine,* Vol. 23, 2005, No. 29, pp. 3800–3807.

[29] Kost, J., et al., "Transdermal Monitoring of Glucose and Other Analytes Using Ultrasound," *Nat. Med.*, Vol. 6, No. 3, 2000, pp. 347–350.

[30] Zderic V, et al., "Ocular Drug Delivery Using 20-kHz Ultrasound," *Ultrasound Med. Biol.*, Vol. 28, No. 6, 2002, pp. 823–829.

[31] Zderic, V., et al., "Ultrasound-Enhanced Transcorneal Drug Delivery," *Cornea*, Vol. 23, No. 8, 2004, pp. 804–811.

[32] Zderic, V., J. I. Clark, and S. Vaezy, "Drug Delivery into the Eye with the Use of Ultrasound," *J. Ultrasound Med.*, Vol. 23, No. 10, 2004, pp. 1349–1359.

[33] Mitragotri, S., and J. Kost, "Low-Frequency Sonophoresis: A Review," *Adv. Drug Deliv. Rev.*, Vol. 56, No. 5, 2004, pp. 589–601.

[34] Clement, G. T., "Perspectives in Clinical Uses of High-Intensity Focused Ultrasound," *Ultrasonics*, Vol. 42, No. 10, 2004, pp. 1087–1093.

[35] Jolesz, F. A., and N. McDannold, "Current Status and Future Potential of MRI-Guided Focused Ultrasound Surgery," *J. Magn. Reson. Imaging*, Vol. 27, No. 2, 2008, pp. 391–399.

[36] Mesiwala, A. H., et al., "High-Intensity Focused Ultrasound Selectively Disrupts the Blood Brain Barrier In Vivo," *Ultrasound Med. Biol.*, Vol. 28, No. 3, 2002, pp. 389–400.

[37] McDannold, N., N. Vykhodtseva, and K. Hynynen, "Targeted Disruption of the Blood-Brain Barrier with Focused Ultrasound: Association with Cavitation Activity," *Phys. Med. Biol.*, Vol. 51, No. 4, 2006, pp. 793–807.

[38] McDannold, N., and K. Hynynen, "Quality Assurance and System Stability of a Clinical MRI-Guided Focused Ultrasound System: Four-Year Experience," *Med. Phys.*, Vol. 33, No. 11, 2006, pp. 4307–4313.

[39] Kinoshita, M., et al., "Noninvasive Localized Delivery of Herceptin to the Mouse Brain by MRI-Guided Focused Ultrasound-Induced Blood-Brain Barrier Disruption," *Proc. Natl. Acad. Sci. USA*, Vol. 103, No. 31, 2006, pp. 11719–11723.

[40] Treat, L. H., et al., "Transcranial MRI-Guided Focused Ultrasound-Induced Blood-Brain Barrier Opening in Rats," *IEEE Ultrasonics Symposium*, Montreal, 2004.

[41] Hynynen, K., "Focused Ultrasound for Blood-Brain Disruption and Delivery of Therapeutic Molecules into the Brain," *Expert Opin. Drug Deliv.*, Vol. 4, No. 1, 2007, pp. 27–35.

[42] Pfaffenberger, S., et al., "Ultrasound Thrombolysis," *Tromb. Haemost.*, Vol. 94, 2005, pp. 26–36.

[43] Atar, S., et al., "The Use of Transducer-Tipped Ultrasound Catheter for Recanalization of Thrombotic Arterial Occlusions," *Echocardiography*, Vol. 18, No. 3, 2001, pp. 233–237.

[44] Alexandrov, A. V., et al., "Ultrasound-Enhanced Systemic Thrombolysis for Acute Ischemic Stroke," *N. Engl. J. Med.*, Vol. 351, 2004, pp. 2170–2178.

[45] Braaten, J. V., R. A. Gross, and C. W. Francis, "Ultrasound Reversibly Disaggregates Fibrin Fibres," *Thromb. Haemost.*, Vol. 78, 1997, pp. 1063–1068.

[46] Siddiqi, F., et al., "Ultrasound Increases Flow Through Fibrin Gels," *Thromb. Haemost.*, Vol. 73, 1995, pp. 495–498.

[47] Francis, C. W., et al., "Ultrasound Accelerates Transport of Recombinant Tissue Plasminogen Activator into Clots," *Ultrasound Med. Biol.*, Vol. 21, 1995, pp. 419–424.

[48] Siegel, R. J., et al., "Noninvasive Transcutaneous Low Frequency Ultrasound Enhances Thrombolysis in Peripheral and Coronary Arteries," *Echocardiography*, Vol. 18, No. 3, 2001, pp. 247–257.

[49] Datta, S., et al., "Correlation of Cavitation with Ultrasound Enhancement of Thrombolysis," *Ultrasound Med. Biol.*, Vol. 32, No. 8, 2006, pp. 1257–1267.

[50] Culp, W. C., et al., "Microbubble Potentiated Ultrasound as a Method of Stroke Therapy in s Pig Model: Preliminary Findings," *J. Vasc. Interv. Radiol.*, Vol. 14, No. 11, 2003, pp. 1433–1436.

[51] Tiukinhoy-Laing, S. D., et al., "Ultrasound-Facilitated Thrombolysis Using Tissue-Plasminogen Activator-Loaded Echogenic Liposomes," *Thromb. Res.*, Vol. 119, No. 6, 2007, pp. 777–784.

[52] Stone, M. J., et al., "Pulsed-High Intensity Focused Ultrasound (HIFU)-Enhanced Thrombolysis In Vitro: Proof of Concept and Investigation of Mechanism," *Proceedings of the 91st Annual Meeting of the Radiological Society of North America*, Chicago, 2005.

[53] Frenkel, V., et al., "Pulsed-High Intensity Ultrasound (HIFU) Enhances Thrombolysis in and In Vitro Model," *Radiology*, Vol. 239, No. 1, 2006, pp. 86–93.

[54] Stone, M. J., et al., "Pulsed-High Intensity Focused Ultrasound Enhanced T-PA Mediated Thrombolysis in a Novel In Vivo Clot Model, a Pilot Study," *Thromb. Res.*, Vol. 121, No. 2, 2007, pp. 193–202.

[55] Purves, W. K., G. H. Orians, and H. G. Heller, *Life: The Science of Biology*, 3rd ed., Salt Lake City, UT: W. H. Freeman and Co., 1992.

[56] Fechheimer, M., et al., "Measurement of Cytoplasmic pH in Dictyostelium Discoideum by Using a New Method for Introducing Macromolecules into Living Cells," *Eur. J. Cell Biol.*, Vol. 40, No. 2, 1986, pp. 242–247.

[57] Fechheimer, M., et al., "Transfection of Mammalian Cells with Plasmid DNA by Scrape Loading and Sonication Loading," *Proc. Natl. Acad. Sci. USA*, Vol. 84, No. 23, 1987, pp. 8463–8467.

[58] Ohl, C. D., M. Arora, and R. Ikink, "Sonoporation from Jetting Cavitation Bubbles," *Biophys. J.*, Vol. 91, No. 11, 2006, pp. 4285–4295.

[59] van Wamel, A., K. Kooiman, and M. Harteveld, "Vibrating Microbubbles Poking Individual Cells: Drug Transfer into Cells Via Sonoporation," *J. Control Release*, Vol. 112, No. 2, 2006, pp. 149–155.

[60] Deng, C. X., et al., "Ultrasound-Induced Cell Membrane Porosity," *Ultrasound Med. Biol.*, Vol. 30, No. 4, 2004, pp. 519–526.

[61] Huber, P. E., and P. Pfisterer, "In Vitro and In Vivo Transfection of Plasmid DNA in the Dunning Prostate Tumor R3327-AT1 Is Enhanced by Focused Ultrasound," *Gene Ther.*, Vol. 7, No. 17, 2000, pp. 1516–1525.

[62] Rahim, A. A., et al., "Spatial and Acoustic Pressure Dependence of Microbubble-Mediated Gene Delivery Targeted Using Focused Ultrasound," *J. Gene Med.*, Vol. 8, No. 11, 2006, pp. 1347–1357.

[63] Mansouri, S., et al., "Chitosan-DNA Nanoparticles as Non-Viral Vectors in Gene Therapy: Strategies to Improve Transfection Efficacy," *Eur. J. Pharm. Biopharm.*, Vol. 57, No. 1, 2004, pp. 1–8.

[64] Hashiya, N., et al., "Local Delivery of E2F Decoy Oligodeoxynucleotides Using Ultrasound with Microbubble Agent (Optison) Inhibits Intimal Hyperplasia After Balloon Injury in Rat Carotid Artery Model," *Biochem. Biophys. Res. Commun.*, Vol. 317, No. 2, 2004, pp. 508–514.

[65] Huber, P. E., et al., "Focused Ultrasound (HIFU) Induces Localized Enhancement of Reporter Gene Expression in Rabbit Carotid," *Gene Ther.*, Vol. 10, 2003, pp. 1600–1607.

[66] Unger, E. C., et al., "Gene Delivery Using Ultrasound Contrast Agents," *Echocardiography*, Vol. 18, No. 4, 2001, pp. 355–361.

[67] Hynynen, K., "The Threshold for Thermally Significant Cavitation in Dog's Thigh Muscle In Vivo," *Ultrasound Med. Biol.*, Vol. 17, No. 2, 1991, pp. 157–169.

[68] Stride, E., and N. Saffari, "The Potential for Thermal Damage Posed by Microbubble Ultrasound Contrast Agents," *Ultrasonics*, Vol. 42, 2004, pp. 907–913.

[69] Miller, D. L., "Ultrasound-mediated gene therapy," in *Emerging Therapeutic Ultrasound*, J. Wu and W. L. Nyborg, (eds.), New York: World Scientific Publishing Co., 2006.

[70] Schratzberger, P., et al., "Transcutaneous Ultrasound Augments Naked DNA Transfection Of Skeletal Muscle," *Mol. Ther.*, Vol. 6, No. 5, 2002, pp. 576–583.

[71] Miao, C. H., et al., "Ultrasound Enhances Gene Delivery of Human Factor IX Plasmid," *Hum. Gene Ther.*, Vol. 16, 2005, pp. 893–905.

[72] Lake, R. A., and B. W. Robinson, "Immunotherapy and Chemotherapy—A Practical Partnership," *Nat Rev Cancer* 2005, Vol. 5, No. 5, pp. 397–405.

[73] Minchinton, A. I., and I. F. Tannock, "Drug Penetration in Solid Tumors," *Nat. Rev. Cancer*, Vol. 6, No. 8, 2006, pp. 583–592.

[74] Wang, Y., and F. Yuan, "Delivery of Viral Vectors to Tumor Cells: Extracellular Transport, Systemic Distribution, and Strategies for Improvement," *Ann. Biomed. Eng.*, Vol. 34, No. 1, 2006, pp. 114–127.

[75] Galmarini, C. M., and F. C. Galmarini, "Multidrug Resistance in Cancer Therapy: Role of the Tumor Microenvironment," *Curr. Opin. Investig. Drugs*, Vol. 4, No. 12, 2003, pp. 1416–1421.

[76] McKee, T. D., et al., "Degradation of Fibrillar Collagen in a Human Melanoma Xenograft Improves the Efficacy of an Oncolytic Herpes Simplex Virus Vector," *Cancer Res.*, Vol. 66, No. 5, 2006, pp. 2509–2513.

[77] Kong, G., and M. W. Dewhirst, "Hyperthermia and Liposomes," *Intl. J. Hyperthermia*, Vol. 15, 1999, pp. 345–370.

[78] Wang, Y., et al., "Characterisation of Systemic Dissemination of Nonreplicating Adenoviral Vectors from Tumours in Local Gene Delivery," *Br. J. Cancer*, Vol. 92, No. 8, 2005, pp. 1414–1420.

[79] Quijano, J., et al., "Enhanced Regression in a Squamous Cell Carcinoma Murine Tumor Model Using Pulsed-High Intensity Focused Ultrasound (HIFU) and Naked TNF-a Plasmid," *Proceedings of the 4th Annual Meeting of the Society for Molecular Imaging*, Cologne, Germany, 2005.

[80] Bazzoni, F., and B. Beutler, "The Tumor Necrosis Factor Ligand and Receptor Families," *N. Engl. J. Med.*,Vol. 334, No. 26, 1996, pp. 1717–1725.

[81] Traughber, B., et al., "Pulsed-High Intensity Focused Ultrasound (HIFU) Exposures Combined with Intratumoral Injection of TNF—A Plasmid Enhance Growth Inhibition in a Murine Squamous Cell Carcinoma Model," *Proceedings of the 6th International Symposium on Therapeutic Ultrasound*, Oxford, 2006.

[82] Patel, P., et al., "Enhancement of AdVgTRAIL Gene Therapy Using Pulsed-High Intensity Focused Ultrasound (HIFU) in a Human Esophageal Carcinoma Model in Mice," *Proceedings of the Meeting of the Radiological Society*, Chicago, 2007.

[83] Miller, D. L., and J. Song, "Tumor Growth Reduction and DNA Transfer by Cavitation-Enhanced High-Intensity Focused Ultrasound In Vivo," *Ultrasound Med. Biol.*, Vol. 29, No. 6, 2003, pp. 887–893.

[84] O'Neill, B. E., et al., "Investigations into the Potential Contribution of a Thermal Mechanism for Pulsed-High Intensity Focused Ultrasound Mediated Delivery," *Proceedings of IEEE Ultrasonics*, New York, October 28–31, 2007.

[85] O'Neill, B. E., et al., "Pulsed HIFU for Enhanced Drug Delivery: A Study of Possible Mechanisms," *Proceedings of the 6th International Symposium on Therapeutic Ultrasound*, Oxford, 2006.

[86] Frenkel, V., et al., "Pulsed-High Intensity Focused Ultrasound (HIFU) Exposures for Enhanced Delivery of Therapeutics: Mechanisms and Applications," *Proceedings of the 5th International Symposium on Therapeutic Ultrasound*, Boston, 2005.

[87] Allen, T. M., "Liposomes: Opportunities in Drug Delivery," *Drugs*, Vol. 54, 1997, pp. 8–14.

[88] Allen, C., et al., "Controlling the Physical Behavior and Biological Performance of Liposome Formulations Through Use of Surface Grafted Poly(Ethylene Glycol)," *Biosci. Rep.*, Vol. 22, No. 2, 2002, pp. 225–250.

[89] Gaber, M. H., et al., "Thermosensitive Liposomes: Extravasation and Release of Contents in Tumor Microvascular Networks," *Int. J. Radiat. Oncol. Biol. Phys.*, Vol. 36, 1996, pp. 1177–1187.

[90] Khoobehi, B., et al., "Hyperthermia and Temperature-Sensitive Liposomes: Selective Delivery of Drugs into the Eye," *Jpn. J. Ophthalmol.*, Vol. 33, 1989, pp. 405–412.

[91] Salomir, R., et al., "Local Delivery of Magnetic Resonance (MR) Contrast Agent in Kidney Using Thermosensitive Liposomes and MR Imaging-Guided Local Hyperthermia: A Feasibility Study In Vivo," *J. Magn. Reson. Imaging*, Vol. 22, 2005, pp. 534–540.

[92] Nishita, T., "Heat-Sensitive Liposomes Containing Cisplatin and Localized Hyperthermia in Treatment of Murine Tumor," *Osaka City Med. J.*, Vol. 44, 1998, pp. 73–83.

[93] Weinstein, J. N., et al., "Treatment of Solid L1210 Murine Tumors with Local Hyperthermia and Temperature-Sensitive Liposomes Containing Methotrexate," *Cancer Res.*, Vol. 40, 1980, pp. 1388–1395.

[94] Kong, G., et al., "Efficacy of Liposomes and Hyperthermia in a Human Tumor Xenograft Model: Importance of Triggered Drug Release," *Cancer Res.*, Vol. 60, 2000, pp. 6950–6957.

[95] McDannold, N., et al., "Heat-Activated Liposomal MR Contrast Agent: Initial In Vivo Results in Rabbit Liver and Kidney," *Radiology*, Vol. 230, 2004, pp. 743–752.

[96] Dromi, S., et al., "Pulsed-High Intensity Focused Ultrasound and Low Temperature Sensitive Liposomes for Enhanced Targeted Drug Delivery and Anti-Tumor Effect," *Clin. Cancer Res.*, Vol. 13, No. 9, 2007, pp. 2722–2727.

[97] Frenkel, V., et al., "Delivery of Liposomal Doxorubicin (Doxil ®) in a Breast Cancer Tumor Model: Investigation of Potential Enhancement by Pulsed-High Intensity Focused Ultrasound Exposure," *Acad. Radiol.*, Vol. 13, No. 4, 2006, pp. 469–479.

[98] Patel, P., et al., "In Vitro and In Vivo Evaluations of Increased Spatial Heat Deposition Using a Split Focus High Intensity Ultrasound (HIFU) Transducer," *Intl. J. Hyperthermia*, 2009.

[99] Iida, A., et al., "Inducible Gene Expression by Retrovirus-Mediated Transfer of a Modified Tetracycline-Regulated System," *J. Virol.*, Vol. 70, No. 9, 1996, pp. 6054–6059.

[100] Szulc, J., et al., "A Versatile Tool for Conditional Gene Expression and Knockdown," *Nat. Methods*, Vol. 3, No. 2, 2006, pp. 109–116.

[101] Clackson, T., "Controlling Mammalian Gene Expression with Small Molecules," *Curr. Opin. Chem. Biol.*, Vol. 1, No. 2, 1997, pp. 210–218.

[102] Rome, C., F. Couillaud, and C. T. Moonen, "Spatial and Temporal Control of Expression of Therapeutic Genes Using Heat Shock Protein Promoters," *Methods*, Vol. 35, No. 2, 2005, pp. 188–198.

[103] Kramer, G., et al., "Response to Sublethal Heat Treatment of Prostatic Tumor Cells and of Prostatic Tumor Infiltrating T-Cells," *Prostate*, Vol. 58, No. 2, 2004, pp. 109–120.

[104] DiDomenico, B. J., G. E. Bugaisky, and S. Lindquist, "Heat Shock and Recovery Are Mediated by Different Translational Mechanisms," *Proc. Natl. Acad. Sci. USA*, Vol. 79, No. 20, 1982, pp. 6181–6185.

[105] Liu, Y., et al., "High Intensity Focused Ultrasound-Induced Gene Activation in Solid Tumors," *J. Acoust. Soc. Am.*, Vol. 120, No. 1, 2006, pp. 492–501.

[106] Guilhon, E., et al., "Spatial and Temporal Control of Transgene Expression In Vivo Using a Heat-Sensitive Promoter and MRI-Guided Focused Ultrasound," *J. Gene Med.*, Vol. 5, No. 4, 2003, pp. 333–342.

[107] Plathow, C., et al., "Focal Gene Induction in the Liver of Rats by a Heat-Inducible Promoter Using Focused Ultrasound Hyperthermia: Preliminary Results," *Invest. Radiol.*, Vol. 40, No. 11, 2005, pp. 729–735.

[108] Silcox, C. E., et al., "MRI-Guided Ultrasonic Heating Allows Spatial Control of Exogenous Luciferase in Canine Prostate," *Ultrasound Med. Biol.*, Vol. 31, No. 7, 2005, pp. 965–970.

[109] Moonen, C. T., "Spatio-Temporal Control of Gene Expression and Cancer Treatment Using Magnetic Resonance Imaging-Guided Focused Ultrasound," *Clin. Cancer Res.*, Vol. 13, No. 12, 2007, pp. 3482–3489.

[110] Kost, J., K. Leong, and R. Langer, "Ultrasound-Enhanced Polymer Degradation and Release of Incorporated Substances," *Proc. Natl. Acad. Sci.*, Vol. 86, No. 20, 1989, pp. 7663–7666.

[111] Zeng, Y., and W. G. Pitt, "A Polymeric Micelle System with a Hydrolysable Segment for Drug Delivery," *J. Biomater. Sci. Polym. Ed.*, Vol. 17, No. 5, 2006, pp. 591–604.

[112] Schroeder, A., et al., "Controlling Liposomal Drug Release with Low Frequency Ultrasound: Mechanism and Feasibility," *Langmuir*, Vol. 23, No. 7, 2007, pp. 4019–4025.

[113] Palumbo, G., "Photodynamic Therapy and Cancer: A Brief Sightseeing Tour," *Expert Opin. Drug Deliv.*, Vol. 4, No. 2, 2007, pp. 131–148.

[114] Yumita, N., et al., "Synergistic Effect of Ultrasound and Hematoporphyrin on Sarcoma 180," *Jpn. J. Cancer Res.*, Vol. 81, No. 3, 1990, pp. 304–308.

[115] Rosenthal, I., J. Z. Sostaric, and P. Riesz, "Sonodynamic Therapy—A Review of the Synergistic Effects of Drugs and Ultrasound," *Ultrason. Sonochem.*, Vol. 11, No. 6, 2004, pp. 349–363.

[116] Mihran, R. T., F. S. Barnes, and H. Wachtel, "Temporally-Specific Modification of Myelinated Axon Excitability In Vitro Following a Single Ultrasound Pulse," *Ultrasound Med. Biol.*, Vol. 16, No. 3, 1990, pp. 297–309.

[117] Dalecki, D., et al., "Effects of Pulsed Ultrasound on the Frog Heart: III. The Radiation Force Mechanism," *Ultrasound Med. Biol.*, Vol. 23, No. 2, 1997, pp. 275–285.

[118] Lizzi, F. L., et al., "Effects of Pulsed Ultrasound on Ocular Tissue," *Ultrasound Med. Biol.*, Vol. 7, No. 3, 1981, pp. 245–252.

[119] Dayton, P. A., J. S. Allen, and K. W. Ferrara, "The Magnitude of Radiation Force on Ultrasound Contrast Agents," *J. Acoust. Soc. Am.*, Vol. 112, No. 5, Pt. 1, 2002, pp. 2183–2192.

[120] Tartis, M. S., et al., "Therapeutic Effects of Paclitaxel-Containing Ultrasound Contrast Agents," *Ultrasound Med Biol* 2006, Vol. 32, No. 11, pp. 1771–1880.

[121] Shortencarier, M. J., et al., "A Method for Radiation-Force Localized Drug Delivery Using Gas Filled Lipospheres," *IEEE Transactions on Ultrasonics, Ferrelectrics and Frequency Control*, Vol. 51, No. 7, 2004, pp. 822–831.

[122] Ferrara, K., R. Pollard, and M. Borden, "Ultrasound Microbubble Contrast Agents: Fundamentals and Application to Gene and Drug Delivery," *Annu. Rev. Biomed. Eng.*, Vol. 9, 2007, pp. 415–447.

[123] Borden, M. A., et al., "Ultrasound Radiation Force Modulates Ligand Availability on Targeted Contrast Agents," *Mol. Imaging*, Vol. 5, No. 3, 2006, pp. 139–147.

[124] Koch, K. O., et al., "Phase I/II Trial of High Intensity Focused Ultrasound for the Treatment of Previously Untreated Localized Prostate Cancer," *J. Urol.*, Vol. 178, No. 6, 2007, pp. 2366–2370.

[125] Wood, B. J., et al., "CT and Ultrasound Guided Stereotactic High Intensity Focused Ultrasound (HIFU)," *Proc. Intl. Sym. Ther. US*, Boston, 2005.

[126] Vo, H., et al., "CT-Guided High Intensity Focused Ultrasound Ablation with Optical 3D Tracking," *Proc. IEEE Ultrasonics*, New York, 2007.

CHAPTER 11

Therapeutic Hyperthermia

Riadh Habash

11.1 Introduction

Hyperthermia is ancient, but these days it is a rapidly developing treatment technique in tumor therapy. Many Greek and Roman physicians thought that if they could simply control body temperature they could cure all diseases. This included cancer, because the pathology of tumor development had been described in the Greek literature [1, 2]. Hyperthermia may be defined also as raising the temperature of a part of or the whole body above normal for a defined period of time. The amount of temperature elevation is on the order of a few degrees above normal temperature (41°C to 45°C). The effect of hyperthermia depends on the temperature and exposure time. First, there is the curative, physiologically based therapy (physiological hyperthermia), which treats aches, pains, strains, and sprains. Hyperthermia is applied in multiple sessions; using low temperature (e.g., below 41°C) for approximately an hour. At temperatures above 42.5°C to 43°C, the exposure time can be halved with each 1°C temperature increase to give an equivalent cell kill [3, 4]. Most normal tissues are undamaged by treatment for 1 h at a temperature of up to 44°C [5]. The main mechanism for cell death is probably protein denaturation, observed at temperatures > 40°C, which leads to, among other things, alterations in multimolecular structures like cytoskeleton and membranes, and changes in enzyme complexes for DNA synthesis and repair [6].

The first paper on hyperthermia was published in 1886 [7]. According to the author, the sarcoma that occurred on the face of a 43-year-old woman was cured when fever was caused by erysipelas. Westermark [8] tried to circulate high-temperature water for the treatment of an inoperable cancer of the uterine cervix and the effectiveness was confirmed. In the early twentieth century applied research was carried out together with basic research; however, since the heating method and temperature-measuring technology, for example, was not sufficiently developed at that time, the positive clinical application of hyperthermia treatment was not carried out. Therefore, surgeries, radiotherapy, chemotherapy, and so on, were the dominant therapy for tumors [9]. Worldwide interest in hyperthermia was initiated by the first international congress on hyperthermic oncology in Washington in 1975. In the United States a hyperthermia group was formed in 1981, and the European Hyperthermia Institute was formed in 1983. In Japan, hyperthermia research started in 1978 and the Japanese Society of Hyperthermia Oncology was established in 1984.

This interest has followed a course that is usual for a new type of treatment. In the first decade there was a growing enthusiasm, reflected by an exponential increase in the number of papers and participants at meetings. Thereafter, the interest waned, due to disappointing clinical results from some of the first randomized studies, accompanied by reluctance among sponsoring authorities and hospital boards to support further research. Currently, there appears to be a renewed interest, thanks to several investigations demonstrating that the improvements in treatment outcome by adjuvant hyperthermia can be very substantial, provided that adequate heating procedures are used [10].

The clinical exploitation of hyperthermia was and still is hampered by technical limitations and the high degree of interdependency between technology, physiology, and biology [11, 12]. Extensive biologic research has shown that there are sound biological reasons for using hyperthermia in the treatment of malignant diseases [13]. The biological rationale for the treatment of malignant disease by heat is mediated by various specific reasons, including the following. (1) The survival of cells depends on the temperature and duration of heating in a predictable and repeatable way. For example, when the temperature increases, the survival rate of the cell becomes lower. (2) Tumor cell environment, such as hypoxia, poor nutrition, and low pH, while detrimental to cell kill by ionizing radiation, is beneficial to heat therapy. (3) Cells may develop a resistance to subsequent heat following previous heat treatment. This condition is known as thermotolerance. (4) The differential sensitivity of normal and tumor cells to heat is dependent on cell type and environmental conditions. (5) Heat treatment enhances the biological effect of both radiation and chemotherapy agents [9, 14].

This chapter outlines and discusses the means by which electromagnetic (EM) energy and other techniques can provide elevation of temperature within the human body. Clinical hyperthermia falls under three major categories: localized, regional, and whole-body hyperthermia (WBH). Because of the individual characteristic of each type of treatment, different types of heating systems have evolved. Hyperthermia may be applied alone or jointly with other modalities such as radiotherapy, chemotherapy, surgical treatment, immunotherapy, and so on. The chapter concludes with a discussion of challenges and opportunities for the future.

11.2 Types of Hyperthermia

Hyperthermia is most often applied within a department of radiation oncology under the authority of a radiation oncologist and a medical physicist. The effectiveness of hyperthermia treatment is related to the temperature achieved during the treatment, as well as the length of treatment, and cell and tissue characteristics [15]. To ensure that the desired temperature is reached, but not exceeded, the temperature of the tumor and surrounding tissues is monitored throughout hyperthermia procedure. Most hyperthermia treatments are applied using external devices, employing energy transfer to tissues by EM technologies [16, 17].

11.2.1 Local Hyperthermia

In local hyperthermia, the aim is to increase the tumor temperature while sparing surrounding normal tissue, using either external or interstitial modalities. Heat is applied to a small area, such as a tumor, using various techniques that can deliver energy to heat the tumor. Local hyperthermia treatment is a well-established cancer treatment method with a simple basic principle: If a rise in temperature to 42°C can be obtained for 1 hour within a cancer tumor, the cancer cells will be destroyed. Primary malignant tumors have poor blood circulation, which makes them more sensitive to changes in temperature.

Local hyperthermia is performed with superficial applicators [radiofrequency (RF), microwave, or ultrasound] of different kinds (waveguide, spiral, current sheet, and so forth) placed on the surface of superficial tumors with a contacting medium (bolus). The resulting specific absorption rate (SAR) distribution is subject to strong physical curtailment resulting in a therapeutic depth of only a few centimeters. The penetration depth depends on the frequency and size of the applicator, and typically the clinical range is not more than 3 to 4 cm. A system for local hyperthermia consisting of a generator, control computer applicator, and a scheme to measure temperature in the tumor is shown in Figure 11.1. The power is increased until the desired temperature is achieved.

The volume that can be heated depends on the physical characteristics of the energy source and on the type of applicator [18]. During local hyperthermia, the tumor temperatures are increased to levels that are as high as possible, as long as the tolerance limits of the surrounding normal tissues are not exceeded [10]. Candidates for local hyperthermia include chest wall recurrences, superficial malignant melanoma lesions, and lymph node metastases of head and neck tumors.

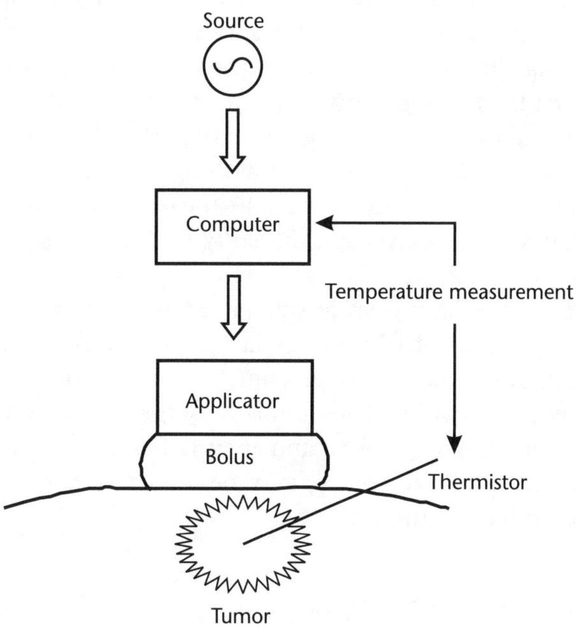

Figure 11.1 Local hyperthermia system.

11.2.1.1 External Local Hyperthermia

Heating of small areas (usually up to 50 cm^2) to treat tumors that are in or just below the skin (up to 4 cm) may be achieved quite easily today. External local hyperthermia therapy may be used alone or in combination with radiation therapy for the treatment of patients with primary or metastatic cutaneous or subcutaneous superficial tumors (e.g., superficial recurrent melanoma, chest wall recurrence of breast cancer, and cervical lymph node metastases from head and neck cancer). Heat is usually applied using high-frequency energy waves generated from a source outside the body (such as a microwave or ultrasound source) [1, 2].

11.2.1.2 Intraluminal Local Hyperthermia

Intraluminal or endocavitary methods may be used to treat tumors within or near body cavities. Endocavitary antennas are inserted in natural openings of hollow organs. These include: (1) gastrointestinal (esophagus, rectum), (2) gynecological (vagina, cervix, and uterus), (3) genitourinary (prostate, bladder), and (4) pulmonary (trachea, bronchus). Very localized heating is possible with this technique by inserting an endotract electrode into lumens of the human body to deliver energy and heat the area directly. Various types of electrodes are available depending on the size of the lumen and the site of the lesion [1, 2].

11.2.1.3 Interstitial Local Hyperthermia

Interstitial techniques are used to treat tumors deep within the body, such as brain tumors. Many types of interstitial hyperthermia equipment are used. These include local current field techniques utilizing RF energy (at a frequency of 0.5 MHz); microwave techniques utilizing small microwave antennas inserted into hollow tubings with frequencies between 300 and 2,450 MHz; ferromagnetic seed implants for delivering thermal energy to deep-seated tumors; hot water tubes; and laser fibers. Interstitial heating allows the tumor to be heated to higher temperatures than external techniques. Other advantages of this technique include better control of heat distributions within the tumor as compared with external hyperthermia, and the sparing of normal tissues, especially the overlaying skin. On the other hand, the disadvantages are invasiveness, difficulty in repeated treatment, and limitation of applicable sites [1, 2].

Under anesthesia, probes or small needles are inserted into the body to produce localized deposition of EM energy in subcutaneous and deep seated tumors. For treatment regions that are large compared to the field penetration depth of frequency used, the required SAR uniformity throughout a tumor volume cannot be achieved with a single antenna, and arrays of antennas are then employed. Imaging techniques, such as ultrasound, may be used to make sure the probe is properly positioned within the tumor.

11.2.2 Regional Hyperthermia

Regional heating suits patients with locally advanced deep-seated tumors such as those in the pelvis or abdomen. The application of regional hyperthermia is, however, more complex than local heating, particularly because of wide variation in physical and physiological properties. It requires more sophisticated planning, thermometry, and quality assurance. Since regional heating techniques apply energy to the adjacent deep-seated tumors in a focused manner, energy is also delivered to the adjacent normal tissues. Under such conditions, selective heating of tumors is only possible when heat dissipation by blood flow in normal tissue is greater than that in tumor tissue. Most clinical trials on regional hyperthermia have used the approach as an adjunct to radiotherapy. Locally advanced and/or recurrent tumors of the pelvis are the major indications for regional hyperthermia, including rectal carcinoma, cervical carcinoma, bladder carcinoma, prostate carcinoma, or soft tissue sarcoma. Some of these indications were validated in prospective studies [1, 2].

11.2.2.1 Deep Regional Hyperthermia

Heat delivery to deep-seated tumors is the most difficult problem and major efforts have been devoted to the development of external deep-heating equipment. The ideal heating device should be capable of raising the whole tumor volume to a therapeutic temperature without overheating adjacent normal tissues. Treatments of deep-seated tumors are difficult because EM energy is rapidly absorbed by human tissue. External applicators are positioned around the body cavity or organ to be treated, and EM energy is focused on the area to raise its temperature. Deep regional hyperthermia is usually performed using arrays of multiple applicators. For example, annular phased-array system delivering EM energy and RF capacitive heating apparatus are examples of regional heating devices. This system has the advantage that subcutaneous fat is not excessively heated, and thus it is suitable for obese patients. However, this method causes systemic symptoms such as tachycardia and malaise, which result from the use of large-sized applicators. Model calculations show significant improvements in control of power distribution by increasing the antenna number, with the assumption of optimum adjustment of phases and amplitudes.

11.2.2.2 Regional Perfusion Hyperthermia

Regional perfusion techniques can be used to treat cancers in the arms and legs, such as melanoma or cancer in some organs, such as the liver or lung. In this procedure, some of the patient's blood is removed, heated, and then pumped (perfused) back into the limb or organ. Anticancer drugs are commonly given during this treatment. Regional hyperthermia is usually applied by perfusion of a limb, organ, or body cavity with heated fluids [1, 2].

Much experience with hyperthermic chemoperfusion has been gained since 1970. In contrast to external heating methods, hyperthermic perfusion techniques carry the risk of severe and persisting adverse effects (for example, neuropathy and amputation of limbs). However, both hyperthermic isolated limb perfusion and hyperthermic intraperitoneal perfusion at different temperatures achieve high response rates in comparison with historical control groups receiving systemic chemotherapy. This success is due to both the homogeneous and well-controlled heat application and the much higher (more than tenfold) drug concentration possible.

Hyperthermic isolated limb perfusion has been mostly used as a melphalan-based induction therapy in advanced stages of nonresectable melanomas and soft-tissue sarcomas (limited to one limb). Trials showed further improvement in response rates with addition of high doses of tumor necrosis factor, whereas application of additional drugs (especially cisplatin) is not beneficial. Because of these high response rates, no prospective randomized trials on induction therapy with hyperthermic isolated limb perfusion have yet been done.

11.2.3 Whole-Body Hyperthermia (WBH)

WBH (to a limit of 42°C) is a distinctive and complex pathophysiological condition that has tremendous impact on tissue metabolism, blood flow, organ function, and tissue repair. It has been investigated since the 1970s as an adjuvant with conventional chemo- or radiotherapy for the treatment of various malignant diseases. WBH is used to treat metastatic cancer that has spread throughout the body. To ensure that the desired temperature is reached, but not exceeded, the temperature of the tumor and surrounding tissue is monitored throughout hyperthermia treatment [1, 2].

Three major methods are now available to achieve reproducible, controlled WBH: thermal conduction (surface heating), extracorporeal induction (blood is pumped out of the patient's body, heated to 42°C or more, then put back in the body while still hot), and radiant or EM induction. The tolerance of liver and brain tissue limits the maximum temperature for using WBH to 41.8°C to 42.0°C, but this temperature may be maintained for several hours.

WBH hyperthermia may also be used to treat AIDS. In a technique called extracorporeal hyperthermia, the blood is pumped out of the patient's body, heated to 42°C or more, then put back in the body while still hot. Extracorporeal hyperthermia treatment of bone followed by its reimplantation may be an optional treatment of bone tumors.

WBH can be applied only to patients in a good general condition, and when combined with drugs the first step must be to demonstrate its safety [10]. The toxicities associated with WBH may be significant; therefore, careful patient selection and supportive care are essential. Sedation or general anesthesia must be used, and continuous monitoring of vital signs, core body temperature, cardiac functions [using electrocardiogram (ECG)], and urine output is necessary.

11.2.4 Extracellular Hyperthermia

The main idea of extracellular hyperthermia (or electro-hyperthermia, oncothermia) is to heat up the targeted tissue by means of an electric field, keeping the energy absorption in the extracellular liquid. Extracellular hyperthermia is devoted to enhancing the efficiency of conventional hyperthermia by additional, nonequilibrium thermal effects with the aim of suppressing the existing disadvantages of the classical thermal treatments. Although this new technique recognizes the benefits of increased tissue temperature and its biological consequences, it also argues that nonequilibrium thermal effects are partially responsible for the observed clinical deviations from the purely temperature-based treatment theory [1, 2].

Extracellular hyperthermia is based on a capacitively coupled energy transfer applied at a frequency that is primarily absorbed in the extracellular matrix due to its inability to penetrate the cell membrane. The energy absorption for these effects is more significant than the temperature; so it is important to characterize the hyperthermia by thermal dose rather than by temperature. Thermal dose changes many energetic processes in the tissue and in their physiology. Most of the desired changes (structural and chemical) involve energy consumption.

11.3 Hyperthermia Devices

Most clinical hyperthermia systems operate by causing a target volume of tissue to be exposed to EM fields or ultrasound radiation. A structure is needed that is capable of transferring energy into biological tissue and getting the best approximation of the area to be treated by 3D distribution of SAR. The majority of the hyperthermia treatments are applied using external devices (applicators), employing energy transfer to the tissue. User needs require that the system be effective, safe, and robust. For a heating system to be effective, it must be able to produce final time and temperature histories that include a set of tumor temperatures that can be maintained for long enough times to result in clinically effective thermal doses without also producing unacceptable normal tissue temperatures.

11.3.1 Techniques

Facilitated by the enormous progression in computational power, the last decade has brought significant advances and innovations in the technology needed to develop RF, microwaves, and ultrasound applicators. Table 11.1 compares these three major hyperthermia techniques. Applicators are positioned around or near the appropriate region, and energy is focused on the tumor to raise its temperature. Currently, hyperthermia systems can be interfaced with magnetic resonance image (MRI) systems, allowing noninvasive temperature monitoring of the treatment.

11.3.1.1 Ultrasound

Sound is vibration. Ultrasound waves involve the propagation of sound waves at a frequency of 2 to 20 MHz through soft tissues. Absorption of ultrasound waves results in heating of the medium. In terms of basic physics, ultrasound has the best combination of small wavelengths and corresponding attenuation coefficient that allow penetration to deep sites with the ability to focus power into regions of small size. The primary limitation of such systems is their inability to penetrate air and the difficulty in penetrating bone [1].

Early ultrasound systems used single-transducer applicators that showed increased tumor temperatures compared with microwave systems. Multiple elements and frequencies can be used in order to increase the focusing of energy while maintaining good penetration depth, thus making SAR shaping by either phasing or mechanical scanning clinically feasible for superficial sites [3].

Table 11.1 Comparison of Major Hyperthermia Techniques

Technique	*Advantages*	*Disadvantages*	*Applications*
Ultrasound	Excellent focus in tissue. No hot spots in fatty tissues. Heating capability up to 5–10-cm depth with single transducer and up to 20-cm depth with multiple transducers. Temperature is easy to measure.	Heating area is small. No penetration of tissue-air interfaces.	Treatment of superficial and deep regional tumors. Examples include surface lesions; head and neck lesions, and lesions in extremities.
Radiofrequency	Simple instrumentation. Large treatment area. Electrodes not limited in size and insulation can be accomplished.	Difficult to control electric fields. Only areas where fat is thin can be treated by capacitive systems. Heating regional with external applicators.	Treatment of large and superficial tumors in neck, limb, chest, brain, abdomen, and so forth.
Microwaves	Heating large volumes is possible. Specific antennas for heating from body cavities have been developed. Multiple applicators, coherent or incoherent, can be used. Can avoid hot spots in fatty tissues.	Limited penetration at high frequencies. Temperature measurement is difficult and thermometry requires noninteracting probes.	Treatment of superficial tumors in breast, limb, prostate, brain, and so forth.

11.3.1.2 Radiofrequency

The early investigation of the use of RF waves in the body is credited to d'Arsonval in 1891, which showed that RF waves that pass through living tissue cause an elevation in tissue temperature without causing neuromuscular excitation. These observations eventually led to the development in the early to mid-1900s of electrocautery and medical diathermy. To heat large tumors at depth, RF fields in the range of 10 to 120 MHz are generally used with wavelengths that are long compared to body dimensions and, thus, deposit energy over a sizeable region. Schematically, a closed-loop circuit is created by placing a generator, a large dispersive electrode (ground pad), a patient, and a needle electrode in series. Both the dispersive electrode and needle electrode are active, while the patient acts as a resistor. Thus, an alternating electric field is created within the tissue of the patient. Given the relatively high electrical resistance of tissue in comparison with the metal electrodes, there is marked agitation of the ions present in the tumor tissue that immediately surrounds the electrode. This ionic agitation creates frictional heating within the body, which can be tightly controlled through modulation of the amount of RF energy deposited.

11.3.1.3 Microwaves

Another promising hyperthermia technique is the use of microwaves. Microwave hyperthermia has been used on thousands of patients suffering from prostate or breast cancer. Microwave-generated heat is used to shrink and/or destroy cancerous tumors. Microwave hyperthermia has generally utilized single-waveguide microwave antennas working at 434, 915, and 2,450 MHz. A hyperthermia system includes the antenna and a noncontacting temperature sensor which scan a predetermined path over the surface of tissue to be treated. The temperature sensor senses temperature of the tissue, and a controller closes a feedback loop which adjusts the microwave power applied to the antenna in a manner which raises the temperature of the tissue uniformly. Microwave hyperthermia is frequently used in conjunction with other cancer therapies, such as radiation therapy. It can increase tumor blood flow, thereby helping to oxygenate poorly oxygenated malignant cells.

The early systems have had the heating disadvantage of having lateral SAR contours that are significantly smaller than the applicator dimensions, thus causing underheating problems in early trials when investigators used applicators that covered the tumors visually but heated only their central region. Also, at the frequency of operation these systems have relatively long wavelengths, limiting their ability to focus on tumors. To overcome these limitations, improved antenna-based systems and multiple-applicator systems have been used clinically for large tumors, and phasing of such systems is a possibility [3].

11.3.2 External RF Applicators

11.3.2.1 Capacitive Heating

This applicator is composed of two-plate capacitor excited by an electric potential between the plates as shown in Figure 11.2. Capacitor-plate applicators are typical electric field (E-type) applicators. These applicators are usually operated at either 13.56 or 27.12 MHz, two of the frequencies assigned to industrial, scientific, and medical use (ISM frequencies). Capacitive hyperthermia equipment generally consists of an RF generator, an RF power meter, an impedance matching network, a set of electrode applicators, a temperature control system for the applicators, a set of connecting cables, and a patient support assembly. The RF energy is transmitted from the generator via coaxial cables to electrodes placed on opposite sides of the body and the power is distributed locally or regionally through interaction of electric (E) fields produced between the parallel-opposed electrodes. The adjustable positions of the electrodes permit heating at different angles and treatment sites [1, 2].

RF-capacitive devices are convenient to apply to various anatomical sites. Tissues can be heated by displacement currents generated between the two capacitor

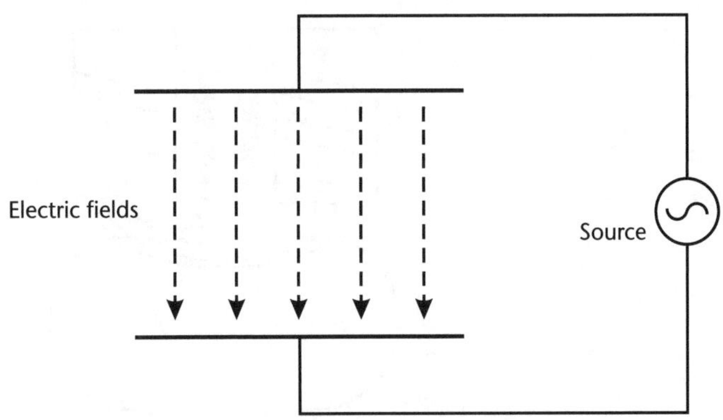

Figure 11.2 Capacitive applicator for hyperthermia.

plates. However, they are not robust in terms of positioning, because currents tend to concentrate around the closer electrode tips when they are nonparallel. Another disadvantage is the excessive heating of subcutaneous fat. This is because electric fields generated are normal to the skin surface and currents must pass through the high-resistance low-blood flow superficial fatty layers causing substantial superficial heating.

11.3.2.2 Inductive Heating

A coupled energy transfer from coil carrying alternating current (ac) surrounding a biological object through air is used to achieve deeper hyperthermia (for example, more than 5 cm). Magnetic fields in RF induction heating can penetrate tissues, such as subcutaneous fat, without excessive heating. Such magnetic fields induce eddy currents inside the tissues. Since the induced E fields are parallel to the tissue interface, heating is maximized in muscle rather than in fat.

The simplest inductive applicator is a single coaxial current loop. Since the coaxial current loop produces eddy currents type E fields that circulate around the axis of the loop, heating in the center of the body is minimal. In general, inductive applicators seem not to couple as strongly to the body as capacitive applicators, and relatively high currents are usually needed to get adequate heating. Subsequent use of these devices shows that they still heat a large amount of normal tissue. These applicators are usually operated at ISM frequencies of 13.56, 27.12, and 40 MHz, with the depth of penetration being a few centimeters.

Induction hyperthermia systems generally consist of an RF power generator, an RF power meter, an impedance matching network, one or more induction coil applicators, a set of connecting cables, and a patient support assembly. An inductive applicator for hyperthermia is shown in Figure 11.3. A pair of cylindrical ferrite cores is used for the applicator. The distance between the pair of ferrite cores is adjustable depending on the size of the region to be heated. The target is placed between or under the pair of ferrite cores. The time-varying magnetic field penetrating the body causes an eddy current. As a result, Joule's heat is produced. To effectively control the heating position vertically or horizontally, conductive plates to shield the magnetic field are introduced.

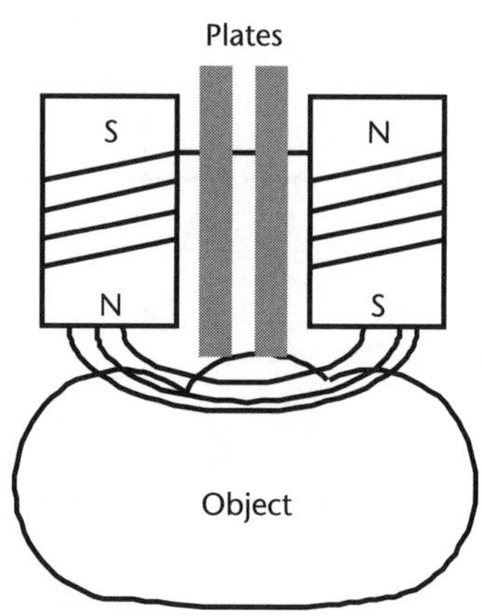

Figure 11.3 Inductive applicator for hyperthermia.

11.3.2.3 Combined Heating Systems

A heating system combining a pair of capacitively coupled electrodes and induction aperture-type applicators is called a hybrid heating system. Figure 11.4 shows schematically the inductive heating system. In this case, the currents produced by the electrodes and applicators are substantially additive in the central region of the phantom but are substantially opposed in the superficial regions beneath the apertures of the applicators.

11.3.3 Radiative EM Devices

One of the major problems of high-frequency EM devices is the limited depth of penetration due to the EM principle of skin-depth. Only tumors located 2 to 3 cm from the skin surface can be heated with conventional surface applicators. Different types of antennas can be used as applicators including waveguides and horns, and microstrip patches.

11.3.3.1 Single Applicators

Early hyperthermia trials were conducted with single aperture devices having no ability to steer or focus energy other than shifting patient position relative to the applicator. Most of the microwave equipment includes a water bolus for surface cooling. Low-profile, light-weight microstrip applicators, which are easier to use clinically, are also used. The type of applicator selected depends on the production of sufficient thermal field distributions at different depths of the tumor in a variety of anatomical sites. Single-element applicators can safely deliver optimum thermal doses to relatively small superficial tumors. Over the years, several types of applicators for external local hyperthermia have been investigated by many researchers based on the principle of dielectric filled waveguide or horn antenna.

11.3.3.2 Array Applicators

To increase the value of SAR at depth relative to the surface SAR in hyperthermia therapy, we must geometrically focus energy deposition from multiple E fields generated

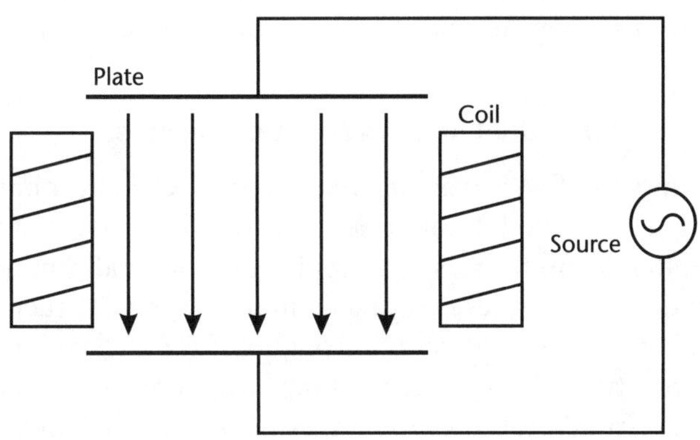

Figure 11.4 Capacitive and inductive applicator for hyperthermia.

by an array of applicators. A basic array for external deep heating will likely consist of an annular ring of radiating apertures. The parameters of interest are an external E field within an array at the surface of the patient's body, the SAR pattern within the target volume, and the radiation leakage levels of the scattered fields around the applicator.

An array of applicators with variations in phase, frequency, amplitude, and orientation of the applied fields can add more dimensions to controlling the heating patterns during hyperthermia cancer therapy. Because of constructive interference of E fields at the intended focus and destructive interference of E fields away from the focus, multichannel coherent phased-array applicators can theoretically provide deeper tissue penetration and improved localization of the absorbed energy in deep-seated tumor regions without overheating the skin and superficial healthy tissues compared to single or incoherent array applicators.

When comparing array applicators with a single applicator, array applicators provide deeper tissue penetration, reduce undesired heating of normal surrounding tissues between the applicator and tumor, and improve local control of the tumor temperature distribution. Heat generated by RF devices is delivered regionally across a much larger area. However, microwave array system requires target compression because of the shallow penetration of the higher microwave frequencies. RF array applicators surrounding the body are used in attempting to heat deep tumors. However, studies in external RF array thermotherapy have shown the difficulty of localizing RF energy in malignant tissue deep within the human body without damaging superficial healthy tissue due to hot spots. Improvements in RF energy deposition are achieved when the RF phased array is controlled by an adaptive algorithm to focus the RF energy in the tumor and tumor margins, while the superficial RF fields are nullified.

Clinically, the use of phased arrays as heating applicators has several advantages. Phased arrays can easily compensate for the effects of inhomogeneities of the treatment volume (which includes the tumor and the surrounding tissues). The heating pattern can be controlled electronically, thus eliminating the need for mechanical movement of the applicator head. This simplifies the machine patient interface and allows for better use of the available power. Also, electronic switching can be performed rapidly, thus enabling a swift response to changes in the tumor environment. Nevertheless, clinicians cannot always accurately predetermine or manually adjust the optimum settings for output power and phase of each antenna to focus heat reliably into deep-seated tumors. Figure 11.5 illustrates the setup that performs hyperthermia using an array of antennas [1, 2].

11.3.4 Interstitial and Intracavitary Devices

As early as 1976 it was suggested that RF currents applied between groups of stainless-steel electrodes could be used to induce elevated temperatures in deep-seated (depth $\geq$ 3 cm) tumors. The application of an alternating voltage of sufficient magnitude across planes comprising multiple pairs of such electrodes is capable of generating electrical currents through the tumor leading to an increase of the tissue temperature. The simplicity of the basic concept accounts for increasing acceptance of interstitial probes by hyperthermia research groups and its application to various anatomical tumor-bearing sites [1, 2].

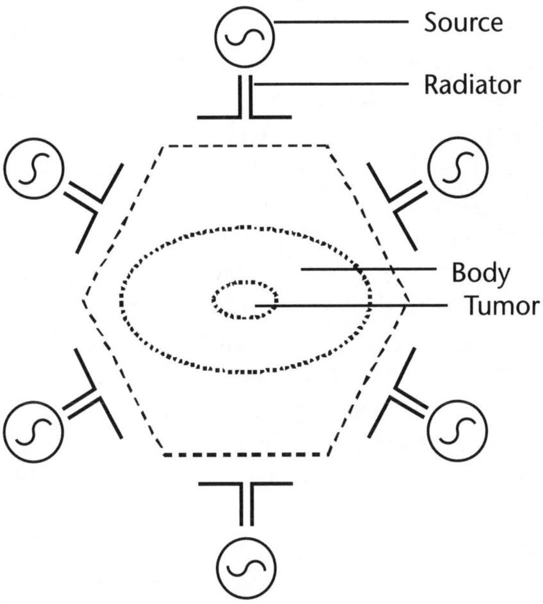

Figure 11.5 A ring of radiating antennas.

Interstitial hyperthermia is an invasive procedure where a single or an array of interstitial antennas or electrodes is implanted in accessible tumors which might be located in deep or superficial tissues. The invasiveness gives interstitial systems the clear advantage of being potentially effective, and therefore, potentially maximizing the tumor temperature while minimizing thermal damage to normal tissue. In addition to electrodes, the interstitial hyperthermia system includes a generator controlled with an automatic tuning system and temperature limitation system. Temperature measurements must be performed at the antennas and between them. In most systems, every single antenna is controlled by its own generator. Dedicated systems have in addition two or more segments per antenna or electrode controlled in phase and/or amplitude. One limitation of the interstitial heating approach is the inability of the system to vary the power deposition along the radial direction [1, 2].

Although often compared to interstitial systems, intracavitary systems are really interior versions of superficial systems that, by using the appropriate body cavities, minimize both the amount of intervening normal tissue between the applicator and the tumor (compared with using a superficial system for the same tumor) and the amount of tissue trauma (compared with the more invasive interstitial system). Intracavitary systems are quite promising for a few important sites such as the prostate and the esophagus. More advances systems have been developed recently including multiple applicators in a segmented, phased array ultrasound system [3].

11.3.5 Nanotechnology-Based Hyperthermia

The major problem of applied hyperthermia treatments is achieving a homogenous heat distribution in the treated tissue. The currently available modalities of hyperthermia are often limited by their inability to selectively target tumor tissue and, hence, they carry a high risk of collateral organ damage, or they deposit heat in a much localized manner which can result in under-treatment of a tumor. The nanotechnology-based cancer therapy is a special form of interstitial thermotherapy with the advantage of selective heat deposition to the tumor cells. This new therapy is one of the first applications of nanotechnology in medicine and based on heating of ferric oxide nanoparticles in an ac magnetic field. The method is also known as magnetic fluid hyperthermia (MFH) or nanocancer therapy. This technique meets the requirement of maximal deposition of heat within the targeted region under maximal protection of the surrounding healthy tissue at the same time.

Deep local inductive heating can be achieved by using an implant material, which generates heat by its interaction with the magnetic field. However, since eddy currents are predominantly induced near the surface of the human body, the result is that both the implanted region and the superficial normal tissues are being heated. Eddy current absorbers consisting of silicon rubber containing a fine carbon powder are used.

For clinical applications, magnetic materials should present low levels of toxicity, as well as a high saturation magnetic moment in order to minimize the doses required for temperature increase. Currently, magnetite (Fe_3O_4) is used in this process because it presents a high Curie temperature, high saturation magnetic moment (90 to 98 emu/g, or ~450 to 500 emu/cm^3), and has shown the lowest toxicity index in preclinic tests [1, 2].

11.4 Hyperthermia with Other Modalities

Hyperthermia has been used for the treatment of resistant tumors of many kinds, but still with unsatisfactory results. Hyperthermia can be used by itself, and results in shrinkage and sometimes complete eradication of tumors. Yet, these results may not last, and the tumors regrow. Most tumor sites are unreachable with the present interstitial, superficial, and regional hyperthermia techniques; while for those limited sites which are heatable, all dosimetry studies indicate that the temperature distribution reached is highly inhomogeneous and that it is almost impossible to obtain the protocol temperature goals. Accordingly, the most beneficial contribution of hyperthermia for oncological treatments will be based on enhancing the effectiveness of other treatment modalities (radiotherapy, chemotherapy, radiochemotherapy, gene therapy, immune therapy, and so forth).

The biological rationale for hyperthermia applied in combination with radiotherapy or chemotherapy is well established and extremely promising; in particular, the sensitivity of hypoxic cells to heating makes hyperthermia an ideal additive to standard radiotherapy. Hyperthermia produces direct injury by damaging the entire cellular machinery, including nucleic acids, cytoskeleton, and cell membranes. Radiotherapy and many chemotherapeutic agents have similar mechanisms of action. There are reports of synergistic effects of regional or WBH for cancer treatments that include radiotherapy, bleomycin, mitomycin C, Adriamycin, 5-flurourical, cisplatin, and carboplatin [1, 2].

11.4.1 Hyperthermia and Radiation

The synergistic effects of hyperthermia combined with radiation have been investigated and reported to yield higher complete and durable responses than radiation alone in superficial tumors. Several mechanisms are responsible for the supra-additive effect of the combination of radiotherapy and hyperthermia. The additive complementary effect comes from the sensitivity of cells in the hypoxic, low pH areas, and the cells in S-phase, which are both relatively radioresistant [4]. Hyperthermia may cause an increased blood flow, which may result in an improvement in tissue oxygenation, which then results in a temporally increased radiosensitivity. Clinical data and experiments in vivo show hyperthermia at mild temperatures to be easily achievable with the use of presently available clinical hyperthermia devices, which increases perfusion in the tumor region, leading to a higher oxygen concentration. Higher perfusion can increase drug delivery and reoxygenation.

Combined hyperthermia and radiation offers potential clinical advantages for treatment of tumors. Importantly, the synergy between radiation and heat is highly dependent on the order of application and highest when given simultaneously. It has been reported by many clinical trials that hyperthermia therapy has been shown to substantially improve local control of cancer, tumor clinical response, and survival rates when added to radiation treatments.

A disadvantage intrinsically associated with hyperthermia is that the heat treatment can cause a transient resistance against a subsequent treatment (thermotolerance). In radiotherapy, a standard treatment regimen consists of a 6-week course of radiation doses. If one would like to apply hyperthermia with each of these radiation treatments, this thermotolerance would certainly negatively interfere with the effectiveness of the treatment. Therefore, the mechanisms underlying thermotolerance are being extensively explored to find ways to minimize its development [1, 2].

11.4.2 Hyperthermia and Chemotherapy

In clinical practice, it is difficult to deliver therapeutic amounts of infused chemotherapy to solid tumors deep in the body without incurring toxic effects in healthy body organs. Only limited amounts of free chemotherapy infused into the bloodstream reach the tumor due to damaged vasculature in the vicinity of the tumor and due to tumor cell pressure which blocks the chemotherapy from passing through the cell membrane. A number of clinical studies have established that elevated cell tissue temperature, induced by EM energy absorption, significantly enhances the effectiveness of chemotherapy in the treatment of malignant tumors in the human body without increasing the infused amount of drug.

For the combination of hyperthermia and chemotherapy, spatial cooperation can again explain the additive effects. Drug concentration will be less in the insufficiently perfused tumor regions. When it comes to chemotherapy, there are indications that some chemo can be potentiated by hyperthermia. This can, in some agents, increase toxicities and the incidence of damage associated with them at the usual doses, or it can be taken advantage of in the sense of getting the same results with lower doses of the drug. The important mechanisms for an interactive effect are an increased intracellular drug uptake, enhanced DNA damage, and higher intratumor drug concentrations, resulting from an increase in blood flow. An interactive effect was observed for virtually all cell lines treated at temperatures above 40°C for alkylating agents, nitrosureas, and platin analogs, with enhancement ratios depending on temperature and exposure time. The effect of these drugs can be enhanced by a factor of 1.2 to 10, and an extremely high thermal enhancement ratio of 23 was even observed for in vitro application of melphalan to drug-resistant cells at 44°C. In combination with chemotherapy, the type of drug, dose, temperature and time of administration all play a role [1, 2].

11.4.3 Hyperthermia and Radiochemotherapy

Radiochemotherapy is a widely used means of treatment for patients suffering from primary, locally advanced, or recurrent rectal cancer. The efficacy of treatment can be enhanced by additional application of regional hyperthermia to this conventional therapy regime. Many researchers conducted investigations on the effectiveness of hyperthermia combined with radiochemotherapy in the treatment of cancer.

11.5 Dosimetry for Hyperthermia

Dosimetry means the accurate measurement of doses, especially of radiation. EM dosimetry (i.e., measurement or calculation of the EM radiation absorbed by humans in radiation fields) has become increasingly important as the use of EM devices in our society has increased. Additionally, dosimetry considers the measurement or determination by calculation of induced current density, specific absorption (SA), or specific absorption rate (SAR) distributions in objects like models (phantoms), animals, humans, or even parts of human body exposed to EM fields [19]. At lower frequencies (below approximately 100 kHz), many biological effects are quantified in terms of the current density in tissue, and this parameter is most often used as a dissymmetric quantity. At higher frequencies, many (but not all) interactions are due to the rate of energy deposition per unit mass. This is why SAR is used as the dissymmetric measure at those frequencies [9].

11.5.1 Modeling Power Deposition

Living systems have a large capacity for compensating for the effects induced by external influences, in particular EM sources. This is very often overlooked, which serves as one more reason why conclusions derived from models have to be taken with precautions. Physiological compensation means that the strain imposed by external factors is fully compensated and the organism is able to perform normally. Pathological compensation means that the imposed strain leads to the appearance of disturbances within the functions of the organism and even structural alterations may result. The border line between these two types of compensation is obviously not always easy to determine [19].

To obtain the solution for the equations of EM deposition inside biological systems it is required to choose a calculation method. Sometimes, the geometry of the model is simple enough (one-dimensional models), and these equations can be solved by analytic methods. However, most models have a complex geometry (especially those based on a very realistic anatomy), with regions of different characteristics, and a numerical method has to be employed. Analytical techniques may be used to predict EM fields deposited inside modeled tissues by solving Maxwell's equations for general source configurations of canonical homogenous bodies. For inhomogeneous bodies, one must resort to numerical analysis. The use of numerical modeling techniques has improved the understanding of power deposition in human bodies with EM energy. Several numerical techniques have been investigated over the past several years. The finite-difference time-domain (FDTD) method is extremely versatile for bioelectromagnetic problems. The FDTD has been used for modeling whole-body or partial-body EM exposures. The human body is modeled as a nonmagnetic, isotropic, linear EM material at the frequencies of interest. Another numerical technique that is usually applied to bioelectromagnetic problems is the finite element method (FEM). FEM requires the complete volume of the configuration to be meshed as opposed to surface integral techniques, which only require surfaces to be meshed. Each mesh element can have different material properties from those of neighboring elements. The aim of the FET analysis is to determine the field quantities at the nodes (corners of the elements). The drawback of this method is that for complicated bodies it will be very difficult and sometimes impossible to carry out the integration procedure over the entire body.

When considering EM interaction with biological systems, it is important to distinguish between levels of fields outside the body (the exposure), and field levels or absorbed energy within body tissues (the dose). The exposure is measured in terms of the electric (E) or magnetic (H) field strength, or power density incident on the body. The dose depends on the exposure, as well as on body geometry, size, its orientation with respect to the field, and other factors. The central issue concerning the dissymmetric assessment of the absorption of EM energy by biological bodies is how much is absorbed and where it is deposited. This is usually quantified SAR, which is the mass-normalized rate at which EM energy is absorbed by the object at a specific location and thus is a good predictor of thermal effects. In the context of RF or microwaves, two alternatives are used, allowing the SAR evaluation from either electric field or temperature measurement. Accordingly, SAR is defined as

$$\text{SAR} = \frac{\sigma|\text{E}|^2}{\rho} = c\frac{dT}{dt} \tag{11.1}$$

where, σ is the electrical conductivity in siemens per meter (S/m), ρ is the mass density in kilogram per cubic meter (kg/m^3), c is the specific heat in joules per kilogram per Kelvin (J/kg K), and $\frac{dT}{dt}$ is the time derivative of the temperature in Kelvin per second (K/s). The unit of SAR is watts per kilogram (W/kg) [19].

It is clear from (11.1) that the localized SAR is directly related to the internal electric field. Calculation of the internal field is, however, difficult to achieve because it is strongly dependent on many factors. These include the nature (near- or far-field zone) and frequency of the incident field, the shape and dimension of the object, the dielectric properties of the object, and whether or not the object is insulated from earth. SAR is a good dissymmetric quantity between approximately 100 kHz and 10 GHz. At frequencies below about 100 kHz, a more useful measure of dose is often the electric field strength in tissue, in units of volts per meter [20].

There are two major types of SAR: (1) a whole-body average SAR; and (2) a local (spatial) peak SAR when the power absorption takes place in a confined body region, as in the case of a head exposed to mobile phone. Whole body SAR measurements are useful for estimating elevations of the core body temperature. As SAR increases, the possibility for heating and, therefore, tissue damage also rises. The whole-body SAR for a given organism will be highest within a certain resonant frequency range, which is dependent on the size of the organism and its orientation relative to the electric and magnetic field vectors and the direction of wave propagation. For an average human the peak whole-body SAR occurs in a frequency range of 60 to 80 MHz, while the resonant frequency for a laboratory rat is about 600 MHz.

Both types of SAR are averaged over a specific period of time and tissue masses of 1g or 10g (defined as a tissue volume in the shape of a cube). Averaging the absorption over a larger amount of body tissue gives a less reliable result. The 1g SAR is a more precise representation of localized RF energy absorption and a better measure of SAR distribution. Local SAR is generally based on estimates from the whole-body average SAR. It incorporates substantial safety factors (for example, 20).

Deposition of energy, usually stated in terms of SAR, although useful for quality control and intercomparison of equipment, is not necessarily related to tissue temperature and, therefore, not to cytotoxicity [20].

11.5.2 Thermal Modeling

To determine the temperature rise once electric fields are known, one must first choose an appropriate continuum model of the evolution of temperature in a biological system. The temperature rise within a biological system depends on the spatial distribution of the EM fields, the thermal constitutive parameters of the biological system, and the governing thermodynamics [21]. The transfer of thermal energy in living tissues is a complex process involving multiple phenomenological mechanisms including blood perfusion, metabolic heat generation, conduction, convection, radiation, evaporation, and external interactions such as EM radiation from other sources.

Successful thermal treatment of tumors requires understanding the attendant thermal processes in both diseased and healthy tissue. Accordingly, it is essential for developers and users of thermal therapy equipment to predict, measure, and interpret correctly the tissue thermal and vascular response to heating. Modeling of heat transfer in living tissues is a means towards this end. Due to the complex morphology of living tissues, such modeling is a difficult task and some simplifying assumptions are needed [22]. Modeling of the bioheat transfer requires as a first step mathematical techniques for solving Maxwell's equations for reasonably accurate representations of the actual objects. Because of the mathematical difficulties encountered in the process of calculation, a combination of techniques is used for the computation of the absorbed EM power distribution in the tissue. Each technique gives information over a limited range of parameters depending on the chosen model. Such modeling is essential because it allows optimal source configurations and provides results that will serve as input data for developing thermal models [20].

An extremely important study in the modeling of bioheat transfer was reported over half a century ago by Pennes [23]. Pennes developed a cylindrical model of a human limb to simulate first the human forearm but later generalized it to any limb. The model considered all the properties essential for the conduction, thermal storage, and environmental exchange terms to be for the tissue while he referred to the blood properties in the blood perfusion system. Pennes suggested a model in which the net heat transfer from blood to tissue was proportional to the temperature difference between the arterial blood entering the tissue and the venous blood leaving the tissue. Pennes' principal theoretical contribution was his suggestion that the rate of heat transfer between blood and tissue is proportional to the product of the volumetric perfusion rate and the difference between the arterial blood temperature and the local tissue temperature. When most researchers apply Pennes' model, they assume that the temperature of venous blood is in equilibrium with the local tissue temperature, and that the arterial blood temperature T_a is constant. The Pennes model describes blood perfusion with acceptable accuracy, if no large vessels are nearby [22].

Following Pennes' suggestion, the thermal energy balance for perfused tissue is expressed in the following form:

$$\rho c \frac{\partial T}{\partial t} = k\frac{\partial^2 T}{dx^2} + k\frac{\partial^2 T}{dy^2}k\frac{\partial^2 T}{dz^2} + \omega_b c_b \rho_b (T_a - T) + Q_m + Q_r(x, y, z, t) \quad (11.2)$$

where $T = T\,(x, y, z, t)$ is the temperature elevation (°C), ρ and ρ_b are the density of tissue and blood, respectively (kg/m^3), c is the specific heat of the tissue (J/kg/K), k is the tissue thermal conductivity (W/m/K), ω_b is the blood volumetric perfusion rate (kg/m^3/s), c_b is the specific heat of blood (J/kg/K), $T_a = T_a\,(x, y, z, t)$ is the ambient temperature of perfusing blood (°C). Q_m is the heat generation in the body—for example, heat generated by the normal process in the body (W/m^3)—and Q_r is the regional heat delivered by the source (W/m^3).

The term $\omega_b c_b \rho_b (T_a - T)$ in (11.2) models the perfusion heat loss. Vascular tissues generally experience increased perfusion as temperature increases. The above term is always considered in cases of tissues with a high degree of perfusion, such as liver tissue. In general, ω_b is assumed as uniform throughout the tissue. However, its value may increase with heating time because of vasodilatation and capillary recruitment.

Spatially distributed heating occurs in skin exposed to penetrating, dissipative radiation such as microwave, ultrasound, and laser light [24]. These heating methods often involve an exponentially decaying power transmission accompanied by reflection at the interface of regions with different electrical properties. For a uniform plane wave incident normally upon the skin surface, with a layer of air included to model the reflection at the skin/air interface, the average absorbed power density Q_r is given by

$$Q_r = \frac{1}{2}\sigma |E|^2 \quad (11.3)$$

Table 11.2 Approximate Value of Biological Tissue Properties

Properties	*Value*
Arterial temperature T_a(°C)	37
Thermal conductivity of tissue k (W/mK)	0.488
Mass density of tissue ρ (kg/m^3)	1,000
Specific heat capacity of tissue c (J/kg/K)	3,590
Specific heat capacity of blood c_b (J/kg/K)	3,840
Blood perfusion rate ω_b (kg/(m^{3}s)	0.5

At the frequencies employed in RF hyperthermia (300 kHz to 1 MHz) and within the area of interest (it is known that the electrical power is deposited within a small radius around the active electrode), the tissues can be considered purely resistive, because the displacement currents are negligible. For this reason, a quasi-static approach is usually employed to resolve the electrical problem. Then, $Q_r = JE$, where J is the current density (A/m^2) [20].

In order to build a theoretical model, the values of the basic physical characteristics have to be set for all the material of the model: mass density (ρ), specific heat (c), thermal conductivity (k), and electrical conductivity (σ). In general, it is difficult to measure tissue properties because they are spatially, temporally, and even temperature dependent. The above properties, however, are considered to be isotropic and their values are usually taken from the scientific literature as shown in Table 11.2 [25–27].

11.6 Imaging Techniques

Guidance and monitoring of therapy is, in fact, very important for general clinical acceptance. Accurate targeting allows precise delivery of the therapeutic dose to the diseased tissue while avoiding exposure to the adjacent normal tissue. Monitoring allows one to assess the tissue response to the dose. Therefore, a practical guidance and monitoring system will contain the following features: (1) pretreatment imaging of the site and surrounding tissue to identify and target the exact location of the abnormal tissue, (2) imaging of the treatment site during therapy to provide dynamic localization of the abnormal tissue, and (3) post-treatment imaging to map the treated region for follow-up and/or continued therapy [28].

Doctors have imaged the human body using X-rays since the early years of the 1900s. However, X-ray has many disadvantages, including the exposure of the subject to ionizing radiation [29]. Given this fact and the likely other issues related to the quality of X-ray images, the idea of thermal detection had obvious appeal. The first report of the use of temperature measurements to diagnose cancer was published by Lawson [30].

11.6.1 Ultrasound

The history of ultrasound imaging is much more recent than that of X-ray imaging. After the pioneering work of Wild and Reid in the 1950s [31], the image quality of medical ultrasound has advanced slowly from low-resolution, bistable images to images with much greater detail. Currently, ultrasound image quality is sufficient to make it an important and often indispensable imaging modality in disease diagnosis and in obstetrics [32]. Ultrasound imaging is now mature technology, to the extent that it has a well-established place in clinical practice, as confirmed by the fact that it currently accounts for about one in four of all imaging procedures worldwide. However, this does not mean that the pace of development, either of the understanding of the physics of the interaction between ultrasound and tissue or of innovation in techniques, has slowed down. Indeed, the opposite is true [33].

Methods for using ultrasound as a noninvasive thermometer fall into three categories: (1) those based on echo-shifts due to changes in tissue thermal expansion and speed of sound (SOS), (2) those that use the measurement of acoustic attenuation coefficient, and (3) those that exploit the change in backscattered energy from tissue inhomogeneities [34].

Ultrasound uses a nonionizing pressure wave generated by acoustic transducers usually placed on the patient's skin to transmit sound into the body. This represents a convenient and inexpensive modality with relatively simple signal processing requirements. During its transit through the body, the pressure wave loses energy due to both scattering and absorption. Sound scattered out of the main beam may be used to form images; absorbed energy gives rise to tissue heating. Accordingly, ultrasound applications in medicine fall into two principal classes, diagnostic imaging and therapy, which differ in the power, intensity, and duration of the ultrasound. Medical ultrasound is perhaps best known for its diagnostic use in obstetrics. An ultrasound scan is now routinely offered to women early in pregnancy. Ultrasound imaging is used in many other fields of medicine, because it gives effective diagnostic information from a number of anatomical sites. Figure 11.6 shows an ultrasound imaging plane.

The transducer is the most critical component in any ultrasonic imaging system. The trend for many years has been towards broader bandwidth transducers with more elements, since these will provide superior resolution at multiple depths by allowing the best possible compromise between penetration/resolution and attenuation to be made [35]. Nowadays, the transducers which are in clinical use almost exclusively use a piezoelectric material, of which the artificial ferroelectric ceramic, lead zirconate titanate (PZT) is the most common. The ideal transducer for ultrasonic imaging would have characteristic acoustic impedance perfectly matched to that of the human body; have high efficiency as a transmitter and high sensitivity as a receiver, a wide dynamic range and a wide frequency response for pulse operation [33].

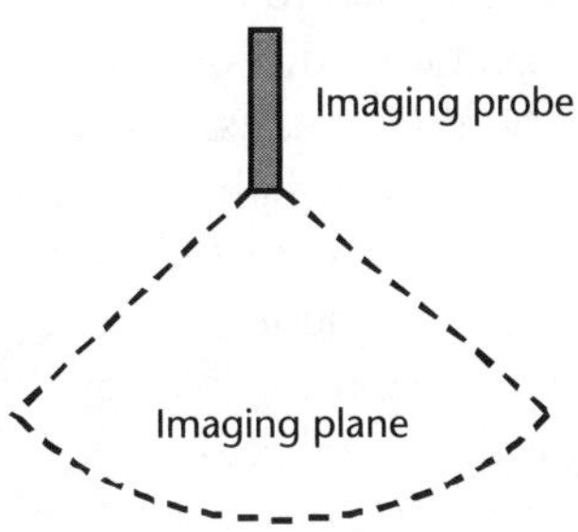

Figure 11.6 Ultrasound imaging plane.

Benefits claimed for ultrasound include the real-time visualization of applicator placement, portability of the technology, nearly universal availability, improved image quality, low cost, and the ability to target and guide therapy with intracavitary endoluminal transducers (for transrectal or transgastric energy application to the prostate and abdominal organs). Because of its ability to obtain blood flow and perfusion information via the Doppler effect, ultrasound is progressively achieving a broader role in radiology, cardiology, and image-guided surgery and therapy.

Ultrasound's limitations come mainly from its rapid attenuation by both bone and gas at the frequencies used, commonly 1 to 20 MHz. Other limitations of ultrasound include occasional poor lesion visualization as a result of overlying bone- or gas-containing structures [36]. These attributes make it an attractive method to use for temperature estimation, if an ultrasonic parameter, which is dependent on temperature, can be found, measured, and calibrated.

11.6.2 Magnetic Resonance Imaging

MRI is a relatively new imaging technique that offers several advantages. It produces no ionizing radiation and provides superior tissue discrimination, lesion definition, an improved anatomic context for surrounding vessels and nerves, and excellent spatial resolution at close to or in real time. MRI also provides the capability of characterizing functional and physiological parameters of tissues, including diffusion, perfusion, flow, and temperature. However, high costs are associated with MRI; it also requires a special environment that can hinder patient accessibility [28].

MRI is based on the principles of nuclear magnetic resonance (NMR), a spectroscopic technique used by scientists to obtain microscopic chemical and physical information about molecules. The technique was called magnetic resonance imaging rather than NMR imaging (NMRI) because of the negative connotations associated with the word nuclear in the late 1970s. MRI started out as a tomographic imaging technique; that is, it produced an image of the NMR signal in a thin slice through the human body. MRI has advanced beyond a tomographic imaging technique to a volume imaging technique [37].

MRI relies on the relaxation properties of excited hydrogen nuclei in tissue water. The object to be examined is positioned in a static external magnetic field, whereupon the spins of the protons align in one of two opposite directions: parallel or antiparallel. The protons process with a frequency determined by the strength of the magnetic field and the gyro-magnetic ratio. The object is then exposed to EM pulses with a frequency identical to the precession frequency in a plane perpendicular to the external magnetic field. For a 1 Tesla (T) scanner, a pulse frequency of 42.58 MHz is used. The pulses cause some of the magnetically aligned hydrogen nuclei to assume a temporary nonaligned high-energy state. As the nuclei realign, they emit energy which can be detected by a receiver coil [38]. Figure 11.7 shows the main components of a magnetic resonance imaging system.

The mechanical integration of any applicator for hyperthermia with MR-tomographs is generally easy to realize. Conversely, interfaces with other methods for noninvasive thermometry (e.g., ultrasound or microwave imaging) are problematic [39]. A particular advantage of MRI is that it not only allows temperature mapping,

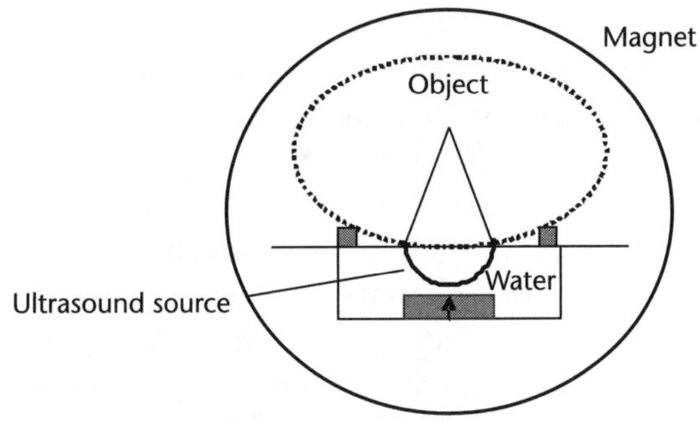

Figure 11.7 Magnetic resonance imaging.

but it can be used as well for target definition and may provide an early evaluation of the therapeutic efficacy [40]. A promising technique for noninvasive thermometry using NMR with computed tomography (CT) has been proposed and studied by Kamimura and Amemiya [41].

Implementing noninvasive monitoring for RF/microwave thermal therapy using the MR technique must solve the problem of EM compatibility: the interference between MR tomography (typically receiving and analyzing low-power signals of mW at 63.9 MHz) and thermal therapy RF applicator (transmitting power signals at therapeutic levels of kW at hundreds of Hz). Both of these systems must be operated simultaneously and without any interaction. In particular, the MR measurements must not be disturbed by any radiation from the thermal therapy system [42].

MRI has demonstrated advantages over other imaging modalities in localizing tissue abnormalities and determining apparent tumor margins. It is therefore ideal for guiding various biopsies and tumor resections. Noninvasive MRI during thermal therapy treatments provides the capability to monitor changes in perfusion, temperature, necrosis, and chemistry. It is unique as an imaging modality in its ability to visualize temperature changes dynamically, therefore providing a mechanism through which thermal therapy can be monitored and controlled. Using the MRI in conjunction with thermal therapy allows the surgeon to view the deposition of energy within the tissues while proceeding with therapy [43, 44]. However, high costs are associated with MRI; it also requires a special environment that can hinder patient accessibility; and minimal use of metal parts in the therapy assembly is necessary to prevent distortion of the MRI trends [28].

11.6.3 Microwave Radiometric Imaging

Biomedical imaging of the human body using microwave technology has been of interest for many years. Microwave images are maps of the electrical property distributions in the body. The electrical properties of various tissues may be related to their physiological state [45]. Because EM radiation can be detected over distance, microwave thermometry can be used to estimate a temperature at depth even if the surface temperature is low. Near-field microwave radiometry and radiometric imaging are noninvasive techniques that are able to provide temperature information at a depth of up to several centimeters in subcutaneous tissues. They are based on the measurement of microwave thermal noise [46]. The principle of microwave radiometer as a tool for biomedical imaging applications is the possibility to monitor a thermal noise produced by objects with temperature above absolute zero. Figure 11.8 shows the principle of imaging by microwave radiometer.

An advantage of the microwave radiometer is the ability to see the temperature increase under the surface of human body. Its main attraction is the innocuous nature of this type of energy at low levels, the relatively low cost of even complex microwave systems compared to the computer-assisted tomography (CAT) and MRI, and the distinctly different permittivity of tumor tissue compared to normal tissue [47, 48].

Current microwave imaging systems image biomedical objects of various sizes, sometimes even the full body. However, despite its unique capabilities, microwave radiometry has so far received only limited acceptance by the medical community, and little commercial success. The chief reasons, we suggest, are the shallow depth of sensing and the difficulty of extracting imaging information from radiometry signals emitted by electrically heterogeneous media. A secondary factor has been the difficulty of validating many proposed clinical applications for the method—in particular, cancer detection. The implementation of a clinically viable microwave imaging system is a technically daunting task since high-resolution imaging requires a sophisticated scanned antenna array.

11.6.4 Terahertz Technology

Terahertz (THz) radiation, which falls between microwaves and infrared light of the EM spectrum, occupies the region between approximately 0.3 and 20 THz. This region of the EM spectrum is sometimes called the "THz-gap" [49]. It is one of the least explored ranges of the EM spectrum. Radiation at these wavelengths is nonionizing and subject to far less Rayleigh scatter than visible or infrared wavelengths, making it suitable for medical applications. Terahertz technology is gaining attention from researchers because it shows great promise for applications to life sciences including medical imaging or even clinical treatment and chemical sensing. The energy levels of this band are very low (1 to 12 meV), and therefore, damage to cells or tissue would be limited to generalized thermal effects (i.e., strong resonant absorption seems unlikely) [50].

THz-ray imaging has several advantages when compared to other sensing and imaging techniques. While microwave and X-ray imaging modalities produce den-

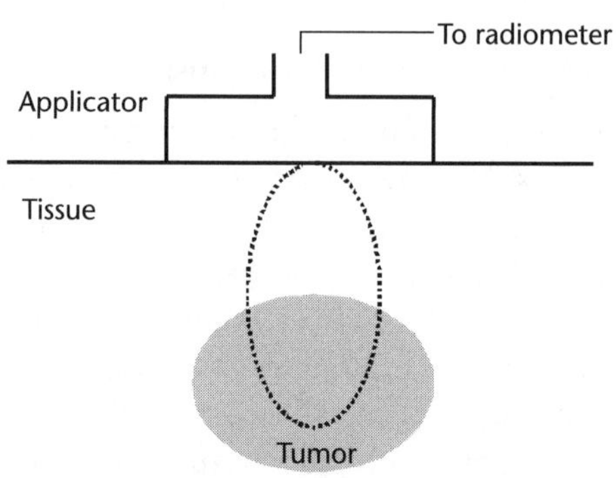

Figure 11.8 Principle of imaging by microwave radiometer.

sity pictures, THz-ray imaging also provides spectroscopic information within the THz range. The unique rotational, vibrational, and translational responses of materials (molecular, radicals, and ions) within the THz range provide information that is generally absent in optical, X-ray, and NMR images [51]. T-ray can also easily penetrate and image inside most dielectric materials, which may be opaque to visible light and low contrast to X-ray, making T-rays a useful and complementary imaging source in this context. The distinctive rotational and vibrational responses of biological tissues within the THz range provide information that can not be offered by optical, X-ray, and MRI techniques.

The excitement about THz imaging stems in part from its degree of penetration. Unlike X-ray, THz radiation is nonionizing. Unlike ultrasound, THz waves can image without contact, and they can go deeper than infrared radiation. THz radiation puts much less energy into biological tissue than the above techniques, which are inadequate. In addition, X-ray raises safety concerns due to the use of ionizing radiation in regular screening. One advantage of THz is the ability to perform spectroscopic measurements at each pixel in an image. This would allow, for example, the use of spectroscopy of tissue to identify regions of disease. Among the challenges to making THz sensing and imaging applications more practical is finding ways to direct the waves to specific targets. Researchers are working to develop THz wave guiding devices that are similar to the waveguides used to channel microwaves and light waves [20].

The challenges in THz imaging appear to lie primarily in the difficulties of fabricating solid-state THz sources. Researchers have focused attention on all-optical techniques of producing THz radiation employing visible/near infrared lasers. Currently, most systems produce THz emissions by either frequency upconversion from the radio wave regime or by frequency downconversion from optical wavelengths. Common downconversion methods include photomixing, notably using semiconductor lasers typical for telecom applications operating around 1.5 μm. An alternative is to irradiate a semiconductor microantenna with the infrared output, typically from a titanium-doped sapphire (Ti: Sapphire) laser with the output wavelength centered around 800 nm [20].

The first THz imaging systems were based on continuous-wave (CW) THz radiation. The setup is less expensive than conventional time-domain imaging systems that comprise femtosecond lasers. CW imaging affords a compact, simple, fast, and relatively low-cost system. The system uses a two-color external-cavity laser diode. Hence it is much more compact as compared to systems based on optically pumped solid-state lasers. The coherent detection scheme is phase sensitive and operates at room temperature. These low-cost, compact systems have image capture rates comparable with those from state-of-the-art pulsed THz systems.

Terahertz time-domain spectroscopy (THz-TDS) based on femtosecond lasers is one of the first and most interesting techniques to generate and detect THz radiation, which is based on frequency conversion using nonlinear optics. Using THz-TDS, the phase and amplitude of the THz pulse at each frequency can be determined. Like radar, THz-TDS also provides time information that allows us to develop various 3D THz tomographic imaging modalities. The key components of a THz-TDS system are a femtosecond laser and a pair of specially designed transducers. By gating these transducers with ultra fast optical pulses, one can generate

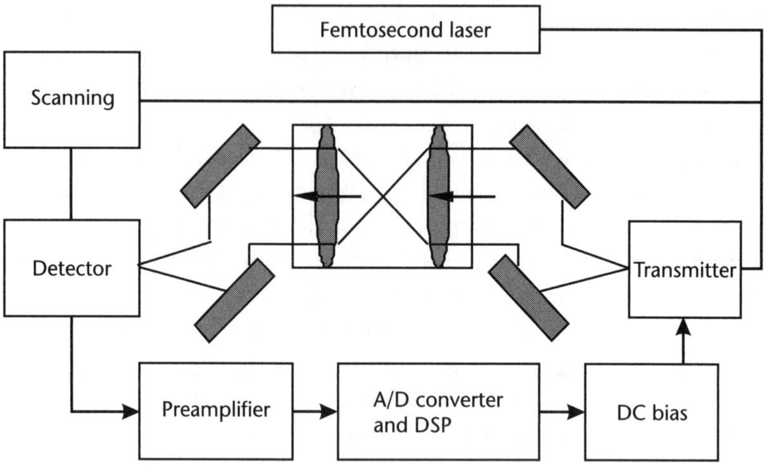

Figure 11.9 Schematic diagram of a THz system.

bursts of THz radiation, and subsequently detect them with high signal-to-noise ratio. These THz transients consist of only one or two cycles of EM field, and they span a very broad bandwidth. Bandwidths extending from 100 GHz to 5 THz can be obtained. Figure 11.9 shows a schematic representation of a THz-ray system. By placing an object at the focus of the THz beam, it is possible to measure the waveform that has traversed through the object. By translating the object, and measuring the transmitted THz waveform for each position of the object, one can build an image pixel by pixel. In order to form images in a reasonable time, the waveforms must be digitized and the desired information extracted on the fly. This can be accomplished using a commercial digital signal processor in a computer, which synchronizes the motion of the object through the focal spot with the waveform acquisition [20].

Scattering is a common problem for many imaging modalities. THz ray exhibits significantly reduced scattering in human tissue compared to near-infrared optical frequencies due to the increased wavelength. Another challenge facing THz imaging in biomedical engineering is the high absorption rate of water and other polar liquids. This strong absorption limits the sensing and imaging in water-rich samples and prohibits transmission-mode imaging through a thick tissue. For this reason, current biomedical THz research has primarily focused on skin conditions [20]. Other disadvantages of a THz system are the size and cost. Current THz-ray imaging systems require areas of a few square meters, most of which is dominated by the ultra-fast laser. In addition, the high cost of the ultrafast laser ($100,000 to $200,000) may impede THz imaging in a number of application settings [51].

11.7 Concluding Remarks

Hyperthermia is an emerging therapy method in oncology. It has been an effective modality of cancer treatments, showing significant improvements in clinical responses for many patients when used alone or in combination with other treatment methods, such as surgery, chemotherapy, radiation therapy, and gene therapy [1, 2]. The clinical exploitation of hyperthermia has been and still is hampered by various challenges, including the high degree of interdependency between physiology and biology, technical and clinical limitations, the lack of standards, and the lack of scientific consensus about its effects on malignant and healthy tissues [20].

An important unresolved factor involves the biological and physiological mechanisms by which hyperthermia works. Although hyperthermic cell killing has been demonstrated in many in vitro studies, the mechanisms underlying cell damage and death have not been fully elucidated. Further work is required towards this end, and information from research studies on the effects of hyperthermia on tumors in vivo will be valuable. Until the underlying mechanisms by which positive clinical results have been obtained are understood and the spatial and temporal distributions of the important biological and physiological variables are known, it will remain impossible to set precise engineering design goals [3].

Realization of the potential of hyperthermia as a primary therapy depends on the advance that must be made in EM heating techniques and imaging. Many major technical advances have been applied in biological and clinical research: the resulting improvements in instrumentation have helped in conducting more accurate and elegant experiments to produce heat for hyperthermia treatment including ultrasound, RF, and microwaves.

Recent developments in hyperthermia have expanded the treatment options of patients with certain types of cancer. The effectiveness of hyperthermia treatment is related to the temperature achieved during the treatment, as well as the length of treatment and cell and tissue characteristics. Control of the heating process as a major part of hyperthermia should be improved to ensure that increased temperature levels can be properly maintained, delivered, and localized within the tumor region. Effectively controlling heating distribution requires: (1) sophisticated controllers that can properly steer the power deposition to achieve close-to-optimal temperatures, and (2) accurate measurements of the spatial and temporal distributions of temperature during the treatment.

The lack of needed engineering tools can be viewed as a major stumbling block to hyperthermia's effective clinical implementation. Developing clinically effective systems will be difficult, however, because it requires solving several complex engineering problems, for which setting appropriate design and evaluation goals is currently difficult owing to a lack of critical biological, physiological, and clinical knowledge, two tasks which must be accomplished within a complicated social/political structure [3].

While hyperthermia requires investments in equipment and personnel training, the same is true for other types of cancer treatment modalities. Another obstacle for the acceptance of hyperthermia may be that it lacks public awareness. Most of the clinical studies are concerned with its combination with radiotherapy. However, the experimental and the few clinical results with combined chemotherapy and hyperthermia make clear that this combination is also worth further testing [10]. Carefully conducted phase III trials with rigorous quality assurance must employ prospective thermal dosimetry to validate the role of hyperthermia in multimodality therapy [52].

A number of challenges must be overcome before hyperthermia can be considered a standard treatment for cancer [2, 10]. Hyperthermia suffers from a lack of dosing and treatment standardization and scientific consensus about its effects on malignant and healthy tissues. In order that hyperthermia will gain widespread approval and clinical use, the technique requires further research and standardization [53]. Standardization of equipment between centers must be achieved before large-scale trials can be realized. Two major factors make hyperthermia difficult. First, there is no clear clinical thermal dose effect relationship, which is coupled with the inability to produce consistently a uniform pattern of heat distribution throughout the tumor mass. Thermal dosimetry is the second major issue; the inability to predict or measure accurately the temperature throughout the tumor mass and the surrounding healthy tissues [20].

Speaking for thermometry and imaging techniques, the future is exciting and challenging for biomedical engineering, and the prospects are certainly brighter than ever before. Techniques and modalities, which were only in the experimental research phase in the early 1970s and 1980s, have now become worldwide accepted clinical procedures. They include CT, MRI, ultrasound, microwave, and THz techniques [54].

Finally, hyperthermia is not yet a fully developed modality; there are still problems with its routine clinical application, and there is still room for further technological improvements. Therefore, the development of hyperthermia is an example of a successful research program which is very important and from which physicians and patients will benefit.

References

[1] Habash, R. W. Y., et al., "Thermal Therapy—Part I: An Introduction to Thermal Therapy," *Critical Reviews in Biomedical Engineering*, Vol. 34, No. 6, 2006, pp. 459–489.

[2] Habash, R. W. Y., et al., "Thermal Therapy-Part II: Hyperthermia Techniques," *Critical Reviews in Biomedical Engineering*, Vol. 34, No. 6, 2006, pp. 491–542.

[3] Roemer, R. B., "Engineering Aspects of Hyperthermia Therapy," *Annual Reviews on Biomedical Engineering*, Vol. 1, 1999, pp. 347–376.

[4] Raaphorst, G. P., "Fundamental Aspects of Hyperthermic Biology," in *An Introduction to the Practical Aspects of Clinical Hyperthermia*, S. B. Field and J. W. Hand, (eds.), London: Taylor & Francis, 1990, pp. 10–54.

[5] Fajardo, L. F., "Pathological Effects of Hyperthermia in Normal Tissues," *Cancer Research*, Vol. 44, 1984, pp. 4826s–4835s.

[6] Dewey, W. C., "Arrhenius Relationships from the Molecule and Cell to the Clinic," *International Journal of Hyperthermia*, Vol. 10, No. 4, 1994, pp. 457–483.

[7] Bush, W., "Uber den Finfluss wetchen heftigere Eryspelen zuweilen auf organlsierte Neubildungen dusuben," *Verh Natruch Preuss Rhein Westphal*, Vol. 23, 1886, pp. 28–30.

[8] Westermark, F., "Uber die Behandlung des ulcerirenden Cervix carcinoma mittels Knonstanter Warme," *Zentralbl Gynkol* 1898, pp. 1335–1339.

[9] Vander Vorst, A., A. Rosen, and Y. Kotsuka, *RF/Microwave Interaction with Biological Tissues*, New York: Wiley-IEEE Press, 2006.

[10] Van der Zee, J., "Heating the Patient: A Promising Approach?" *Annals of Oncology*, Vol. 13, 2002, pp. 1173–1184.

[11] Fiorentini, G., and A. Szasz, "Hyperthermia Today: Electric Energy, A New Opportunity in Cancer Treatment," *Journal of Cancer Research Therapy*, Vol. 2, No. 2, 2006, pp. 41–46.

[12] Gerard, C., V. Rhoon, and P. Wust, "Introduction: Non-Invasive Thermometry for Thermotherapy," *International Journal of Hyperthermia*, Vol. 21, No. 6, 2005, pp. 489–495.

[13] Field, S. B., "1985 Douglas Lea Memorial Lecture. Hyperthermia in the Treatment of Cancer," *Physics in Medicine and Biology*, Vol. 32, No. 7, 1987, pp. 789–811.

[14] Conway, J., and A. P. Anderson, "Electromagnetic Techniques in Hyperthermia," *Clinical Physics and Physiological Measurements*, Vol. 7, 1986, pp. 287–318.

[15] Hildebrandt, B., et al., "The Cellular and Molecular Basis of Hyperthermia," *Critical Reviews on Oncology Hematology*, Vol. 43, No. 1, 2002, pp. 33–56.

[16] Lee, E. R., "Electromagnetic Superficial Heating Technology," in *Thermoradiotherapy and Thermochemotherapy*, M. H. Seegenschmiedt, P. Fessenden, and C. C. Vernon, (eds.), Berlin, Heidelberg: Springer-Verlag, 1995, pp. 193–217.

[17] Wust, P., et al., "Electromagnetic Deep Heating Technology," in *Thermoradiotherapy and Thermochemotherapy*, M. H. Seegenschmiedt, P. Fessenden, and C. C. Vernon, (eds.), Berlin, Heidelberg: Springer-Verlag, 1995, pp. 219–251.

[18] Myerson, R. J., E. Moros, and J. L. Roti Roti, "Hyperthermia," in *Principles and Practice of Radiation Oncology*, C. A. Perez and L. W. Brady, (eds.), Philadelphia, PA: Lippincott-Raven Publishers, 1997, pp. 637–683.

[19] Habash, R. W. H., et al., "Thermal Therapy-Part IV: Electromagnetic and Thermal Dosimetry," *Critical Reviews in Biomedical Engineering*, Vol. 35, No. 1–2, 2007, pp. 123–182.

[20] Habash, R. W. H., *Bioeffects and Therapeutic Applications of Electromagnetic Energy*, Boca Raton, FL: CRC Taylor and Francis, 2007.

[21] Kowalski, M. E., and J.-M., Jin, "A Temperature-Based Feedback Control System for Electromagnetic Phased-Array Thermal Therapy: Theory and Simulation," *Physics in Medicine and Biology*, Vol. 48, No. 5, 2003, pp. 633–651.

[22] Arkin, H., L. X. Xu, and K. R. Holmes, "Recent Developments in Modeling Heat Transfer in Blood Perfused Tissues," *IEEE Transactions on Biomedical Engineering*, Vol. 41, No. 2, 1994, pp. 97–107.

[23] Pennes, H. H., "Analysis of Tissue and Arterial Blood Temperatures in the Resting Human Arm," *Journal of Applied Physiology*, Vol. 1, 1948, pp. 93–122.

[24] Diller, K. R., "Modeling of Bioheat Transfer Processes at High and Low Temperatures," *Advances in Heat Transfer*, Vol. 22, 1992, pp. 157–167.

[25] Vrba, J., M. Lapes, and L. Oppl, "Technical Aspects of Microwave Thermotherapy," *Bioelectrochemistry and Bioenergetics*, Vol. 48, No. 2, 1999, pp. 305–309.

[26] Hardie, D., A. J. Sangster, and N. J. Cronin, "Coupled Field Analysis of Heat Flow in the Near Field of a Microwave Applicator for Tumor Ablation," *Electromagnetic Biology and Medicine*, Vol. 25, No. 1, 2006, pp. 29–43.

[27] Liu, J., "Uncertainty Analysis for Temperature Prediction of Biological Bodies Subject to Randomly Special Heating," *Journal of Biomechanics*, Vol. 34, No. 12, 2001, pp. 1637–1642.

[28] Vaezy, A., M. Andrew, and P. Kaczkowski, "Image-Guided Acoustic Therapy," *Annual Reviews of Biomedical Engineering*, Vol. 3, 2001, pp. 375–390.

[29] Foster, K. R., "Thermographic Detection of Breast Cancer," *IEEE Engineering in Medicine and Biology Magazine*, November/December 1998, pp. 10–14.

[30] Lawson, R. N., "Implications of Surface Temperature in the Diagnosis of Breast Cancer," *Canadian Medical Association Journal*, Vol. 75, No. 4, 1956, pp. 309–310.

[31] Wild, J. J., and J. M. Reid, "Application of Echo-Ranging Techniques to the Determination of the Structure of Biological Tissues," *Science*, Vol. 115, No. 2983, 1952, pp. 226–230.

[32] Fenster, A., and D. B. Downey, "3-D Ultrasound Imaging: A Review," *IEEE Engineering in Medicine and Biology*, Vol. 15, No. 6, 1996, pp. 41–51.

[33] Wells, P. N. T., "Ultrasound Imaging," *Physics in Medicine and Biology*, Vol. 51, 2006, pp. R83–R98.

[34] Arthur, R. M., et al., "Non-Invasive Estimation of Hyperthermia Temperatures with Ultrasound," *International Journal of Hyperthermia*, Vol. 21, No. 6, 2005, pp. 589–600.

[35] Forsberg, F., "Ultrasonic Biomedical Technology; Marketing Versus Clinical Reality," *Ultrasonics*, Vol. 42, No. 1–9, 2004, pp. 17–27.

[36] Goldberg S. N., G. S. Gazelle, and P. R. Mueller, "Thermal Ablation Therapy for Focal Malignancy: A Unified Approach to Underlying Principles, Techniques, and Diagnostic Imaging Guidance," *American Journal of Radiology*, Vol. 174, 2000, pp. 323–331.

[37] Hornak, J. P., *The Basics of MRI*, Online book, 1996, http://www.cis.rit.edu/htbooks/mri/.

[38] Frich, L., "Non-Invasive Thermometry for Monitoring Hepatic Radiofrequency Ablation," *Minimum Invasive Therapy and Allied Technology*, Vol. 15, No. 1, 2006, pp. 18–25.

[39] Van Rhoon, G. C., and P. Wust, "Introduction: Non-Invasive Thermometry for Thermotherapy," *International Journal of Hyperthermia*, Vol. 21, No. 6, 2005, pp. 489–495.

[40] Denis De Senneville, B., B. Quesson, and C. T. W. Moonen, "Magnetic Resonance Temperature Imaging," *International Journal of Hyperthermia*, Vol. 21, No. 4, 2005, pp. 515–531.

[41] Kamimura, Y., and Y. Amemiya, *Automedica*, New York: Gordon and Breach, 1987, pp. 295–313.

[42] Gellermann, J., et al., "A Practical Approach to Thermography in Thermal Therapy/Magnetic Resonance Hybrid System: Validation in a Heterogeneous Phantom," *International Journal of Radiation Oncology Biology Physics*, Vol. 61, 2005, pp. 267–277.

[43] Bleier, A., et al., "Real-Time Magnetic Imaging of Laser Heat Deposition in Tissue," *Magnetic Resonance Medicine*, Vol. 21, No. 1, 1991, pp. 132–137.

[44] Higuchi, N., et al., "MRI of the Acute Effects of Interstitial Neodymium: YAG Laser on Tissues," *Investigative Radiology*, Vol. 27, No. 10, 1992, pp. 814–821.

[45] Fear, E. C., P. M. Meaney, and M. A. Stuchly, "Microwaves for Breast Cancer Detection," *IEEE Potentials*, Vol. 22, 2003, pp. 12–18.

[46] Leroy, Y., B. Bocquet, and A. Mamouni, "Non-Invasive Microwave Radiometry Thermometry," *Physiological Measurement*, Vol. 19, 1998, pp. 127–148.

[47] Rosen, A., and H. D. Rosen, *New Frontiers in Medical Device Technology*, New York: Wiley, 1995.

[48] Rosen, A., M. A. Stuchly, and A. Vander Vorst, "Applications of RF/Microwaves in Medicine," *IEEE Transactions on Microwave Theory and Techniques*, Vol. 50, No. 3, 2002, pp. 963–974.

[49] Smye, S. W., et al., "The Interaction Between Terahertz Radiation and Biological Tissue," *Physics in Medicine and Biology*, Vol. 46, No. 9, 2001, pp. R101–R112.

[50] Mittleman, D. M., et al., "Recent Advances in Terahertz Technology," *Applied Physics* B, Vol. 68, 1999, pp. 1085–1094.

[51] Zhang, X.-C., "Terahertz Wave Imaging: Horizons and Hurdles," *Physics in Medicine and Biology*, Vol. 47, No. 21, 2002, pp. 3667–3677.

[52] Jones, E., et al., "Prospective Thermal Dosimetry: The Key to Hyperthermia's Future," *International Journal of Hyperthermia*, Vol. 22, No. 3, 2006, pp. 247–253.

[53] Durney, C. H., "Electromagnetic Dosimetry for Models of Humans and Animals: A Review of Theoretical and Numerical Techniques," *Proceedings of the IEEE*, Vol. 68, No. 1, 1980, pp. 33–40.

[54] Habash, R. W. Y., et al., "Therapy-Part IV: Electromagnetic and Thermal Dosimetry," *Critical Reviews in Biomedical Engineering*, Vol. 35, Nos. 1–2, 2006, pp. 123–182.

PART III

Image-Guided Therapy

CHAPTER 12

Image-Guided High Intensity Focused Ultrasound

David Goertz, Rajiv Chopra, and Kullervo Hynynen

There is growing interest in the use of minimally invasive or noninvasive thermal ablation techniques. The appeal of such approaches is to achieve rapid, irreversible, and localized tissue damage, though monitoring and control can be limiting factors in many applications. While the ability of high intensity focused ultrasound (HIFU) to heat and ablate tissue has been recognized for more than a half a century [1], it was not until it was employed in conjunction with modern medical imaging systems that it began to emerge as a viable alternative or adjunct to conventional therapeutic approaches. Similar to other ablative techniques, the goal of HIFU is to selectively target specific regions of tissue while sparing and minimizing damage to surrounding tissue and structures. The capacity to guide, monitor, and evaluate HIFU treatments is critical to accomplishing these objectives and thereby ensuring patient safety as well as increasing procedural effectiveness. The two primary imaging modalities currently used for HIFU therapy guidance are diagnostic ultrasound (US) and magnetic resonance imaging (MRI).

Since the development of the initial experimental and commercial integrated HIFU imaging systems in the 1990s, the pace of both technical advances and clinical use has accelerated. With either experimental or commercial systems, HIFU now has the flexibility to be delivered under image guidance using a range of extracorporeal, intracavitary, and interstitial devices. It is poised to play an increasingly significant clinical role in the treatment of solid tumors, and has developing applications ranging from cardiac arrhythmia treatment, to hemostasis, nerve ablation and thrombolysis. In this chapter we provide a brief overview of basic HIFU principles, and survey current and developing image-guided HIFU systems and applications.

12.1 Basic Principles

Conceptually, the way in which HIFU is used to ablate tissue is relatively simple: an ultrasound radiator (transducer) is used to focus energy within a region of tissue, which in turn results in a localized elevation of temperature and/or cavitation. However, in many circumstances the propagation of ultrasound through intervening layers of tissue can lead to significant distortions of the focal zone in terms of its amplitude, location, shape, and size [2]. Variability in local tissue properties can result in further uncertainties in predictions of local temperature rise [3]. On the short time scales employed for HIFU ablation, the effects of tissue perfusion are generally considered to be of lesser significance [4]. These factors, along with the need to ensure that unintended thermal damage does not occur outside of the focal region, make guidance and monitoring essential elements of HIFU therapy. Before considering these points further in the context of practical HIFU systems and applications, it is useful to provide a brief overview of ultrasound, ultrasound-bioeffects, and HIFU transducers.

12.1.1 Ultrasound Principles

Ultrasound is a pressure wave that propagates at a velocity c, and has a wavelength λ inversely related to the ratio of the velocity over frequency. The product of density and velocity is a material property referred to as the acoustic impedance that determines the amount of reflected ultrasound energy at the interface of two tissue layers. Waves impinging upon boundaries between materials with different acoustic impedances will have a portion of their energy reflected, and the transmitted component will undergo refraction. In soft tissues, velocities average approximately 1,550 m/s, with fat being on the low end at 1,480 m/s. In bone, velocities vary between 1,800 to 3,700 m/s [5]. Acoustic impedances in soft tissues are on the order of $1.6 \cdot 10^6$ kg·m^{-2}s^{-1} although bone is significantly higher. Transmission through bone is therefore challenging, which has implications for trancranial applications and in targeting tissue lying underneath ribs, for example. Similarly, the presence of air (low acoustic impedance) that causes complete reflection of an ultrasound beam has effectively prohibited applications in the lungs and bowels.

As ultrasound waves propagate they undergo attenuation, through absorption and scattering mechanisms [6]. Absorption in tissue arises from both viscous forces between moving particles as well as relaxation mechanisms, which ultimately cause a portion of the incident ultrasound wave energy to be converted to heat. Typical attenuation values at 1 MHz are in the range of 5 to 40 Np/m for soft tissues, and are significantly higher in bone. It is notable that attenuation increases as a function of frequency, with an exponent generally in the range of 1 to 1.2 [7]. This has significant implications for HIFU thermal applications in that the frequency must be high enough to cause absorption and focus, yet low enough to achieve sufficient penetration without excessive heating prior to the focus. In practice, frequencies in the range of 0.5 to 4 MHz are used for most applications. Tissue properties, including speed of sound and absorption, also exhibit nonlinear and often irreversible changes with temperature and thermal coagulation, which adds further complexity to HIFU treatment predictions.

While at lower pressures linear wave propagation is a valid assumption, as transmit intensities are raised nonlinearities become increasingly significant [8]. This is largely due to the speed of sound being inversely dependant upon density, which is modulated by the successive compression and rarefactional cycles of an US wave. A pulse will thereby distort with propagation which has the effect of coupling energy into higher harmonics (integral multiples) of the transmit frequency and consequently increasing absorption. For tightly focused transducers, nonlinear propagation effects are concentrated near the focal zone [9].

Cavitation, a process involving the interaction between a pressure wave and a small gas body, can play an important role in HIFU [10, 11]. Gas cavitation nuclei may be present in normal tissue [12], and may also be introduced in the form of encapsulated microbubble contrast agents [13]. Gas body oscillations can occur in a stable manner (stable cavitation), or in an unstable and violent manner, referred to as inertial cavitation [14]. Energy is absorbed and reradiated by these processes which results in increased local energy deposition and therefore thermal damage. The violent collapse of bubbles during inertial cavitation can also result in extremely high local temperatures, light emission, the formation of free radicals, and cause more direct mechanical tissue damage [15].

12.1.2 Mechanisms of Bioeffects

HIFU is capable of inducing tissue damage through several mechanisms. The primary mechanism exploited is temperature elevation, which is associated with absorption effects. With mild to moderate hyperthermia, therapeutic effects can be achieved in the absence of ablation [16]. At higher temperatures, irreversible coagulative necrosis of cells occurs. The threshold for this occurring is dependant upon the absolute temperature attained as well as the duration and temperature trajectory [17]. For example, elevating temperatures to near 60°C and above for in excess of 1 second is sufficient to achieve thermal coagulation. The resulting lesions are ellipsoidal in shape and have clearly demarcated boundaries [18, 19]. Vascular damage within thermal lesions has been observed [20, 21]. It is also possible to thermally induce apoptosis, which evolves at longer time scales than coagulative necrosis [22].

Aside from thermal effects, the radiation pressure of HIFU beams will induce tissue displacements, acoustic streaming, and can create standing wave patterns. These effects have been reported to induce bioeffects [23]. An additional mechanism for inducing tissue damage is through cavitation. Thermal lesions associated with cavitation tend to develop more rapidly, are larger, and have a different shape ("tadpole" like) due to the complex deposition and attenuation patterns that evolve during lesion formation [13]. Cavitation occurring at very high intensities associated with collapsing bubbles under violent inertial cavitation can cause the disintegration of tissue, leaving a fluid filled cavities containing tissue debris. This process has been referred to as *histotripsy* [24].

12.1.3 Transducers and Ultrasound Fields

In the context of HIFU, ultrasound is generated by transducers that are capable of concentrating ultrasound energy into highly localized regions (typically 1 to 3 mm laterally by 0.5 to 3 cm in depth). Generally these transducers are air backed piezo-ceramic (e.g., PZT) or piezocomposite devices that are stimulated with single frequency sinusoidal driving pulses. In its simplest form, a HIFU system employs a high gain spherically focused single element transducer [Figure 12.1(a)]. With this approach, the energy present along the path length prior to the focus is low, thereby reducing exposure in intervening tissue layers [Figure 12.1(b)]. As the target volumes are generally much larger than the focal size, such beams require mechanical scanning, which has a significant impact on treatment times.

Ultrasound beams can also be focused by using one- or two-dimensional arrays of smaller transducer elements. In this case electronic control of the relative transmit

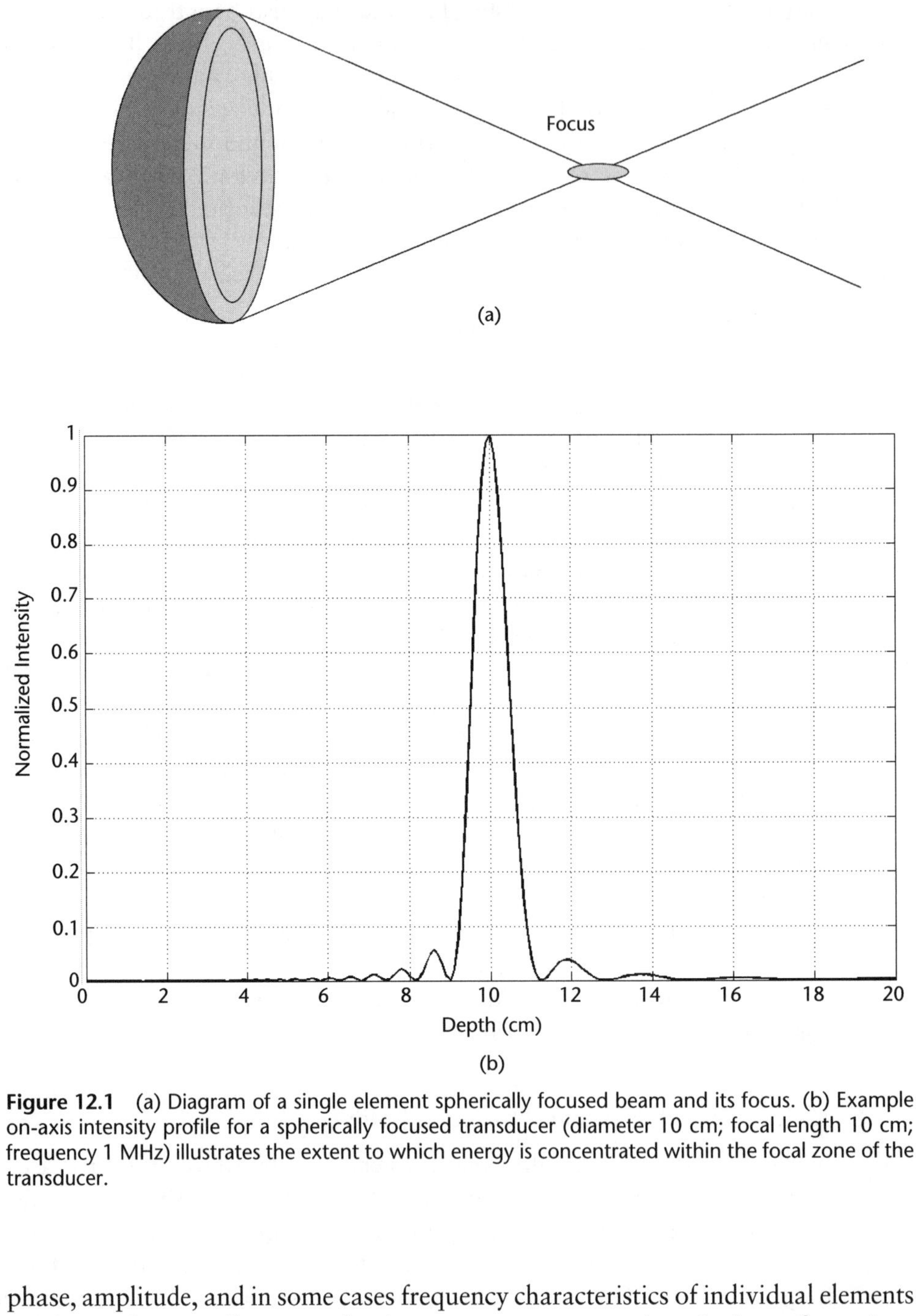

Figure 12.1 (a) Diagram of a single element spherically focused beam and its focus. (b) Example on-axis intensity profile for a spherically focused transducer (diameter 10 cm; focal length 10 cm; frequency 1 MHz) illustrates the extent to which energy is concentrated within the focal zone of the transducer.

phase, amplitude, and in some cases frequency characteristics of individual elements can be used to rapidly scan a focal zone over a target region. Such configurations permit not only axial scanning, but 2D arrays can also achieve degrees of off-axis focusing. This approach has been widely employed in diagnostic ultrasound for more than two decades, but has only somewhat recently been effectively realized in the context of therapeutic ultrasound [25, 26]. Therapeutic phased arrays and their associated driving systems began with smaller numbers of elements in experimental systems before increasing the array sizes and transitioning to commercial devices such as the first ~200 element extracorporeal system. There is a trend to increase the number of elements in order to achieve increased electronic focusing range, which is an active and challenging area of research and development at present.

For therapeutic applications, the increased speed of focal region scanning offered by these approaches reduces and in some circumstances eliminates the need for mechanical scanning. These factors improve treatment times considerably, which is a key factor in making practical many applications. In addition to improving scan times, having transmit control of individual elements also allows for the compensation of aberrations introduced by intervening tissue layers that act to distort and displace the focal spot of the transducer. This can be a significant effect in many soft tissue applications, and may be critical to target sights that lie beneath bone, such as the brain and the subcostal aspects of kidney and liver [27, 28].

12.2 Treatment Approach and Systems

The basic approach for HIFU therapy is to scan a small focal zone over a target region, thereby accumulating damage conformally over the entire region of interest [18, 29]. At each location a dwell time is on the order of 1 to 30 seconds, with intensities ranging between 10^3 to 10^4 W/cm^2. The treatment process involves components of targeting, monitoring, and treatment evaluation. For targeting, or guidance, imaging ideally should be able to clearly delineate the target region, identifying an appropriate acoustic window for the beam path through intervening tissue, and locating the focal zone within tissue. For monitoring, it is necessary to detect or predict tissue damage and lesion formation as it occurs in the target zone, and provide feedback with regards to potential unintended heating or tissue damage outside the intended target zone. Finally, there should be the ability to evaluate the treatment after completion.

12.2.1 MRI Guidance

MRI has two primary advantages for guiding HIFU therapy [30]. First, it has excellent soft tissue contrast, which in many circumstances enables it to accurately delineate and map the boundaries of the intended treatment region as well as the subsequent ablation volume. Second, it is generally able to detect and monitor local temperature elevations with a high degree of sensitivity. This can be used to ensure an accurate prediction of the treated area, as well as detecting heating in unintended regions. At present, only MRI has been shown to be capable of quantitative temperature monitoring during treatments in animal and clinical studies [31, 32]. This is usually accomplished with imaging protocols that exploit temperature-dependent proton resonance frequency (PRF) shifts [33]. This approach has been shown to have good temperature sensitivity and linearity in most tissue types [34], though its performance can be degraded by tissue motion and in the presence of significant concentrations of fat [35]. The focal location is initially determined using anatomic MR images, assuming that its position relative to the transducer face has not been altered by propagation through tissue. Pilot mild heating exposures can then be conducted to confirm the focal location with thermometry, which can also be used to compare with predicted heating results. In practice, MRI guided systems can also have a cavitation monitoring transducer, as well as capabilities to perform pulse echo measurements to detect gas along the path length of the therapy transducer [30].

Lesion formation is determined primarily based on monitoring the time history of temperature rise at a target location. The manner in which individual lesions are used to cover the treatment volume can vary from inducing sequential, partially overlapping lesions to more complex patterns that permit cooling of tissue between sonications. Initial implementations of MRI thermometry monitored therapy required operators to obtain direct feedback of the temperature at each location to ensure sufficient heating occurred and to permit adjustment of sonications between locations. The detection of ablated tissue at the end of the treatment can be aided by the use of gadolinium injections, which are evident as perfusion deficient regions [36]. An example of the use of temperature monitoring to determine the ablation region, followed by confirmation with MRI contrast images, is shown in Figure 12.2.

A number of more sophisticated closed-loop feedback control approaches have been proposed and demonstrated in animal experiments and are being or will be implemented in commercial systems. These can incorporate elements of feedback control theory to adhere to predetermined temperature trajectories as well as modeling to account for energy deposition and thermal conduction effects. The 2D MRI thermometry control has been reported by [37], for example, whose authors employed sequential spiral patterns incorporating temperature feedback to determine transducer speed on subsequent passes. In the context of transurethral MRI, active temperature feedback is used to achieve conformal ablation to comply with prostate geometry [38].

The original experimental MRI guided extracorporeal HIFU systems employed single element transducers, which were supplanted in subsequent experimental and commercial systems by array-based approaches. The first commercial extracorporeal system uses ~200 elements, operates at frequencies between 0.9 and 1.3 MHz, and is compatible for use with breast, abdomen, pelvic, and limb tissue [39]. A system recently developed for transcranial applications is currently undergoing clinical trials using ~500 elements. Other experimental systems include transrectal [40, 41] and transurethral [38, 42] approaches for prostate therapy, which employ smaller array sizes.

12.2.2 Ultrasound

Ultrasound imaging guidance offers the advantages of reduced equipment and operating costs as well as being more compact in size. These factors may facilitate a more widespread adoption of HIFU therapy worldwide. At present, its primary disadvantages relative to MRI lie in its limitations in achieving comparable soft tissue contrast to define target sights, and in monitoring the formation of lesions. During the targeting stage, diagnostic US is well suited to identify an acoustic window for treatment and the possible presence of gas along the beam path. During treatment, US approaches are well suited to detect potential cavitation arising during the treatment procedure, as well as to monitor patient motion. Thermometry approaches for treatment monitoring are not effectively employed with US due to its current inability to reliably estimate temperatures in vivo. Ultrasound thermometry

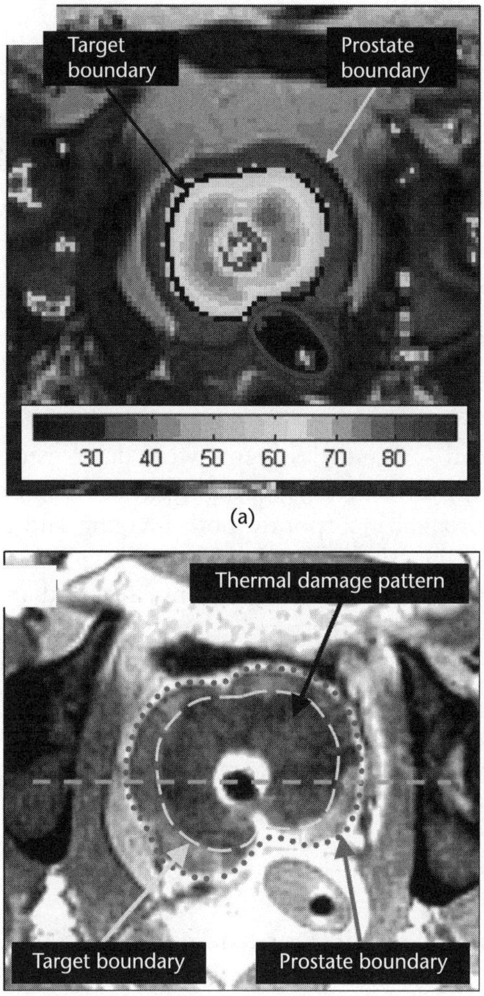

(b)

Figure 12.2 (a) Overlay of the maximum temperature distribution measured during transurethral ultrasound therapy (for T>55°C) within the target region in a canine prostate gland. (b) Axial T1-weighted contrast-enhanced MR image of the treated region of the prostate gland. The agreement between the MR thermometry and contrast enhanced images can be seen in the panels. (Courtesy of R. Chopra.)

is, however, actively being investigated [43], by, for example, monitoring changes in attenuation [44, 45] or speed of sound. Direct lesion detection through observations of tissue hyperechogenicity is the main approach employed at present, though this is not always a reliable indictor of ablation. Other methods of direct lesion detection are also being investigated such as attenuation, speed of sound, reflection coefficients, and elastography [46, 47]. Similar to the use of gadolinium with MRI, the use of microbubble ultrasound contrast agents may aid in both the target volume definition, as well as in mapping the ablated volume based on perfusion defects [48]. It should also be noted that post-treatment evaluation of treated volumes may also be conducted with a range of other imaging modalities [49], though issues of registration, precision, and ease of use can be confounding factors.

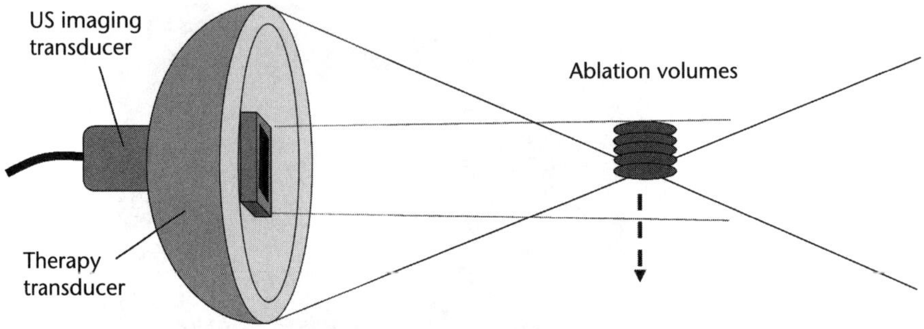

Figure 12.3 Schematic of diagnostic US imaging of HIFU therapy.

Commercial US guided systems were developed in the 1990s for transrectal prostate therapy and extracorporeal applications. Two prostate systems, relatively similar in approach, incorporate both imaging and therapy transducers into one probe, which takes the form of a truncated spherical shape [50]. Current extracorporeal commercial systems are comprised of diagnostic US imaging transducers mounted within the aperture of highly focused large aperture (typically 12-cm diameter) therapy transducer (Figure 12.3). The use of array transducer technology is now also beginning to be employed. As discussed later, dual functionality therapy/imaging arrays are under development. Experimental interstitial probes are also being investigated.

12.3 Applications

The large majority of HIFU procedures to date have focused upon the ablation of solid tumors, for which a considerable body of clinical data has now accumulated. Other notable applications include arterial occlusion, hemostasis, thrombolysis, and the delivery of drugs and genes. A brief overview of some of the relevant results will now be presented, with an emphasis on applications that have had at least initial clinical exposure.

12.3.1 Solid Tumors

12.3.1.1 Uterine Fibroids

Uterine fibroids (leiomyomas) are benign and frequently bulky tumors that give rise to clinical symptoms in approximately 25% of all women. Surgical approaches to management are associated with significant morbidity rates [51]. Following extensive feasibility studies [32], HIFU ablation of uterine fibroids became the first MRI guided application to receive FDA approval and has now received approval and is being conducted in several countries. It has been shown to be a promising technique for debulking these tumors with minimal side effects and rapid recovery times.

Initial clinical work has been reported for US guided uterine fibroid ablation [48, 52] with 1.0-MHz treatment transducers and a 5-MHz imaging transducers.

The results indicated the potential to ablate tissue and did not report adverse side effects.

12.3.1.2 Prostate

Prostate cancer is the most prevalent cancer type diagnosed in men and is a leading cause of death from cancer. The most widely used radical therapies (surgical excision and external beam radiotherapy) achieve effective local control of the disease, but these are associated with significant side effects. Transrectal US guided HIFU has been clinically investigated as an alternative means of treating prostate cancer and benign prostate hyperplasia for more than a decade. Transrectal systems have been most successful in performing whole gland ablation [53], both as a primary treatment and salvage operations. Evidence to date indicates that survival improvement outcomes are generally comparable to those achieved with standard therapies, though with improved side effect results [54, 55].

MRI compatible experimental transrectal systems have also been reported and tested in animal experiments [41]. MRI guided transurethral systems have been developed over the last decade which have shown considerable promise in animal studies [38, 42]. This approach has implemented sophisticated feedback approaches [56] and array-based technology for conformal mapping and will begin clinical trials in the near future.

12.3.1.3 Breast

Breast tissue is readily accessible by ultrasound, without bone or air lying in intervening tissue layers along the beam path. Initial clinical trials have been conducted with both US and MRI guidance for the ablation of both benign and malignant tumors. MRI guided HIFU feasibility tests were conducted on breast fibroadenomas, followed by limited clinical studies on breast cancer patients which confirmed its ability to ablate tumor tissue [57]. Subsequent work has shown the approach to be well tolerated, and capable of ablating a high percentage of tumor volume [58]. Clinical studies are ongoing. Significant work has also been conducted for US guided HIFU breast tumor ablation [59]. The ability to achieve ablation of the majority of tumor tissue was reported.

12.3.1.4 Liver

Primary and metastatic liver tumors are an increasingly prevalent cause of death worldwide. This, coupled with the limitations of existing treatments, has generated considerable interest in the use of HIFU for liver lesion ablation. Several studies have reported the successful and efficient ablation of hepatocellular carcinoma and metastatic liver tumors with extracorporeal US guided devices [60]. Improved survival times have been reported when HIFU was combined with transarterial chemoembolization (TACE) [61]. As a palliative treatment in advanced liver cancer, symptomatic improvements were reported in the majority of recipients. Issues of ultrasound access through ribs and the requirement of breathing control are limiting factors with current systems and are an active area of research. Interstitial devices for use in percutaneous or laparoscopic focal liver ablation are being developed, which combine US guidance with a high frequency ablation elements [62]. Focal liver ablation is also of interest in the context of extracorporeal MRI guided HIFU [63].

12.3.1.5 Renal

HIFU clinical treatment of renal tumors is at an early stage. Several US guided extracorporeal studies have been reported involving the ablation of renal cell carcinomas, and have indicated that the current approaches have limitations in terms of ablation efficacy, more so than in liver. This has been attributed to the effects of respiratory motion (even with breathing control) coupled with the effects of acoustical complexities introduced by the abdominal wall and ribs [60, 64].

12.3.1.6 Pancreatic

Pancreatic cancer has up to 200,000 diagnoses annually worldwide and is characterized by very low (5%) 5-year survival rates. HIFU is currently under investigation to provide palliative treatment for pancreatic tumors. Several studies have reported that HIFU can reduce tumor size in advanced pancreatic cancer, and can achieve positive palliative results and increase survival times [65]. It should be noted that prospective randomized controlled studies to quantitatively evaluate these factors remain to be carried out.

12.3.1.7 Bone

HIFU is under investigation and holds considerable promise for the treatment of osteosarcoma and metastatic bone tumors. Metastatic bone tumors arise in over 50% of cancer patients, and are associated with persistent and disabling pain that is frequently refractory to radiotherapy, chemotherapy, and analgesics. The high attenuation and acoustic impedance of bone makes penetration and focusing challenging, but at the same time high absorption permits the rapid elevation of temperature. Primary neoplasms may also be associated with cortical degradation which can facilitate ultrasound access. Results have been reported for osteosarcoma ablation under US guidance in combination with neoadjuvant therapy for limb salvage and well as for palliative purposes [49].

Clinical studies employing MRIgFUS for the palliative treatment of bone metastases are underway, where periosteal nerve destruction is sought for metastases present in the superficial aspects of bone. Initial results for a small number trial indicated a high rate of success at achieving improvements in pain scores, with no adverse events reported [66].

12.3.1.8 Other Malignancies

HIFU has been shown to be successful based on 5-year follow-ups for treating testicular cancer using transrectal probes [67]. The feasibility of biliary duct cancer ablation using 10-MHz interstitial HIFU has been experimentally demonstrated

[68]. This probe is positioned under fluoroscopy guidance. Interstitial high frequency probes are also being developed for the purposes of esophageal tumor ablation [69].

12.3.2 Other Applications

12.3.2.1 Vascular Occlusion

Techniques for achieving nonsurgical deep blood vessel occlusion are at present limited, and improved approaches would be of benefit to a significant number of patients for the treatment of tumors, hemorrhage, or arteriovenous malformations. Ultrasound cessation of flow in small and large vessels in superficial and deeper locations has been reported. Permanent vessel occlusion of larger arteries under high flow conditions was achieved under MRI guidance [20] and US guidance [70]. The control of hemorrhage due to the puncture of larger vessels is also being investigated, which is of particular relevance to trauma applications [71]. Early clinical results have been obtained for catheter wound closure using a superficial US guided system.

12.3.2.2 Ophthalmology

Some of the most substantial early clinical work with HIFU was conducted in ophthalmology. Experimental models demonstrated the feasibility of inducing lesions in the vitreous, lens, retina, choroids, as well as in intraocular tumors [72, 73]. Clinical work conducted on glaucoma patients was found to be successful in reducing intraocular pressures in the majority of cases [74]. Despite these successes, the technique has not emerged as a widespread tool, as laser approaches have.

12.4 Future Developments and Trends

12.4.1 Technical Developments

From a technical perspective, there continues to be considerable effort focused on reducing treatment times and increasing the precision of ultrasound energy delivery. This entails work on a spectrum of technical aspects ranging from array development to improved monitoring and treatment planning. Two particular areas of current interest are cavitation enhanced HIFU and motion compensation.

12.4.1.1 Cavitation

It has been known for some time that the presence of cavitation can increase the rate of temperature elevation in tissues [29]. While it has been previously considered that cavitation is desirable to avoid in HIFU therapy, there is increasing interest in controlling it to exploit its potential to reduce treatment times [13]. This would have significant implications for a range of applications, such as those involving tissue motions, transcranial applications that can induce inadvertent skull heating, and large tumors. The use of preformed microbubble contrast agents may be of particular interest in this context, as they lower the threshold for cavitation considerably relative to native tissue, and provide a potentially high density of cavitation sights. Research is ongoing to optimize this technique, and to ensure sufficient control of the spatial extent and locations of the resulting lesions [75, 76]. Also related is the use of histotripsy to perform tissue destruction through cavitation. This has been demonstrated in a number of applications, and it is an active area of research.

12.4.1.2 Motion Tracking and Compensation

Tissue motion effects pose a considerable challenge for many target tissues such as kidneys, liver, and heart, and can lead to either inaccuracies in targeting or, with respiratory control approaches, greatly extended treatment times. Active motion tracking and beam guidance approaches are currently being pursued by several groups with both MRI and US imaging. Recent reports have demonstrated the feasibility of real-time US guided motion compensation in animal studies for liver ablation [28].

12.4.2 Developing Applications

Section 12.3 highlighted a range of applications that have been clinically investigated with HIFU, with an emphasis on work directed towards the ablation of solid tumors where a clear acoustic window is generally available. In addition to these applications, we will now discuss several emerging areas in more detail.

12.4.2.1 Cardiac Arrhythmia

Atrial fibrillation is the most common type of cardiac arrhythmia, affecting approximately 2% of adults [77], with the majority of cases thought to be initiated by the pulmonary vein. The primary therapy for atrial fibrillation at present is percutaneous RF catheter ablation, which is used to modify electrical conduction paths within tissue to restore cardiac synchronization. The invasive nature of this approach is less desirable, and has limitations in terms of trade-offs between lesion penetration depth and catheter dimension. The use of HIFU for ablating myocardial tissue is being investigated using extracardiac [78], intracardiac [79, 80], and transesopageal approaches [81]. Pulsed transmission schemes have been investigated for ablating cardiac tissue [82] in the beating heart with extracardiac sources. Real-time US motion tracking and lesion monitoring techniques treatments have also been reported for extracardiac cardiac ablation [83]. Transesophageal HIFU, while at an earlier stage of development [81] may offer a balance between the invasiveness of intracardiac and technical challenges of extracardiac approaches.

12.4.2.2 Nerves

The suppression of nerve function by HIFU is under investigation [84], which has potential for applications in pain management or in reducing muscle spasticity associated with, for example, multiple sclerosis. Results to date have been achieved in animal experiments for superficial nerves under US guidance [85].

12.4.2.3 Brain

One of the most promising applications of focused ultrasound is for transcranial brain therapy. Ablative thermal therapy of brain tissue is one of the oldest goals of HIFU [86], yet it has been perhaps the most technically challenging one to achieve. Earlier HIFU investigations focused on tumors and neurological disorders such as Parkinson's disease [87]. More recent work conducted at lower intensities in combination with microbubble contrast agents shows the considerable promise of focused ultrasound for transiently breaking down the blood brain barrier [31] in order to achieve drug delivery [88]. Noninvasive ultrasound treatment of the brain presents a distinct advantage over surgical techniques, which invariably disrupt overlying tissue structures and can disturb functionality. Due to the highly attenuating nature for bone, the majority of early experiments were conducted through skull windows [89], a factor which, along with issues of guidance, has prohibited its potential for widespread use.

The recent development of phased array technology for therapeutic ultrasound offers the possibility of focusing through the intact skull by correcting for aberrations [90, 91]. While initial experimental work required the use of hydrophones or reflectors to determine the phase correction for the array focusing, it has since been shown that this can be achieved noninvasively [92, 93]. These approaches require the use of CT data to extract bone density maps and thereby acoustic impedances. These data can then be used in conjunction with beam modeling approaches to select array transmission parameters (e.g., delays and amplitudes) that are then used to compensate for aberrations introduced by propagation through the skull and restore the focus.

A 500-element transcranial MRI guided system was developed [94] and evaluated using both hydrophone and model-based approaches to focus through ex vivo human skulls and expose rabbit brains [95]. A commercial system based on these approaches was then developed (Exablate 3000, InSightech, Haifa, Israel), which underwent feasibility tests on Rhesus monkeys to verify operation and achieve temperature elevation [96]. This system now in clinical trials for transcranial treatment of malignant brain tumors [27].

In separate experiments, a 300-element ultrasound guided array was developed [97] and used to achieve trans-skull thermal ablation of brain tissue in sheep [98], and subsequently in monkeys [28, 99].

References

[1] Kremkau, F. W., "Cancer Therapy with Ultrasound: A Historical Review," *J. Clin. Ultrasound*, Vol. 7, No. 4, 1979, pp. 287–300.

[2] Liu, H. L., N. McDannold, and K. Hynynen, "Focal Beam Distortion and Treatment Planning in Abdominal Focused Ultrasound Surgery," *Med. Phys.*, Vol. 32, No. 5, 2005, pp. 1270–1280.

[3] Dorr, L. N., and K. Hynynen, "The Effects of Tissue Heterogeneities and Large Blood Vessels on the Thermal Exposure Induced by Short High-Power Ultrasound Pulses," *Int. J. Hyperthermia*, Vol. 8, No. 1, 1992, pp. 45–59.

[4] Kolios, M. C., M. D. Sherar, and J. W. Hunt, "Blood Flow Cooling and Ultrasonic Lesion Formation," *Med. Phys.*, Vol. 23, No. 7, 1996, pp. 1287–1298.

[5] Bamber, J. C., "Speed of Sound," in *Physical Principles of Medical Ultrasonics*, C. R. Hill, J. C. Bamber, and G. R. ter Haar, (eds.), New York: Wiley, 2004, pp. 167–190.

[6] Cobbold, R. S. C., *Foundations of Biomedical Ultrasound*, Biomedical Engineering Series, New York: Oxford University Press, 2007.

[7] Goss, S. A., R. L. Johnston, and F. Dunn, "Comprehensive Compilation of Empirical Ultrasonic Properties of Mammalian Tissues," *J. Acoust. Soc. Am.*, Vol. 64, No. 2, 1978, pp. 423–457.

[8] Hamilton, M. F., and D. T. Blackstock, *Nonlinear Acoustics, Vol. XVIII*, San Diego, CA: Academic Press, 1998, Chapter 8.

[9] Hallaj, I. M., R. O. Cleveland, and K. Hynynen, "Simulations of the Thermo-Acoustic Lens Effect During Focused Ultrasound Surgery," *J. Acoust. Soc. Am.*, Vol. 109, No. 5, Pt. 1, 2001, pp. 2245–2253.

[10] Carstensen, E. L., and H. G. Flynn, "The Potential for Transient Cavitation with Microsecond Pulses of Ultrasound," *Ultrasound Med. Biol.*, Vol. 8, No. 6, 1982, pp. L720–L724.

[11] Holt, R. G., R. A. Roy, and P. A. Edson, "Bubbles and HIFU: The Good, the Bad, and the Ugly," *Proceedings of the 2nd International Symposium on Therapeutic Ultrasound*, Seattle, WA, University of Washington, 2002.

[12] Fry, F. J., et al., "Ultrasound and Microbubbles: Their Generation, Detection and Potential Utilization in Tissue and Organ Therapy—Experimental," *Ultrasound Med. Biol.*, Vol. 21, No. 9, 1995, pp. 1227–1237.

[13] Sokka, S. D., R. King, and K. Hynynen, "MRI-Guided Gas Bubble Enhanced Ultrasound Heating in In Vivo Rabbit Thigh," *Phys. Med. Biol.*, Vol. 48, No. 2, 2003, pp. 223–241.

[14] Leighton, T. G., *The Acoustic Bubble*, London: Academic Press, 1994, pp. 319–320.

[15] Margulis, M. A., *Sonochemistry and Cavitation*, London: Gordon and Breach, 1996.

[16] Dewhirst, M. W., et al., "Carcinogenic Effects of Hyperthermia," *Int. J. Hyperthermia*, Vol. 19, No. 3, 2003, pp. 236–251.

[17] Dewhirst, M. W., et al., "Basic Principles of Thermal Dosimetry and Thermal Thresholds for Tissue Damage from Hyperthermia," *Int. J. Hyperthermia*, Vol. 19, No. 3, 2003, pp. 267–294.

[18] Fry, W. J., et al., "Production of Focal Destructive Lesions in the Central Nervous System with Ultrasound," *J. Neurosurg.*, Vol. 11, No. 5, 1954, pp. 471–478.

[19] Lele, P. P., "A Simple Method for Production of Trackless Focal Lesions with Focused Ultrasound: Physical Factors," *J. Physiol.*, Vol. 160, 1962, pp. 494–512.

[20] Hynynen, K., et al., "Potential Adverse Effects of High-Intensity Focused Ultrasound Exposure on Blood Vessels In Vivo," *Ultrasound Med. Biol.*, Vol. 22, No. 2, 1996, pp. 193–201.

[21] Wu, F., et al., "Tumor Vessel Destruction Resulting from High-Intensity Focused Ultrasound in Patients with Solid Malignancies," *Ultrasound Med. Biol.*, Vol. 28, No. 4, 2002, pp. 535–542.

[22] Vykhodtseva, N., et al., "Apoptosis in Ultrasound-Produced Threshold Lesions in the Rabbit Brain," *Ultrasound Med. Biol.*, Vol. 27, No. 1, 2001, pp. 111–117.

[23] Martin, C. J., B. M. Pratt, and D. J. Watmough, "Observations of Ultrasound-Induced Effects in the Fish Xiphophorous Maculatus," *Ultrasound Med. Biol.*, Vol. 9, No. 2, 1983, pp. 177–183.

[24] Xu, Z., J. B. Fowlkes, and C. A. Cain, "A New Strategy to Enhance Cavitational Tissue Erosion Using a High-Intensity, Initiating Sequence," *IEEE Transactions on Ultrasonics, Ferroelectrics and Frequency Control*, Vol. 53, No. 8, 2006, pp. 1412–1424.

[25] Daum, D. R., and K. Hynynen, "A 256-Element Ultrasonic Phased Array System for the Treatment of Large Volumes of Deep Seated Tissue," *IEEE Transactions on Ultrasonics, Ferroelectrics, and Frequency Control*, Vol. 46, No. 5, 1999, pp. 1254–1268.

[26] Wan, H., et al., "Ultrasound Surgery: Comparison of Strategies Using Phased Array Systems," *IEEE Transactions on Ultrasonics, Ferroelectrics and Frequency Control*, 43, No. 6, 1996, pp. 1085–1098.

[27] Hynynen, K., and G. Clement, "Clinical Applications of Focused Ultrasound—The Brain," *Int. J. Hyperthermia*, Vol. 23, No. 2, 2007, pp. 193–202.

[28] Tanter, M., et al., "Compensating for Bone Interfaces and Respiratory Motion in High-Intensity Focused Ultrasound," *Int. J. Hyperthermia*, Vol. 23, No. 2, 2007, pp. 141–151.

[29] Lele, P. P., "Cavitation and Its Effects on Organized Mammalian Tissues, A Summary," in *Ultrasound: Its Application in Medicine and Biology*, Part 2, F. J. Fry, (ed.), Amsterdam: Elsevier Scientific Pub. Co., 1978, pp. 737–741.

[30] Hynynen, K., and N. McDannold, "MRI Guided and Monitored Focused Ultrasound Thermal Ablation Methods: A Review of Progress," *Int. J. Hyperthermia*, Vol. 20, No. 7, 2004, pp. 725–737.

[31] Hynynen, K., et al., "Noninvasive MR Imaging-Guided Focal Opening of the Blood-Brain Barrier in Rabbits," *Radiology*, Vol. 220, No. 3, 2001, pp. 640–646.

[32] Tempany, C. M., et al., "MR Imaging-Guided Focused Ultrasound Surgery of Uterine Leiomyomas: A Feasibility Study," *Radiology*, Vol. 226, No. 3, 2003, pp. 897–905.

[33] Ishihara, Y., et al., "A Precise and Fast Temperature Mapping Using Water Proton Chemical Shift," *Magn. Reson. Med.*, Vol. 34, No. 6, 1995, pp. 814–823.

[34] Peters, R. D., R. S. Hinks, and R. M. Henkelman, "Ex Vivo Tissue-Type Independence in Proton-Resonance Frequency Shift MR Thermometry," *Magn. Reson. Med.*, Vol. 40, No. 3, 1998, pp. 454–459.

[35] de Zwart, J. A., et al., "Fast Lipid-Suppressed MR Temperature Mapping with Echo-Shifted Gradient-Echo Imaging and Spectral-Spatial Excitation," *Magn. Reson. Med.*, Vol. 42, No. 1, 1999, pp. 53–59.

[36] Hynynen, K., et al., "The Usefulness of a Contrast Agent and Gradient-Recalled Acquisition in a Steady-State Imaging Sequence for Magnetic Resonance Imaging-Guided Noninvasive Ultrasound Surgery," *Invest. Radiol.*, Vol. 29, No. 10, 1994, pp. 897–903.

[37] Salomir, R., et al., "Local Hyperthermia with MR-Guided Focused Ultrasound: Spiral Trajectory of the Focal Point Optimized for Temperature Uniformity in the Target Region," *J. Magn. Reson. Imaging*, Vol. 12, No. 4, 2000, pp. 571–583.

[38] Chopra, R., et al., "MRI-Compatible Transurethral Ultrasound System for the Treatment of Localized Prostate Cancer Using Rotational Control," *Medical Physics*, Vol. 35, No. 4, 2008, pp. 1346–1357.

[39] Hynynen, K. H., and N. McDannold, "Integrated Therapy Systems," in *MRI-Guided Focused Ultrasound Surgery*, F. A. Jolesz and K. H. Hynynen, (eds.), New York: Informa Healthcare, 2008.

[40] Hutchinson, E. B., and K. Hynynen, "Intracavitary Ultrasound Phased Arrays for Prostate Thermal Therapies: MRI Compatibility and In Vivo Testing," *Med. Phys.*, Vol. 25, No. 12, 1998, pp. 2392–2399.

[41] Sokka, S. D., and K. H. Hynynen, "The Feasibility of MRI-Guided Whole Prostate Ablation with a Linear Aperiodic Intracavitary Ultrasound Phased Array," *Phys. Med. Biol.*, Vol. 45, No. 11, 2000, pp. 3373–3783.

[42] Diederich, C. J., et al., "Catheter-Based Ultrasound Applicators for Selective Thermal Ablation: Progress Towards MRI-Guided Applications in Prostate," *Int. J. Hyperthermia*, Vol. 20, No. 7, 2004, pp. 739–756.

[43] Rivens, I., et al., "Treatment Monitoring and Thermometry for Therapeutic Focused Ultrasound," *Int. J. Hyperthermia*, Vol. 23, No. 2, 2007, pp. 121–139.

[44] Clarke, R. L., N. L. Bush, and G. R. Ter Haar, "The Changes in Acoustic Attenuation Due to In Vitro Heating," *Ultrasound Med. Biol.*, Vol. 29, No. 1, 2003, pp. 127–135.

[45] Bevan, P. D., and M. D. Sherar, "B-Scan Ultrasound Imaging of Thermal Coagulation in Bovine Liver: Frequency Shift Attenuation Mapping," *Ultrasound Med. Biol.*, Vol. 27, No. 6, 2001, pp. 809–817.

[46] Shi, X. G., et al., "Detection of High-Intensity Focused Ultrasound Liver Lesions Using Dynamic Elastometry," *Ultrasonic Imaging*, Vol. 21, No. 2, 1999, pp. 107–126.

[47] Souchon, R., et al., "Visualisation of Hifu Lesions Using Elastography of the Human Prostate In Vivo: Preliminary Results," *Ultrasound in Medicine and Biology*, Vol. 29, No. 7, 2003, pp. 1007–1015.

[48] Zhou, X. D., et al., "Therapeutic Response Assessment of High Intensity Focused Ultrasound Therapy for Uterine Fibroid: Utility of Contrast-Enhanced Ultrasonography," *Eur. J. Radiol.*, Vol. 62, No. 2, 2007, pp. 289–294.

[49] Wu, F., "Extracorporeal High Intensity Focused Ultrasound in the Treatment of Patients with Solid Malignancy," *Minimally Invasive Therapy & Allied Technologies*, Vol. 15, No. 1, 2006, pp. 26–35.

[50] Sanghvi, N. T., et al., "Noninvasive Surgery of Prostate Tissue by High-Intensity Focused Ultrasound," *IEEE Transactions on Ultrasonics Ferroelectrics and Frequency Control*, Vol. 43, No. 6, 1996, pp. 1099–1110.

[51] Sawin, S. W., et al., "Comparability of Perioperative Morbidity Between Abdominal Myomectomy and Hysterectomy for Women with Uterine Leiomyomas," *Am. J. Obstet. Gynecol.*, Vol. 183, No. 6, 2000, pp. 1448–1455.

[52] Fruehauf, J. H., et al., "High-Intensity Focused Ultrasound for the Targeted Destruction of Uterine Tissues: Experiences from a Pilot Study Using a Mobile HIFU Unit," *Arch. Gynecol. Obstet.*, Vol. 277, No. 2, 2008, pp. 143–150.

[53] Madersbacher, S., et al., "Effect of High-Intensity Focused Ultrasound on Human Prostate Cancer in Vivo," *Cancer Res.*, Vol. 55, No. 15, 1995, pp. 3346–3351.

[54] Blana, A., et al., "Morbidity Associated with Repeated Transrectal High-Intensity Focused Ultrasound Treatment of Localized Prostate Cancer," *World J. Urol.*, Vol. 24, No. 5, 2006, pp. 585–590.

[55] Poissonnier, L., et al., "Control of Prostate Cancer by Transrectal HIFU in 227 Patients," *Eur. Urol.*, Vol. 51, No. 2, 2007, pp. 381–387.

[56] Tang, K., et al., "Conformal Thermal Therapy Using Planar Ultrasound Transducers and Adaptive Closed-Loop MR Temperature Control: Demonstration in Gel Phantoms and Ex Vivo Tissues," *Phys. Med. Biol.*, Vol. 52, No. 10, 2007, pp. 2905–2919.

[57] Gianfelice, D., et al., "MR Imaging-Guided Focused US Ablation of Breast Cancer: Histopathologic Assessment of Effectiveness—Initial Experience," *Radiology*, Vol. 227, No. 3, 2003, pp. 849–855.

[58] Furusawa, H., et al., "Magnetic Resonance-Guided Focused Ultrasound Surgery of Breast Cancer: Reliability and Effectiveness," *J. Am. Coll. Surg.*, Vol. 203, No. 1, 2006, pp. 54–63.

[59] Wu, F., et al., "'Wide Local Ablation' of Localized Breast Cancer Using High Intensity Focused Ultrasound," *J. Surg. Oncol.*, Vol. 96, No. 2, 2007, pp. 130–136.

[60] Illing, R. O., et al., "The Safety and Feasibility of Extracorporeal High-Intensity Focused Ultrasound (HIFU) for the Treatment of Liver and Kidney Tumours in a Western Population," *Br. J. Cancer*, Vol. 93, No. 8, 2005, pp. 890–895.

[61] Wu, F., et al., "Advanced Hepatocellular Carcinoma: Treatment with High-Intensity Focused Ultrasound Ablation Combined with Transcatheter Arterial Embolization," *Radiology*, Vol. 235, No. 2, 2005, pp. 659–667.

[62] Makin, I. R., et al., "Miniaturized Ultrasound Arrays for Interstitial Ablation and Imaging," *Ultrasound Med. Biol.*, Vol. 31, No. 11, 2005, pp. 1539–1550.

[63] Daum, D. R., et al., "In Vivo Demonstration of Noninvasive Thermal Surgery of the Liver and Kidney Using an Ultrasonic Phased Array," *Ultrasound Med. Biol.*, Vol. 25, No. 7, 1999, pp. 1087–1098.

[64] Marberger, M., "Ablation of Renal Tumours with Extracorporeal High-Intensity Focused Ultrasound," *BJU Int.*, Vol. 99, No. 5, Pt. B, 2007, pp. 1273–1276.

[65] Wu, F., et al., "Feasibility of US-Guided High-Intensity Focused Ultrasound Treatment in Patients with Advanced Pancreatic Cancer: Initial Experience," *Radiology*, Vol. 236, No. 3, 2005, pp. 1034–1040.

[66] Catane, R., et al., "MR-Guided Focused Ultrasound Surgery (MRGFUS) for the Palliation of Pain in Patients with Bone Metastases—Preliminary Clinical Experience," *Annals of Oncology*, Vol. 18, No. 1, 2007, pp. 163–167.

[67] Kratzik, C., et al., "Transcutaneous High-Intensity Focused Ultrasonography Can Cure Testicular Cancer in Solitary Testis," *Urology*, Vol. 67, No. 6, 2006, pp. 1269–1273.

[68] Prat, F., et al., "Endoscopic Treatment of Cholangiocarcinoma and Carcinoma of the Duodenal Papilla by Intraductal High-Intensity US: Results of a Pilot Study," *Gastrointest. Endosc.*, Vol. 56, No. 6, 2002, pp. 909–915.

[69] Melodelima, D., et al., "Intraluminal High Intensity Ultrasound Treatment in the Esophagus Under Fast MR Temperature Mapping: In Vivo Studies," *Magn. Reson. Med.*, Vol. 54, No. 4, 2005, pp. 975–982.

[70] Rivens, I. H., et al., "Vascular Occlusion Using Focused Ultrasound Surgery for Use in Fetal Medicine," *Eur. J. Ultrasound*, Vol. 9, No. 1, 1999, pp. 89–97.

[71] Vaezy, S., R. Martin, and L. Crum, "High Intensity Focused Ultrasound: A Method of Hemostasis," *Echocardiography—A Journal of Cardiovascular Ultrasound and Allied Techniques*, Vol. 18, No. 4, 2001, pp. 309–315.

[72] Lavine, O., et al., "Effects of Ultrasonic Waves on the Refractive Media of the Eye," *AMA Arch. Ophthalmol.*, Vol. 47, No. 2, 1952, pp. 204–219.

[73] Lizzi, F. L., et al., "Experimental, Ultrasonically Induced Lesions in the Retina, Choroid, and Sclera," *Invest. Ophthalmol. Vis. Sci.*, Vol. 17, No. 4, 1978, pp. 350–360.

[74] Silverman, R. H., et al., "Therapeutic Ultrasound for the Treatment of Glaucoma," *Am. J. Ophthalmol.*, Vol. 111, No. 3, 1991, pp. 327–337.

[75] McDannold, N. J., N. I. Vykhodtseva, and K. Hynynen, "Microbubble Contrast Agent with Focused Ultrasound to Create Brain Lesions at Low Power Levels: MR Imaging and Histologic Study in Rabbits," *Radiology*, Vol. 241, No. 1, 2006, pp. 95–106.

[76] Coussios, C. C., et al., "Role of Acoustic Cavitation in the Delivery and Monitoring of Cancer Treatment by High-Intensity Focused Ultrasound (HIFU)," *Int. J. Hyperthermia*, Vol. 23, No. 2, 2007, pp. 105–120.

[77] Huang, S. K. S., and M. A. Wood, *Pulmonary Vein Isolation for Atrial Fibrillation*, Philadelphia, PA: Saunders, 2006, pp. 269–288.

[78] Cain, C. A., "Phased Array Ultrasound System and Method for Cardiac Ablation," *The Journal of the Acoustical Society of America*, Vol. 102, No. 2, 1997, p. 687.

[79] Hynynen, K., et al., "Cylindrical Ultrasonic Transducers for Cardiac Catheter Ablation," *IEEE Transactions on Biomedical Engineering*, Vol. 44, No. 2, 1997, pp. 144–151.

[80] Gentry, K. L., and S. W. Smith, "Integrated Catheter for 3-D Intracardiac Echocardiography and Ultrasound Ablation," *IEEE Transactions on Ultrasonics, Ferroelectrics and Frequency Control*, Vol. 51, No. 7, 2004, pp. 800–808.

[81] Yin, X. T., L. M. Epstein, and K. Hynynen, "Noninvasive Transesophageal Cardiac Thermal Ablation Using a 2-D Focused, Ultrasound Phased Array: A Simulation Study," *IEEE Transactions on Ultrasonics, Ferroelectrics and Frequency Control*, Vol. 53, No. 6, 2006, pp. 1138–1149.

[82] Engel, D. J., et al., "Myocardial Lesion Formation Using High-Intensity Focused Ultrasound," *J. Am. Soc. Echocardiogr.*, Vol. 19, No. 7, 2006, pp. 932–937.

[83] Sanghvi, N. T., et al., "Cardiac Ablation Using High Intensity Focused Ultrasound: A Feasibility Study," *Proceedings of the IEEE Ultrasonics Symposium*, 1997.

[84] Lele, P., "Effects of Focused Ultrasonic Radiation on Peripheral Nerve, with Observations on Local Heating," *Experimental Neurology*, Vol. 8, No. 1, 1963, p. 47.

[85] Foley, J. L., et al., "Image-Guided HIFU Neurolysis of Peripheral Nerves to Treat Spasticity and Pain," *Ultrasound Med. Biol.*, Vol. 30, No. 9, 2004, pp. 1199–1207.

[86] Lynn, J. G., et al., "A New Method for the Generation and Use of Focused Ultrasound in Experimental Biology," *J. Gen. Physiol.*, Vol. 26, No. 2, 1942, pp. 179–193.

[87] Fry, W. J., and F. J. Fry, "Fundamental Neurological Research and Human Neurosurgery Using Intense Ultrasound," *IRE Transactions on Medical Electronics*, Vol. 7, No. 3, 1960, pp. 166–181.

[88] Hynynen, K., "Focused Ultrasound for Blood-Brain-Barrier Disruption and Delivery of Therapeutic Molecules into the Brain," *Expert Opinion on Drug Delivery*, Vol. 4, No. 1, 2007, pp. 27–35.

[89] Fry, F. J., and L. K. Johnson, "Tumor Irradiation with Intense Ultrasound," *Ultrasound Med. Biol.*, Vol. 4, No. 4, 1978, pp. 337–341.

[90] Thomas, J. L., and M. A. Fink, "Ultrasonic Beam Focusing Through Tissue Inhomogeneities with a Time Reversal Mirror: Application to Transskull Therapy," *IEEE Transactions on Ultrasonics, Ferroelectrics and Frequency Control*, Vol. 43, No. 6, 1996, pp. 1122–1129.

[91] Hynynen, K., and F. A. Jolesz, "Demonstration of Potential Noninvasive Ultrasound Brain Therapy Through an Intact Skull," *Ultrasound Med. Biol.*, Vol. 24, No. 2, 1998, pp. 275–283.

[92] Clement, G. T., and K. Hynynen, "A Non-Invasive Method for Focusing Ultrasound Through the Human Skull," *Phys. Med. Biol.*, Vol. 47, No. 8, 2002, pp. 1219–1236.

[93] Aubry, J. F., et al., "Experimental Demonstration of Noninvasive Transskull Adaptive Focusing Based on Prior Computed Tomography Scans," *J. Acoust. Soc. Am.*, Vol. 113, No. 1, 2003, pp. 84–93.

[94] Clement, G. T., et al., "A Magnetic Resonance Imaging-Compatible, Large-Scale Array for Trans-Skull Ultrasound Surgery and Therapy," *J. Ultrasound Med.*, Vol. 24, No. 8, 2005, pp. 1117–1125.

[95] Hynynen, K., et al., "500-Element Ultrasound Phased Array System for Noninvasive Focal Surgery of the Brain: A Preliminary Rabbit Study with Ex Vivo Human Skulls," *Magn. Reson. Med.*, Vol. 52, No. 1, 2004, pp. 100–107.

[96] Hynynen, K., et al., "Pre-Clinical Testing of a Phased Array Ultrasound System for MRI-Guided Noninvasive Surgery of the Brain—A Primate Study," *Eur. J. Radiol.*, Vol. 59, No. 2, 2006, pp. 149–156.

[97] Pernot, M., et al., "High Power Transcranial Beam Steering for Ultrasonic Brain Therapy," *Phys. Med. Biol.*, Vol. 48, No. 16, 2003, pp. 2577–2589.

[98] Pernot, M., et al., "In Vivo Transcranial Brain Surgery with an Ultrasonic Time Reversal Mirror," *Journal of Neurosurgery*, Vol. 106, No. 6, 2007, pp. 1061–1066.

[99] Marquet, F., et al., "Non-Invasive Transcranial Ultrasound Therapy Guided by CT-Scans," *28th Annual International Conference of the IEEE Engineering in Medicine and Biology Society, 2006, EMBS '06*, 2006.

CHAPTER 13

3D Visualization and Guidance

Daniel F. Leotta

The three-dimensional nature of the targets for image-guided therapy has driven computer visualization tools increasingly toward realistic 3D renderings that can guide the user during procedures. Three-dimensional representations of targeted sites are designed to provide more natural and intuitive guidance than can be achieved with 2D views. The evolution of 3D medical imaging modalities, spatial tracking systems, and computing capabilities has made it possible to present real-time 3D displays during procedures. Modern imaging methods acquire 3D anatomic datasets, and spatial tracking systems are used to measure the 3D locations of the devices used during image-guided procedures. Computer processing allows the combination of these datasets, and it can produce multiple formats for visualization of 3D data. Displays include surface renderings that produce realistic solid representations of objects of interest, and volume renderings that depict selected parameters throughout the field of view. Interactive computer graphics let the user adjust the views and rendering to suit a particular procedure and enhance their interpretation. Spatial tracking systems in the operating room allow real-time visualization of instruments in the context of the 3D image space. Advanced display systems incorporate stereoscopy, augmented reality, and virtual reality for navigation of the 3D datasets.

13.1 Background

Three-dimensional displays are tools that are used to improve some aspect of image-guided surgical procedures. The technological overhead in cost and complexity must be offset by a concrete gain in performance, for instance in improved treatment outcomes or in time saved during a procedure. The three-dimensional nature of the targets for image-guided therapy has driven computer visualization tools increasingly toward realistic 3D renderings that can guide the user during procedures. Three-dimensional representations of targeted sites are designed to provide more natural and intuitive guidance than can be achieved with 2D views. The evolution of 3D medical imaging modalities, spatial tracking systems, and computing capabilities has made it possible to present real-time 3D displays during procedures. Modern imaging methods acquire 3D anatomic datasets, and spatial tracking systems are used to measure the 3D locations of the devices used during image-guided procedures. Computer processing allows the combination of these datasets, and it can produce multiple formats for visualization of 3D data.

The earliest example of the application of 3D methods for procedure guidance is stereotactic surgery. Stereotaxy was developed before the availability of modern 3D medical imaging modalities, but it demonstrates the benefit of procedure planning using a 3D coordinate system. This method relies on the rigid attachment of a 3D reference frame to the patient. Image data acquired with the frame in place provides a quantitative positioning method during surgery. These methods were developed in the context of neurosurgery because of the critical nature of the brain tissue and the lack of clear visual anatomic landmarks that relate to the function of the brain. Stereotactic frames allow the surgeon to plan a procedure using preoperative images, and then follow that plan with confidence by using tools whose positions are registered with the frame.

The first 3D visualization technique to be applied in medical imaging was stereoscopic viewing. Like stereotaxy, stereoscopic viewing was developed prior to the availability of true 3D image sets in medical imaging. However, by capturing simultaneous 2D images that mimic the natural separation of the human eyes, viewing devices can produce the sensation of depth in an image. While not a standard practice in the medical field, this method has been experimented with for many years. The potential for true 3D visualization and guidance in surgical procedures was realized with the advent of medical imaging modalities that capture 3D datasets. The multislice tomographic images produced by CT and MRI scanners opened the field of image guidance to the application of 3D techniques. With the capture of volume datasets and the evolution of powerful computing for processing and visualization, realistic real-time depiction of 3D anatomy has become widely available.

The general expansion of computing and 3D visualization in other fields has benefited the medical field. Medical imaging has benefited from computer graphics advances associated with industries as diverse as gaming, film, and defense. Methods to track objects in 3D space have been developed for military, manufacturing, and entertainment applications. These methods have been incorporated into practical systems that can be used in the operating room to provide real-time guidance and feedback during surgical procedures.

Three-dimensional guidance for surgical procedures involves acquisition of 3D image data, visualization of the data, and interactive display tools for use in the operating room. Medical imaging modalities that produce 3D datasets are discussed in other chapters, so they will not be presented in detail here. This chapter will focus on display techniques developed specifically for 3D image data and the interactive guidance techniques that use the 3D image sets for procedure guidance.

13.2 3D Visualization

Given the availability of 3D image data from modern medical imaging devices, a key component of 3D image-guided therapy is the presentation of this 3D information to the user [1, 2]. The challenge is to convey the 3D data in an efficient and intuitive format so that the procedure is enhanced without adding an interpretive burden for the operator. An inherent challenge is the presentation of 3D data through two-dimensional devices. The complexity of the data also presents challenges regarding data processing speed.

13.2.1 3D Coordinate System

Three-dimensional imaging for image-guided therapy requires that a 3D coordinate system be established for the surgical space. Within this coordinate system, the position and orientation of tools and targets can then be tracked. The standard 3D coordinate system is described by three orthogonal axes (x, y, z). The position of an object is expressed as the distance along each axis of a reference point from the origin of the 3D coordinate system. The orientation can be described in several different formats, including Euler angles, a matrix of angle cosines, and quaternions [3, 4]. The motion of a rigid body is described as a three degree-of-freedom translation and a three degree-of-freedom rotation; a rigid body has no deformation.

13.2.2 3D Medical Imaging

Three-dimensional guidance for image-guided therapy has been driven by the availability of 3D medical imaging modalities. Modern imaging modalities such as computed tomography (CT), magnetic resonance imaging (MRI), and positron emission tomography (PET) produce 3D image sets as part of their standard protocols. Ultrasound has traditionally operated as a 2D modality, but methods have been developed to acquire 3D information from ultrasound also.

CT captures images as a series of tomographic slices, so the dataset is inherently 3D. CT is particularly useful for applications involving bone because X-rays, on which CT imaging is based, provide high contrast between bone and soft tissue. Like CT, MRI is an inherently 3D imaging modality, obtaining data over a volume as a series of tomographic slices. MRI can provide high contrast between different soft tissue types, and image characteristics can be varied depending on pulse sequences of the magnetic fields applied to the tissue. It can also provide functional imaging, including brain activity and blood flow. PET and single photon emission computed tomography (SPECT) use the uptake of radioisotopes to provide images related to function. The detectors are arranged so that they acquire 3D image sets, although not at the high spatial resolution that is possible with CT and MRI.

Ultrasound uses echoes from high-frequency sound waves to create tomographic images of tissue. The majority of standard ultrasound instruments provide images of a single 2D plane in real time. Newer ultrasound technology can provide 3D images either by using spatial trackers as adjunct devices, or with 2D transducer arrays [5]. Ultrasound has the advantages of patient safety, low cost, real-time user interaction, and high temporal resolution. It can provide images of both anatomic structure and also function by using Doppler shift detection to quantify blood flow and tissue motion.

13.2.3 3D Reconstruction

Most 3D medical imaging modalities collect 3D image data as a set of 2D planes. The most basic method of viewing the data is as a series of 2D images (Figure 13.1). Reconstruction is the processing of the raw image data into a 3D format that is representative of the true target. The two major formats for 3D reconstruction are surface reconstruction and volume reconstruction [2].

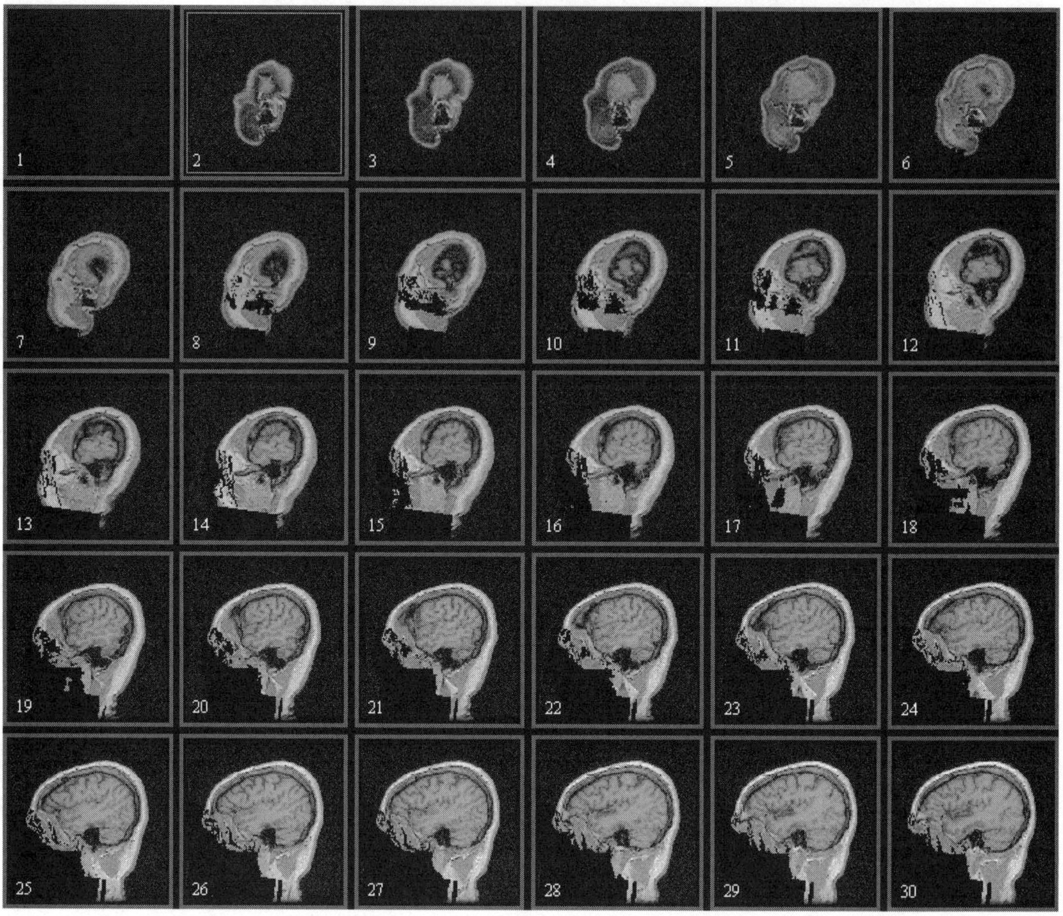

Figure 13.1 A series of 2D images from a 3D MRI dataset. Figure generated with MIPAV (Medical Image Processing, Analysis, and Visualization) software (MIPAV 4.0.1, Center for Information Technology, National Institutes of Health, Bethesda, Maryland).

13.2.3.1 Surface Reconstruction

Surface reconstruction expresses specific objects as a group of connected points that form a surface in space (Figure 13.2). This method of reconstruction relies on the identification of objects of interest by segmentation. Segmentation methods will be discussed below. Once an object of interest has been segmented, its surface can be represented by a set of points. Connection of neighboring points to create polygons produces a faceted model that approximates the surface in 3D space. The density of points can be changed depending on data storage constraints, computation time related to display, and the fidelity of the surface reconstruction required for a given application. Subdividing a surface mesh provides a smoother surface and can result in more realistic displays.

13.2.3.2 Volume Reconstruction

Volume reconstruction is based on a regular 3D grid of voxels (Figure 13.3). A voxel is a volume element, analogous to pixels in a 2D image. In volume reconstruction,

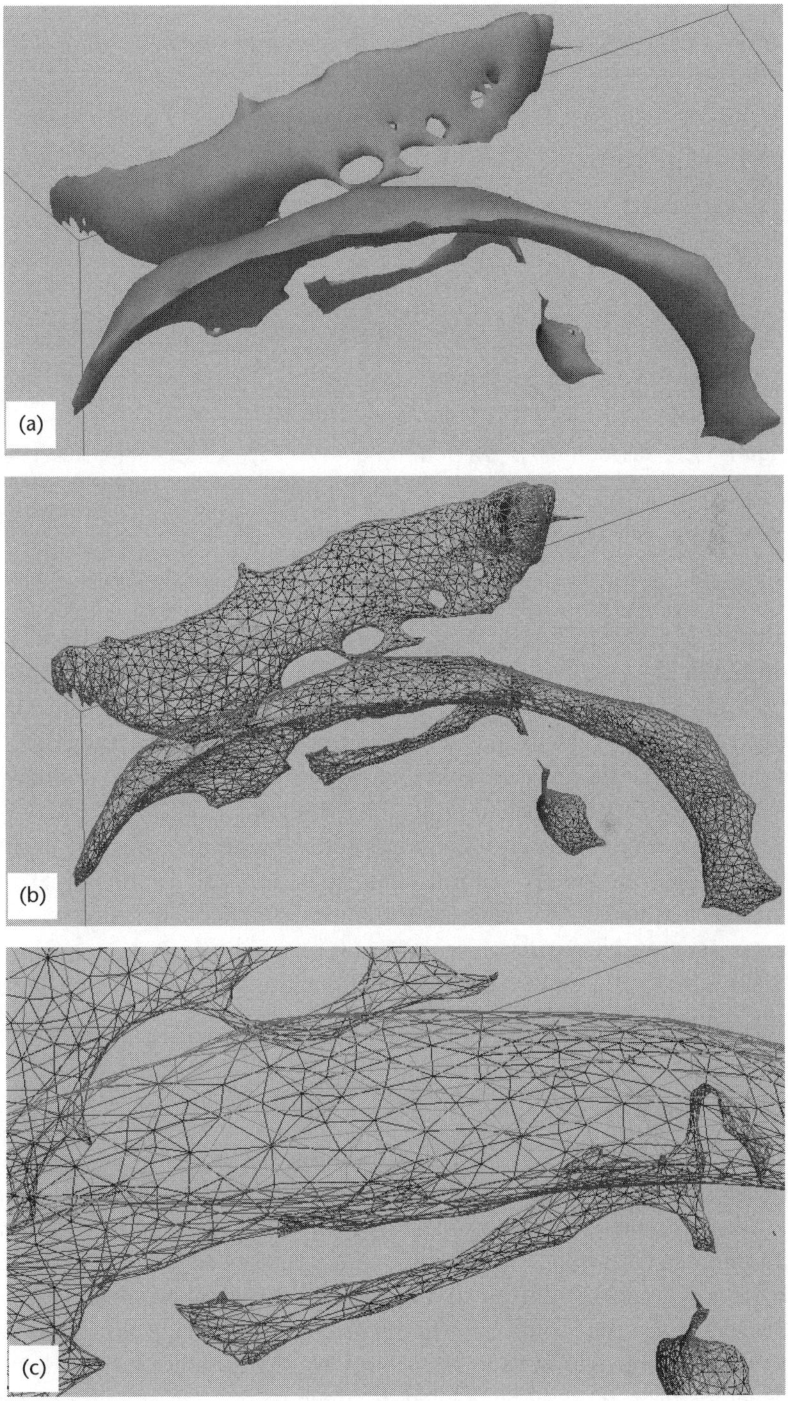

Figure 13.2 Surface reconstruction of the ventricles of the brain. (a) Rendering as a solid surface with shading. (b) Wireframe representation showing the connections of neighboring points that define the surface. (c) Zoom of the center region of (b) showing the polygon structure of the surface. Figure generated with Slicer software and demonstration data (Slicer 2.6, National Alliance for Medical Computing).

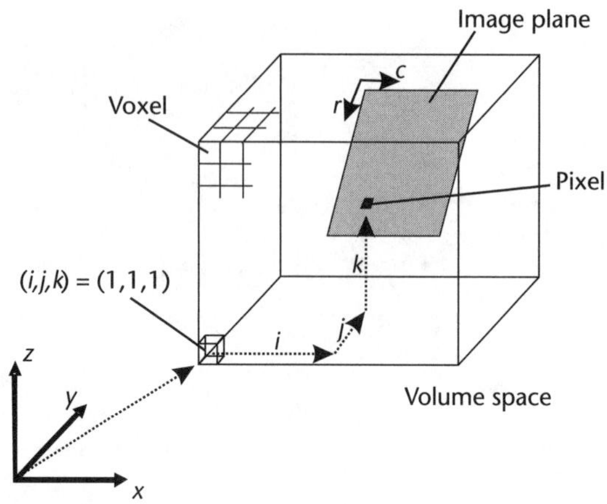

Figure 13.3 Relationship between the origin of the global 3D coordinate system (*x*, *y*, *z*), the 2D image coordinate system (*r*, *c*), and the reconstructed volume coordinate system (*i*, *j*, *k*). Each pixel from the 2D image is mapped to a location in the 3D volume based on the position and orientation of the image within the global coordinate system.

a value is associated with every voxel in the 3D grid. The size of the grid depends on the field of view of interest for a specific case and the resolution desired. Interpolation between voxels may be required if images were acquired at a low density or irregular intervals [6]. The parameters represented by the voxel values can vary depending on the imaging modality that is used. Individual anatomic structures are not explicitly distinguished within the volume.

Volume reconstruction requires more computer memory resources than surface reconstruction. A volume reconstruction can retain all of the image information acquired. To reduce the memory overhead the size of the voxels can be increased, which requires combination of neighboring voxels and loss of some of the original data. Data compression algorithms can also be used to reduce the storage requirements.

13.2.4 3D Image Display

Three-dimensional datasets contain a large amount of information, so the goal of the display is to convey the most useful components to the user in an efficient and intuitive manner. This becomes especially critical when the displays are part of an interactive system for guidance during a procedure. The data display must not require so much attention that the time and effort required or the efficacy of the procedure is compromised. The most common device for display of the 3D data to the end user is a 2D screen. Therefore, the majority of the display methods for developed for 3D data have been designed to present 3D data in a 2D view.

13.2.4.1 Rendering Methods

Rendering refers to the generation of an image from the 3D data. Different rendering methods can be used to emphasize particular aspects of the data [1, 2, 7–9]. Rendering methods may be specified for certain applications based on general consensus in the field, or selected by the user depending on preference or the particular target of interest.

Surface Rendering

If objects have been segmented and converted to surface representations as described above, the objects can be displayed with different characteristics using surface rendering methods. Surface rendering is a highly developed field of computer graphics with wide-ranging applications outside of medical imaging [10]. Therefore, only a brief summary of issues relating to surface rendering will be summarized here.

The surface model is composed of a wireframe (Figure 13.2), and textures are applied to the surface patches to customize the visual characteristics of the surface [7]. The character of the surface display is also affected by lighting and perspective. The rendering software specifies a virtual point of observation in the 3D coordinate system and a virtual light source. Light rays are assumed to strike the surface and reflect, depending on the surface orientation and its reflective properties. Surfaces can be made to appear as specular or diffuse reflectors, which affects their appearance to the user. Shading can be used to indicate depth or provide realism.

Surfaces can be displayed simply as points or a wireframe (Figure 13.2), or as solids with varying transparency (Figure 13.4). User interaction options typically include rotation, translation, and zooming of the view. Because of the efficiency of the representation of the object as a set of points, the speed of updating the view is generally not an issue with current computers.

Multiplanar Reformatting

A common rendering method for 3D medical image data is multiplanar reformatting, in which the 3D volume is intersected by a 2D plane. Other terms for this rendering method include multiplanar reconstruction and volume reslicing. This method produces 2D views of the data in planes that were not originally acquired by the imaging device. Interpolation between the original pixels of the dataset is generally required to fill in gaps in the data. A standard format for display is three orthogonal views at intersecting locations in the transverse (or axial), sagittal, and coronal directions (Figure 13.5). Display software for multiplanar rendering gener-

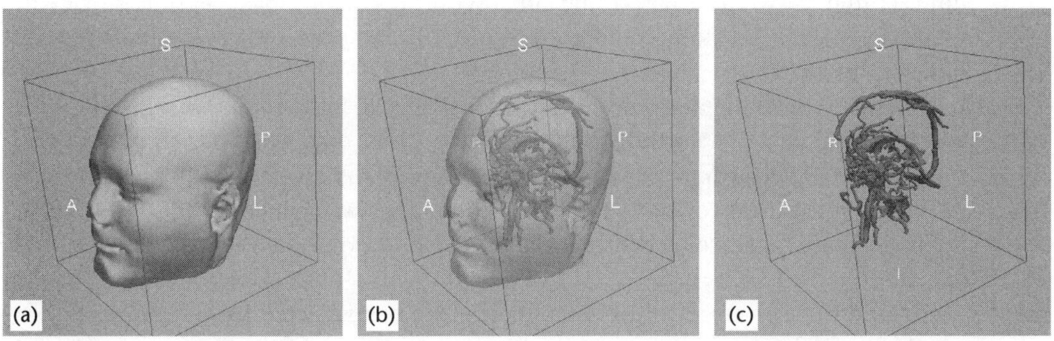

Figure 13.4 Surface displays. (a) Skin surface shown as a solid object. (b) Skin surface with transparency. (c) Skin surface is hidden to show surface reconstructions of the vessels and ventricles in the brain. Figure generated with Slicer software and demonstration data.

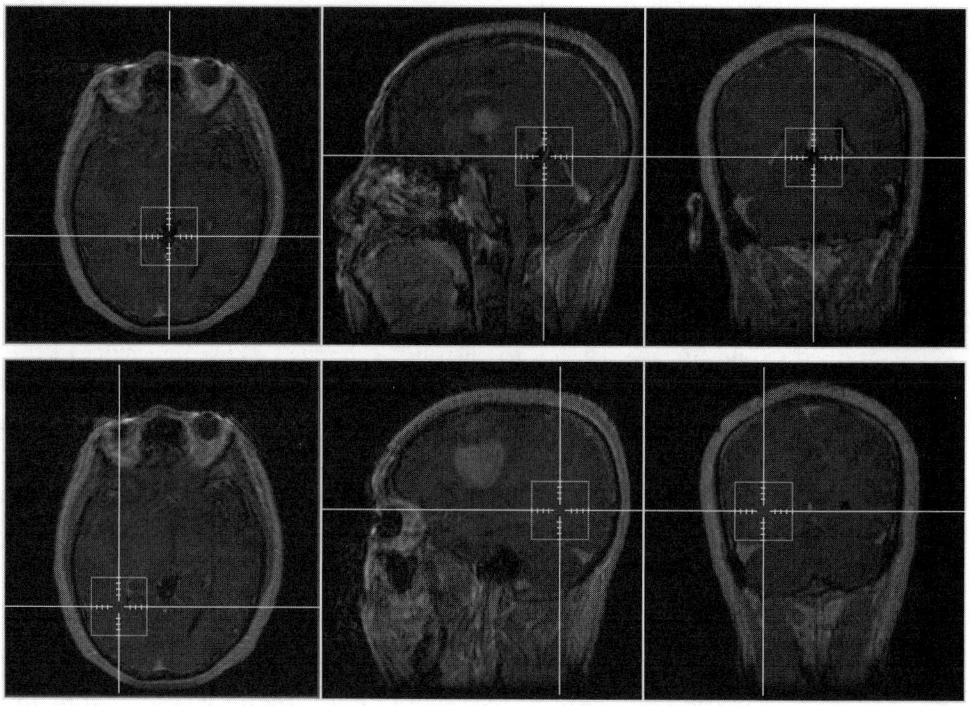

Figure 13.5 Orthogonal views of a 3D dataset. The views from left to right are transverse, sagittal, and coronal planes. The top row shows the intersecting planes at the point selected in the transverse slice. In the bottom row the selected point in the transverse slice has been moved, and the intersecting views are updated in the sagittal and coronal views. [Figure generated with 3DMed software (3DMed 2.1.0, Medical Image Processing Group, Institute of Automation, Chinese Academy of Sciences).]

ally includes interactive controls that allow the user to adjust the locations of the individual viewing planes in real time.

Multiplanar displays can include several features to help the user navigate through the 3D dataset. Planes are often framed in unique colors and projected into the other views as lines with the corresponding color. A selected point in a specific plane can be highlighted in the other two views. A 3D view of the entire data volume is often shown as a wireframe cube, with the current location of each viewing plane displayed. A volume rendering of the full dataset may also be included as a navigation aid.

There are several variations on the multiplanar display available in most display software packages. The orthogonal planes may all be displayed in their correct positions in the 3D coordinate system (Figure 13.6). This display explicitly shows the intersection locations of each plane, but the planes will generally obscure some of the image data. Surface reconstructions can also be combined with the image plane display [Figure 13.7(a)].

In addition, arbitrary or oblique planes may be extracted from the dataset [Figure 13.7(b)]. This operation requires interpolation to fill in the image values at points that were not necessarily acquired by the imaging system itself. Specification of arbitrary planes allows a user to see structures from perspectives that are not ex-

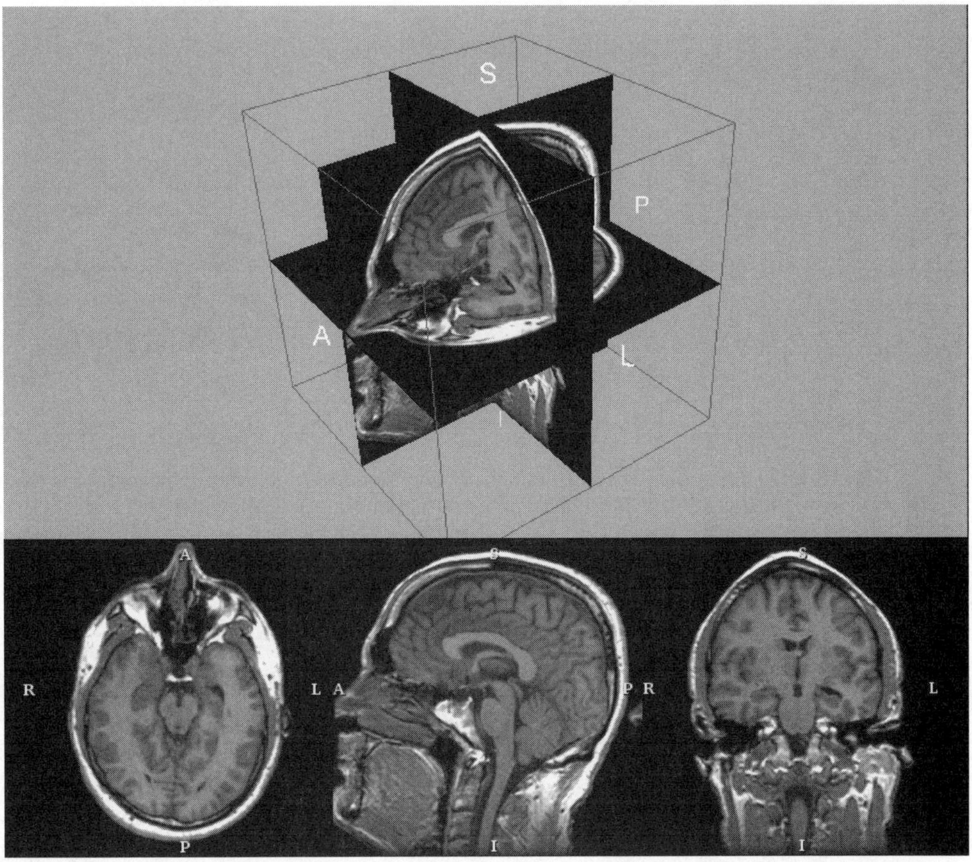

Figure 13.6 Intersecting orthogonal planes displayed in 3D space. Figure generated with Slicer software and demonstration data.

plicitly acquired by the imaging system. Many users are most comfortable viewing the standard orthogonal planes because of their familiarity with standard 2D slices. However, the arbitrary slice function can be useful to show the maximum dimension of a tumor, for instance. An extension of the arbitrary slice display is the curved plane [1]. A user can draw a curve in one of the orthogonal slices, and the image can be reformatted to show this curve as a 2D image. This function can be used for instance to show the entire lumen of a curved vessel such as the aorta.

Volume Rendering

Volume rendering refers to projection of the 3D dataset onto a 2D plane for display. A viewing direction is defined by the location of a virtual camera in 3D space, and each voxel is assigned an opacity and color. Virtual rays are projected through the volume data, and values are assigned to the points on the 2D viewing plane depending on the voxels encountered by each ray. Many different specific algorithms for volume rendering are available, with various trade-offs in speed and appearance [2, 9, 11–13].

Volume rendering does not require explicit segmentation of anatomic structures, since it uses the original values in the 3D voxel grid to generate a display. However,

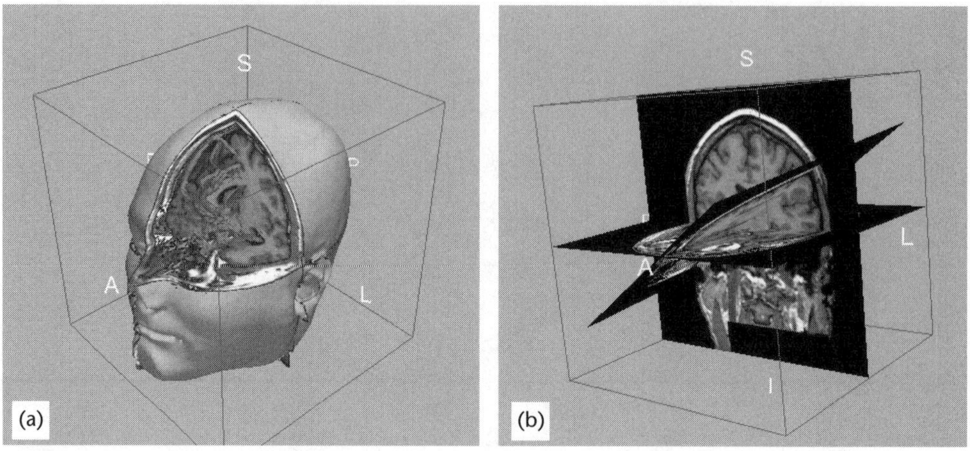

Figure 13.7 (a) Surface reconstructions are combined with an orthogonal image plane display. In this case, the image plane locations clip the outer skin surface to show the gray scale image data and the reconstructed vessels and ventricles. (b) Oblique slice through the 3D dataset. Figures generated with Slicer software and demonstration data.

variations in the display methods can be used to highlight inherent features that may be relevant for a given application. In particular, the transfer function that assigns the color and opacity to each voxel is chosen to emphasize different features of the data [1].

For example, the first value encountered by the ray (above a certain threshold) will display an outer surface of the data. If the volume of interest encompasses the full field of view of a standard CT or MRI dataset, rendering of the first value will display the skin surface [Figure 13.8(a)]. Other surfaces can be preferentially selected for display by choosing a threshold and creating an isosurface. An isosurface displays those points in the 3D dataset that have the same intensity value. Changing the intensity value of interest can selectively highlight structures or tissue types in the dataset.

The rays can also be allowed to traverse the entire volume, and the average value (or sum) of all voxels encountered along each ray can be displayed. This generally produces a display similar in appearance to an X-ray image [Figure 13.8(b)]. Unlike a standard X-ray, however, the viewing position can be changed to allow views of the data from any direction. Alternatively, the maximum value encountered by each ray can be assigned to each pixel in the display to generate a maximum intensity projection (MIP) [Figure 13.8(c)]. This display method is particularly useful to display bones in CT data, or vascular contrast in MRI data. Magnetic resonance angiography (MRA) relies heavily on the MIP display to show vascular structures that appear bright in the images because of contrast agents or pulse sequences that are sensitive to flow. MIP rendering is also useful for CT angiography if the vessels of interest are not obscured by bone.

Accumulation or compositing allows selective highlighting of different tissue types based on the values encountered in each voxel along the ray. For example, a CT volume will contain Hounsfield Units as the voxel values. The assignment of

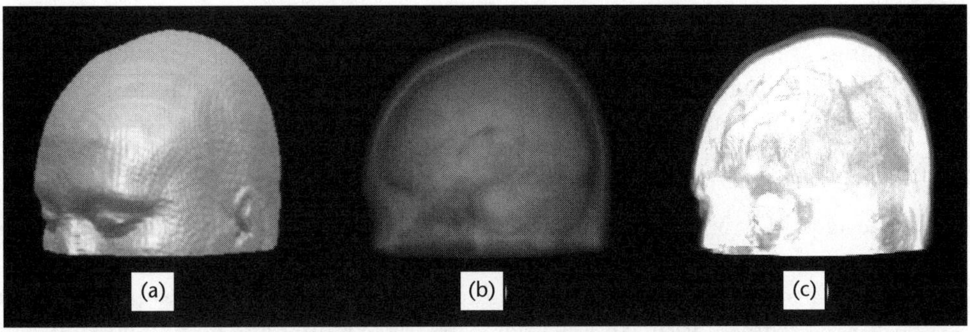

Figure 13.8 Volume rendering. (a) Isosurface display of the outer surface of a 3D scan of the brain. (b) Rendering of the data set in (a) with opacity to show the brain. (c) Maximum intensity projection of the data set in (a). Figures generated with MRIcro software and demonstration data (MRIcro 1.38, www.mricro.com).

opacities and grayscale values or colors can then be adjusted based on the specific value of each voxel [1]. For CT, voxels within a selected range of Hounsfield Units can be displayed or hidden, which can preferentially choose between displays of soft tissue and bone.

Volume rendering requires intensive computer processing for interactive viewing, since the full 3D grid data is used and the processing must be performed as the user changes views. Specification of a volume of interest for a particular application helps to reduce the computational overhead. Development of efficient computational algorithms for volume rendering is an active field of research [14–16].

13.2.4.2 Segmentation

Segmentation is the identification and labeling of objects in an image. It requires the accurate separation and grouping of structures so that they can be treated as units in the display. Construction of the surface of an object from a medical imaging dataset requires segmentation. Volume rendering can be optimized to display certain tissue types of interest by applying segmentation algorithms. Segmentation methods, and the difficulty associated with the task, vary depending on the imaging modality used. Segmentation can be performed through fully manual interaction. However, for practical display of large 3D datasets, semi- or fully automated segmentation algorithms are generally required.

A full discussion of image segmentation is beyond the scope of this chapter; reviews of image segmentation algorithms are found in the literature [2, 17]. Some standard methods for automated or assisted segmentation are described next.

Thresholding

The most straightforward method of segmentation is thresholding [18]. Simple thresholding displays all pixels or voxels in a dataset that are above a specified value as white, and all others as black. This produces a binary representation of the data. Thresholding can also be made more flexible by specifying a range of image values of interest, so that values within the selected range are white and those outside the range are black. The binary result can be used as a mask to select or exclude regions from the original dataset. Connected regions that result from the threshold operation can be classified as objects [19]. Additional image processing methods can be applied to the thresholded data to achieve desired results if the simple threshold does not segment the data completely. For example, morphological operators are designed for binary data and respond to the shape of borders. Morphological operations can expand, reduce, smooth, and separate regions [19].

Clustering is a method related to thresholding, but it uses multiple parameters for the segmentation. In MRI datasets, for example, the combined values of multiple pulse sequences may be used to isolate data points corresponding to specific tissue types [2]. The selection of those voxels whose values in different pulse sequences cluster into groups can segment out particular anatomic structures.

Edge Detection

The detection of edges is an important tool in image segmentation. Contrast between regions is generally indicative of different tissue types in medical images, so identifying the border between regions can extract anatomic structures. Edge detection is often based on intensity gradients in the image, using well-developed image processing techniques [20]. Extracted edges can be connected in three dimensions to produce a surface.

Guided Methods

It is extremely difficult to implement fully automated segmentation algorithms that can perform perfectly across all cases. This is especially true of medical images, where variability between patients is expected. Given the importance of accurate segmentation when planning and performing image-guided interventions, most practical segmentation algorithms for medical imaging incorporate some degree of user interaction. An automated segmentation may be modified by an expert based on their anatomic knowledge, or an expert can interactively guide the segmentation algorithm.

For example, the "live wire" method is a computer-assisted segmentation algorithm [21]. The user sets the starting point by clicking at a location of interest in the image. As the cursor is moved along the general direction of a boundary of interest, a path is automatically drawn from the initial point based on a cost function. The path is continually updated as the user moves the cursor. The user can enter additional points to select the current path determined by the cost algorithm. The user can choose different paths if the boundary is deemed incorrect, or manually enter additional points to guide the segmentation. Active contours (also known as snakes) are based on a rough delineation of edges by several points at or near borders of interest, or specification of a bounding box to restrict the region of interest. A boundary is then computed based on image gradients that minimize an energy function [22–24].

Region growing uses seed points specified by the user to initiate the segmentation of structures of interest [19]. Similarity measures of neighboring voxels are then used to select voxels to be included in an object. Contiguous image regions with similar characteristics are grouped into objects. How much a region is allowed to grow can be controlled by a tolerance setting. The inclusion criteria and tolerance can be set for different tissues based on past knowledge, or it can be set interactively. Region growing is more robust than thresholding in that it uses more information than just intensity level to group an object. Texture is one method, which takes into account the statistical variation of neighboring voxels to make decisions of inclusion or exclusion. Similarly, level set methods use initial points to compute an evolving curve or surface based on constraints defining regions with consistent properties [25–27]. The end result can then delineate structures of interest (Figure 13.9).

Model-Based Methods

Previously segmented models can be applied to new image datasets by registering the models with the current data of interest [28]. For instance, structures segmented in a CT dataset of a given patient could be used to segment an MRI dataset of the same patient. A more general application is the use of an image atlas, which is a generic model that is applied to independent datasets. Brain atlases are the most common example of this approach to segmentation, in which brain components that cannot be explicitly identified can instead be defined in relation to other anatomic structures in the brain. The Talairach atlas is one of the most widely used examples of atlas-based segmentation [29]. The Talairach atlas uses a three-dimensional proportional grid system to identify and measure brains from any number of patients despite the variability of brain sizes and proportions [30]. Registration of an individual dataset with the Talairach atlas requires two transformations: a rigid alignment and a piecewise linear deformation [30]. An example of the registration of a segmented brain atlas [31] with a patient scan is shown in Figure 13.10.

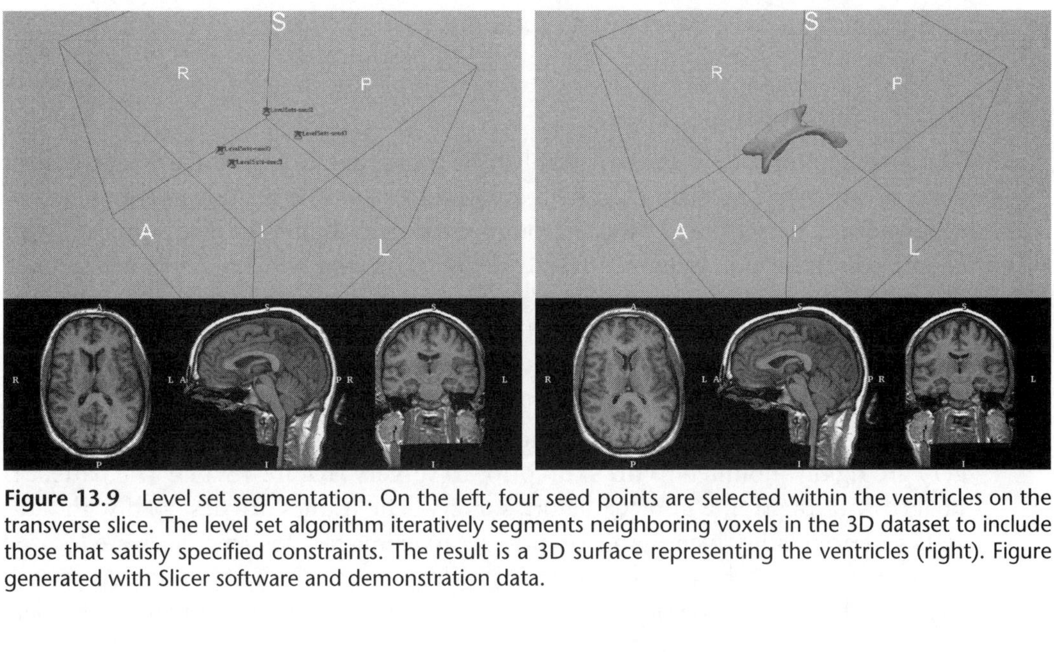

Figure 13.9 Level set segmentation. On the left, four seed points are selected within the ventricles on the transverse slice. The level set algorithm iteratively segments neighboring voxels in the 3D dataset to include those that satisfy specified constraints. The result is a 3D surface representing the ventricles (right). Figure generated with Slicer software and demonstration data.

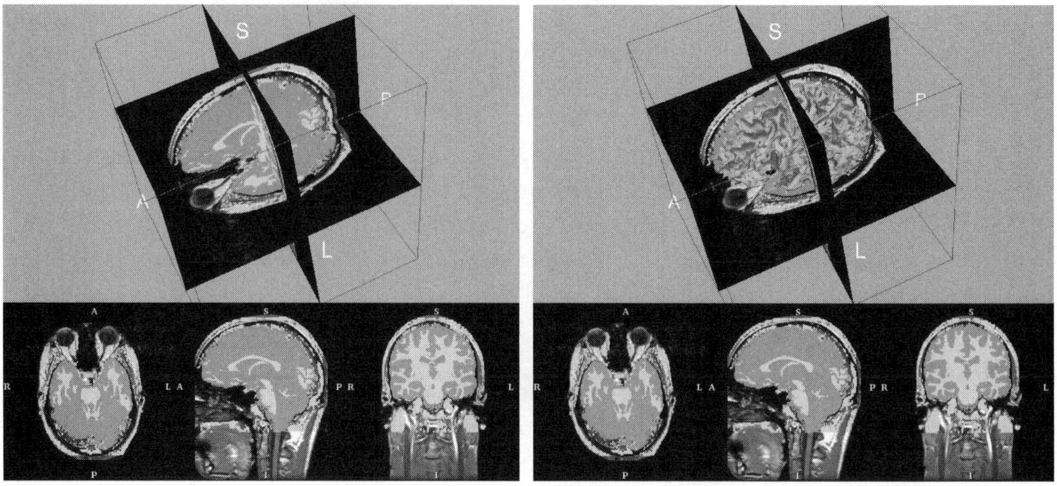

Figure 13.10 Brain atlas segmentation. On the left, a brain atlas compiled from multiple patient datasets is fit to a patient-specific MRI scan. The atlas has been segmented to classify white matter, gray matter, cerebrospinal fluid, and background. On the right, a surface reconstruction is generated for the segmented white matter. Figure generated with Slicer software and demonstration data.

13.3 3D Guidance

The benefits of 3D imaging techniques for therapy guidance are based on the integration of the 3D image data with real-time tracking of surgical tools in 3D space. The 3D features of the guidance must provide the user with real advantages, such as time saved or better outcomes due to increased accuracy and precision of the targeting. Note that when discussing system performance, "accuracy" refers to the ability to locate the true position of a target in 3D space, while "precision" refers to the repeatability of the localization. This section reviews methods for applying 3D imaging methods to guidance of a procedure.

13.3.1 Stereotactics

The first method widely used to establish a 3D coordinate system for image-guided therapy was stereotactics [32, 33]. Stereotactics rely on a rigid frame attached to the patient to define the 3D space around the target of interest. The surgical target is located within this reference frame by imaging, and surgical tools are tracked during the procedure.

Stereotactic surgery was originally developed for neurosurgery, and this remains its main application area. Stereotactics was motivated by the need for surgical methods that could accurately target specific regions of the brain with minimal disruption of intervening and surrounding tissues. Stereotactic frames for neurosurgery are rigidly mounted to the skull prior to surgery (Figure 13.11). The patient is imaged with the frame in place before surgery. The frames are designed with fiducials that are readily identifiable on preoperative images. Target tissues are located in the images, and their locations are recorded relative to the fiducials. Approach paths can be planned to minimize damage to intervening tissue. Instrument holders

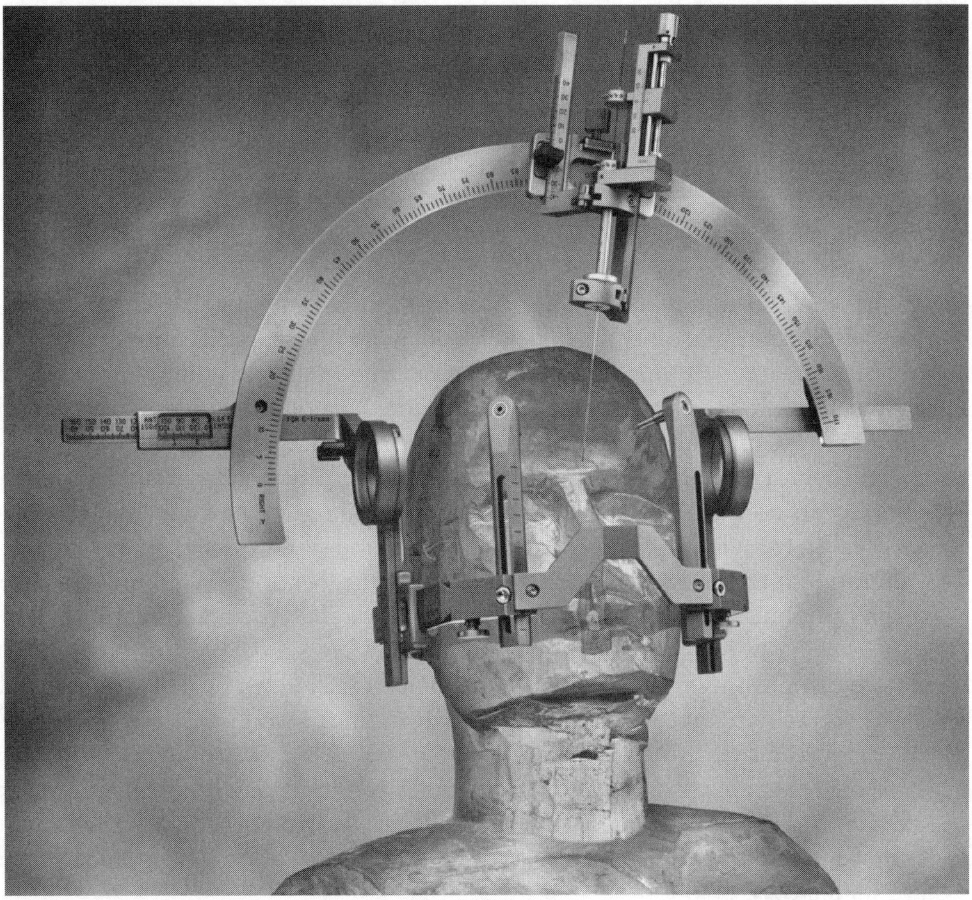

Figure 13.11 Stereotactic head frame (Leksell Stereotactic System, Elekta AB, Stockholm, Sweden). (Photograph courtesy of Elekta AB.)

attached to the stereotactic frame allow access to specific points in the 3D coordinate system defined by the frame.

Stereotactic frames are commercially available for specific imaging modalities, or for use with multiple imaging modalities. The fiducial material and size/shape are chosen to assure visibility in the images. Stereotactic frames provide registration between the images and the target with an accuracy and precision on the order of 1 mm [34].

The simplest version of stereotactic surgery assumes that there is no significant tissue motion or deformation at the time of the procedure. Therefore, the preoperative planning is considered to be accurate and the surgery proceeds using the fixed tool positions. For neurosurgery this assumption may be reasonably accurate if the procedure is minimally invasive, with tools introduced through small holes in the skull. However, if the procedure requires a craniotomy, significant shifts of the brain can be expected. Accurate adjustment of preoperative plan to compensate for intraoperative tissue changes requires an update of the images of the target [35]. Intraoperative imaging is possible with fluoroscopy, CT, MRI, and ultrasound.

13.3.2 Spatial Tracking Systems

The concept of stereotactics can be extended by establishing the 3D coordinate system of the patient without relying on a rigid external frame. Instead, a spatial tracking system establishes the coordinates of the patient and surgical tools and devices. Preoperative images are registered with this intraoperative coordinate system so that preoperative plans can be accurately transferred to the operating room. This method is sometimes referred to as *frameless stereotaxy.*

Spatial tracking systems use a coordinate system origin that is not attached to the patient, allowing more flexibility during the procedure than a stereotactic frame. In addition, multiple objects can be tracked, including surgical tools, catheters, and displays, creating a dynamic 3D environment in which real-time guidance is possible. Motion of the patient, however, becomes a potential source of error when the frameless approach is used. The patient must remain immobile, or the patient's position must be tracked or remeasured if movement occurs. Calibration of the instruments used with the tracking system is also a requirement, so that objects can be accurately registered in the tracking coordinate system [36, 37]. For instance, a calibration transformation is needed to specify the location of a pointer tip in space given position and orientation of the tracking system sensor (Figure 13.12).

Tracking systems may operate with three, five, or six degrees-of-freedom. Three degree-of-freedom systems only track a point (translation). Five degree-of-freedom systems track an axis (translation and two rotational angles), as in tracking of a device tip aligned with an axis. Six degree-of-freedom systems describe the full 3D coordinate system (translation in x, y, and z, and rotation about each of the three axes). Various methods for spatial tracking are available, each with their own advantages and disadvantages [38]. The main methods used in image-guided therapy are summarized below.

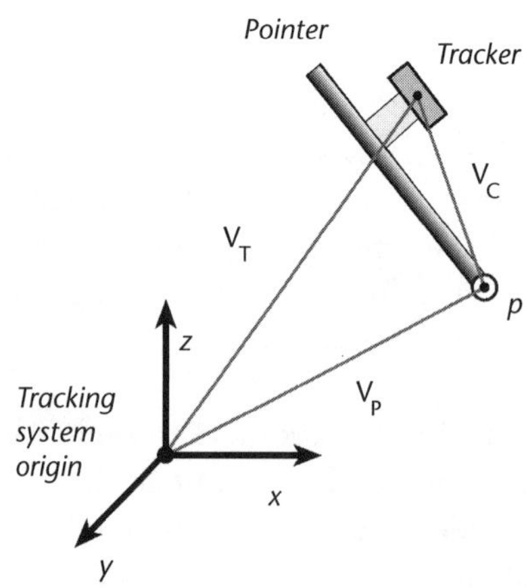

Figure 13.12 Schematic diagram of the vector relationship between the tracking system origin, the tracking device, and a point of interest in space located by a calibrated pointer. The vector V_P (the 3D location of the point of interest) is the sum of the tracker measurement V_T and the calibration vector V_C. The spatial relationship between the tracking device and the tip of the pointer (V_C) must be accurately known in order to reliably locate individual points in space.

13.3.2.1 Mechanical

The most common mechanical tracking devices for image-guided therapy are articulated arms [Figure 13.13(a)]. Articulated arms have multiple joints whose positions are tracked by potentiometers or optical encoders. From a standard resting position, the location and orientation of the arm tip can be tracked, given accurate measurement of each joint's motion.

Articulated arms are a mature technology that was developed in large part for measurements in manufacturing. A wide range of models are available, varying in size and quality, but in general they achieve high accuracy (resolution less than 1 mm) in tracking the arm tip [39]. In medical applications, however, they can be cumbersome to use, with the rigid link of the arm restricting motion and physically interfering with other instruments in the operating field.

13.3.2.2 Acoustic

The first freehand spatial tracking devices used in the operating room were acoustic trackers. These devices use a series of ultrasonic pulses from a group of emitters to track the position and orientation of an object. Ultrasonic emitters, usually small spark gaps that fire in succession, are mounted on the object to be tracked in a known configuration [40]. A set of microphones is mounted at some distance from the active work area, usually on the ceiling. Time-of-flight measurements for pulses from each emitter to each microphone are used to calculate the object's distance and orientation relative to a stationary reference point.

While these acoustic systems free the user from the rigid constraints of the articulated arm, they have their own limitations. First, the spatial measurements are subject to errors in the sound time-of-flight. Differences in the speed of sound from the standard value assumed by the system will result in errors in the calculated spatial coordinates. Second, the emitters on the object cannot fire simultaneously, so motion of the object during a measurement cycle can produce tracking errors. Third, blocking of a clear line-of-sight to the microphones can produce erroneous results.

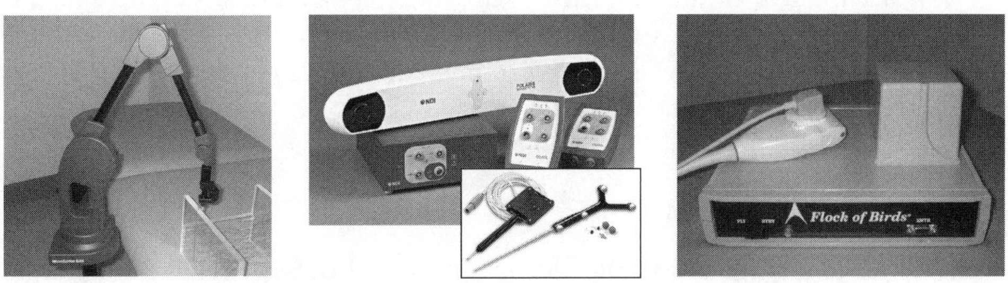

(a) (b) (c)

Figure 13.13 Spatial tracking devices. (a) Articulated arm (Microscribe G2X, Immersion Corporation, San Jose, California). (b) Optical tracking system (Polaris Spectra, Northern Digital, Inc., Waterloo, Ontario, Canada). (c) Magnetic tracking system (Flock of Birds, Ascension Technology Corporation, Burlington. Vermont). [Photographs for (b) courtesy of Northern Digital, Inc.]

13.3.2.3 Optical

Optical tracking systems use an array of cameras to detect either active or passive markers mounted on an object [Figure 13.13(b)]. Active markers emit visible or infrared light; passive markers are reflectors that are used with an infrared light source. Similar to the acoustic systems, the configuration of the markers is known, so the relative pattern viewed by multiple cameras allows the calculation of the object's location and orientation in the system's 3D coordinate system. They are able to simultaneously track multiple objects.

The performance of optical systems typically varies with their price, but in general they can achieve very accurate (submillimeter) localization [39]. If price is not a concern, then the major drawback with optical systems is the line-of-sight constraint between the cameras and the markers. If an object has the minimum number of markers, then all must be visible to the cameras for proper localization. This can restrict the permitted orientations of the object during a procedure. More than three markers can be mounted on an object to allow a wider range of orientations, but the system is still susceptible to blocking by personnel or other objects in the working area. In addition, tracking of devices within the patient, which is needed for guidance of minimally invasive procedures, is not possible.

13.3.2.4 Magnetic

Magnetic tracking systems use electromagnetic fields generated by a stationary transmitter and a set of detecting coils mounted on an object to track the object's position and orientation in space [Figure 13.13(c)]. Magnetic tracking systems are generally not as accurate as optical systems, with accuracy on the order of 1 mm [37, 41], but they tend to be considerably less expensive. Their main disadvantage is susceptibility to electromagnetic interference and distortions due to ferromagnetic materials in the vicinity. Because the magnetic field strength decreases with distance from the transmitter, their performance can also vary within the working space. While their operating range may be limited compared with optical systems, their main advantage is that they are not limited by direct line-of-sight constraints relative to the transmitter. This gives them the unique capability to track instruments inside the patient. In fact, sensors are available that are less than 1 mm in diameter and can be placed inside endoscopes and catheters [42, 43]. The construction of electromagnetic systems that are immune to distortion from metals is also an area of current activity in the industry.

13.3.3 Registration

Three-dimensional guidance for image-guided therapy relies on the accurate registration of the coordinate systems associated with the tracking system, pre- and intraoperative images, and the patient. Registration aligns the multiple datasets associated with a particular procedure within a common coordinate system.

Some applications of 3D visualization in image-guided therapy rely on the combined display of several medical imaging datasets. Image fusion refers to the simultaneous display of multiple image datasets within a common 3D coordinate system. One motivation for image fusion is the combination of anatomic and functional data to improve targeting. A second application is the combination of preoperative and intraoperative images.

Registration is also necessary when atlases are used for procedure guidance. In this case a general atlas that maps functional areas of interest must be applied to a specific patient. The reference atlas must be registered so that the general functional segmentation is applicable to the specific case. The most common use of guidance based on an atlas is in neurosurgery. Because many of the features of interest in the brain are functional and do not include readily identifiable anatomic landmarks, a predefined atlas of brain functional regions is used to guide procedure planning and execution. Deformable registration warps the standard atlas to help identify functional regions in the brain on a patient's image data.

13.3.3.1 Registration Methods

Registration of preoperative images and the intraoperative coordinate system can be accomplished using several different approaches [44]. Methods used for a particular application depend on the image data available and the targets of interest.

Point Matching

Point matching relies on the identification of homologous points on the preoperative images and the patient in the operating room [45, 46]. The points used for registration can be intrinsic or extrinsic [28]. Intrinsic points are anatomical landmarks that are identified both in the image data and on the patient. For neurosurgery, these points are often distinct landmarks such as the nasion and zygomatic arch. Registration is performed by using a stylus or pointer that is tracked by the spatial tracking system in the operating room and has been calibrated so that the location of the pointer tip is known in the 3D coordinate system of the tracking system. The pointer tip is touched to the external physical landmarks on the patient, and the 3D location of each landmark is recorded. The corresponding points are identified on the images, and a point-matching algorithm (discussed in the next section) is used to calculate the transformation between the two sets of points. Identification of homologous points can also be used to register preoperative images with intraoperative images if they are available.

The accuracy of registration using intrinsic points is limited by the ability to identify corresponding points in the images and on the patient. Exact correspondence can be difficult to achieve for enough points to establish an accurate transformation between the images and the patient. For CT and MRI images, the partial volume effect can make exact identification of landmarks difficult. There is also some variability in pointer placement on the patient.

Extrinsic points are markers that are placed on the patient before the preoperative imaging study so that they appear in the images and are easily identifiable in the operating room (Figure 13.14). Extrinsic markers can be placed on the skin or attached to bone. Skin markers do not require an invasive procedure, but their location can change between the time of the imaging study and the procedure. Changes in swelling can move the markers radially, or skin stretching can shift their position

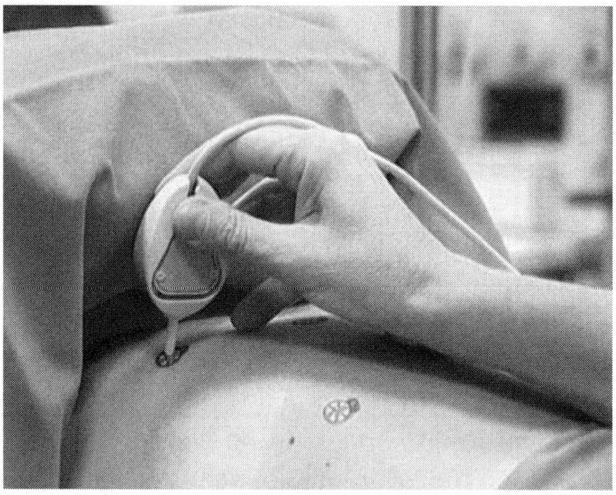

Figure 13.14 Extrinsic points specified by markers placed on a patient, located in 3D space with a pointer and a magnetic tracking system (NaviSuite, MedCom GmbH, Darmstadt, Germany). (Photograph courtesy of MedCom GmbH.)

tangentially. Extrinsic markers rigidly attached to bone are more accurate than skin markers, but their placement requires a surgical procedure. Still, if the accuracy is needed for the procedure, then the minimally invasive surgery to place the markers is generally considered acceptable.

Surface Matching

When only a few points are available for matching, an error in locating one of the points can lead to a significant error in the overall coordinate system registration. The number of intrinsic points available for matching is generally limited by the number of landmarks that can be reliably identified in both the preoperative image set and on the patient. The number of extrinsic points is limited by the number of markers that can be attached.

An alternative to the matching of discrete points for registration is surface matching. In this case, surface reconstructions of regions of interest are generated from the preoperative images. The reconstructed surfaces are then matched with a digitized surface of the patient in the operating room, or with surfaces extracted from intraoperative image data. Direct digitization of the body surface can be performed using a pointer tip in contact with the skin, or with a laser scanner [47–50] (Figure 13.15). A geometric pattern can also be projected on the surface of interest and stereo cameras can be used to reconstruct the surface. As an alternative to registration of external surfaces, bone surfaces can be extracted from pre- and intraoperative image sets by segmentation. Surfaces provide a more robust dataset for registration than the discrete points used for point matching. Sources of error in surface matching include segmentation errors and surface deformation.

Volume Matching

Direct matching of volume image data can be accomplished by using algorithms such as Mutual Information, where voxel values over a volume of interest are

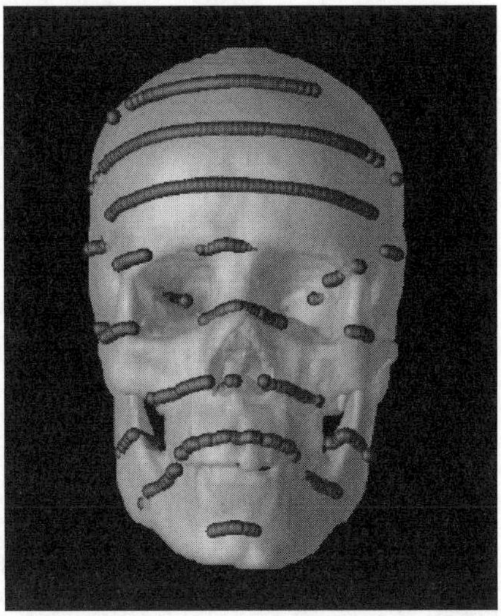

Figure 13.15 Points from a laser range scanner are registered with a reconstructed CT scan of a plastic skull. (Reprinted from [48], © 1996 IEEE, with permission from IEEE.)

aligned such that an error function is minimized [51]. In this case markers, segmentation, and surface reconstruction are not required.

13.3.3.2 Coordinate System Transformations

Registration between preoperative and intraoperative image sets draws on extensive work in image processing [44]. Methods from image processing can also be applied to the image-to-patient matching of points and surface. Transformations between coordinate systems for registration can be rigid or deformable. Rigid transformations perform translation and rotation to match the corresponding points. A common method for matching is to minimize the least squares difference between the points or surfaces.

For direct point matching, a translation and rotation is computed that merges at least three noncollinear points [52, 53]. The ordered point sets are translated to their centers of mass, and the optimum rotation is found to match the points. The Iterative Closest Point algorithm is an example of a surface-matching algorithm for nonordered points; with this method direct correspondence of point pairs is not required [54, 55].

Rigid registration is the most common method for matching of pre- and intraoperative coordinate systems. However, in some cases the assumption that there is no tissue deformation between the time of the preoperative image study and the procedure in the operating room is not true. As noted previously, significant tissue deformation is expected for neurosurgical procedures involving craniotomy. Endoscopic procedures in the abdomen also include tissue deformation, because the abdominal cavity is often inflated with air to allow room for instruments and cameras during the procedure. In these cases, deformable registration algorithms are required to assure accurate registration of the intraoperative images and surgical tools with the preoperative images [56–58]. Deformable registration is also required for procedures that rely on atlases for planning and guidance, because the general atlas anatomy cannot be expected to match the anatomy of a specific patient. Deformable registration techniques remain an area of active research.

Registration of deformable tissues during a procedure generally requires the availability of an intraoperative imaging modality, so that the preoperative images can be warped to match the actual intraoperative configuration. An area of ongoing research is the use of biomechanical tissue models that predict tissue deformation and adjust the preoperative images without relying on intraoperative imaging [59, 60].

13.3.3.3 Registration Accuracy and Precision

System accuracy must be assessed to assure that the guidance is, in fact, of benefit to the procedure. Overall registration performance depends on a combination of tracker performance, tracker calibration, image resolution, identification of matching points and surfaces, registration algorithms, and target motion or deformation. These results will vary across systems with differences in components, approaches, and individual experience. Detailed analysis of several systems can be found in the literature which provide a guide to the methods of system evaluation [42, 45, 61–63]. In general, acceptable registration performance for the localization of arbitrary objects is on the order of several millimeters [28].

13.3.3.4 Registration Applications

Tools and Images

The most basic registration task for 3D image guidance is the registration of the intraoperative surgical tools with the preoperative planning images [64, 65]. The position and orientation of the tools used during surgery must be tracked in the same coordinate system as the images. An optical tracker deployed in the operating room is shown in Figure 13.16. An example of a software user interface showing a tracked pointer is shown in Figure 13.17.

Atlases and Images

Standard atlases can be a useful tool for 3D guidance of surgical procedures. As mentioned previously, neurosurgery is the most common example of atlases used for surgical guidance. With the availability of 3D image data of patient-specific cases, standard 3D atlas data can be projected into the 3D reconstruction for individual cases (Figure 13.10). Atlases of functional regions of the brain are important for neurosurgery because of the critical nature of all of the tissues traversed during the intervention. Knowledge of the functional regions both during planning and the procedure itself helps the surgeon to minimize collateral damage and functional deficits that could result from accessing the site of the actual lesion.

Multimodality Images

Multimodality imaging is becoming more common as a general diagnostic procedure. Functional imaging combined with anatomic images can be a powerful tool

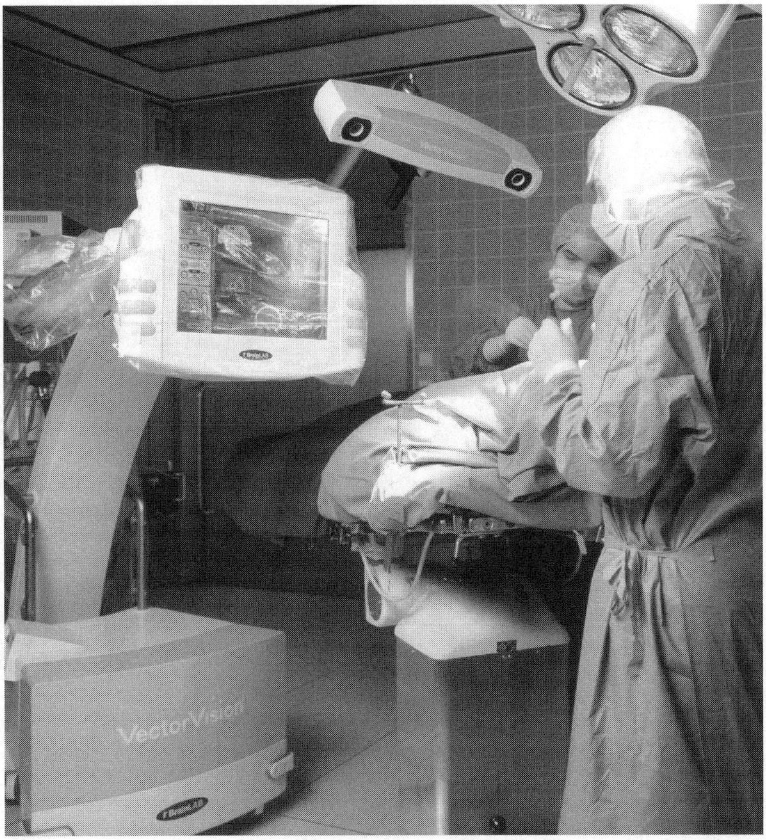

Figure 13.16 Optical tracking system (VectorVision², BrainLAB AG, Feldkirchen, Germany) in use in the operating room. (Photograph courtesy of BrainLAB AG.)

for 3D image guidance. While the brain atlases described in the previous section can provide useful guidance for gross guidance of functional regions, they can never be a perfect guide due to both registration errors and variability across patients. Functional imaging that pinpoints brain activity for individual cases provides a more accurate map of the regions of interest for a particular procedure.

Preoperative multimodality imaging most often involves CT for anatomy and PET/SPECT for function [66]. In addition, functional MRI techniques for the brain are becoming more practical [67]. Functional MRI for the brain has the advantage of inherent registration between the anatomic and functional data, since both are acquired at the same time (Figure 13.18). Fluoroscopy and ultrasound are also often used intraoperatively, and their images must be registered with preoperative CT or MRI data [35, 68].

Another application of multimodality image registration is the combination of preoperative images with intraoperative images. Often the imaging modality available in the operating room is not the same as that used for preoperative planning. Even when the imaging modalities are the same, the equipment used in the operating room is generally not the same as that used preoperatively. For instance, open MRI instruments that are becoming available for use in the operating room generally have lower resolution than the diagnostic instruments. The field strength

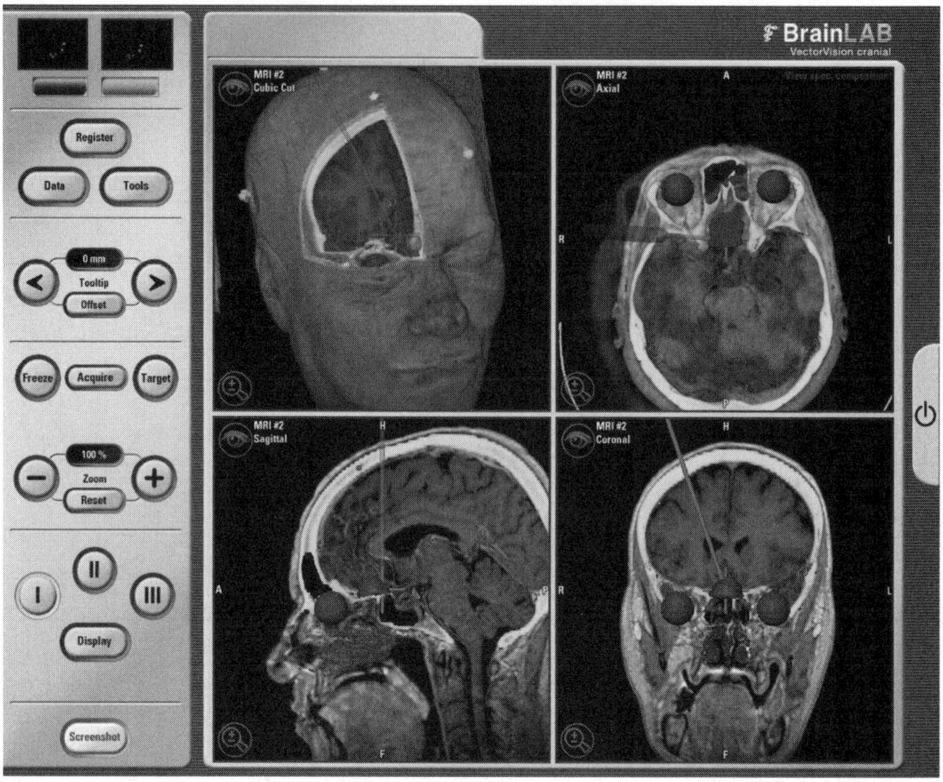

Figure 13.17 Software display of a surgical pointer in 3D space registered with a rendered model of the head (upper left). The location of the pointer tip is also shown in orthogonal views of the MRI data. (Image courtesy of BrainLAB AG.)

of the MRI scanners that can be used intraoperatively is less than that used for high-resolution diagnostic scans. Therefore, pre- and intraoperative MRI images still require registration for accurate guidance (Figure 13.19).

13.3.4 Devices for Display of 3D Data

Display devices are an important component of a 3D image guidance system. Effective display of 3D datasets is a challenge, particularly when these displays are needed in the operating room to guide procedures. Different physical devices can be used to display the processed image data. The most basic is the standard 2D screen, which presents the rendered data as a projected image. In this case, the rendering methods alone are the means for conveying 3D relationships of the original objects. Lighting, perspective, and shading are used to simulate a 3D object as a 2D projection. More advanced display systems have been developed to enhance the perception of the 3D nature of the data.

A standard function provided by image guidance systems is the display of patient images with a real-time display of instrument locations (Figure 13.17). User interaction with the display must be considered in terms of the constraints of the operating room environment and the attention requirements of the operator. Interaction can not be so burdensome as to compromise technical aspects of a proce-

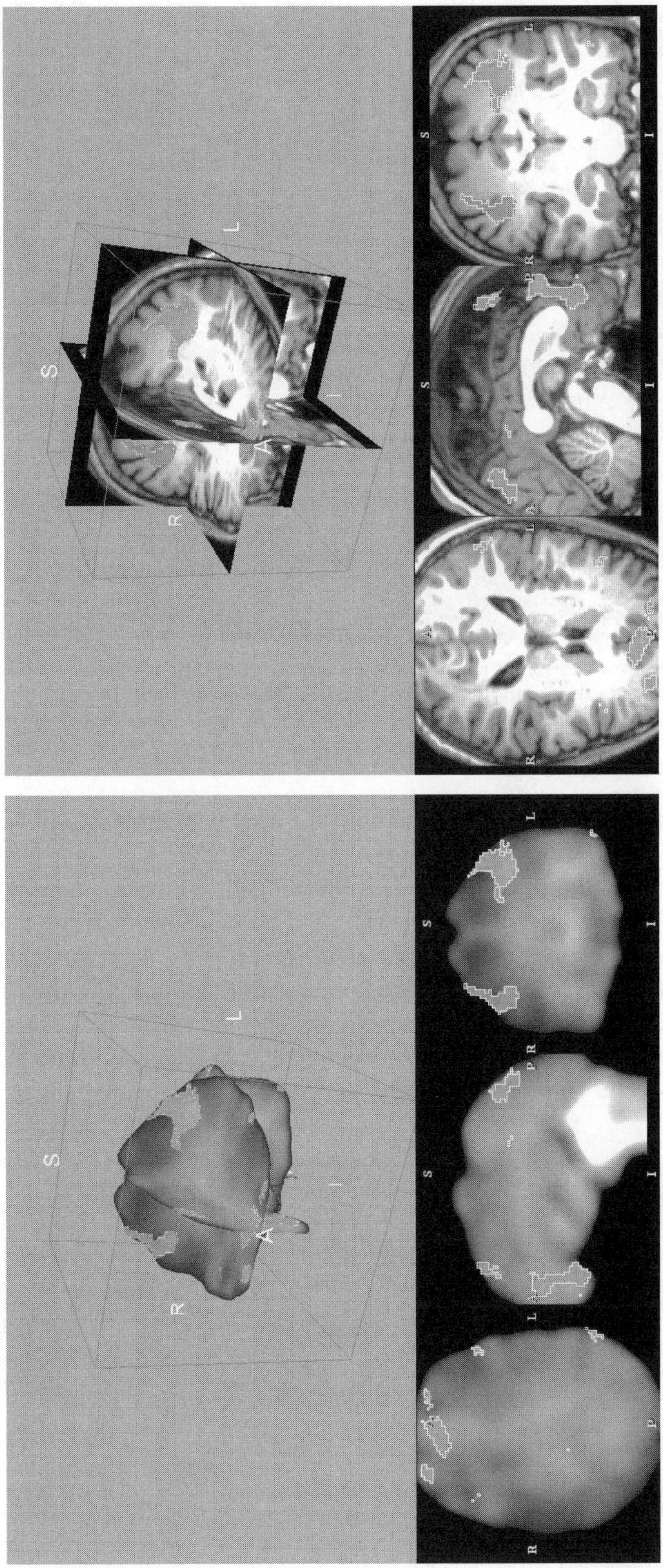

Figure 13.18 Functional MRI. Brain regions activated by a finger-tapping exercise are shown in the left figure. The activated regions are superimposed on the anatomic MRI data on the right. Figure generated with Slicer software and demonstration data.

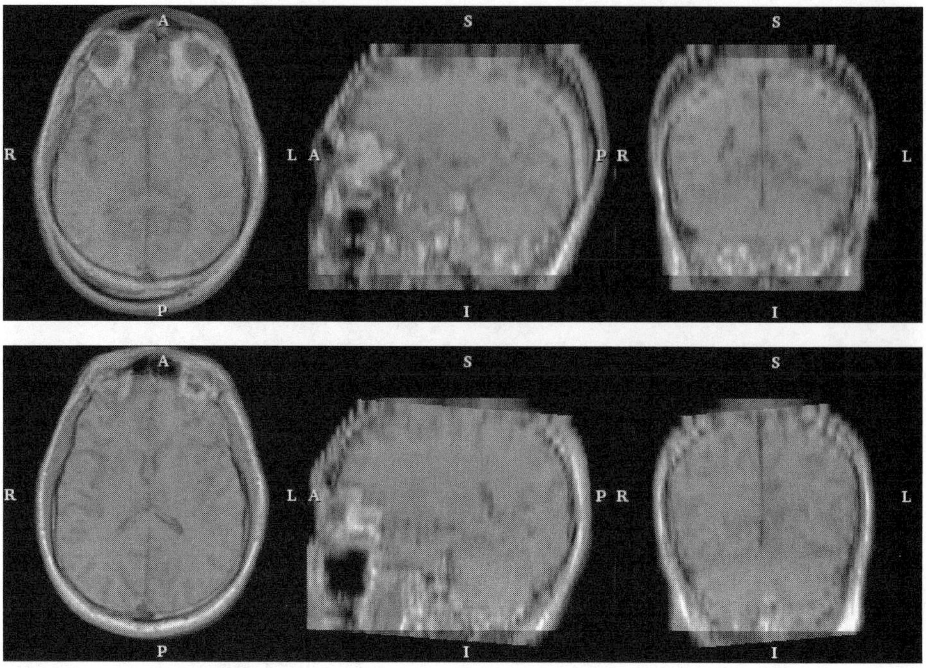

Figure 13.19 Data registration. The top row demonstrates the misregistration of a high- and low-resolution MRI scan superimposed on one another. The bottom row shows the two datasets after registration by a combination of manual and automatic algorithms. Figure generated with Slicer software and demonstration data.

dure. Strategies for user interaction with the display include pointers, foot switches, hand tracking, and voice commands.

Display techniques have also been developed to provide more realistic and intuitive 3D information to the user [69]. Stereo viewing is the most common technique used to produce more realistic 3D views [70–74]. Two separate rendered views of the dataset are produced to simulate the separation of the eyes. Presenting these views separately to each eye produces the perception of a 3D object in space. Stereoscopic viewing has a long history in medical imaging, although it has not been used extensively. The most common method for stereo viewing is to use glasses to

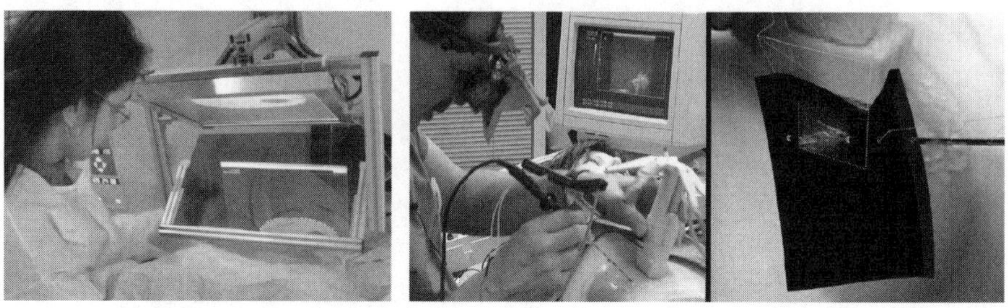

(a) (b)

Figure 13.20 Examples of augmented reality displays. (a) Transparent panel showing a CT image overlay during a needle insertion procedure. (Reprinted from [77], © 2006 IOS Press, with permission from IOS Press.) (b) See-through head-mounted display (left) showing an ultrasound image projected into a synthetic opening in a phantom (right) during insertion of a radio frequency ablation probe. (Reprinted from [71], © 2008 IOS Press, with permission from IOS Press.)

present the two different views to separate eyes. However, stereoscopic glasses can be bulky and distracting.

Another class of display systems is known as augmented reality. These methods use specialized display devices to incorporate computer reconstructions of relevant structures into the surgeon's natural field of view. In one approach a semi-transparent mirror is mounted over the region of interest, and images from a computer monitor are reflected so that the operator can see both the patient and the computer image [75–77]. With this method, tomographic slices from preoperative or intraoperative imaging scans can be projected into their actual location relative to the patient [Figure 13.20(a)]. In addition, 3D surface reconstructions of objects of interest can be displayed such that they appear in their correct anatomic locations.

Augmented reality can also make use of head-mounted displays to add 3D objects or scenes to the user's field of view [71, 78] [Figure 13.20(b)], or it can be applied to operating microscopes [56]. In the case of operating microscopes, the introduction of a 3D image is less intrusive because standard procedure already calls for the surgeon to use an eyepiece or a video screen. Additional tracking devices attached to the user and the display devices make it possible for the physician's head to move and maintain registration of the images, or for the actual display device to be moved [71, 79].

Finally, some procedures may be able to make use of virtual reality, in which the user is immersed in a computer-generated environment [80]. This approach can be used for endoscopic or laproscopic procedures, where the surgeon's standard interface with the target tissue is already removed from direct physical interaction. Since these procedures already rely on a video screen for feedback to the operator, it is a more natural step to replace the 2D video image with a 3D reconstruction. Technological challenges for both augmented and virtual reality include latency of the display, display quality, tracking, and acceptance by the user.

13.3.5 Systems and Applications

Finally, this section will present an overview of system approaches that utilize the techniques described previously to incorporate 3D image guidance in surgical procedures. This is not an exhaustive review, however, as the field of 3D image guidance is continuously evolving.

13.3.5.1 System Configurations

The simplest configurations for 3D image guidance rely on preoperative images. Preoperative image guidance assumes that tissue deformation during a procedure is negligible. Surgical tools are registered with the patient, and their position is displayed in real time in the context of the preoperative image set. While the assumption of target stability may not always be true, this approach does not require the availability of additional imaging instruments in the operating room. Imaging in the operating room adds considerable complexity and expense to facility, so there is a practical benefit if a procedure can be performed without additional imaging.

The more complex approach to 3D guidance incorporates intraoperative imaging into the procedure. Currently, fluoroscopy is the most common imaging modality used for intraoperative guidance. Fluoroscopy is a 2D imaging method, but it is able to provide real-time images of instrument locations during a procedure [68]. Benefits of fluoroscopy for image guidance are the availability of the equipment, which is relatively common, and the familiarity of the surgeons with this modality. Major drawbacks of fluoroscopy are the exposure of both the patient and the surgical team to radiation, and the inherent 2D nature of the images.

Ultrasound is an alternative intraoperative imaging modality that does not use ionizing radiation. Ultrasound instruments are relatively inexpensive and they are also now available as compact portable devices. Ultrasound can be used in its standard 2D imaging mode, with the real-time position of the ultrasound image plane displayed in 3D space [65, 72]. Alternatively, image reconstruction can be applied to a tracked ultrasound probe so that 3D views of target tissues can be generated during a procedure. High-end clinical ultrasound systems are also available that image a 3D volume in real time. These instruments use a 2D transducer array to interrogate a volume of tissue and produce real-time 3D images. Note, however, that ultrasound images do not have a precise correspondence with the preoperative image sets, which are usually CT or MRI. In addition, they can require more training to interpret and the images can be operator dependent.

Intraoperative MRI systems are becoming increasingly available [81, 82]. Manufacturers are designing MRI systems specifically for use in the operating room. Designs include instruments that are open on one side, or short-bore instruments that allow access from the ends. These instruments are designed with a lower magnetic field strength than those used for standard diagnostic imaging. Although their image resolution is not as good as that achieved preoperatively, they can be readily matched with the preoperative images since they are acquired with the same modality. Intraoperative MRI instruments, however, still represent a significant expense and they are not currently in widespread use.

Intraoperative CT has also become available recently, although it is mostly limited to research at this time [28]. It is useful when the preoperative images were acquired with CT, so that the pre- and intraoperative images can be more accurately matched. However, it has the drawback of additional radiation exposure to the patient.

13.3.5.2 Applications

Applications of 3D image guidance can be found across numerous disciplines [28, 32, 33]. Neurosurgery represents perhaps the most widespread use of 3D image guidance to date [83, 84]. Endoscopic methods with image guidance are also being applied to ear, nose, and throat procedures so that critical structures can be avoided during the intervention [85]. Cranio-facial surgery procedures employing 3D image guidance include osteotomy, bone grafts, and implants [86]. Three-dimensional imaging is also useful for planning and guidance of procedures for correction of asymmetries and deformities of the maxilla and mandible, and for angulation of dental implants [61, 87]. Orthopedic surgery applications include spinal, hip, and knee implants [88–90]. Image-guided radiation therapy (IGRT) uses treatment plans devised with the help of 3D reconstructions to focus the radiation beam at the proper location and minimize exposure to intervening tissues [91]. Other specialties using 3D image guidance include laparoscopic surgery [50], radiofrequency ablation [92], and needle guidance [75, 76, 78].

References

[1] Lucchichenti, G., et al., "3D Reconstruction Techniques Made Easy: Know-How and Pictures," *European Radiology*, Vol. 15, 2005, pp. 2146–2156.

[2] Udupa, J. K., "3D Imaging: Principles and Approaches," in *3D Imaging in Medicine*, J. K. Udupa and G. T. Herman, (eds.), Boca Raton, FL: CRC Press, 1999, pp. 1–73.

[3] Rogers, D. F., and J. A. Adams, *Mathematical Elements for Computer Graphics*, New York: McGraw-Hill, 1990.

[4] Shepperd, S. W., "Quaternion from Rotation Matrix," *AIAA Journal of Guidance, Control and Dynamics*, Vol. 1, No. 3, 1978, pp. 223–224.

[5] Nelson, T. R., and D. H. Pretorius, "Three-Dimensional Ultrasound Imaging," *Ultrasound in Medicine and Biology*, Vol. 24, No. 9, 1998, pp. 1243–1270.

[6] Solberg, O. V., et al., "Freehand 3D Ultrasound Reconstruction Algorithms—A Review," *Ultrasound in Medicine and Biology*, Vol. 33, No. 7, 2007, pp. 991–1009.

[7] Barillot, C., "Surface and Volume Rendering Techniques to Display 3-D Data," *IEEE Engineering in Medicine and Biology*, Vol. 12, No. 1, 1993, pp. 111–119.

[8] Pelizzari, C. A., "Image Processing in Stereotactic Planning: Volume Visualization and Image Registration," *Medical Dosimetry*, Vol. 23, No. 3, 1998, pp. 137–145.

[9] Robb, R. A., and C. Barillot, "Interactive Display and Analysis of 3-D Medical Images," *IEEE Transactions on Medical Imaging*, Vol. 8, No. 3, 1989, pp. 217–226.

[10] Foley, J. D., et al., *Computer Graphics: Principles and Practice*, Reading, MA: Addison-Wesley, 1995.

[11] Birkfellner, W., et al., "Wobbled Splatting – A Fast Perspective Volume Rendering Method for Simulation of X-Ray Images from CT," *Physics in Medicine and Biology*, Vol. 50, 2005, pp. N73–N84.

[12] Drebin, R. A., L. Carpenter, and P. Hanrahan, "Volume Rendering," *Computer Graphics*, Vol. 22, No. 4, 1988, pp. 65–74.

[13] Steen, E., and B. Olstad, "Volume Rendering of 3D Medical Ultrasound Data Using Direct Feature Mapping," *IEEE Transactions on Medical Imaging*, Vol. 13, 1994, pp. 517–525.

[14] Lacroute, P., and M. Levoy, "Fast Volume Rendering Using a Shear-Warp Factorization of the Viewing Transformation," *Proc. SIGGRAPH 94*, Orlando, FL, July 24–29, 1994, pp. 451–458.

[15] Levoy, M., "Efficient Ray Tracing of Volume Data," *ACM Transactions on Graphics*, Vol. 9, No. 3, 1990, pp. 245–261.

[16] Levoy, M., "Volume Rendering, a Hybrid Ray Tracer for Rendering Polygon and Volume Data," *IEEE Computer Graphics and Applications*, Vol. 10, 1990, pp. 33–40.

[17] Pham, D. L., C. Xu, and J. L. Prince, "Current Methods in Medical Image Segmentation," *Annual Review of Biomedical Engineering*, Vol. 2, No. 1, 2000, pp. 315–337.

[18] Russ, J. C., "Thresholding Images," *Journal of Computer-Assisted Microscopy*, Vol. 7, No. 3, 1995, pp. 141–164.

[19] Haralick, R. M., and L. G. Shapiro, *Computer and Robot Vision*, Reading, MA: Addison-Wesley, 1992.

[20] Gonzalez, R. C., and R. E. Woods, *Digital Image Processing*, Reading, MA: Addison-Wesley, 1992.

[21] Falcão, A. X., and J. K. Udupa, "A 3D Generalization of User-Steered Live-Wire Segmentation," *Medical Image Analysis*, Vol. 4, No. 4, 2000, pp. 389–402.

[22] Kass, M., A. Witkin, and D. Terzopoulos, "Snakes: Active Contour Models," *International Journal of Computer Vision*, Vol. 1, No. 4, 1988, pp. 312–331.

[23] Xu, C., D. L. Pham, and J. L. Prince, "Image Segmentation Using Deformable Models," in *Handbook of Medical Imaging*, M. Sonka and J. M. Fitzpatrick, (eds.), Bellingham, WA: SPIE Press, 2000, pp. 129–174.

[24] Yushkevich, P. A., et al., "User-Guided 3D Active Contour Segmentation of Anatomical Structures: Significantly Improved Efficiency and Reliability," *NeuroImage*, Vol. 31, 2006, pp. 1116–1128.

[25] Fan, S., L. K. Voon, and N. W. Sing, "3D Prostate Surface Detection from Ultrasound Images Based on Level Set Method," *Proc. 5th Int. Conference on Medical Image Computing and Computer-Assisted Intervention*, Tokyo, Japan, September 25–28, 2002, pp. 389–396.

[26] Whitaker, R., et al., "A Framework for Level Set Segmentation of Volume Datasets," *Proc. ACM Int. Workshop on Volume Graphics*, Stony Brook, NY, June 21–22, 2001, pp. 159–168.

[27] Zhukov, L., et al., "Level Set Modeling and Segmentation of DT-MRI Brain Data," *Journal of Electronic Imaging*, Vol. 12, No. 1, 2003, pp. 125–133.

[28] Yaniv, Z., and K. Cleary, *Image-Guided Procedures: A Review*, Image Science and Information Systems Center, Georgetown University, Washington, D.C., Technical Report CAIMR TR-2006-3, 2006.

[29] Talairach, J., and P. Tournoux, *Co-Planar Stereotaxic Atlas of the Human Brain*, New York: Thieme Medical Publishers, 1988.

[30] Bazin, P.-L., et al., "Volumetric Neuroimage Analysis Extensions for the MIPAV Software Package," *Journal of Neuroscience Methods*, Vol. 165, 2007, pp. 111–121.

[31] Pohl, K. M., et al., "Anatomical Guided Segmentation with Non-Stationary Tissue Class Distributions in an Expectation-Maximization Framework," *Proc. IEEE International Symposium on Biomedical Imaging: From Nano to Macro*, Arlington, VA, April 15–18, 2004, pp. 81–84.

[32] Peters, T. M., "Image-Guided Surgery: From X-Rays to Virtual Reality," *Computer Methods in Biomechanics and Biomedical Engineering*, Vol. 4, No. 1, 2000, pp. 27–57.

[33] Galloway, R. L., Jr., "The Process and Development of Image-Guided Procedures," *Annual Review of Biomedical Engineering*, Vol. 3, 2001, pp. 83–108.

[34] Galloway, R. L., Jr., R. J. Maciunas, and J. W. Latimer, "The Accuracies of Four Stereotactic Frame Systems: An Independent Assessment," *Biomedical Instrumentation & Technology*, Vol. 25, 1991, pp. 457–460.

[35] Comeau, R. M., et al., "Intraoperative Ultrasound for Guidance and Tissue Shift Correction in Image-Guided Neurosurgery," *Medical Physics*, Vol. 27, No. 4, 2000, pp. 787–800.

[36] Birkfellner W., et al., "Calibration of Tracking Systems in a Surgical Environment," *IEEE Transactions on Medical Imaging*, Vol. 17, No. 5, 1998, pp. 737–742.

[37] Leotta, D. F., P. R. Detmer, and R. W. Martin, "Performance of a Miniature Magnetic Sensor for Three-Dimensional Ultrasound Imaging," *Ultrasound in Medicine and Biology*, Vol. 23, 1997, pp. 597–609.

[38] Welch, G., and E. Foxlin, "Motion Tracking: No Silver Bullet, but a Respectable Arsenal," *IEEE Computer Graphics and Applications*, Vol. 22, No. 6, 2002, pp. 24–38.

[39] Martelli, S., et al., "Comparison of an Optical and a Mechanical Navigation System," *Proc. 6th Int. Conference on Medical Image Computing and Computer-Assisted Intervention*, Montreal, Canada, November 15–18, 2003, pp. 303–310.

[40] Reinhardt, H. F., and H. J. Zweifel, "Interactive Sonar-Operated Device for Stereotactic and Open Surgery," *Stereotactic and Functional Neurosurgery*, Vol. 54–55, 1990, pp. 393–397.

[41] Birkfellner, W., et al., "Systematic Distortions in Magnetic Position Digitizers," *Medical Physics*, Vol. 25, 1998, pp. 2242–2248.

[42] Hummel, J., et al., "Evaluation of a New Electromagnetic Tracking System Using a Standardized Assessment Protocol," *Physics in Medicine and Biology*, Vol. 51, 2006, pp. N205–N210.

[43] Schicho, K., et al., "Stability of Miniature Electromagnetic Tracking Systems," *Physics in Medicine and Biology*, Vol. 50, No. 9, 2005, pp. 2089–2098.

[44] Maintz, J. B. A., and M. A. Viergever, "A Survey of Medical Image Registration," *Medical Image Analysis*, Vol. 2, No. 1, 1998, pp. 1–36.

[45] Knott, P. D., et al., "Contour and Paired-Point Registration in a Model for Image-Guided Surgery," *The Laryngoscope*, Vol. 116, 2006, pp. 1877–1881.

[46] Nottmeier, E. W., and T. L. Crosby, "Timing of Paired Points and Surface Matching Registration in Three-Dimensional (3D) Image-Guided Spinal Surgery," *Journal of Spinal Disorders & Techniques*, Vol. 20, No. 4, 2007, pp. 268–270.

[47] Fleute, M., S. Lavallée, and L. Desbat, "Integrated Approach for Matching Statistical Shape Models with Intra-Operative 2D and 3D Data," *Proc. 5th Int. Conference on Medical Image Computing and Computer-Assisted Intervention*, Tokyo, Japan, September 25–28, 2002, pp. 364–372.

[48] Grimson, W. E. L., et al., "An Automatic Registration Method for Frameless Stereotaxy, Image Guided Surgery, and Enhanced Reality Visualization," *IEEE Transactions on Medical Imaging*, Vol. 15, No. 2, 1996, pp. 129–140.

[49] Miga, M. I., et al., "Cortical Surface Registration for Image-Guided Neurosurgery Using Laser-Range Scanning," *IEEE Transactions on Medical Imaging*, Vol. 22, No. 8, 2003, pp. 973–985.

[50] Rauth, T. P., et al., "Laparoscopic Surface Scanning and Subsurface Targeting: Implications for Image-Guided Laparoscopic Liver Surgery," *Surgery*, Vol. 142, 2007, pp. 207–214.

[51] Wells, W. M., et al., "Multi-Modal Volume Registration by Maximization of Mutual Information," *Medical Image Analysis*, Vol. 1, No. 1, 1996, pp. 35–51.

[52] Arun, K. S., T. S. Huang, and S. D. Blostein, "Least-Squares Fitting of Two 3-D Point Sets," *IEEE Transactions on Pattern Analysis and Machine Intelligence*, Vol. PAMI-9, No. 5, 1987, pp. 698–700.

[53] Horn, B. K. P., "Closed-Form Solution of Absolute Orientation Using Unit Quaternions," *Journal of the Optical Society of America A*, Vol. 4, No. 4, 1987, pp. 629–642.

[54] Besl, P. J., and N. D. McKay, "A Method for Registration of 3-D Shapes," *IEEE Transactions on Pattern Analysis and Machine Intelligence*, Vol. 14, No. 2, 1992, pp. 239–256.

[55] Zhang, Z., "Iterative Point Matching for Registration of Free-Form Curves and Surfaces," *International Journal of Computer Vision*, Vol. 13, No. 2, 1994, pp. 119–152.

[56] Hawkes, D. J., et al., "Measuring and Modeling Soft Tissue Deformation for Image Guided Interventions," *Proc. IS4TM*, Juan-Les-Pins, France, June 12–13, 2003, pp. 1–14.

[57] Lester, H., and S. R. Arridge, "A Survey of Hierarchical Non-Linear Medical Image Registration," *Pattern Recognition*, Vol. 32, No.1, 1999, pp. 129–149.

[58] Sarrut, D., "Deformable Registration for Image-Guided Radiation Therapy," *Zeitschrift für Medizinische Physik (Medical Physics)*, Vol. 16, 2006, pp. 285–297.

[59] Foskey, M., et al., "Large Deformation Three-Dimensional Image Registration in Image-Guided Radiation Therapy," *Physics in Medicine and Biology*, Vol. 50, 2005, pp. 5869–5892.

[60] Wittek, A., et al., "Patient-Specific Model of Brain Deformation: Application to Medical Image Registration," *Journal of Biomechanics*, Vol. 40, 2007, pp. 919–929.

[61] Birkfellner, W., et al., "In-Vitro Assessment of a Registration Protocol for Image Guided Implant Dentistry," *Clinical Oral Implants Research*, Vol. 12, No. 1, 2001, pp. 69–78.

[62] Maurer, C. R., Jr., et al., "Registration of Head Volume Images Using Implantable Fiducial Markers," *IEEE Transactions on Medical Imaging*, Vol. 16, No. 4, 1997, pp. 447–462.

[63] Wiles, A. D., D. G. Thompson, and D. D. Frantz, "Accuracy Assessment and Interpretation for Optical Tracking Systems," *Proc. of SPIE Medical Imaging 2004: Visualization, Image-Guided Procedures, and Display*, San Diego, CA, February 14–19, 2004, pp. 421–432.

[64] Grimson, W. E. L., et al., "Utilizing Segmented MRI Data in Image-Guided Surgery," *International Journal of Pattern Recognition and Artificial Intelligence*, Vol. 11, No. 8, 1997, pp. 1367–1397.

[65] Hernes, T. A. N., et al., "Computer-Assisted 3D Ultrasound-Guided Neurosurgery: Technological Contributions, Including Multimodal Registration and Advanced Display, Demonstrating Future Perspectives," *The International Journal of Medical Robotics and Computer Assisted Surgery*, Vol. 2, 2006, pp. 45–59.

[66] Ratib, O., "PET/CT Image Navigation and Communication," *The Journal of Nuclear Medicine*, Vol. 45, 2004, pp. 46S–55S.

[67] Gering, D. T., et al., "An Integrated Visualization System for Surgical Planning and Guidance Using Image Fusion and an Open MR," *Journal of Magnetic Resonance Imaging*, Vol. 13, 2001, pp. 967–975.

[68] Eyke, J. C., et al., "Computer-Assisted Virtual Fluoroscopy," *The University of Pennsylvania Orthopedic Journal*, Vol. 15, 2002, pp. 53–59.

[69] McAllister, D. F., (ed.), *Stereo Computer Graphics and Other True 3D Technologies*, Princeton, NJ: Princeton University Press, 1993.

[70] Birkfellner, W., et al., "Computer-Enhanced Stereoscopic Vision in a Head-Mounted Operating Binocular," *Physics in Medicine and Biology*, Vol. 48, 2003, pp. N49–N57.

[71] Fuchs, H., et al., "Optimizing a Head-Tracked Stereo Display System to Guide Hepatic Tumor Ablation," *Proc. Medicine Meets Virtual Reality 16*, Newport Beach, CA, January 29–February 1, 2008.

[72] Hernes, T. A. N., et al., "Stereoscopic Navigation-Controlled Display of Preoperative MRI and Intraoperative 3D Ultrasound in Planning and Guidance of Neurosurgery: New Technology for Minimally Invasive Image-Guided Surgery Approaches," *Minimally Invasive Neurosurgery*, Vol. 46, 2003, pp. 129–137.

[73] Peters, T. M., et al., "Integration of Stereoscopic DSA and 3D MRI for Image-Guided Neurosurgery," *Computerized Medical Imaging and Graphics*, Vol. 18, 1994, pp. 289–299.

[74] Peters, T. M., "Image Guidance for Surgical Procedures," *Physics in Medicine and Biology*, Vol. 51, 2006, pp. R505–R540.

[75] Fischer, G. S., et al., "MRI Image Overlay: Application to Arthrography Needle Insertion," *Computer Aided Surgery*, Vol.12, No. 1, 2007, pp. 2–14.

[76] Fichtinger, G., et al., "Image Overlay for CT-Guided Needle Insertions," *Computer Aided Surgery*, Vol. 10, No. 4, 2005, pp. 241–255.

[77] Fischer, G. S., et al., "MRI Image Overlay: Applications to Arthrography Needle Insertion," *Proc. Medicine Meets Virtual Reality 14*, Long Beach, CA, January 24–27, 2006, pp. 150–155.

[78] State, A., et al., "Technologies for Augmented-Reality Systems: Realizing Ultrasound-Guided Needle Biopsies," *Proc. ACM SIGGRAPH 96*, New Orleans, LA, August 4–9, 1996, pp. 439–446.

[79] Wacker, F. K., et al., "An Augmented Reality System for MR Image-Guided Needle Biopsy: Initial Results in a Swine Model," *Radiology*, Vol. 238, No. 2, 2006, pp. 497–504.

[80] Hart, R., and K. Karthigasu, "The Benefits of Virtual Reality Simulator Training for Laparoscopic Surgery," *Current Opinion in Obstetrics and Gynecology*, Vol. 19, 2007, pp. 297–302.

[81] Lewin, J. S., et al., "Intraoperative MRI with a Rotating, Tiltable Surgical Table: A Time-Use Study and Clinical Results in 122 Patients," *AJR*, Vol. 189, 2007, pp. 1096–1103.

[82] Moche, M., et al., "Navigation Concepts for MR Image-Guided Interventions," *Journal of Magnetic Resonance Imaging*, Vol. 27, 2008, pp. 276–291.

[83] DiMaio, S. P., et al., "Image-Guided Neurosurgery at Brigham and Women's Hospital: The Integration of Imaging, Navigation and Interventional Devices," *IEEE Engineering in Medicine and Biology*, Vol. 25, No. 5, 2006, pp. 67–73.

[84] Kansy, K., et al., "LOCALITE—A Frameless Neuronavigation System for Interventional Magnetic Resonance Imaging," *Proc. Medical Image Computing and Computer Assisted Intervention*, Cambridge, U.K., September 19–22, 1999, pp. 832–841.

[85] Olson, G., and M. J. Citardi, "Image-Guided Functional Endoscopic Sinus Surgery," *Otolaryngology: Head and Neck Surgery*, Vol. 123, No. 3, 2000, pp. 188–194.

[86] Nijmeh, A. D., et al., "Image-Guided Navigation in Oral and Maxillofacial Surgery," *British Journal of Oral and Maxillofacial Surgery*, Vol. 43, 2005, pp. 294–302.

[87] Casap, N., et al., "Navigation Surgery for Dental Implants: Assessment of Accuracy of the Image Guided Implantology System," *Journal of Oral and Maxillofacial Surgery*, Vol. 62, 2004, pp. 116–119.

[88] Cleary, K., et al., "Technology Improvements for Image-Guided and Minimally Invasive Spine Procedures," *IEEE Transactions on Information Technology in Biomedicine*, Vol. 6, No. 4, 2002, pp. 249–261.

[89] DiGioia, A., et al., (eds.), *Computer and Robotic Assisted Hip and Knee Surgery*, Oxford, England: Oxford University Press, 2004.

[90] Resnick, D. K., "Prospective Comparison of Virtual Fluoroscopy to Fluoroscopy and Plain Radiographs for Placement of Lumbar Pedicle Screws," *Journal of Spinal Disorders & Techniques*, Vol. 16, No. 3, 2003, pp. 254–260.

[91] Verellen, D., et al., "Innovations in Image-Guided Radiotherapy," *Nature Reviews Cancer*, Vol. 7, 2007, pp. 949–960.

[92] Dickfeld, T., et al., "Stereotactic Magnetic Resonance Guidance for Anatomically Targeted Ablations of the Fossa Ovalis and the Left Atrium," *Journal of Interventional Cardiac Electrophysiology*, Vol. 11, 2004, pp. 105–115.

CHAPTER 14

Optical Coherence Tomography

Jason Zara

14.1 Introduction

Optical coherence tomography (OCT) is an optical imaging technique analogous to ultrasound that uses partially coherent infrared light to interrogate a target and the resulting echoes to produce images of subsurface microscopic structures. The origin of the received echoes is detected with interferometry, so a map of reflectivity versus optical depth can be created. OCT has been shown to produce images with a spatial resolution of 10 to 20 μm or less [1].

While OCT is able to produce images with high spatial resolution, the tissue penetration of OCT is limited to only 1 to 2 mm [2] due to the high level of scattering of infrared light in biological tissues. However, for many applications, such as evaluation of epithelial tissues, the depth penetration of OCT is more than sufficient. In addition, recent advances in OCT technology allow for image acquisition rates that approach video speed giving OCT the potential to act as the basis for an "optical biopsy" that could provide immediate feedback to the physician. OCT has demonstrated great promise in applications ranging from eye and skin imaging to intravascular imaging, imaging of the bladder and urinary tract, and imaging of the lining of the gastrointestinal tract.

The main advantages of OCT are its resolution, speed, size, and cost. OCT systems can image at a resolution significantly higher than imaging modalities such as ultrasound and X-ray, and the new spectral domain systems allow for acquisition rates that approach video speed. In addition, OCT systems can be built using fiber optics, which reduces the costs of the systems and also enables them to be used for endoscopic and catheter-based imaging applications.

14.2 OCT System Configuration

The primary functional units of an OCT system are the light source that is used to illuminate the target, the interferometer used to detect the location of the received optical reflections, and the methods used to image the lateral dimensions of the target object. In the following three sections, more detail will be provided regarding the light source, the interferometer, and the lateral scanning mechanisms commonly used in OCT imaging systems. These sections will investigate various different technologies that can be used for each of these portions of the OCT imaging system.

14.2.1 OCT Light Sources

OCT uses partially coherent infrared light to interrogate imaging targets. The wider the bandwidth of the light used in the OCT system, the better the axial resolution of the system will be. The most commonly used wavelengths of light in OCT are 830, 980, and 1,310 nm in the near-infrared. There are trade-offs between depth of penetration and resolution for these wavelengths that will be discussed in more detail in Section 14.3. There are various light sources that have been utilized for OCT imaging, including super-luminescent diodes (SLDs), femtosecond lasers, white light sources, and tunable narrowband sources.

SLDs and femtosecond lasers produce broadband partially coherent light, while white light sources produce very broadband light, but with lower intensities compared to SLDs or femtosecond lasers. For swept-source OCT (Section 14.2.2) tunable narrowband sources are used. Due to issues of costs and the small size of the packaging, the most commonly used light sources in OCT systems are super-luminescent diodes. However, femtosecond lasers and tunable sources have some distinct advantages over SLDs. These advantages include broader bandwidths for femtosecond lasers compared to SLDs and the very high imaging speeds that can be achieved using SS-OCT systems that require tunable sources.

14.2.2 Interferometer Configurations

The interferometer in an OCT system is used to detect the location in the target object from which the returning infrared light was reflected. A majority of OCT systems use Michelson interferometers, but systems that use a common-path interferometer configuration are also prevalent. Figure 14.1 is a schematic of a time domain OCT imaging system. The core of the imaging system is a Michelson interferometer. The light from the optical source is split into two paths by an optical coupler (50/50 in this configuration). One of the paths, the reference arm, consists of a delay line that varies the path length to create the depth information of the image. The other path directs light towards the imaging target. When the optical path lengths of the light returning to each of the two arms are equal, the returning light will constructively interfere at the detector.

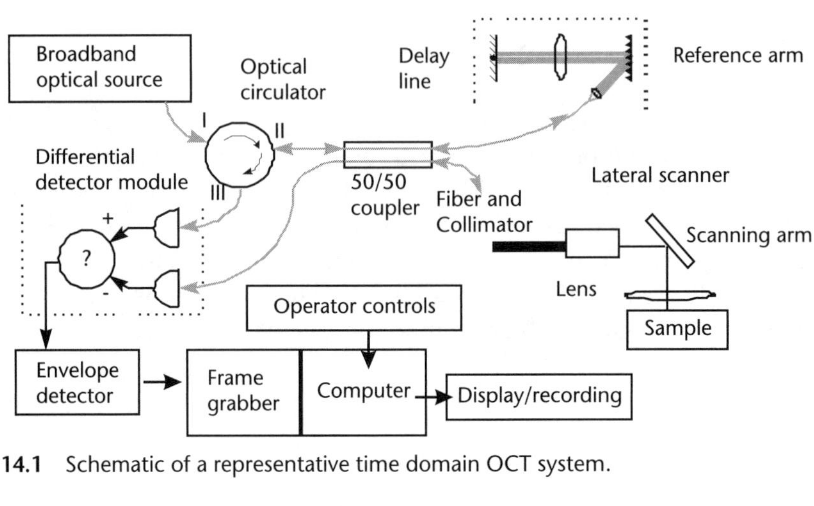

Figure 14.1 Schematic of a representative time domain OCT system.

The acquisition rate of time domain OCT systems depends on the rate at which the reference arm path length can be modified. The first OCT systems utilized varying methods to modify the reference arm path length, including using galvanometers coupled with corner cube mirrors, piezoelectric fiber stretchers, and diffraction gratings with resonant scanners. However, mechanical inertia for these systems limits the resulting scanning speeds.

Advances in spectral domain OCT [3, 4] have resulted in OCT systems that scan at much faster line rates and have much higher signal-to-noise ratios than time domain systems.

Unlike time domain systems, which use a variable group delay in the reference arm to modify the depth being interrogated, spectral domain OCT systems use a fixed group delay but acquire the data at different wavelengths. There are two primary methods of acquiring the data at different wavelengths, swept-source and Fourier domain OCT. Swept-source (SS) OCT uses a tunable narrowband source and rapidly sweeps the optical wavelengths while using the same single optical detector used in time domain systems. Fourier domain (FD) OCT uses a broadband light source similar to that used in time domain systems, but uses a spectrometer in the detector arm to recognize the different wavelengths.

A schematic of a representative FD OCT imaging system is depicted in Figure 14.2. In this system, an SLD provides broadband near-infrared light that is passed through an optical circulator and a 90/10 fiber optic coupler to illuminate the sample. The light returning from the sample arm is coupled with light returning from the stationary reference arm and then passed to a spectrometer through the optical circulator. The spectrometer consists of a diffraction grating and a line-scan CCD camera that reads out the spectrum of the interference pattern. A discrete Fourier transform is then performed on the output of the CCD array to produce an axial depth profile of the optical reflections from the sample. A galvanometer moves under the control of the computer to produce scans across the lateral dimension of the sample to produce a two-dimensional image. A similarly configured system was reported in [5].

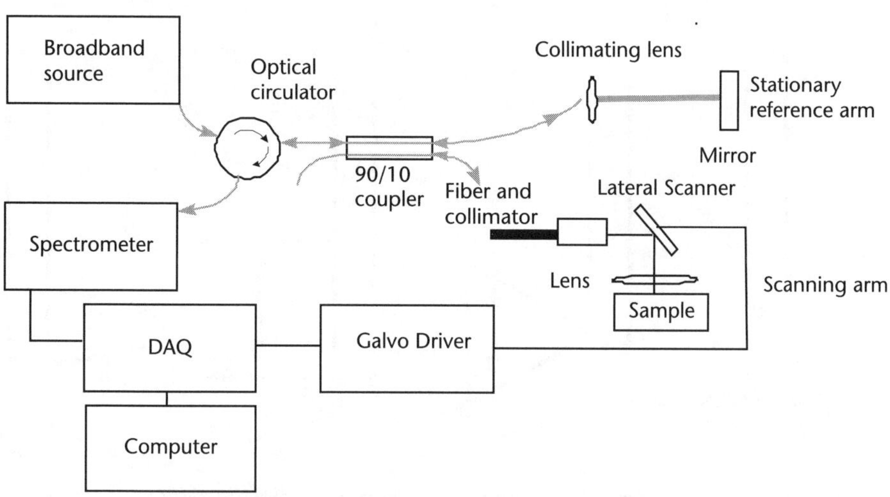

Figure 14.2 Schematic of a representative FD OCT imaging system.

14.2.3 Beam Scanning Techniques

Most OCT systems generate a single line of axial data through the target at a time. It is necessary to steer the infrared beam laterally across the target and compile the individual axial scan lines to form two- or three-dimensional images. This makes the lateral beam scanning method one of the most critical aspects of an OCT system. This is particularly true for endoscopic OCT applications, where the imaging probe must be small enough to be inserted into the body and placed in close proximity to the tissues of interest.

The most common scanning methods for nonendoscopic OCT systems are mechanical and use galvanometers and other actuation techniques to steer the infrared beam across the target. However, these methods are not practical for endoscopic systems. For minimally invasive endoscopic imaging interventions, it is most desirable for the OCT imaging probe to be inserted through the accessory ports of conventional endoscopes. For this reason, compact scanning methods are of the utmost importance.

There are several scanning geometries that are utilized for endoscopic OCT scanning probes. These include scanning towards the front or side of the probe in a sector scanning configuration, scanning from the side of the probe in a linear scanning configuration, or scanning around the circumference of the probe in a circumferential scanning configuration. Figure 14.3 is a schematic showing various scanning configurations.

Sector scanning probes generally utilize either a stationary fiber in conjunction with a tilting mirror to scan the optical beam, or actuation methods that scan the optical fiber itself in a sector motion. Linear scanning probes push and pull the optical fiber to move the focal spot across the imaging target. This pushing and pulling is generally accomplished using an external precision actuator. Circumferential scanning probes commonly use an external motor coupled via a connecting wire to the distal end of the probe tip to steer the OCT imaging beam. It is, of course, possible to combine these methods in a single probe to either produce an

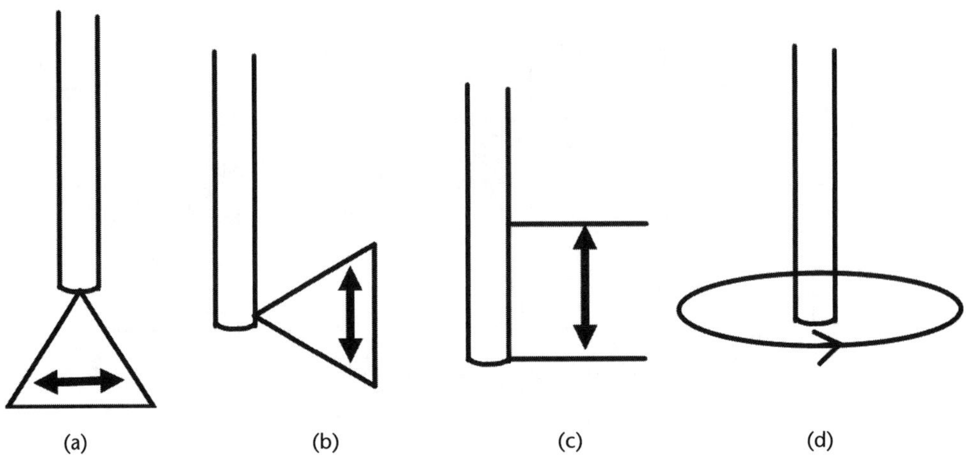

Figure 14.3 Endoscopic OCT scanning configurations: (a) forward sector scan; (b) side sector scan; (c) side linear scan; and (d) circumferential scan.

imaging probe with varying scan geometries, or even to produce three-dimensional scans.

Each of the scanning configurations has specific advantages and disadvantages. For example, a circumferential scanning probe has an ideal imaging geometry for a small circular lumen (arterial imaging) but can image only perpendicular to the imaging probe and cannot image structures or interventional procedures occurring out of this plane. A sector scanning device, while it may have a smaller field of view than a circumferential scanner, can image structures or interventional procedures occurring in the area to the side or front of the probe.

The most common external scanning endoscopic OCT system design, which has been used in many clinical trials in the digestive tract, utilizes a spinning reflective element to scan the infrared beam across the tissue in a circular side-scanning configuration [6, 7]. In addition, several studies have been conducted that use linear-scanning probes that rely on an external precision linear actuator to pull the optical fiber back along the bore of the endoscopic probe to produce two-dimensional images. In addition, there is a great deal of research being conducted to develop new types of scanning mechanisms with the goal of creating small imaging probes that can imaging large areas of tissue at real-time imaging speeds [8–14].

An alternative method to illuminate the imaging target is to expose the entire imaging area to the light source at the same instant and use and array of detectors (such as a CCD array) to detect the returning light in a two-dimensional configuration. Rather than generating an image of a slice through the tissue, these types of systems generate an en face image, or an image parallel to the surface of the catheter. The depth of these en face images can be varied by changing the reference arm path length in the system.

14.3 System Specifications

14.3.1 Resolution—Axial and Lateral

The axial and lateral resolutions of an OCT imaging system are decoupled. The lateral resolution is determined by the optics in the scanning arm, and the axial resolution is determined by the coherence length of the light source used. Equations (14.1) and (14.2) give expressions for the lateral resolution (*lr*) and coherence length (*cl*) (which determines the axial resolution) for an OCT imaging system (assuming a Gaussian source spectrum) [15]. In these equations, λ is the center wavelength of the light source, $\Delta\lambda$ is the bandwidth of the light source, d is the focal spot size on the objective lens, and f is the focal length of the objective lens in the scanning arm.

$$lr = \left(\frac{4\lambda}{\pi}\right)\left(\frac{f}{d}\right) \tag{14.1}$$

$$cl = \frac{2\ln(2)}{\pi}\frac{\lambda^2}{\Delta\lambda} \tag{14.2}$$

14.3.2 SNR

The dynamic range (DR) of an OCT system has been reported to be as high as 90 to 140 dB and is directly determined by the minimal reflectivity, R_{min}, of the object beam as shown in (14.3) [16]:

$$DR = -10\log(R_{\min}) \tag{14.3}$$

These very high dynamic range systems enable the detection of reflected light energy with much smaller power than the incident light. OCT systems with incident optical powers of 20 μW have shown the ability to detect reflected signals with 5×10^{-10} of the incident power resulting in a dynamic range of 93 dB [17]. This high sensitivity enables the small amounts of scattered light returning to the system to be used to make OCT images of tissue.

14.3.3 Imaging Depths

Tissue penetration depth in OCT is also a function of the wavelength of light used. For optical energy, the tissue preferentially absorbs some wavelengths of light, while having very little effect on others. For instance, at a wavelength of 830 nm, there is very little absorption in tissue. For this reason, certain windows of wavelengths are more useful for optical reflection imaging. For frequencies that are not absorbed, scattering is the primary limitation of penetration depth. Optical scattering also decreases with increasing wavelength, so longer wavelengths are scattered less. OCT imaging has been investigated at different infrared wavelengths (830, 980, and 1,300 nm), depending on whether the emphasis is on resolution or tissue penetration.

14.4 Current Applications of OCT

OCT was originally developed for use on transparent tissue, but in recent years has been investigated for use on nontransparent tissue due to its potential advantages over conventional biopsy, which were studied and described in [16]. This study, one of the first studies of OCT in nontransparent tissues, identified three areas where OCT could be beneficial: guidance of microsurgical procedures, situations where a biopsy could be hazardous or difficult such as in the examination of vascular tissue, and areas with high false negative rates such as early cancer detection. OCT has since been investigated for use in eye imaging, intravascular imaging, and endoscopic imaging of epithelial tissues, among other uses.

14.4.1 Ophthalmology

OCT imaging in ophthalmology has been by far the most successful application to date. Clinical systems are being routinely used to image both the anterior segment of the eye and the retina. The systems can be used to image conditions such as glaucoma, macular degeneration, and retinal detachments. Due to the fact that a large portion of the eye contains optically transparent tissues and fluids, the eye is an ideal target for an optical imaging system. Figure 14.4 shows images obtained using an SD-OCT system at Duke University that demonstrate the usefulness of OCT imaging when evaluating the retina in patients.

14.4.2 Intra-Arterial Imaging

Researchers have noted that the most common cause of myocardial infarction and unstable angina is the rupture of plaque. However, not all plaques or even plaque ruptures lead to problems, leading to the search for so-called *unstable plaques*. Previously, attempts have been made to recognize these unstable plaques using intravascular ultrasound and ultrasound elastography, but the attempts have suffered from the lack of resolution offered by ultrasound. Due to its high resolution, OCT is now being studied as a means of characterizing intravascular plaque [18, 19]. In a comparison of the use of OCT and ultrasound [20] when studying atherosclerotic

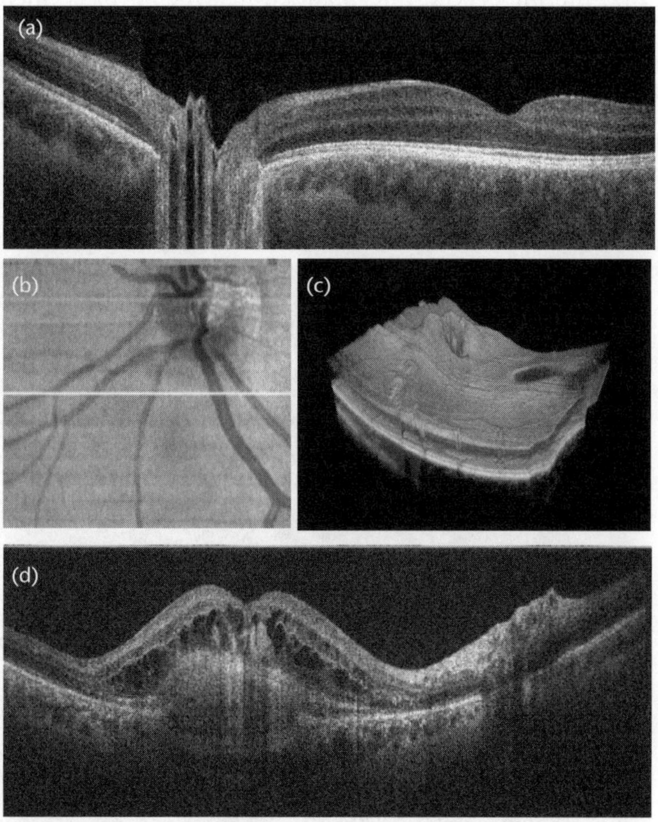

Figure 14.4 (a–c) Images of a normal human retina acquired using a retinal SD-OCT scanner at Duke University. (a) Normal retina image with 11-mm lateral scan, axial range 1.8 mm. (b) "OCT Fundus Image" constructed entirely from OCT volumetric data obtained in a single eye blink interval over 5.7 sec, consisting of 100 laterally displaced B-scans, data summed axially. (c) Volumetric rendering of 3D retinal SD-OCT dataset. (d) SD-OCT B-scan of a patient with neovascular age-related macular degeneration. (Image courtesy of Joseph A. Izatt and Cynthia Toth, Duke University, 3D rendering software courtesy of IDAV Laboratory, UC Davis.)

plaques, it was demonstrated that not only did OCT provide better resolution, it provided more structural detail as well.

Figure 14.5 shows an intravascular OCT image of a patient with an atherosclerotic plaque.

14.4.3 Endoscopic Imaging

The application of OCT to the recognition of precancerous and cancerous conditions in different mucosal tissues has been an active area of research since the mid-1990s. The first results of in vivo endoscopic OCT imaging of human mucosa were reported in 1997 [21]. The study used a forward-scanning endoscopic OCT system to image healthy and cancerous mucosal tissue of the esophagus, larynx, stomach, uterine cervix, and bladder. They concluded that the well-defined stratified structure of healthy tissue was no longer apparent in images of cancerous tissue, making OCT a promising diagnostic tool. In a follow-up study done by the same group [22], OCT was integrated with laparoscopy and used to study a variety of mucosal tissues. It was concluded that OCT is more useful when applied to organs, such as the larynx, uterine cervix, and bladder, in which a basal membrane separates the epithelial layer from the underlying stroma.

More recently, OCT has been studied for the diagnosis of many types of cancer including cancer of the digestive tract [23, 24], the breast [25], the esophagus [26, 27], and the prostate [28]. The course of research in most of these systems has been very similar. Initial studies began by imaging the microstructure of in vitro tissues

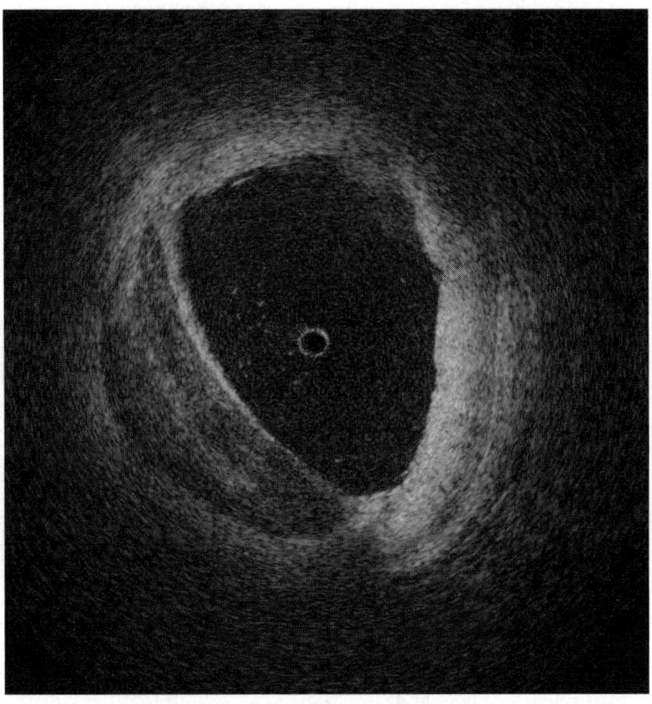

Figure 14.5 In vivo intravascular OCT image showing a atherosclerotic plaque in the lower left quadrant of the image. (Image courtesy of LightLab Imaging.)

in each of the systems. This early work has then been followed in all of the systems by in vivo studies conducted on the most easily accessible tissues in each system. A review of studies to detect cancer using endoscopic OCT is contained in [29]. Figure 14.6 contains OCT images of in vivo bladder tissue showing the difference in appearance of OCT images for healthy and cancerous bladder tissue.

14.5 New Directions

While OCT has been very successful in many areas of the clinic, there are several areas of research that are currently underway that promise to significantly improve the clinical impact of OCT. These include the development of three-dimensional OCT imaging technology, the development computer-aided diagnosis (CAD) algorithms for OCT imaging, and the investigation of OCT as an imaging modality to guide surgical procedures.

14.5.1 3D OCT

The previously mentioned imaging devices result in the formation of two-dimensional images. Two different methods for creating three-dimensional OCT systems have been reported, but neither appears to be applicable for delivery to the target via a cystoscope or endoscope. One of these techniques uses two galvanometers to scan the beam in two orthogonal dimensions, while the reference arm of the scanning system provides the information for the third dimension of the image [30, 31]. Another method, referred to as "full-field" or "parallel" OCT, makes use of a wide-field illumination of the target and an array of optical detectors to create an image parallel to the face of the system. The target can then be moved through the image field to create a three-dimensional image [32, 33].

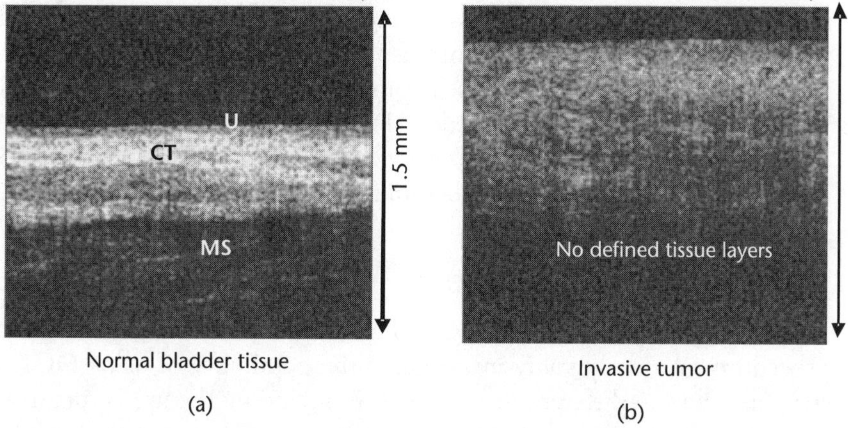

Figure 14.6 In vivo OCT images of normal and cancerous bladder tissue during clinical collaboration between George Washington University and Imalux Corporation showing (a) normal bladder wall and (b) an invasive bladder tumor.

While both of these methods have shown great promise for three-dimensional imaging, the systems tend to be large, and the optical beam cannot be delivered through an optical fiber to the internal lumens of the body. Micromachined two-dimensional scanners offer unique advantages in three-dimensional OCT scanning. A silicon micromachined two-dimensional scanner has recently been reported for three-dimensional OCT applications, but the devices are too large for many imaging applications (over 5 mm in diameter) and have reported limited scan angles (around 5°) [34, 35]. Many endoscopic probes have access ports with diameters of 2.8 mm, so the scanning device must be this size or smaller for optimum utility. Also, a two-axis electrothermal scanning mirror has also been proposed for OCT [36], but the devices have a moving optical pivot, which changes the path length throughout the scan and makes design of the imaging system more complicated. Work in the area of 3D endoscopic OCT is ongoing and is an active area of interest in the field.

14.5.2 Computer-Aided Diagnosis

The automated diagnosis of OCT images is a relatively new area of interest that has the potential to greatly increase the diagnostic ability of OCT images. Currently, OCT is a new technology and there are few experts qualified to interpret the results of OCT imaging. Consequently, in order to allow the medical community to benefit from this new technology, systems are needed which will automatically read the OCT images and provide suggested diagnosis. These systems, once verified, would provide reliable, user-independent, real-time results to the physicians operating the OCT systems.

The first published study that used measures of texture in OCT images to classify tissue investigated differences between mouse skin, testicular fat, and lung [8]. Each 1,024 × 256-pixel original image, acquired at a 1 × 1-μm pixel size, was down-sampled to 4 × 4 μm by averaging; the resulting 256 × 64-pixel image was used as a unit for feature extraction. Three features were chosen from a set of 24 texture descriptors and used in minimum-distance classifiers to distinguish between mouse skin and testicular fat (accuracy greater than 97%), between normal and abnormal mouse lung (64% to 89% accuracy), and between the three classes of skin, fat, and normal lung (37% to 95% accuracy). Other interesting studies have been published recently that developed algorithms for tissue diagnosis in OCT images: one focused on using texture analysis and optical phantoms [36]; one used novel scattering models for in vivo image analysis [37]; one used computer-aided diagnosis to detect dysplasia in the esophagus [38]; and one used CAD to investigate OCT images of breast tissue [39]. These preliminary results are very encouraging and suggest that OCT diagnosis can be greatly improved via further image analysis algorithm development.

14.5.3 Guiding Surgery with OCT

As early as 1997, OCT was being studied as a possible tool in guiding microsurgical procedures. An early study investigated the possibility of using OCT to recognize structures within different urologic tissues including the ureter, prostrate, prostatic urethra, and bladder [40]. The study concluded that it was possible to identify structures such as prostatic glandular secretions, ureteral muscular layers, and peri-urethral exocrine ducts. In addition, the study concluded that the ability to delineate borders such as the prostate-capsule border and to recognize neurovascular bundles would make OCT a valuable guidance tool for urologic microsurgery.

In addition, OCT has the potential to image vessel lumens during vascular surgery to determine if newly created lumens are patent and eventually to someday possibly allow the surgeon to determine the margins of cancerous lesions in real time during excision to greatly improve the success of these procedures.

14.6 Summary

In summary, OCT is an imaging modality that inhabits a unique niche in the world of imaging. This uniqueness is a result of being able to produce images with very high resolution at real-time imaging speeds. While these are significant advantages, the uses of OCT are constrained by the limited penetration of infrared light in non-transparent tissue. These capabilities make OCT imaging ideal for the detection and diagnosis of conditions that occur near the surface of tissues but may not be evident at the tissue surface. This includes conditions such as macular degeneration in the retina, or early cancer development in epithelial tissues. OCT is a powerful imaging modality that combines high resolution with the ability to couple the imaging energy into the body with optical fibers which enables numerous catheter and endoscopic-based applications.

References

[1] Fercher, A. F., "Optical Coherence Tomography," *Journal of Biomedical Optics*, Vol. 1, No. 3, 1996, pp. 157–173.

[2] Fujimoto, J. G., et al., "Optical Biopsy and Imaging Using Optical Coherence Tomography," *Nature Medicine*, Vol. 1, No. 9, 1995, pp. 970–972.

[3] Yun, S. H., et al., "High-Speed Optical Frequency-Domain Imaging," *Optics Express*, Vol. 11, No. 22, 2003, pp. 2953–2963.

[4] Choma, M. A., et al., "Sensitivity Advantage of Swept Source and Fourier Domain Optical Coherence Tomography," *Optics Express*, Vol. 11, No. 18, 2003, pp. 2183–2189.

[5] Yun, S. H., et al., "High-Speed Spectral-Domain Optical Coherence Tomography at 1.3 μm Wavelength," *Optics Express*, Vol. 11, No. 26, 2003, pp. 3598–3604.

[6] Boppart, S. A., et al., "Forward-Imaging Instruments for Optical Coherence Tomography," *Optics Letters*, Vol. 22, 1997, pp. 1618–1620.

[7] Pan, Y., H. Xie, and G. K. Fedder, "Endoscopic Optical Coherence Tomography Based on a Microelectromechanical Mirror," *Optics Letters*, Vol. 26, 2001, pp. 1966–1968.

[8] Bouma, B. E., and G. J. Tearney, "Power-Efficient Nonreciprocal Interferometer and Linear-Scanning Fiber-Optic Catheter for Optical Coherence Tomography," *Optics Letters*, Vol. 24, 1999, pp. 531–533.

[9] Liu, X., et al., "Rapid-Scanning Forward-Imaging Miniature Endoscope for Real-Time Optical Coherence Tomography," *Optics Letters*, Vol. 29, No. 15, 2004, pp. 1763–1765.

[10] Zara, J. M., et al., "Electrostatic MEMS Actuator Scanning Mirror for Optical Coherence Tomography," *Optics Letters*, Vol. 28, No. 8, 2003, pp. 628–630.

[11] Zara, J. M., and P. E. Patterson, "Polyimide Amplified Piezoelectric Scanning Mirror for Spectral Domain Optical Coherence Tomography," *Applied Physics Letters*, Vol. 89, 2006, p. 263901.

[12] Tran, P. H., et al., "In Vivo Endoscopic Optical Coherence Tomography by Use of a Rotational Microelectromechanical System Probe," *Optics Letters*, Vol. 29, No. 11, 2004, pp. 1236–1238.

[13] Su, J., et al., "In Vivo Three-Dimensional Micromechanical Endoscopic Swept Source Optical Coherence Tomography," *Optics Express*, Vol. 15, No. 16, 2007, pp. 10390–10396.

[14] Aguirre, A. D., et al., "Two-Axis MEMS Scanning Catheter for Ultrahigh Resolution Three-Dimensional and En Face Imaging," *Optics Express*, Vol. 15, No. 5, 2007, pp. 2445–2453.

[15] Fercher, A. F., et al., "Optical Coherence Tomography—Principles and Applications," *Reports on Progress in Physics*, Institute of Physics Publishing, 2003, pp. 239–303.

[16] Brezinski, M. E., and J. G. Fujimoto, "Optical Coherence Tomography: High-Resolution Imaging in Nontransparent Tissue," *IEEE Journal of Selected Topics in Quantum Electronics*, Vol. 5, No. 4, July/August 1999, pp. 1185–1192.

[17] Huang, D., et al., "Optical Coherence Tomography," *Science*, Vol. 254, August 1991, pp. 1178–1181.

[18] Patel, N. A., D. L. Stamper, and M. E. Brezinski, "Review of the Ability of Optical Coherence Tomography to Characterize Plaque, Including a Comparison with Intravascular Ultrasound," *Cardiovascular & Interventional Radiology*, Vol. 28, No. 1, 2005, pp. 1–9.

[19] Stamper, D., N. J. Weissman, and M. Brezinski, "Plaque Characterization with Optical Coherence Tomography," *Journal of the American College of Cardiology*, Vol. 47, No. 8, Suppl. C, 2005, pp. C69–C79.

[20] Jang, I. K., et al., "Visualization of Coronary Atherosclerotic Plaques in Patients Using Optical Coherence Tomography: Comparison with Intravascular Ultrasound," *Journal of the American College of Cardiolology*, Vol. 39, 2002, pp. 604–609.

[21] Sergeev, A. M., et al., "In Vivo Endoscopic OCT Imaging of Precancer and Cancer States of Human Mucosa," *Optics Express*, Vol. 1, No. 13, December 1997, pp. 432–440.

[22] Feldchtein, F. I., et al., "Endoscopic Applications of Optical Coherence Tomography," *Optics Express*, Vol. 3, No. 6, September 1998, pp. 257–270.

[23] Pfau, P. R., et al., "Criteria for the Diagnosis of Dysplasia by Endoscopic Optical Coherence Tomography," *Gastrointestinal Endoscopy*, Vol. 58, No. 2, 2003, pp. 196–202.

[24] Westphal, V., et al., "Correlation of Endoscopic Optical Coherence Tomography with Histology in the Lower-GI Tract," *Gastrointestinal Endoscopy*, Vol. 61, No. 4, 2005, pp. 537–546.

[25] Zysk, A. M., and S. A. Boppart, "Computational Methods for Analysis of Human Breast Tumor Tissue in Optical Coherence Tomography Images," *Journal of Biomedical Optics*, Vol. 11, No. 5, September/October 2006.

[26] Isenberg, G., et al., "Accuracy of Endoscopic Optical Coherence Tomography in the Detection of Dysplasia in Barrett's Esophagus: A Prospective, Double-Blinded Study," *Gastrointestinal Endoscopy*, Vol. 62, No. 6, 2005, pp. 825–831.

[27] Qi, X., et al., "Computer-Aided Diagnosis of Dysplasia in Barrett's Esophagus Using Multiple Endoscopic OCT Images," *Proceedings of SPIE*, Vol. 6079, 2006.

[28] D'Amico, A. V., et al., "Optical Coherence Tomography as a Method for Identifying Benign and Malignant Microscopic Structures in the Prostrate Gland," *Urology*, Vol. 55, No. 5, 2000, pp. 783–787.

[29] Zara, J. M., and A. Lingley-Papadopoulos, "Endoscopic OCT Approaches Towards Cancer Diagnosis," *IEEE Journal of Selected Topics in Quantum Electronics*, Vol. 14, No. 1, 2008, pp. 70–81.

[30] Beaurepaire, E., et al., "Full-Field Optical Coherence Tomography," *Optics Letters*, Vol. 23, 1998, pp. 244–246.

[31] Laubscher, M., et al., "Video-Rate Three-Dimensional Optical Coherence Tomography," *Optics Express*, Vol. 10, 2002, pp. 429–435.

[32] Schneider, I., "2-D OCT Scanner Promises In-Situ Diagnosis," *Laser Focus World*, July 2004, pp. 47–50.

[33] Piyawattanametha, W., et al., "A 2D Scanner by Surface and Bulk Micromachined Angular Vertical Comb Actuators," *Proceedings of Optical MEMS Conference*, 2003.

[34] Jain, A., et al., "A Two-Axis Electrothermal Micromirror for Endoscopic Optical Coherence Tomography," *IEEE Journal of Selected Topics in Quantum Electronics*, Vol. 10, No. 3, 2004, pp. 636–642.

[35] Gossage, K. W., and T. S. Tkaczyk, "Texture Analysis of Optical Coherence Tomography Images: Feasibility for Tissue Classification," *Journal of Biomedical Optics*, Vol. 8, No. 3, July 2003, pp. 570–575.

[36] Gossage, K. W., et al., "Texture Analysis of Speckle in Optical Coherence Tomography Images of Tissue Phantoms," *Physics in Medicine and Biology*, Vol. 51, 2006, pp. 1563–1575.

[37] Turchin, I. V., et al., "Novel Algorithm of Processing Optical Coherence Tomography Images for Differentiation of Biological Tissue Pathologies," *Journal of Biomedical Optics*, Vol. 10, No. 6, November/December 2005.

[38] Qi, X., et al., "Computer-Aided Diagnosis of Dysplasia in Barrett's Esophagus Using Endoscopic Optical Coherence Tomography," *Journal of Biomedical Optics*, Vol. 11, No. 4, July/August 2006.

[39] Zysk, A. M., and S. A. Boppart, "Computational Methods for Analysis of Human Breast Tumor Tissue in Optical Coherence Tomography Images," *Journal of Biomedical Optics*, Vol. 11, No. 5, 2006.

[40] Tearney, G. J., et al., "Optical Biopsy in Human Urologic Tissue Using Optical Coherence Tomography," *The Journal of Urology*, Vol. 157, May 1997, pp. 1915–1919.

CHAPTER 15

Advanced Cardiac Imaging for Evaluation, Diagnosis, and Treatment of Arrhythmias

Matthew Kay and Marco Mercader

Normal contraction of the heart is dependent upon an ordered progression of electrical excitation that is carried by propagating action potentials. Action potentials originate from the sino-atrial node, propagate through the atria, pass into the atrioventricular (AV) node and bundle of His, and are then distributed to the ventricular muscle by the Purkinje system. Action potentials that emanate from Purkinje-myocardial junctions form waves of electrical excitation that spread through the surrounding myocardial tissue. The waves coalesce and are self-extinguished a few milliseconds after the beginning of systole. This process maintains synchronized contraction for efficient pumping of blood. In cardiac arrhythmias, such as tachycardia or fibrillation, the ordered progression of action potentials through the myocardium is interrupted by abnormal pathways that allow the electrical waves to reexcite myocardial tissue at very high rates, a process called *reentry*. Identifying these pathways, or *reentrant circuits*, and understanding the anatomic and electrophysiologic mechanisms that cause them is crucial for treating cardiac arrhythmias.

Abnormal pathways are often identified by tracking the position of electrical waves as they propagate through myocardial tissue. This is a process called *cardiac mapping* and is usually accomplished by measuring extracellular potentials at multiple sites using electrodes or by using optical techniques to record the fluorescence of tissue stained with a voltage-sensitive dye. Clinical cardiac mapping systems use minimally invasive catheter techniques to record extracellular potentials (electrograms) from many sites on the endocardial surface of the heart. The electrograms are analyzed to identify the depolarization time (i.e., the action potential upstroke) at each site to reveal the location of an electrical wave front. These times are rendered as an *activation map* and show the progression of electrical waves. Abnormal electrical pathways can be identified using activation maps. Ablation therapy is then applied to interrupt the abnormal pathways. This type of image-guided therapy has cured many patients suffering from cardiac arrhythmias.

Anatomic and electrophysiologic mechanisms of arrhythmias can be studied in great detail by recording the fluorescence of myocardial tissue stained with a voltage-sensitive dye. Action potentials are represented by changes in the tissue fluorescence at each recording site. Simultaneously recording such fluorescence from many sites is one mode of *fluorescence imaging*, a technique that is often used in animal heart preparations for arrhythmia research in the laboratory. Clinical cardiac mapping techniques and laboratory fluorescence imaging techniques provide complimentary information for elucidating arrhythmia mechanisms and for perfecting therapies.

One example of this is the treatment of supraventricular tachycardias that have a point of origin in the atrioventricular node [1]. AV nodal reentrant tachycardia (AVNRT) is the most common supraventricular tachycardia. Clinical mapping of this arrhythmia using catheter electrode arrays has shown that it is most often caused by a reentrant circuit conducted along fast and slow pathways within the AV node. Ablating one of the pathways can stop the reentry and cure the arrhythmia [2–4]. In some patients, supraventricular tachycardia may be caused by increased automaticity of tissue within the AV node that discharges spontaneously at high rates [5], a phenomenon called an *ectopic focus*. Other types arrhythmia can be caused by ectopic foci in other areas of the heart and these sources of spontaneous electrical excitation are also targeted in ablation procedures [6–8].

While clinical mapping provides activation times for identifying AV node reentry in patients, it does not provide action potentials or the anatomical details of conduction within the AV node, which are crucial for understanding the mechanisms of the arrhythmia. These weaknesses of clinical mapping are strengths of fluorescence imaging. With fluorescence imaging, the heterogeneity of action potential morphology within the AV node itself, as well as AV node anatomy, can be simultaneously studied at high spatiotemporal resolution [9, 10]. Fluorescence imaging has provided detailed descriptions of conduction delay within the AV node [11] and its pacemaker activity [9], two of the primary functions of the AV node. Conduction pathways and reentrant circuits within the AV node have also been described using fluorescence imaging [12] to explain the mechanisms of AVNRT and how appropriate ablation therapy cures it.

In this chapter, the basic concepts of cardiac mapping will be introduced from the perspective of fluorescence imaging in the laboratory and mapping with catheter electrode arrays in the clinic. First, the three main modes of fluorescence imaging of cardiac tissue will be explained and instrumentation for two-dimensional and panoramic fluorescence imaging will be described. Typical fluorescence signals during regular rhythms and arrhythmias, and the maps generated from them, will be presented. Current clinical techniques will then be described with a focus on three-dimensional mapping, including noncontact endocardial mapping and electroanatomical mapping. The use of these techniques for image-guided ablation for arrhythmia therapy will be explained using images recently acquired from clinical procedures.

15.1 Fluorescence Imaging of Cardiac Tissue

Fluorescence imaging is a powerful tool for studying mechanisms of cardiac arrhythmias [13, 14]. It has been especially useful in revealing how a dispersion of tissue function can lead to the formation of functionally reentrant circuits, known as electrical *rotors* [15, 16]. Rotor breakup and the reformation of rotors is a main mechanism of ventricular fibrillation [17, 18]. Defibrillation studies using fluorescence imaging have shown how rotors are extinguished when defibrillation is successful and how a rotor may be reinitiated when it is unsuccessful [19].

Multiple modes of fluorescence imaging can be combined for acquisition of separate physiological processes from the same recording sites [20, 21]. Such multiple-process imaging may provide spatiotemporally coupled data that is essential for understanding complex arrhythmias, and will be discussed below. The three main modes of fluorescence imaging of cardiac tissue are: (1) transmembrane potential imaging, (2) intracellular calcium ($[Ca^{+2}]_i$) transient imaging, and (3) imaging of the reduced form of nicotinamide adenine dinucleotide (NADH), an important molecule during aerobic metabolism. The transduction of cellular processes (action potentials, $[Ca^{+2}]_i$ transients, and cellular metabolism) by changes in fluorescence is summarized in Figure 15.1.

15.1.1 Transmembrane Potential Imaging

In transmembrane potential imaging, often referred to as *optical mapping*, the tissue is stained with a voltage-sensitive fluorescent dye (e.g., di-4-ANEPPS or RH-237). Such dyes are lipid soluble and are incorporated into the plasma membrane of cardiac myocytes [22]. The dye is energized by illuminating the tissue with light that contains the peak *excitation* wavelength of the dye. The peak of the *emission* spectrum of the dye occurs at wavelengths longer than the peak of the excitation spectrum (Stokes shift), allowing the two light bands (excitation and emission) to

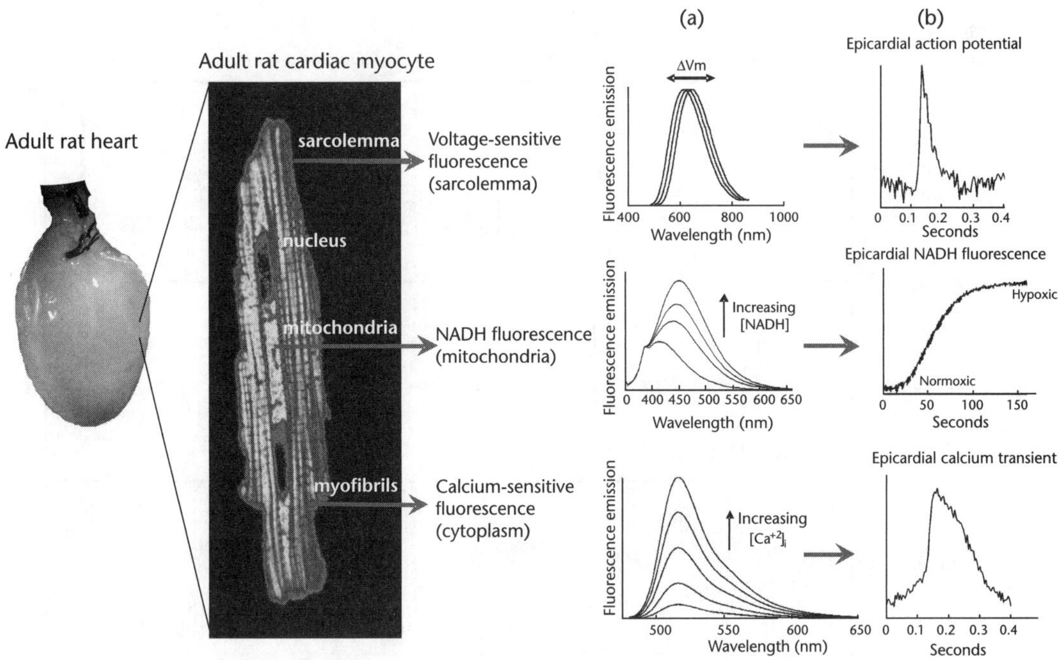

Figure 15.1 Three main modes of fluorescence imaging of cardiac tissue. The transduction of cellular processes by changes in fluorescence is illustrated for action potentials, $[Ca^{+2}]_i$ transients, and mitochondrial redox state (amount of NADH). (a) Representative emission spectra are shown. (b) Fluorescence signals from isolated perfused rat heart preparations are shown. The electromechanical uncoupler blebbistatin (10 mM) was to minimize motion artifacts.

be separated with appropriate optical filters. Changes in transmembrane potential shift the emission spectrum of the dye [22, 23], which changes the amount of emitted light passing through an emission filter (Figure 15.1). Filtered emitted light is then recorded using CCD video cameras [17, 24], photodiode arrays [25, 26], or photomultiplier tubes [27] to reproduce the time course of action potentials.

Transmembrane potential imaging offers several advantages over conventional electrical mapping techniques, in which signals are recorded from electrodes that contact the tissue. One advantage is that signals represent the time course of an action potential, allowing for analysis of repolarization and refractoriness—even during tachyarrhythmias when the T-wave is not visible in electrical recordings. This is illustrated in Figure 15.2, which shows temporally synchronized recordings of electrograms using a bipolar electrode and fluoresced action potentials from the epicardium of a rat heart for three different rhythms. The time course of repolarization that is provided by fluoresced action potentials is critical for understanding reentrant arrhythmias, especially fibrillation. Another advantage of transmembrane potential imaging is that signals are not contaminated by electrical artifacts that may result from pacing stimuli and defibrillation shocks. This is important for studying mechanisms of defibrillation because the spatial distribution of the shock-induced changes in transmembrane potentials can be observed.

15.1.2 Intracellular Calcium Transient Imaging

Calcium is a ubiquitous cytosolic messenger. In myocytes, cytosolic calcium is required for *excitation-contraction coupling*, the process by which contraction fol-

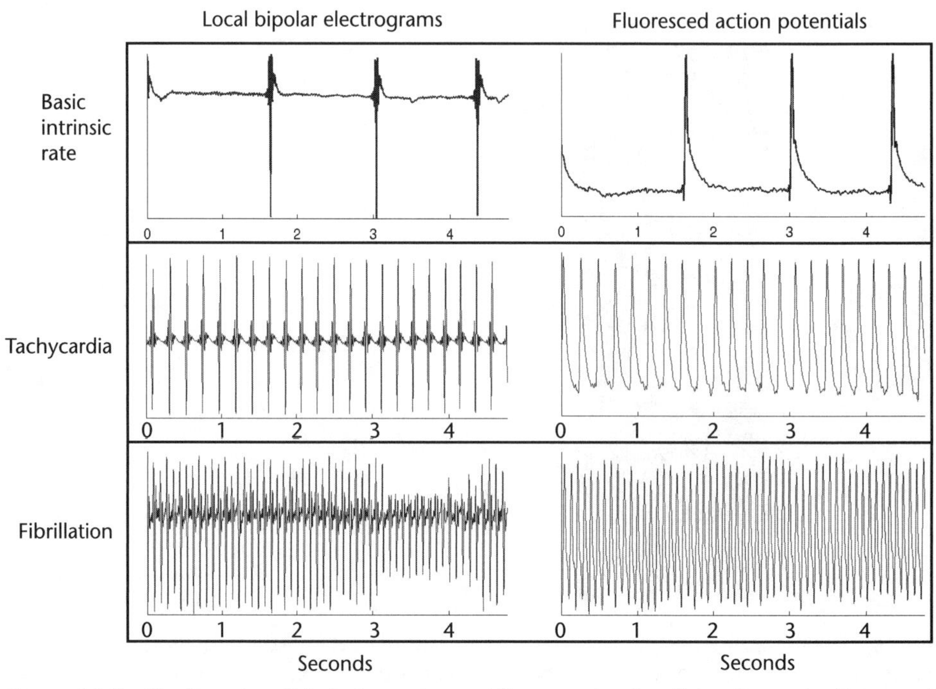

Figure 15.2 Bipolar epicardial electrograms and fluoresced epicardial action potentials acquired during three different rhythms in isolated perfused rat heart preparations. The acquisition of electrograms and fluoresced signals was temporally synchronized.

lows the upstroke of an action potential [28]. At rest, myocytes store a large amount of calcium in an organelle called the sarcoplasmic reticulum (SR). When excited, the cell depolarizes and voltage-gated calcium ion channels within the T-tubules open to allow a small amount of extracellular calcium to enter the cell. Those calcium ions then trigger a large amount of calcium to be released from the SR, a process called *calcium-induced calcium release*. Once calcium is released from the SR it activates cross-bridge cycling in the sarcomeres, which shorten the cell and cause contraction. At the same time, cytosolic calcium is actively resequestered by the SR to prepare for the next contraction. This sequence of a rise and fall of cytolic calcium during contraction is called an *intracellular calcium transient*. Disturbances in cycling of cytosolic calcium can cause loss of contractile force as well as altered electrical activity, such as focal arrhythmias. The details of many of these concepts are explained in the classical book by Donald Bers [29].

Changes in the cycling of cytosolic calcium can be studied by recording intracellular calcium ($[Ca^{+2}]_i$) transients [30, 31]. Fluorescence imaging of $[Ca^{+2}]_i$ transients is accomplished using techniques similar to those for imaging transmembrane potential, except that tissue is stained with a *cell-permeant* calcium-sensitive fluorescent dye (e.g., Rhod-2AM or Fluo-4AM). The fluorescence of a calcium-sensitive dye increases when it binds with calcium, therefore its fluorescence reflects local calcium concentration [32, 33] (Figure 15.1). Although protocols for loading the cytosol of myocytes with a calcium-sensitive dye may vary, each protocol typically includes 10 to 20 minutes of incubating myocytes with a solution of the dye plus Pluronic (a detergent), followed by a period of washout to remove any unhydrolyzed dye.

We typically use Rhod-2AM to image $[Ca^{+2}]_i$ transients from excised animal hearts. To energize the dye the epicardium is illuminated using LEDs with a peak wavelength of 530 nm and a spectral half-width of 35 nm (530/35 nm). Rhod-2AM fluorescence is band-pass filtered at 585/20 nm and imaged using a high speed CCD camera to record epicardial $[Ca^{+2}]_i$ transients. We also image $[Ca^{+2}]_i$ transients from monolayers of rat neonatal myocytes, as shown in Figure 15.3. A mechanism of successful anti-tachycardia pacing has been recently described using these techniques [34].

Unlike action potentials, $[Ca^{+2}]_i$ transients typically do not propagate from cell to cell. However, an action potential normally elicits a $[Ca^{+2}]_i$ transient, so propagation can usually be tracked by imaging $[Ca^{+2}]_i$ transients [35, 36]. This is illustrated in Figure 15.3 for a reentrant circuit in a myocyte monolayer. The position of the wave front is tracked by approximating the activation time at each pixel as the time that the first derivative of the $[Ca^{+2}]_i$ transient exceeds a threshold [Figure 15.3(b)]. The image of these times is displayed as an *activation map* [Figure 15.3(d)]. A contour plot of activation times is displayed as an *isochronal map* and clearly shows the progression of the reentrant wave [Figure 15.3(e)]. Activation and isochronal maps are most often generated from electrode mapping data and transmembrane potential images to reveal propagation pathways. They are especially important for visualizing clinical mapping data, as described in later sections of this chapter.

15.1.3 NADH Imaging

Myocardial ischemia is caused by loss of coronary blood flow and is a major cause of arrhythmias and sudden cardiac death [37]. During ischemia there is a rapid

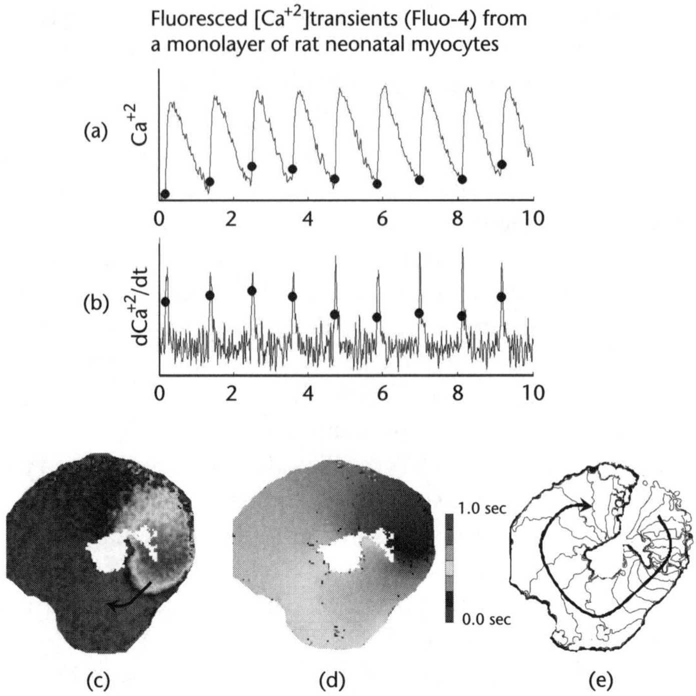

Figure 15.3 Intracellular calcium transient imaging of monolayers of rat neonatal myocytes. (a) Fluoresced calcium transients recorded from one site using Fluo-4AM. Solid dots indicate the approximated activation times. (b) The first derivative of the calcium transients shown in (a). Activation times (solid dots) can be approximated as the time that the derivative exceeds a threshold. (c) An image of the fluorescence of Fluo-4AM shows a reentrant wave front. (d) An activation map of the reentrant wave front shown in (c). (e) An isochronal map of the reentrant wave front shown in (c).

decline of contractile performance and an increased incidence of reentrant arrhythmias caused by slowing of conduction [38] and ectopic arrhythmias caused by increased tissue automaticity [39, 40]. Ischemia-induced hypoxia severely reduces aerobic metabolism, cellular ATP levels decline, and oxidation of NADH in the electron transport chain is lost, causing NADH to accumulate in the mitochondria. NADH is autofluorescent with an emission peak at 460 nm (Figure 15.1). Its fluorescence provides a rapid, direct measure of oxygen-limited mitochondrial activity [41, 42]. For these reasons it is commonly used as a metabolic metric of acute ischemia [43, 44] and can be used to accurately identify the location and progression of hypoxia [45].

In our studies, NADH is imaged at frequent intervals to identify the epicardial border between hypoxic and normoxic tissue caused by the total occlusion of a major coronary [46], as shown in Figure 15.4. This is done by illuminating the heart with ultraviolet light from a mercury lamp that has been band-pass filtered at a peak wavelength of 360 nm and a spectral half-width of 50 nm (360/50 nm). The emitted NADH fluorescence is bandpass filtered (475/50 nm) and imaged with a CCD camera at 2 frames per second (fps). During acute local ischemia, NADH fluorescence homogeneously increases and plateaus (Figure 15.4). When a total occlusion is partially relieved, resulting in low-flow reperfusion, NADH fluorescence becomes patchy as NADH is oxidized in the areas of tissue that receive the limited

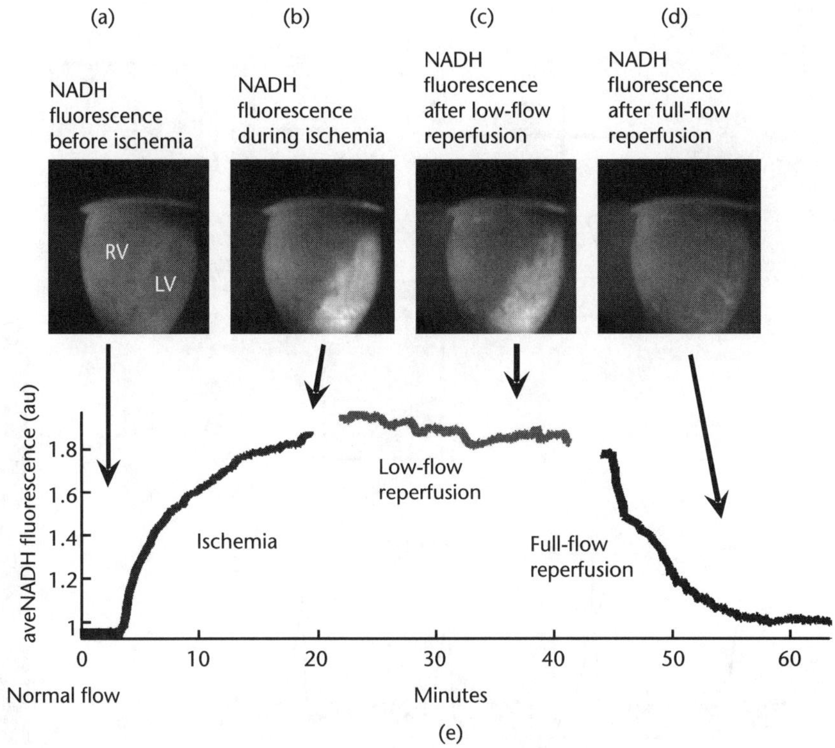

Figure 15.4 (a–d) NADH images during acute local ischemia and reperfusion in an isolated perfused rat heart. Ischemia was induced by occluding a major coronary artery. White areas indicate elevated levels of NADH (e.g., hypoxic tissue). (e) Average level of NADH within the ischemic region. The electromechanical uncoupler blebbistatin (10 mM) was used to minimize motion artifacts.

amount of flow. During full-flow reperfusion, NADH fluorescence homogeneously returns to its preischemic levels, indicating complete oxidation of NADH and relief of the coronary occlusion. Recent studies using dual imaging of NADH and transmembrane potential have provided new insights into the cause of ectopic arrhythmias during acute local ischemia [47].

15.1.4 Dual Imaging of the Same Field of View

Dual-mode fluorescence imaging systems are currently used by multiple laboratories to study cardiac electrophysiology [20, 48, 49]. Our dual-mode system is capable of high-resolution imaging using two high-speed CCD cameras (Andor IXON DV860s) that are positioned to image the same field of view with an error of less than 70 μm [46, 47]. The cameras are coupled to a dual port adapter (Andor CSU Adapter Dual Cam) that contains a dichroic mirror (610 nm) and lenses, as shown in Figure 15.5. At low magnification this system can image the entire anterior surface of small animal hearts at a spatial resolution of ~150 μm (128 × 128 pixels). At high magnification the field of view is ~3 × 3 mm with a spatial resolution of 25 μm (128 × 128 pixels). The system is typically operated at frame rates between 250 and 500 fps. Frame rates up to 1,000 fps are possible.

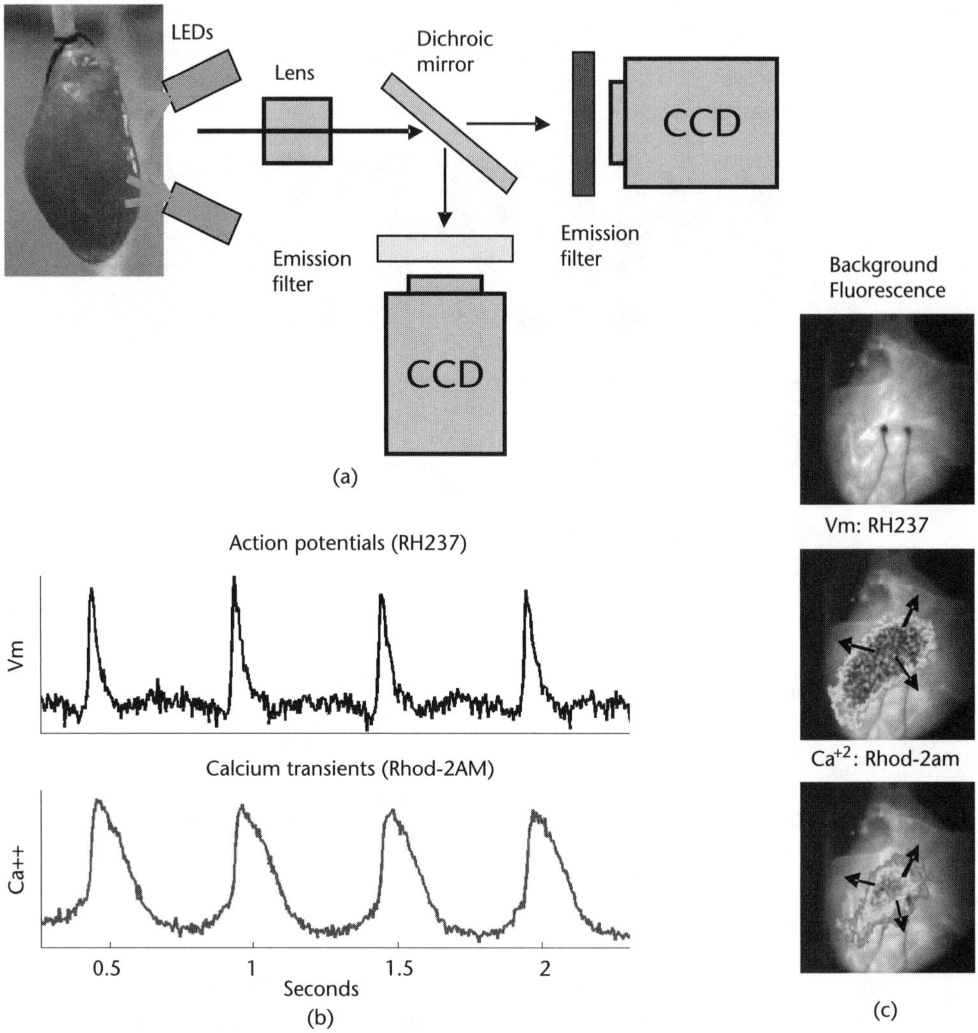

Figure 15.5 Dual fluorescence imaging of the same field of view. (a) Schematic of the imaging system. (b) Fluoresced signals acquired during pacing using simultaneous dual imaging of transmembrane potential and $[Ca^{+2}]_i$ transients. (c) Images of the initial sequence of one paced beat shown in (b).

Transmembrane potential and $[Ca^{+2}]_i$ transients are imaged *simultaneously* by staining the tissue with both RH237 and Rhod-2AM, as shown in Figure 15.5. Such simultaneous imaging is feasible because the two dyes can be energized using light of one wavelength band (530/35 nm) and the emitted light can be separated into each camera without crosstalk using a 610-nm dichroic mirror [25]. In this mode, the cameras are precisely synchronized in time so that the time course of fluoresced action potentials and fluoresced $[Ca^{+2}]_i$ transients can be accurately compared (Figure 15.5).

Transmembrane potential and NADH are *sequentially* imaged by selective illumination of the tissue using two light sources, one to energize a voltage-sensitive dye and ultraviolet light to energize NADH [46]. Such sequential imaging is feasible because the time course of changes in NADH is much longer than that of transmembrane potential. Examples of datasets acquired from excised rat heart preparations before and after acute local ischemia are illustrated in Figure 15.6.

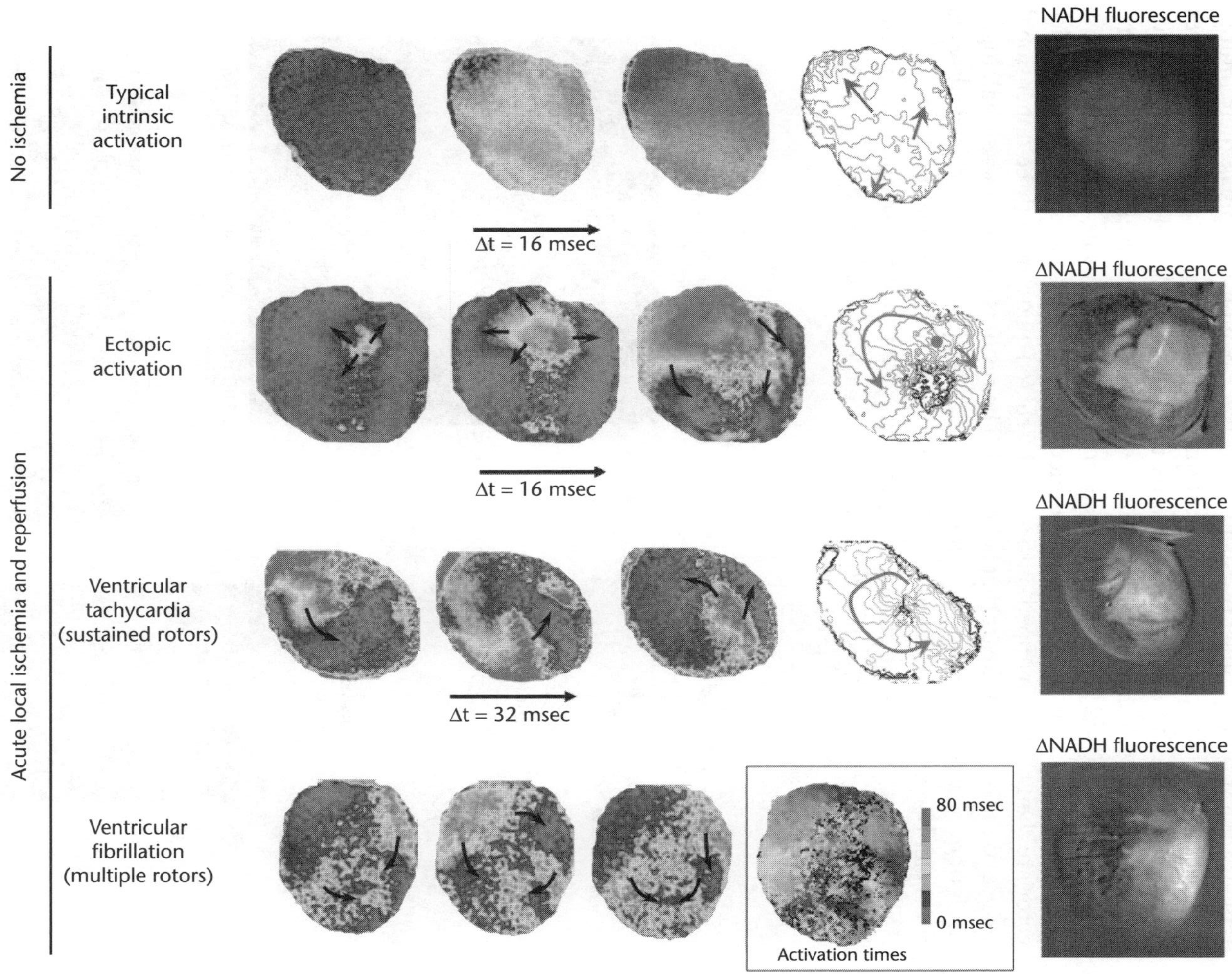

Figure 15.6 Dual sequential imaging of transmembrane potential and NADH in isolated perfused rat hearts before and after acute local ischemia. Sequences of fluoresced transmembrane potential (RH237) and changes in NADH fluorescence during typical intrinsic activation before ischemia (first row) and during three main arrhythmias resulting from reperfusion after ischemia (rows 2 to 4) are shown.

Conduction sequences and changes in NADH fluorescence during typical intrinsic activation before and after ischemia are shown.

15.1.5 Panoramic Fluorescence Imaging

A main limitation of conventional fluorescence imaging systems is their limited field of view. This is particularly important when reentrant pathways or sources of ectopic beats cannot be studied because they originate outside the field of view. Panoramic fluorescence imaging systems have recently been developed to overcome this limitation [50–52]. These systems record fluorescence using multiple detectors positioned around the heart. The two-dimensional fluorescence data from each detector are then texture-mapped onto a reconstructed anatomical three-dimensional surface of the particular heart that is imaged. The result is a four-dimensional, high-resolution, spatially contiguous, dataset [x, y, z, $F(t)$] from which electrical wave fronts can be visualized and tracked over most of the epicardial surface.

The panoramic system shown in Figure 15.7 can image transmembrane potential from nearly the entire epicardial surface of large animal hearts [50]. The goal

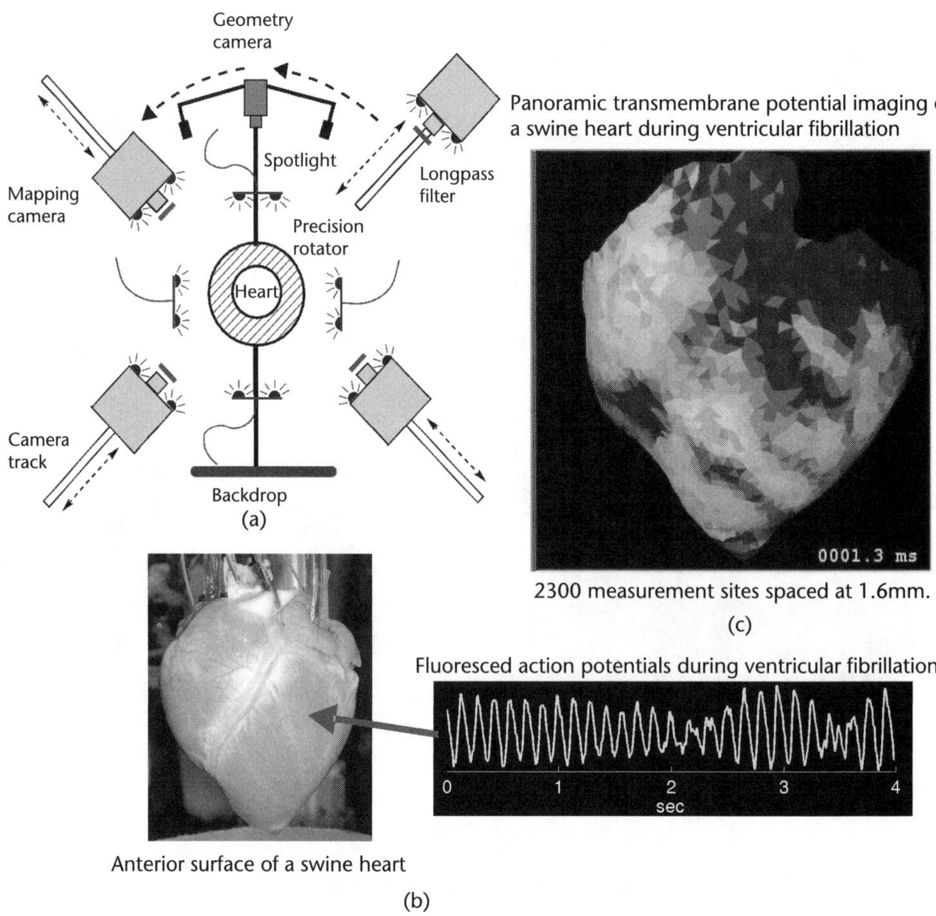

Figure 15.7 Panoramic fluorescence imaging of transmembrane potential in large animal hearts. (a) A diagram of the system. (b) A typical isolated perfused swine heart. (c) A panoramic image of transmembrane potential during ventricular fibrillation in a swine heart.

for developing this system was to study electrical rotor formation in hearts similar in size to those of humans [53, 54]. Four high-speed CCD cameras image fluorescence from viewpoints spaced every 90 degrees around the heart. A geometrical model of the epicardial surface for each heart is generated using images of the heart obtained every 5 degrees from a conventional CCD camera that rotates around the heart, also shown in Figure 15.7. Custom software is an essential component of the system. This includes algorithms to create the geometrical model and use it to combine fluorescence images from each camera into one dataset. A calibration algorithm generates the mathematical transforms that register all images to a common coordinate frame [50].

Panoramic imaging has revealed the first complete picture of epicardial rotors during ventricular fibrillation in healthy swine hearts [17, 53, 55]. The main conclusion of these studies was that ventricular fibrillation was not maintained by stable, persistent rotors that are visible on the epicardium. Instead, the many electrical wave fronts that are characteristic of ventricular fibrillation are maintained by many transient and widely scattered rotors [55]. The epicardial trajectories of rotors imaged in those studies and their anatomic locations are shown in Figure 15.8. These panoramic imaging studies suggest that new rational antifibrillation therapies should focus on preventing the formation of new rotors and not on extinguishing existing rotors, because they will eventually terminate by themselves [17].

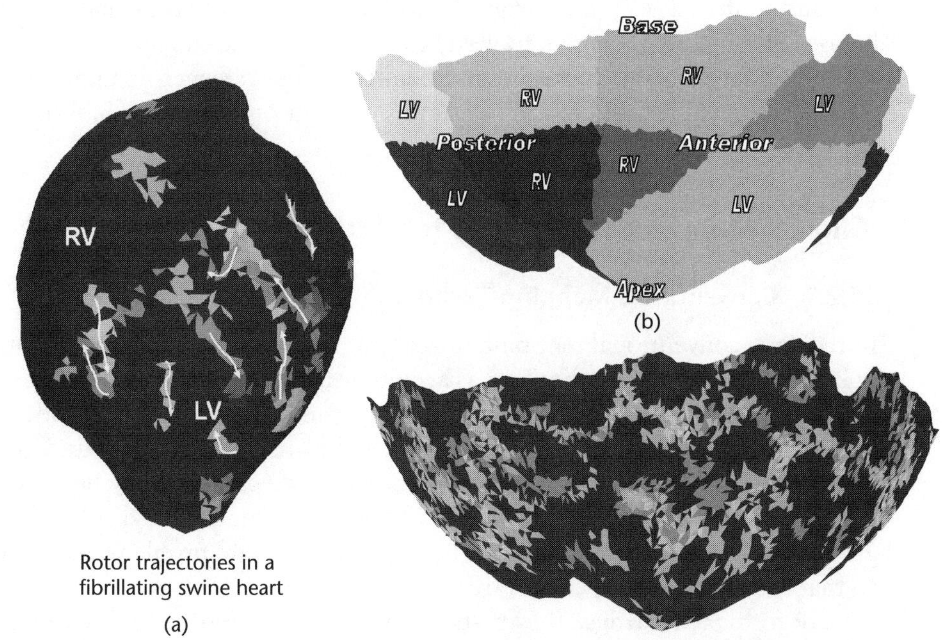

Rotor trajectories in a fibrillating swine heart

(a)

(b)

Trajectories of all rotors identified in a 4 second interval during ventricular fibrillation in a swine heart.

(c)

Figure 15.8 Results from panoramic fluorescence imaging of a fibrillating healthy swine heart. (a) Trajectories of multiple rotors identified during ventricular fibrillation. (b) Specific anatomic regions can be identified from each heart studied. (c) Trajectory pathways for all rotors identified in a four second interval of ventricular fibrillation. Rotors are scattered over the entire epicardium, indicating that, in healthy swine hearts, they are not localized to specific anatomic regions.

15.1.6 Motion Artifact in Fluoresced Signals

Fluorescence data can be confounded by mechanical contraction, which causes loss of signal registration between the imaging device and the heart [56]. The result is signals contaminated with "motion artifact" [44, 57]. When imaging transmembrane potential, distortions primarily occur in the plateau and repolarization phases of the action potential because contraction begins during those phases. Therefore, to record during those phases, hearts are typically immobilized. In most situations, however, the depolarization phase of the action potential can be recorded without motion artifact and used to identify excitation wave fronts [57, 58]. In our recent studies, we are successfully using the depolarization phase to track ectopic wave fronts without completely immobilizing the heart.

There are several ways to immobilize the heart to record fluoresced action potentials without motion artifact: (1) reduce the concentration of Ca^{+2} in the purfusate; (2) administer electromechanical uncoupling agents such as 2,3-butanedione monoxime (DAM or BDM) [59], cytochalasin-D [60], or blebbistatin [61]; or (3) constrain the heart mechanically [44, 62, 63]. Typically, methods (1) and (2) are avoided due to their potential to suppress some arrhythmias [64] and/or disturb $[Ca^{+2}]_i$ dynamics, the conductance of ion channels, and coronary smooth muscle tone. In method (3), motion artifact is minimized by applying gentle mechanical constraint to each side of the heart. This can usually be done without causing ischemia, as has been demonstrated in the labs of Salama [64, 65], Rosenbaum [63, 66], and Jalife [62, 67]. Background fluorescence levels of epicardial NADH could be used as an internal control to verify that constraints do not cause local ischemia. With both mechanical constraint and dual-mode fluorescence imaging, signal ratio techniques could be used to remove almost all motion artifacts [68, 69].

15.2 Clinical Mapping Techniques for Arrhythmia Therapy

15.2.1 Conventional Mapping Techniques

In the past, conventional mapping of reentrant and ectopic foci for patients undergoing treatment for arrhythmias was accomplished using single point contact catheter mapping techniques. For conventional mapping, quadripolar electrode catheters may be positioned high in the right atrium, in the His bundle region, and in the right ventricular apex. In addition, a multipolar electrode catheter may be positioned in the coronary sinus. Surface and intracardiac electrograms are displayed and programmed electrical stimulation can be applied to initiate problematic tachycardias so that they can be mapped and treated.

For focal tachycardias, the ablation catheter can be moved to different positions to identify the earliest site of electrical activation. For reentrant tachycardias, activation sequences can be determined with the use of the multiple catheter recordings available during the study. The mechanisms responsible for the tachycardia can be determined using information gained from programmed stimulation and recordings of the tachycardia behavior during the procedure.

The main limitations of conventional mapping result from having a limited number of recording electrodes. Limitations include difficulties in accurately mapping unstable tachycardias as well as in identifying an early site of activation or a reentrant circuit. This can lead to low success rates and unnecessarily prolong procedure time or increase the use fluoroscopy.

Fluoroscopy is an essential part of all clinical cardiac mapping and ablation procedures. It requires a single or biplane fluoroscopy system. The radiographic images are used to aid both in the placement of catheters and in moving them during mapping and ablation. Radiation exposure can be limited by the use of lead shielding, lead aprons, lead glasses, and thyroid shields. However, reducing the use of X-rays provides the greatest reduction of radiation exposure and this is the main advantage of three-dimensional clinical cardiac mapping systems.

15.2.2 Three-Dimensional Clinical Cardiac Mapping Systems

With current mapping and catheter techniques, complex cardiac arrhythmias in humans can be visualized in three dimensions. This section covers a few of the most commonly used methods for clinical mapping of cardiac arrhythmias, including electroanatomical and noncontact endocardial techniques. A theme of this book is image-guided therapy; as such, cardiac ablation procedures performed using three-dimensional mapping systems serve as an excellent example of the use of images for the guidance of therapy in patients.

15.2.2.1 Nonfluoroscopic Electro-Anatomical Cardiac Mapping

The CARTO system (Biosense, Diamond Bar, California) is a clinical mapping system that is currently the leading platform for three-dimensional electro-anatomical mapping. This system uses electrodes that contact the endocardium to sense local electrograms. Activation maps are generated by acquiring electrograms from multiple points and displaying the activation times measured from those electrograms in three dimensions at high resolution. Essentially, the activation maps provide local activation times and their three-dimensional coordinates within in the heart. The quality of each measured data point and the number of points acquired enhances the accuracy of the three-dimensional activation map. The main advantage of the system is that by using the location of the electrode at the catheter tip, together with its local electrogram, an electroanatomical map of the heart can be generated in real time without the use of X-rays [70].

The CARTO system uses a small magnetic field sensor (the *location sensor*) and an external ultra-low magnetic field emitter (the *location pad*) with a processing unit. The location sensor is integrated into end of a standard deflectable tip electrophysiological catheter. A low level magnetic field (0.05 to 0.5 gauss) is generated by three separate coils in the location pad, which is placed beneath the table supporting the patient. The field strength from each coil is measured by the location sensor and its position relative to each coil is triangulated. This allows the position and orientation of the catheter tip to be determined with 6 degrees of freedom [70, 71].

Methods

First, the anatomical source of an arrhythmia is estimated using standard chest electrocardiograms (i.e., left or right atrium, left or right ventricle). The mapping catheter is then positioned inside the chamber of interest. Electrograms from the distal catheter electrodes are recorded through the entire cardiac cycle. The catheter tip is then moved over the endocardium to acquire multiple electrograms and tip locations. The local activation times from each measurement site are then color coded to generate an activation map that shows the progression of activation. An example is shown in Figure 15.9 for the right atrium during atrial tachycardia.

A separate reference catheter is usually placed in a stable position within the heart, such as the coronary sinus. An electrode on this catheter is used as a reference to correct for movement of the heart and motion of the patient. The operator can then navigate the mapping catheter without fluoroscopy to acquire multiple points that enhance the electrophysiological features and/or representation of the endocardial anatomy. In vitro tests have shown that endocardial positions can be resolved with an accuracy of 0.16 ± 0.02 mm, with the maximal range being 0.55 ± 0.07 mm. In vivo tests in swine showed that mapping points in the left ventricular endocardium were resolved with an accuracy of 0.54 ± 0.05 mm, with a maximal range of 1.26 ± 0.08 mm [72].

The CARTO system requires a stable rhythm and a stable reference point. If the reference point moves then the entire surface must be remapped. Because of this, unstable arrhythmias can be extremely difficult to map.

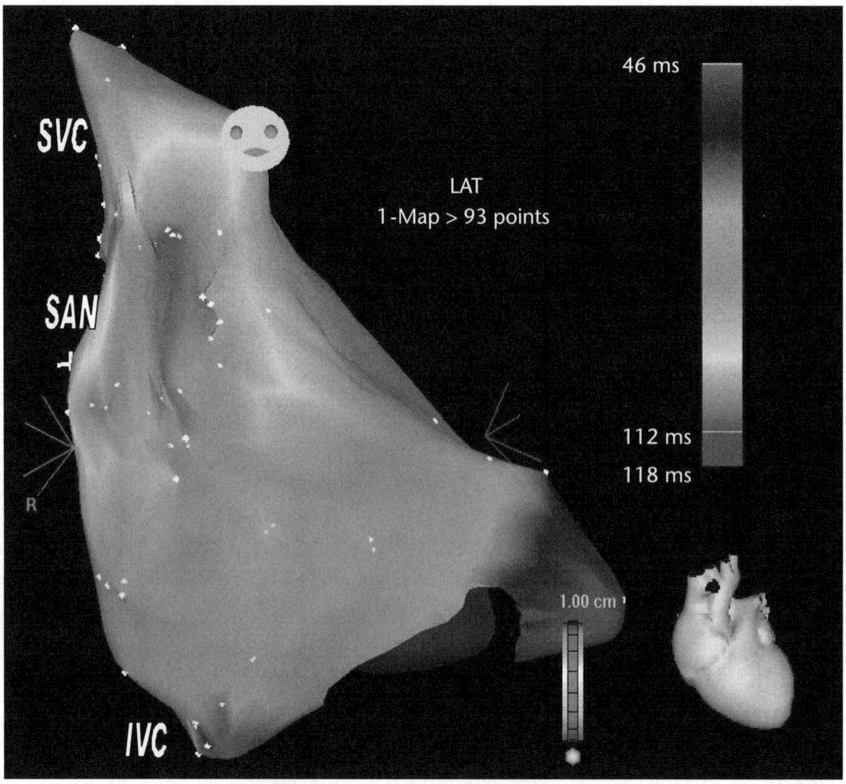

Figure 15.9 Three-dimensional map of the right atrium during atrial tachycardia originating near the sinus node. The top of the figure represents the superior vena cava and the bottom represents the inferior vena cava. SAN: sino-atrial node; IVC: inferior vena cava; SVC: superior vena cava.

Clinical Applications

Electro-anatomical mapping systems are often used to enhance the success of ablation therapy, particularly in cases of complex cardiac arrhythmias or when cardiac anatomy makes it difficult for a catheter to reach an ablation target. For example, Figure 15.10 shows an atypical atrial flutter in a pediatric patient that could not be ablated using conventional techniques. The flutter was successfully treated using the CARTO system to accurately map scar tissue to identify the critical isthmus of conduction that was causing the atrial flutter. This isthmus was then successfully ablated to eliminate the arrhythmia.

Another example is shown in Figure 15.11, which illustrates a junctional tachycardia originating near the AV node. The CARTO system provided accurate electroanatomical mapping and helped identify the earliest activation of the tachycardia in relationship to the AV node and His bundle using 3D images. This is very useful to perform the ablation and successfully eliminate the tachycardia without damaging the AV node or His bundle. Keeping track of the location of earliest activation in relationship to the other structures is of greatest importance and key to the success of the procedure.

Many clinical arrhythmias have been successfully mapped using the CARTO system. This system has consistently reduced the time of fluoroscopy and therefore the amount of radiation exposed to a patient, as well as the overall time of a procedure with the outcome still remaining excellent [73, 74]. In one study, ablations of four different tachycardias (AV node reentrant tachycardia, atrial tachycardia/

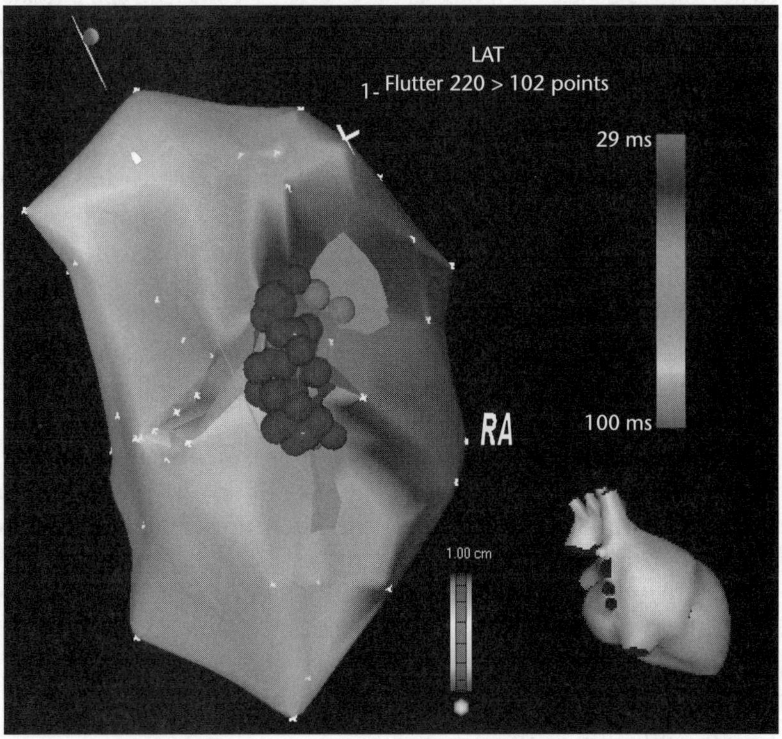

Figure 15.10 Atypical atrial flutter. The map shows the critical isthmus of a reentrant tachycardia between two areas of scar tissue. The scar tissue is shown as gray areas above and below the ablation sites (dark balls), which are placed within the critical isthmus. Right atrial anatomy is depicted and rotated to show a caudal view to reveal the isthmus. RA: right atrium.

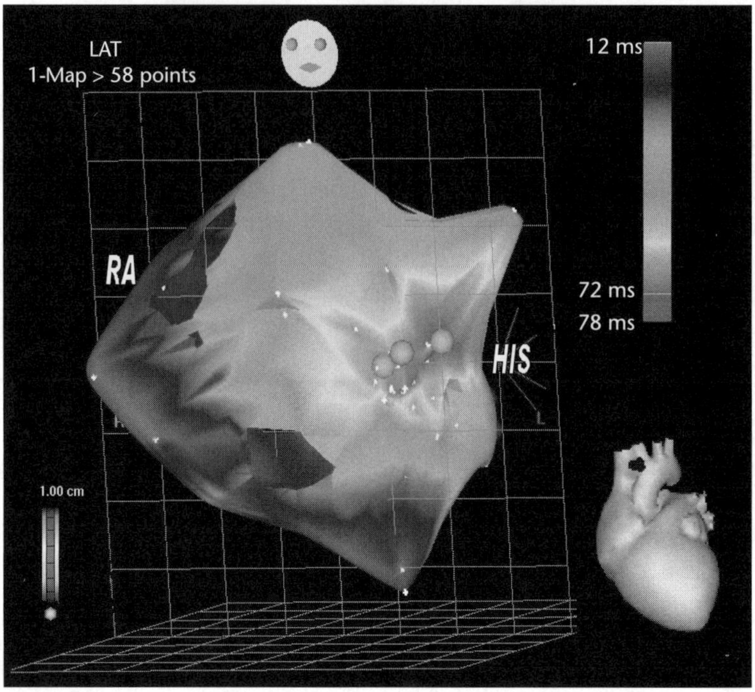

Figure 15.11 Electro-anatomical map of the right atrium. This patient had a focal atrial tachycardia originating near the AV node. Using conventional mapping, the early site of activation was identified near the HIS bundle but it was difficult to determine where to apply ablation therapy without damaging the bundle. This was clarified using electro-anatomical mapping because the early site of activation and the location of the His bundle location were clearly identified. Tissue near the early site of activation, but not exactly on top of the His bundle, could then be ablated. RA: right atrium, HIS: His bundle location.

flutter, ventricular tachycardia, and bypass tract tachycardia) that were either augmented by conventional mapping or with the CARTO system were compared. Fluoroscopy time was shorted overall using the CARTO system: 10 ± 7 minutes versus 27 ± 15 minutes for AV node reentrant tachycardia ($p < 0.01$), 15 ± 12 minutes versus 34 ± 31 minutes for VT ($p < 0.05$), and 21 ± 14 min versus 53 ± 32 minutes for bypass tract tachycardia ($p < 0.01$). Procedure times were similar, except for cases of bypass tract tachycardia, which was shorter in the CARTO group, 4 ± 1.3 hours versus 5.5 ± 2.5 hours ($p < 0.01$) [74].

Electro-anatomical mapping seems to provide the greatest benefit for ablation procedures that electrically isolate the pulmonary veins for the treatment of atrial fibrillation. Pappone recently reported a new anatomic approach for curing atrial fibrillation using the CARTO system [75]. Since then, multiple investigators have published studies describing the effectiveness of electroanatomical mapping systems. Most recently, patients with chronic atrial fibrillation have been treated with circumferential pulmonary vein ablation using electro-anatomical mapping with a high therapeutic success rate: 74% of patients remained in normal sinus rhythm 1 year after ablation [76].

Substrate mapping can also be performed using the CARTO system. Areas with complex fractionated atrial electrograms represent a defined electrophysiologic substrate and are ideal ablation sites to eliminate atrial fibrillation and maintain normal sinus rhythm. Substrates for complex fractionated atrial electrograms can be mapped to identify ablation targets in patients with atrial fibrillation. The success of substrate mapping has recently been reported to be 81.4% in selected high-risk patients with atrial fibrillation [77].

15.2.2.2 Noncontact Endocardial Mapping Systems

Advanced three-dimensional mapping systems are currently being used in clinics for diagnosing and treating complex and sporadic arrhythmias. One such system has been developed by Endocardial Solutions (St. Jude Medical, Inc., St. Paul, Minnesota). It is known as the EnSite 3000 system and uses noncontact technology for sensing local electrograms from endocardial tissue.

Noncontact mapping was first described by Taccardi and colleages in 1987. That group used arrays of unipolar electrodes deployed freely within a canine cardiac chamber to record electrograms [78]. The technique to detect such far-field potentials is based on an inverse solution of Laplace's equation using a boundary element method. To compensate for potential distortions in the detected electrograms, stability was provided by applying a mathematical constraint, which has a physiological basis, to the solution using a customized version of a technique called *regularization* [79]. Such noncontact mapping technology has been developed to augment cardiac ablation therapy.

Conventional techniques for clinical cardiac mapping involve advancing several catheters into the chambers of the heart and maneuvering them to map the local activation sequences of the cardiac muscle. Using a single-point contact catheter mapping technique to map certain arrhythmias can be time-consuming and the acquired data has limited spatial resolution. The high-resolution, three-dimensional, color display provided by the EnSite 3000 provides for faster recognition of complex cardiac arrhythmias. Essentially, the system provides a real-time virtual image of the electrical activity of the heart without contacting the heart's surface. The system is able to reconstruct electrograms for up to 3,000 sites, if specified by the electrophysiologist, and display them as three-dimensional maps of the heart.

Methods

The EnSite 3000 system has a locator known as EnGuide that provides a real-time display of the precise location of the ablation catheter during the procedure. The main catheter used for mapping is the EnSite Array catheter, shown in Figure 15.12. This is a noncontact, single-use, multielectrode array that can be placed transvenously into the chamber of interest, usually the right atrium. The EnSite Array catheter is comprised of an inflatable polyurethane balloon (1.8 × 4.5 cm, 7.5 ml) within a mechanically expandable multielectrode array. The multielectrode array contains a wire braid of 64 electrodes. The catheter is inserted over a standard guide-wire into a chamber of the heart. The wire braid is then mechanically expanded and the balloon residing under the wire braid is inflated with a radio-opaque solution to form an ellipsoidal multielectrode array.

A single-point diagnotic EnSite catheter is also inserted into the chamber to aide in establishing the chamber's spatial boundaries. The multielectrode braid array collects data used to compute more than 3,000 points of the heart chamber's

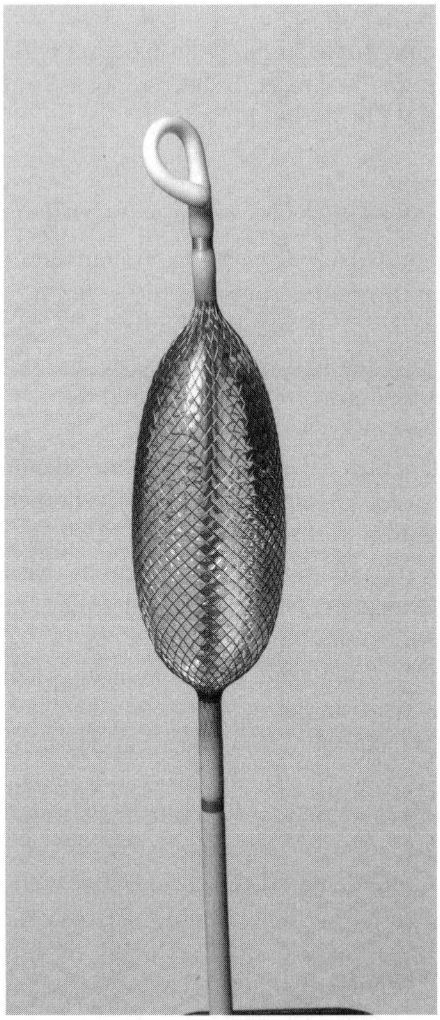

Figure 15.12 The EnSite Array. This multielectrode braid array is used to record electrical potentials within a chamber of the heart. Those recordings are processed by the EnSite 3000 Electrophysiology Workstation to reconstruct electrical activity for more than 3,000 points on the inner surface of the chamber. (Image used with permission from St. Jude Medical.)

electrical activity in the span of a few heartbeats by gathering a large amount of the electrical conduction information from the entire chamber and transmitting this information through the wire braid back down the catheter shaft to the EnSite 3000 Electrophysiology Workstation [79].

The main advantage of using this system is that relatively high-density mapping can be generated, even from a single beat of tachycardia. This feature is particularly helpful when mapping fast activation sequences of atrial tachycardias as well as sporadic ventricular tachycardias.

15.2.2.3 Potential Adverse Events Using Three-Dimensional Mapping Systems

Adverse complications with noncontact mapping and electro-anatomical mapping systems have been reported to include thromboembolic events, damage to blood vessels or valves, hematoma at the site of entry, infection, cardiac tamponade, cardiac irritability, hemothorax, and hypotension. These complications may arise using either conventional mapping catheters or 3D mapping catheters. The catheters could also perforate a wall of the heart or cause cardiac arrhythmias if they are not properly positioned during the procedure. In addition, simply inserting catheters into the body could result in thrombus formation, injury to blood vessels, and create an entry point for infection. Many techniques are used to minimize the above complications and they are explained in Josephson's textbook *Clinical Cardiac Electrophysiology, Techniques and Interpretations*, Third Edition [80].

15.2.3 Image-Guided Therapy for Cardiac Arrhythmias

15.2.3.1 Atrial Flutter

Atrial flutter is a common arrhythmia typically caused by large reentrant circuits in the right atrium. An example of successful treatment of atrial flutter using catheter ablation is shown in Figure 15.13. An area of slow conduction was identified in the lower right atrium at the inferior vena cava-tricuspid annulus (IVC-TA) isthmus. This particular area was the target for ablation, which was successful in terminating the reentrant activity and cured the atrial flutter.

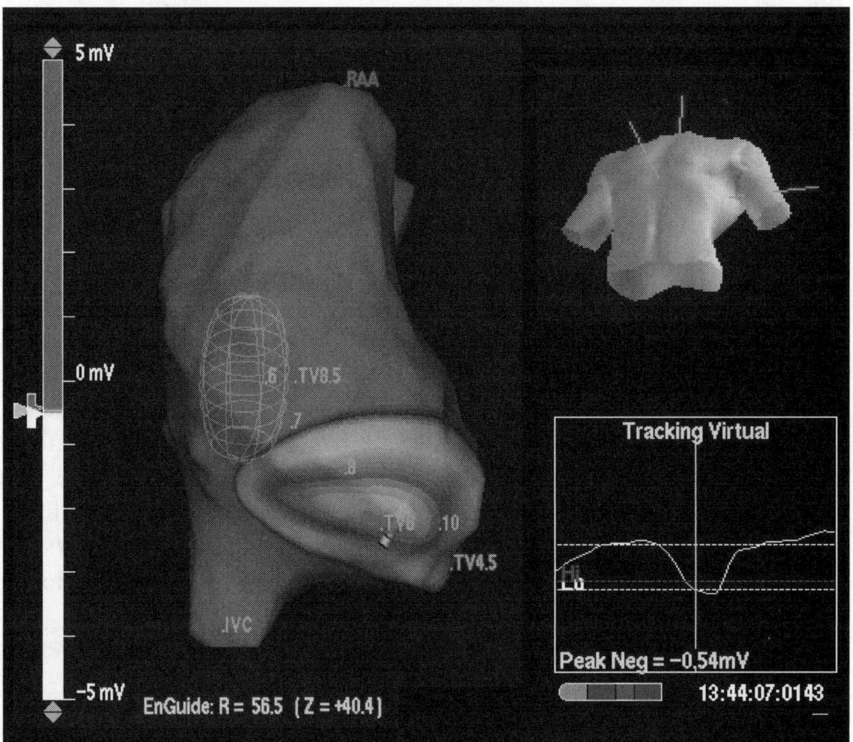

Figure 15.13 Noncontact mapping during atrial flutter. An activation map shows that electrical activation occurs at the tricuspid valve/inferior vena cava isthmus. This is the area where successful ablation was performed to terminate the tachycardia. The patient had no recurrences after 6 months of follow up. IVC: inferior vena cava, RAA: right atrial appendage, TV6: tricuspid valve at the 6 o'clock position in a left anterior oblique view obtained by fluoroscopy.

The success rate of treatment using catheter ablation at the IVC-TA isthmus using noncontact mapping has been reported to be 97% [81]. The three-dimensional activation sequence and isthmus conduction were delineated during ongoing atrial flutter and paced rhythms. During follow-up after 15.9 ± 5.9 months, two atrial flutter recurrences (5.8%) occurred. A gap of the resumed conduction through the IVC-TA isthmus was delineated as a mechanism of recurrence and was ablated. Noncontact mapping allowed for reconstruction of the global activation patterns in typical and atypical atrial flutter [81].

15.2.3.2 Focal Atrial Tachycardia

Focal atrial tachycardia originates from small areas in the atrium, such as the crista terminalis, triangle of Koch, and right atrial free wall. It can be treated with radiofrequency ablation using single catheter techniques. Radiofrequency energy is usually applied at the earliest activation site or at the proximal portion of preferential conduction from the origin of the tachycardia. Using noncontact mapping, Higa et al. reported a 91.7% success rate of therapy for a variety of atrial tachycardias, with a mean follow-up time per patient of 8 ± 5 months [82].

15.2.3.3 Ventricular Tachycardia

Monomorphic ventricular tachycardias can be ablated using catheter techniques. Some patients with ventricular tachycardia originating within the right ventricular outflow tract (RVOT) are difficult to treat because of difficulties in mapping the outflow tract to identify the reentrant pathway. Noncontact mapping has been useful in this situation to safely and effectively guide ablation therapy in patients with difficult to treat RVOT ventricular tachycardia. The main reason that noncontact maps are effective is that 3,000 points of activation can be instantaneously visualized as a 3D image, rather than one point at a time being compared to the electrocardiograms of the tachycardia. At times, the tachycardia is nonsustained and mapping point by point may take hours. However, with 3D noncontact mapping, a single beat of tachycardia can be used to map its point of origin. Using noncontact mapping, Friedman et al. reported a 90% success rate in 10 patients with RVOT ventricular tachycardia that was difficult to treat using conventional mapping. With a mean follow-up time of 11 months, seven of nine patients were cured of the arrhythmia. Both patients in whom a blinded reviewer predicted failure had arrhythmia recurrence: one due to an epicardial origin with multiple endocardial exit sites and the other due to discordance between the site of lesion placement and the site of early activation in the noncontact map [83].

A three-dimensional map of a premature ventricular contraction originating from the RVOT of a patient suffering from ventricular tachycardia is shown in Figure 15.14. This particular site was the source of multiple episodes of ventricular tachycardia and was the target for ablation therapy. The patient was quite symptomatic prior to the procedure, despite treatment with a high dosage of beta-blockers. The patient was cured of the ventricular tachycardia after ablating tissue at the early site of activation shown in the image. Noncontact mapping reduced the time of the

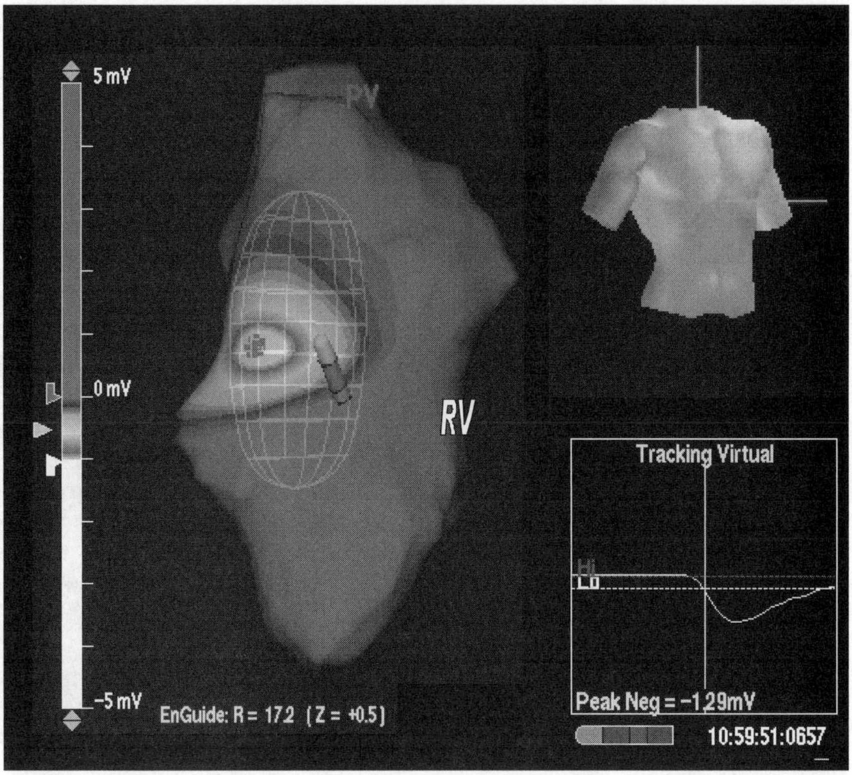

Figure 15.14 Noncontact right ventricular map during a premature ventricular contraction. The site of earliest activation denotes origin of the premature ventricular contractions. The ablation of tissue at this site was successful in eliminating the tachycardia. The use of noncontact mapping minimized patient exposure to radiation during the procedure. PV: pulmonic valve; RV: right ventricle.

procedure and enhanced the efficacy of the ablation by providing high-resolution mapping for accurate localization of the arrhythmia source.

15.2.3.4 Atrial Fibrillation

Atrial fibrillation is the arrhythmia most often treated by cardiologists. Catheter ablation techniques to cure the arrhythmia are currently being performed throughout the world. In a majority of cases, the origin of atrial fibrillation is located within the pulmonary veins [7]. Ectopic beats originating from the pulmonary veins initiate frequent paroxysms of atrial fibrillation and can be treated using radiofrequency ablation. The success of the ablation therapy is dependent upon the accuracy of representing both the anatomy of the left atrium and the location of the pulmonary veins. The EnSite NavX system (Endocardial Solutions, St. Jude Medical, Inc., St. Paul, Minnesota) is an advanced navigation and visualization system that is widely used for this particular purpose.

An EnSite NavX map acquired during an ablation procedure for atrial fibrillation is shown in Figure 15.15. Ablation lesions were circumferentially placed to electrically isolate the pulmonary veins from the left atrium. One advantage of the

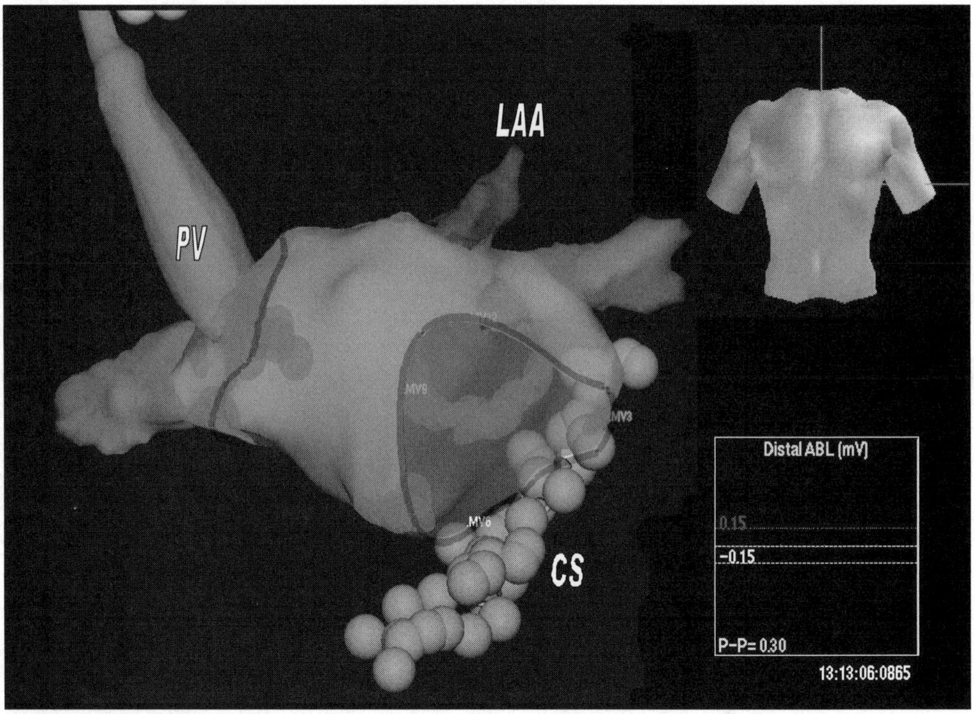

Figure 15.15 A three-dimensional map generated during an ablation procedure for atrial fibrillation using EnSite NavX Navigation and Visualization Technology (St. Jude Medical).

EnSite NavX system is that it is compatible with any electrophysiological catheter available to the operator [84].

The EnSite NavX system displays the three-dimensional position of multiple mapping catheters using triangulation. Essentially, multiple orthogonally located skin electrodes are placed on the patient and a low-level 5.6-kHz current is applied through them. The voltage generated by this current and impedance is recorded by each electrode on the catheter. This data, plus data from a reference electrode, allows the distance of each electrode from each skin patch to be determined by triangulation. The three-dimensional geometry of an endocardial surface can be mapped by moving the catheter along the surface. Three-dimensional images of the surface are then rendered and displayed. Additional detail can be obtained by correlating the mapped geometry with a previously acquired three-dimensional image generated by CT or MRI. With this imaging technology ablation therapy can be accurately applied to the left atrium and/or pulmonary veins for effective treatment of atrial fibrillation [84].

15.3 Summary

Fluorescence imaging is a proven experimental tool for recording the dynamics of electrical excitation in cardiac tissue at high spatiotemporal resolution. Critical details regarding the mechanistic influence of ectopic foci, reentrant circuits, and local ischemia during arrhythmias can be obtained using the fluorescence techniques described in this chapter. Although, for now, the development of transmembrane potential imaging and $[Ca^{+2}]_i$ transient imaging for clinical use would be very difficult. These modes are used primarily for laboratory research, where animal tissue can be exposed and stained with fluorescent probes in nonsurvival studies. On the other hand, NADH imaging records endogenous tissue fluorescence and recent work has developed fiber optic probes for measuring levels of NADH in vivo from small areas within various organs, including the heart [85, 86].

Whole-heart fluorescence imaging of explanted human hearts, obtained at the time of cardiac transplantation, can provide critical information for understanding clinically relevant phenomena. Tissue for these studies is very difficult to obtain, but recent transmembrane potential imaging of human hearts has recently explained a mechanism of AVNRT [9]. Other recent studies have described rotor formation, wave breaks, and fibrillatory conduction in human ventricles [87].

In the clinic, three-dimensional mapping systems are frequently used to visualize electrical excitation in patients suffering from arrhythmias to enhance the success of ablation procedures. Each mapping system has a primary application and they all have particular strengths and weaknesses, as discussed above. When planning an ablation procedure, an imaging system is selected by the type of arrhythmia to be targeted. Clinical mapping systems provide a wealth of data and can substantially facilitate mapping efforts, reduce procedure time, and reduce exposure of the patient to radiation during fluoroscopy. However, careful interpretation of the data and strict adherence to basic electrophysiological principles are still required to ensure successful cardiac ablation therapy.

Acknowledgments

This work was supported in part by a Biomedical Engineering Research grant from the Whitaker Foundation (Matthew W. Kay), an American Heart Association Beginning-Grant-In-Aid (Matthew W. Kay), National Institutes of Health grant HL76722 (Narine A. Sarvazyan), and National Institutes of Health grant HL64184 (Jack M. Rogers).

References

[1] Goldreyer, B. N., and J. T. Bigger, Jr., "Site of Reentry in Paroxysmal Supraventricular Tachycardia in Man," *Circulation*, Vol. 43, 1971, pp. 15–26.

[2] Krahn, A. D., et al., "Progressive Anterior Ablation in the Coronary Sinus Region: Evidence to Support the Presence of a 'Slow Pathway' Input in Normal Patients?" *Circulation*, Vol. 96, 1997, pp. 3477–3483.

[3] Eisenberger, M., et al., "Atrioventricular Node Reentrant Tachycardia Ablation in a Patient with Congenitally Corrected Transposition of the Great Vessels Using the CARTO Mapping System," *J. Interv. Card. Electrophysiol.*, Vol. 19, 2007, pp. 129–132.

[4] Akhtar, M., et al., "Atrioventricular Nodal Reentry. Clinical, Electrophysiological, and Therapeutic Considerations," *Circulation*, Vol. 88, 1993, pp. 282–295.

[5] Ruder, M. A., et al., "Clinical and Electrophysiologic Characterization of Automatic Junctional Tachycardia in Adults," *Circulation*, Vol. 73, 1986, pp. 930–937.

[6] Nattel, S., "Basic Electrophysiology of the Pulmonary Veins and Their Role in Atrial Fibrillation: Precipitators, Perpetuators, and Perplexers," *J. Cardiovasc. Electrophysiol.*, Vol. 14, 2003, pp. 1372–1375.

[7] Haissaguerre, M., et al., "Spontaneous Initiation of Atrial Fibrillation by Ectopic Beats Originating in the Pulmonary Veins," *N. Engl. J. Med.*, Vol. 339, 1998, pp. 659–666.

[8] Jais, P., et al., "A Focal Source of Atrial Fibrillation Treated by Discrete Radiofrequency Ablation," *Circulation*, Vol. 95, 1997, pp. 572–576.

[9] Hucker, W. J., et al., "Images in Cardiovascular Medicine. Optical Mapping of the Human Atrioventricular Junction," *Circulation*, Vol. 117, 2008, pp. 1474–1477.

[10] Hucker, W. J., V. P. Nikolski, and I. R. Efimov, "Optical Mapping of the Atrioventricular Junction," *J. Electrocardiol.*, Vol. 38, 2005, pp. 121–125.

[11] Choi, B. R., and G. Salama, "Optical Mapping of Atrioventricular Node Reveals a Conduction Barrier Between Atrial and Nodal Cells," *Am. J. Physiol.*, Vol. 274, 1998, pp. H829–H845.

[12] Wu, J., et al., "Mechanisms Underlying the Reentrant Circuit of Atrioventricular Nodal Reentrant Tachycardia in Isolated Canine Atrioventricular Nodal Preparation Using Optical Mapping," *Circ. Res.*, Vol. 88, 2001, pp. 1189–1195.

[13] Rosenbaum, D. S., and J. Jalife, *Optical Mapping of Cardiac Excitation and Arrhythmias*, Armonk, NY: Futura Publishing Company, Inc., 2001.

[14] Efimov, I. R., V. P. Nikolski, and G. Salama, "Optical Imaging of the Heart," *Circ. Res.*, Vol. 95, 2004, pp. 21–33.

[15] Gray, R. A., A. M. Pertsov, and J. Jalife, "Spatial and Temporal Organization During Cardiac Fibrillation," *Nature*, Vol. 392, 1998, pp. 75–78.

[16] Witkowski, F. X., et al., "Spatiotemporal Evolution of Ventricular Fibrillation," *Nature*, Vol. 392, 1998, pp. 78–82.

[17] Kay, M. W., et al., "Lifetimes of Epicardial Rotors in Panoramic Optical Maps of Fibrillating Swine Ventricles," *Am. J. Physiol. Heart Circ. Physiol.*, Vol. 291, 2006, pp. H1935–H1941.

[18] Choi, B. R., et al., "Life Span of Ventricular Fibrillation Frequencies," *Circ. Res.*, Vol. 91, 2002, pp. 339–345.

[19] Cheng, Y., et al., "Virtual Electrode-Induced Reexcitation: A Mechanism of Defibrillation," *Circ. Res.*, Vol. 85, 1999, pp. 1056–1066.

[20] Laurita, K. R., and A. Singal, "Mapping Action Potentials and Calcium Transients Simultaneously from the Intact Heart," *Am. J. Physiol. Heart Circ. Physiol.*, Vol. 280, 2001, pp. H2053–H2060.

[21] Kay, M., et al., "Locations of Ectopic Beats Coincide with Spatial Gradients of NADH in a Regional Model of Low-Flow Reperfusion," *Am. J. Physiol. Heart Circ. Physiol.*, Vol. 294, 2008, pp. H2400–H2405.

[22] Salama, G., and M. Morad, "Merocyanine 540 as an Optical Probe of Transmembrane Electrical Activity in the Heart," *Science*, Vol. 191, 1976, pp. 485–487.

[23] Morad, M., and G. Salama, "Optical Probes of Membrane Potential in Heart Muscle," *J. Physiol.*, Vol. 292, 1979, pp. 267–295.

[24] Vetter, F. J., et al., "Epicardial Fiber Organization in Swine Right Ventricle and Its Impact on Propagation," *Circ. Res.*, Vol. 96, 2005, pp. 244–251.

[25] Fast, V. G., "Simultaneous Optical Imaging of Membrane Potential and Intracellular Calcium," *J. Electrocardiol.*, Vol. 38, 2005, pp. 107–112.

[26] Mills, W. R., et al., "Optical Mapping of Late Myocardial Infarction in Rats," *Am. J. Physiol. Heart Circ. Physiol.*, Vol. 290, 2006, pp. H1298–H1306.

[27] Himel, H. D., and S. B. Knisley, "Imaging of Cardiac Movement Using Ratiometric and Nonratiometric Optical Mapping: Effects of Ischemia and 2, 3-Butaneodione Monoxime," *IEEE Transactions on Medical Imaging*, Vol. 25, 2006, pp. 122–127.

[28] Bers, D. M., "Cardiac Excitation-Contraction Coupling," *Nature*, Vol. 415, 2002, pp. 198–205.

[29] Bers, D. M., *Excitation-Contraction Coupling and Cardiac Contractile Force*, 2nd ed., New York: Springer, 2001.

[30] Litwin, S. E., D. Zhang, and J. H. Bridge, "Dyssynchronous ca(2+) Sparks in Myocytes from Infarcted Hearts," *Circ. Res.*, Vol. 87, 2000, pp. 1040–1047.

[31] Katra, R. P., and K. R. Laurita, "Cellular Mechanism of Calcium-Mediated Triggered Activity in the Heart," *Circ. Res.*, Vol. 96, 2005, pp. 535–542.

[32] MacGowan, G. A., et al., "Rhod-2 Based Measurements of Intracellular Calcium in the Perfused Mouse Heart: Cellular and Subcellular Localization and Response to Positive Inotropy," *J. Biomed. Opt.*, Vol. 6, 2001, pp. 23–30.

[33] Del Nido, P. J., et al., "Fluorescence Measurement of Calcium Transients in Perfused Rabbit Heart Using Rhod 2," *Am. J. Physiol.*, Vol. 274, 1998, pp. H728–H741.

[34] Agladze, K., et al., "Interaction Between Spiral and Paced Waves in Cardiac Tissue," *Am. J. Physiol. Heart Circ. Physiol.*, Vol. 293, 2007, pp. H503–H513.

[35] Arutunyan, A., et al., "Behavior of Ectopic Surface: Effects of Beta-Adrenergic Stimulation and Uncoupling," *Am. J. Physiol. Heart Circ. Physiol.*, 2003.

[36] Arutunyan, A., L. M. Swift, and N. Sarvazyan, "Initiation and Propagation of Ectopic Waves: Insights from an In Vitro Model of Ischemia-Reperfusion Injury," *Am. J. Physiol. Heart Circ. Physiol.*, Vol. 283, 2002, pp. H741–H749.

[37] Janse, M. J., and A. L. Wit, "Electrophysiological Mechanisms of Ventricular Arrhythmias Resulting from Myocardial Ischemia and Infarction," *Physiol. Rev.*, Vol. 69, 1989, pp. 1049–1169.

[38] Kleber, A. G., et al., "Changes in Conduction Velocity During Acute Ischemia in Ventricular Myocardium of the Isolated Porcine Heart," *Circulation*, Vol. 73, 1986, pp. 189–198.

[39] Kaplinsky, E., et al., "Two Periods of Early Ventricular Arrhythmia in the Canine Acute Myocardial Infarction Model," *Circulation*, Vol. 60, 1979, pp. 397–403.

[40] Coronel, R., et al., "Heterogeneities in [K+]o and TQ Potential and the Inducibility of Ventricular Fibrillation During Acute Regional Ischemia in the Isolated Perfused Porcine Heart," *Circulation*, Vol. 92, 1995, pp. 120–129.

[41] Chance, B., "Pyridine Nucleotide as an Indicator of the Oxygen Requirements for Energy-Linked Functions of Mitochondria," *Circ. Res.*, Vol. 38, 1976, pp. I31–I38.

[42] Barlow, C. H., D. A. Rorvik, and J. J. Kelly, "Imaging Epicardial Oxygen," *Ann. Biomed. Eng.*, Vol. 26, 1998, pp. 76–85.

[43] Barlow, C. H., and B. Chance, "Ischemic Areas in Perfused Rat Hearts: Measurement by NADH Fluorescence Photography," *Science*, Vol. 193, 1976, pp. 909–910.

[44] Salama, G., R. Lombardi, and J. Elson, "Maps of Optical Action Potentials and NADH Fluorescence in Intact Working Hearts," *Am. J. Physiol.*, Vol. 252, 1987, pp. H384–H394.

[45] Steenbergen, C., et al., "Heterogeneity of the Hypoxic State in Perfused Rat Heart," *Circ Res.*, Vol. 41, 1977, pp. 606–615.

[46] Swift, L., et al., "Controlled Regional Hypoperfusion in Langendorff Heart Preparations," *Physiol. Meas.*, Vol. 29, 2008, pp. 269–279.

[47] Kay, M., et al., "Locations of Ectopic Beats Coincide with Spatial Gradients of NADH in a Regional Model of Low-Flow Reperfusion," *Am. J. Physiol. Heart Circ. Physiol.*, Vol. 294, 2008, pp. 2400–2405.

[48] Tang, L., et al., "Intracellular Calcium Dynamics at the Core of Endocardial Stationary Spiral Waves in Langendorff-Perfused Rabbit Hearts," *Am. J. Physiol. Heart Circ. Physiol.*, 2008.

[49] Saba, S., et al., "Dual-Dye Optical Mapping After Myocardial Infarction: Does the Site of Ventricular Stimulation Alter the Properties of Electrical Propagation?" *J. Cardiovasc. Electrophysiol.*, Vol. 19, 2008, pp. 197–202.

[50] Kay, M. W., P. M. Amison, and J. M. Rogers, "Three-Dimensional Surface Reconstruction and Panoramic Optical Mapping of Large Hearts," *IEEE Transactions on Biomedical Engineering*, Vol. 51, 2004, pp. 1219–1229.

[51] Bray, M. A., S. F. Lin, and J. P. Wikswo, Jr., "Three-Dimensional Surface Reconstruction and Fluorescent Visualization of Cardiac Activation," *IEEE Transactions on Biomedical Engineering*, Vol. 47, 2000, pp. 1382–1391.

[52] Qu, F., et al., "Three-Dimensional Panoramic Imaging of Cardiac Arrhythmias in Rabbit Heart," *J. Biomed. Opt.*, Vol. 12, 2007.

[53] Rogers, J. M., et al., "Panoramic Optical Mapping Reveals Continuous Epicardial Reentry During Ventricular Fibrillation in the Isolated Swine Heart," *Biophys. J.*, Vol. 92, 2007, pp. 1090–1095.

[54] Kay, M., et al., "Lifetimes of Epicardial Rotors in Panoramic Optical Maps of Fibrillating Swine Ventricles," *Am. J. Physiol. Heart Circ. Physiol.*, Vol. 291, 2006, pp. H1935-41.

[55] Rogers, J., et al., "Epicardial Wavefronts Arise from Widely Distributed Transient Sources During Ventricular Fibrillation in the Isolated Swine Heart," *New Journal of Physics*, Vol. 10, 2008, pp. 1–14.

[56] Kay, M. W., and J. M. Rogers, "Mapping a Moving Target," *J. Cardiovasc. Electrophysiol.*, Vol. 14, 2003, pp. 1085–1086.

[57] Girouard, S. D., K. R. Laurita, and D. S. Rosenbaum, "Unique Properties of Cardiac Action Potentials Recorded with Voltage-Sensitive Dyes," *J. Cardiovasc. Electrophysiol.*, Vol. 7, 1996, pp. 1024–1038.

[58] Efimov, I. R., et al., "Activation and Repolarization Patterns Are Governed by Different Structural Characteristics of Ventricular Myocardium: Experimental Study with Voltage-Sensitive Dyes and Numerical Simulations," *J. Cardiovasc. Electrophysiol.*, Vol. 7, 1996, pp. 512–530.

[59] Banville, I., and R. A. Gray, "Effect of Action Potential Duration and Conduction Velocity Restitution and Their Spatial Dispersion on Alternans and the Stability of Arrhythmias," *J. Cardiovasc. Electrophysiol.*, Vol. 13, 2002, pp. 1141–1149.

[60] Wu, J., et al., "Cytochalasin D as Excitation-Contraction Uncoupler for Optically Mapping Action Potentials in Wedges of Ventricular Myocardium," *J. Cardiovasc. Electrophysiol.*, Vol. 9, 1998, pp. 1336–1347.

[61] Fedorov, V. V., et al., "Application of Blebbistatin as an Excitation-Contraction Uncoupler for Electrophysiologic Study of Rat and Rabbit Hearts," *Heart Rhythm*, Vol. 4, 2007, pp. 619–626.

[62] Zaitsev, A. V., et al., "Wavebreak Formation During Ventricular Fibrillation in the Isolated, Regionally Ischemic Pig Heart," *Circ. Res.*, Vol. 92, 2003, pp. 546–553.

[63] Laurita, K., et al., "Modulated Dispersion Explains Changes in Arrhythmia Vulnerability During Premature Stimulation of the Heart," *Circulation*, Vol. 98, 1998, pp. 2774–2780.

[64] Baker, L. C., et al., "Effects of Mechanical Uncouplers, Diacetyl Monoxime, and Cytochalasin-D on the Electrophysiology of Perfused Mouse Hearts," *Am. J. Physiol. Heart Circ. Physiol.*, Vol. 287, 2004, pp. H1771–H1779.

[65] Baker, L. C., et al., "Enhanced Dispersion of Repolarization and Refractoriness in Transgenic Mouse Hearts Promotes Reentrant Ventricular Tachycardia," *Circ. Res.*, Vol. 86, 2000, pp. 396–407.

[66] Girouard, S. D., et al., "Optical Mapping in a New Guinea Pig Model of Ventricular Tachycardia Reveals Mechanisms for Multiple Wavelengths in a Single Reentrant Circuit," *Circulation*, Vol. 93, 1996, pp. 603–613.

[67] Liu, Y., et al., "Effects of Diacetyl Monoxime on the Electrical Properties of Sheep and Guinea Pig Ventricular Muscle," *Cardiovasc. Res.*, Vol. 27, 1993, pp. 1991–1997.

[68] Knisley, S. B., et al., "Ratiometry of Transmembrane Voltage-Sensitive Fluorescent Dye Emission in Hearts," *Am. J. Physiol. Heart Circ. Physiol.*, Vol. 279, 2000, pp. H1421–H1433.

[69] Kong, W., et al. "Emission Ratiometry for Simultaneous Calcium and Action Potential Measurements with Coloaded Dyes in Rabbit Hearts: Reduction of Motion and Drift," *J. Cardiovasc. Electrophysiol.*, Vol. 14, 2003, pp. 76–82.

[70] Bhakta, D., and J. M. Miller, "Principles of Electroanatomic Mapping," *Indian Pacing Electrophysiol. J.*, Vol. 8, 2008, pp. 32–50.

[71] Ben-Haim, S. A., "Non-Fluoroscopic Electroanatomical Cardiac Mapping," in D. P. Zipes and J. Jalife, (eds.), *Cardiac Electrophysiology: From Cell to Bedside, Vol. 92*, 3rd ed., Philadelphia, PA: Saunders, 2000, pp. 834–839.

[72] Gepstein, L., G. Hayam, and S. A. Ben-Haim, "A Novel Method for Nonfluoroscopic Catheter-Based Electroanatomical Mapping of the Heart. In Vitro and In Vivo Accuracy Results," *Circulation*, Vol. 95, 1997, pp. 1611–1622.

[73] Rotter, M., et al., "Reduction of Fluoroscopy Exposure and Procedure Duration During Ablation of Atrial Fibrillation Using a Novel Anatomical Navigation System," *Eur. Heart J.*, Vol. 26, 2005, pp. 1415–1421.

[74] Khongphatthanayothin, A., E. Kosar, and K. Nademanee, "Nonfluoroscopic Three-Dimensional Mapping for Arrhythmia Ablation: Tool or Toy?" *J. Cardiovasc. Electrophysiol.*, Vol. 11, 2000, pp. 239–243.

[75] Pappone, C., et al., "Circumferential Radiofrequency Ablation of Pulmonary Vein Ostia: A New Anatomic Approach for Curing Atrial Fibrillation," *Circulation*, Vol. 102, 2000, pp. 2619–2628.

[76] Oral, H., et al., "Circumferential Pulmonary-Vein Ablation for Chronic Atrial Fibrillation," *N. Engl. J. Med.*, Vol. 354, 2006, pp. 934–941.

[77] Nademanee, K., et al., "Clinical Outcomes of Catheter Substrate Ablation for High-Risk Patients with Atrial Fibrillation," *J. Am. Coll. Cardiol.*, Vol. 51, 2008, pp. 843–849.

[78] Taccardi, B., et al., "A New Intracavitary Probe for Detecting the Site of Origin of Ectopic Ventricular Beats During One Cardiac Cycle," *Circulation*, Vol. 75, 1987, pp. 272–281.

[79] Peters, N. S., R. J. Schilling, and D. W. Davies, "Non-Contact Endocardial Activation Mapping," in D. P. Zipes and J. Jalife, (eds.), *Cardiac Electrophysiology: From Cell to Bedside, Vol. 93*, 3rd ed., Philadelphia, PA: Saunders, 2000, pp. 839–843.

[80] Josephson, M. E., *Clinical Cardiac Electrophysiology: Techniques and Interpretations*, 3rd ed., Baltimore, MD: Lippincott Williams and Wilkins, 2002.

[81] Schneider, M. A., et al., "Noncontact Mapping-Guided Ablation of Atrial Flutter and Enhanced-Density Mapping of the Inferior Vena Caval-Tricuspid Annulus Isthmus," *Pacing Clin. Electrophysiol.*, Vol. 24, 2001, pp. 1755–1764.

[82] Higa, S., et al., "Focal Atrial Tachycardia: New Insight from Noncontact Mapping and Catheter Ablation," *Circulation*, Vol. 109, 2004, pp. 84–91.

[83] Friedman, P. A., et al., "Noncontact Mapping to Guide Ablation of Right Ventricular Outflow Tract Tachycardia," *J. Am. Coll. Cardiol.*, Vol. 39, 2002, pp. 1808–1812.

[84] Estner, H. L., et al., "Electrical Isolation of Pulmonary Veins in Patients with Atrial Fibrillation: Reduction of Fluoroscopy Exposure and Procedure Duration by the Use of a Non-Fluoroscopic Navigation System (NavX)," *Europace*, Vol. 8, 2006, pp. 583–587.

[85] Mayevsky, A., and B. Chance, "Oxidation-Reduction States of NADH In Vivo: From Animals to Clinical Use," *Mitochondrion*, Vol. 7, 2007, pp. 330–339.

[86] Mayevsky, A., and G. G. Rogatsky, "Mitochondrial Function In Vivo Evaluated by NADH Fluorescence: From Animal Models to Human Studies," *Am. J. Physiol. Cell Physiol.*, Vol. 292, 2007, pp. C615–C640.

[87] Nanthakumar, K., et al., "Optical Mapping of Langendorff-Perfused Human Hearts: Establishing a Model for the Study of Ventricular Fibrillation in Humans," *Am. J. Physiol. Heart Circ. Physiol.*, Vol. 293, 2007, pp. H875–H880.

CHAPTER 16

Percutaneous Image-Guided Needle-Based Procedures

Orpheus Kolokythas and Bill H. Warren

16.1 Introduction

In spite of the significant advances in image-based and other noninvasive diagnostic modalities, a definite diagnosis or verification of a suggested disease can often still only be obtained by chemical, microbiological, or pathologic analysis of fluid or tissue. Image-guided percutaneous procedures such as aspirations and biopsies have gained increased popularity over the last 30 years. Cross-sectional imaging modalities as a standard for needle guidance have widely replaced real-time fluoroscopy or incremental static radiographic imaging. However, selected indications for fluoroscopic guidance or plain film radiography guidance exist. Increased availability of modern imaging systems, better diagnostic image quality, rapid image acquisition and display as well as more sophisticated guidance tools have added to the safety of percutaneous procedures. The increased safety and ease of documentation of image-guided percutaneous nerve blocks (neurolysis) have generally replaced clinically guided approaches, which used to be performed by anatomic landmarks only.

This chapter will give an overview of the technical approaches to percutaneous diagnostic and therapeutic procedures such as aspirations, biopsies, and nerve blocks. Needle devices, guidance tools, and imaging modalities as well as various applications will be described.

16.2 Technical Equipment

For retrieval of fluid collections, needle-based and catheter-based approaches are utilized. For tissue biopsies, fine needle aspiration techniques or core needle devices are being used. Depending on the number of intended biopsy passes, the organ and the location of the lesion, and diagnostic goal, a coaxial versus a noncoaxial technique can be chosen for both fine and core needle biopsies.

Needles for percutaneous retrieval of specimen are available from 9 to 25 gauge (G) in lengths of 6 to 25 cm. So-called "fine needles" are defined as needles of 0.9 mm and smaller external diameter, usually referenced in terms of "gauge." While the metric system correlates ascending numbers with larger calibers of the device, the gauge system has an inverse relationship to the size (Table 16.1). For example, 0.7 mm in the metric system translates to 22G, while 0.9 mm corresponds to 20G.

When gauge numbers are given for a pipe without reference to a system, Birmingham Wire Gauge (BWG) is implied. Needles larger than 20G are usually referred to as "core needle" biopsy devices. However core needle biopsy devices are also available in smaller sizes up to 22G.

16.2.1 Fine Needle Devices

Fine needle devices are used to obtain small amounts of fluid or cells for cytological, microbiological, or chemical analysis. They are usually not sufficient to obtain tissue for histological evaluation. Fine needle devices are also the appropriate tools for nerve blocks, since only small volumes of agents are being injected for diagnostic or therapeutic purposes. While the diagnostic or therapeutic value of these procedures is very high, the small size of these needles yields a low rate of severe complications [1]. Samples of abdominal organs such as the pancreas or kidneys retrieved by fine needle aspirations may provide sensitivity and specificity for a malignant tissue diagnosis as high as 93% and 100%, respectively, by cytological evaluation [2, 3]. However for more challenging procedures such as lung biopsies of small lung nodules, the sensitivity for malignancy is significantly reduced to less than 70% [4].

A large variety of fine needle devices is available for percutaneous aspirations or tissue biopsies—they mostly have in common an outer cannula and an inner stylet. The inner stylet stiffens the hollow needle during the insertion and is helpful in minimizing unintended bending of the needle when transgressing firmer tissues. The hollow cannula contains the specimen when the needle is removed from the target or serves as a conduit to drain fluid.

Table 16.1 Steel Thickness Conversion Table (Gauge, Inches, Millimeters)

	Core Needle Devices					*Fine Needle Devices*			
	*B.W.G.**		*U.S.G***			*B.W.G.**		*U.S.G. ***	
Gauge No.	*inch*	*mm*	*inch*	*mm*	*Gauge No.*	*inch*	*mm*	*inch*	*mm*
6	.203	5.156	.2031	5.16	20	.035	.889	.0375	.953
7	.180	4.572	.1875	4.76	21	.032	.813	.0344	.873
8	.165	4.191	.1719	4.37	22	.028	.711	.0313	.794
9	.148	3.759	.1563	3.97	23	.025	.635	.0218	.714
10	.134	3.404	.1406	3.57	24	.022	.559	.0250	.635
11	.120	3.048	.1250	3.18	25	.020	.508	.0219	.556
12	.109	2.769	.1094	2.78	26	.018	.457	.0188	.478
13	.095	2.413	.0938	2.38	27	.016	.406	.0172	.437
14	.083	2.108	.0781	1.98	28	.014	.356	.0156	.396
15	.072	1.829	.0703	1.79	29	.013	.330	.0141	.358
16	.065	1.651	.0625	1.59	30	.012	.305	.0125	.318
17	.058	1.473	.0563	1.43	31	.010	.254	.0109	.277
18	.049	1.245	.0500	1.27	32	.009	.229	.0102	.259
19	.042	1.067	.0438	1.11	33	.008	.203	.0094	.239
					34	.007	.178	.0086	.218
					35	.005	.127	.0078	.198

*B.W.G = Birmingham Wire Gauge for iron and steel wire. **USG = US Standard Gauge for Stainless Steel.

Some examples of fine needles are given below.

Spinal needles are up to 10 cm long and designed for aspirations and injections of the vertebral canal but are also commonly used for aspirations or injections in other parts of the body, if not too deeply located. For superficial procedures simple needles, commonly used for intramuscular injections, are also used. They have a sharp beveled tip and are usually up to 4 cm long. The tip of both needle types has a coned shape to increase its sharpness (Quincke-type point) [Figure 16.1(a)].

Chiba needles have the same outer caliber as spinal needles, but a thinner outer cannula [Figure 16.1(b)]. They also carry an inner stylet, which is thicker than the one in spinal needles. Because of this design they accommodate a guiding wire if needed, which may be inserted in the same session immediately after diagnostic aspiration of a fluid collection in order to place a larger caliber drain. Chiba needles are more flat beveled than spinal needles, which may pose a challenge for mobile small targets such as lymph nodes in fatty tissue as they tend to bounce off the capsule as one is trying to position the needle inside the node.

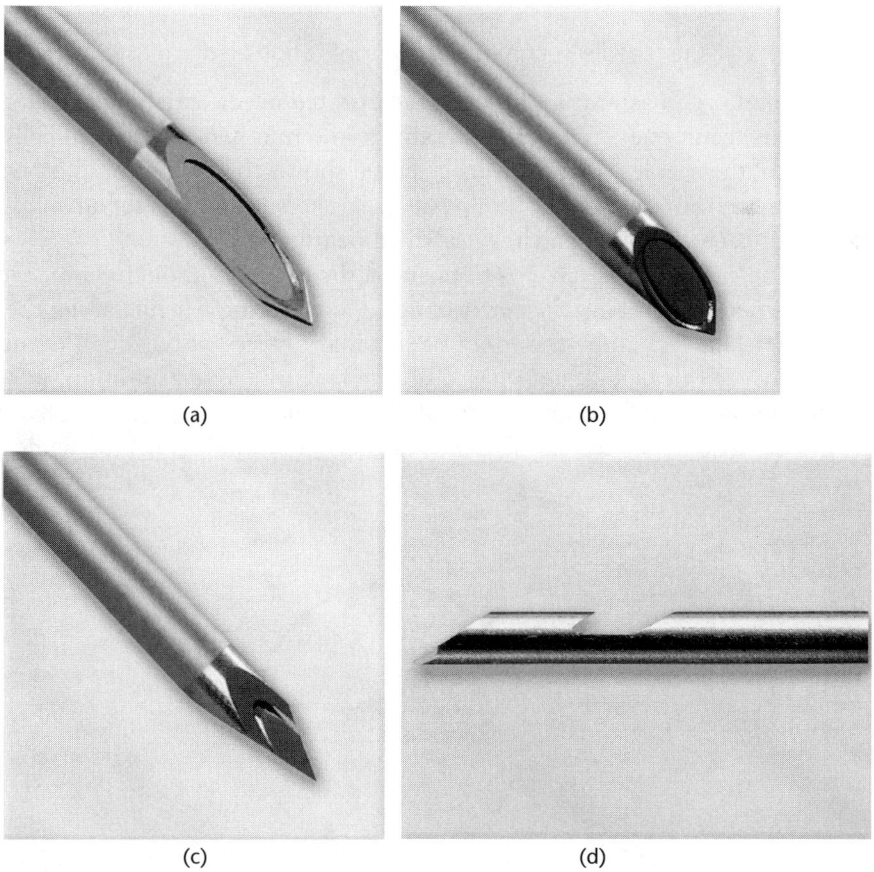

(a) (b) (c) (d)

Figure 16.1 Various tips of fine needles. (a) Spinal needle with Quincke tip; (b) Chiba needle; (c) Franseen needle; and (d) Westcott needle. The surface of needle tips in (a–c) are coated and designed to increase conspicuity when used with ultrasound guidance. (Courtesy of Angiotech Interventional, Gainesville, Florida, USA. © 2008 Medical Device Technologies, Inc. © 2008 Angiotech Pharmaceuticals Inc., All Rights Reserved, with permission.)

The Franseen needle has a very sharp cutting tip and serves almost as a cutting needle [Figure 16.1(c)]. The design of the tip allows for retrieval of a solid tissue block with potential for histopathologic evaluation.

The Westcott needle has a side-notch with the intent to maximize cell harvest on both forward and backward thrust [Figure 16.1(d)]. Its tip is very sharp and beveled.

Recently vacuum fine needles, such as the Sonopsy (Havel's, Inc., Cincinnati, Ohio) have become available, which may increase the number of cells obtained and may also result in small tissue blocks adequate for histological analysis (Figure 16.2).

Once inserted into the target tissue, such as a solid lesion within the breast or thyroid gland, a vacuum is engaged so that constant significant suction is applied as the sampling is carried out.

Other designs of devices and handles with the intent to increase constant vacuum while performing the procedure include specific handles that allow a better grip of the syringe and its plunger. Simpler models offer a built-in stop to hold sustained suction.

16.2.1.1 Fine Needle Techniques and Applications

For solid organ aspiration biopsies the inserted needle can be maneuvered utilizing various techniques in order to maximize the number of retrieved cells. However, none of the needles or maneuvers has been shown to be superior to others according to some authors [5]. Other groups of researchers found a slight advantage using the aspiration technique, which is described below [6].

The simplest maneuver is to position the needle without an attached syringe in the target and obtain cells performing to-and-fro movements along the axis of the needle. This technique uses only the capillary forces of the small needle to obtain cells. Since this technique is based on the lack of active aspiration, it is most commonly used in thyroid and other solid organ biopsies that are usually very cellular and are also very vascular. Absence of suction minimizes hemorrhagic contamina-

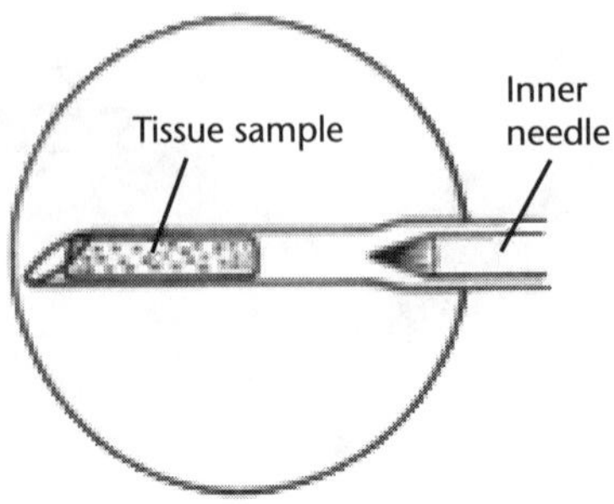

Figure 16.2 Vacuum needle (Sonopsy device). Once the needle is inserted into the target, the needle tip is withdrawn and suction is engaged once the device is cocked; the larger diameter of the needle shaft provides stronger vacuum than a straight shaft would do. (Courtesy of Havel's, Inc., Cincinnati, Ohio, USA, with permission.)

tion of the specimen. Bloody samples compromise the detectability of the cells of interest on the pathology slide and thus decrease the sensitivity and specificity of the cytological evaluation. Depending on the organ of interest, adequate sample results compared to the aspiration technique have been reported with this technique, as described below [5–7].

Higher accuracy has been described by some authors for the aspiration technique over the nonaspiration technique [6, 8, 9]. The aspiration technique uses a syringe attached to the needle in order to create a constant manual suction while the needle is being oscillated the same way it is for the capillary technique. This technique is preferable in pulmonary lesions where it is important to minimize the risk for pneumothorax by using a needle with an attached syringe. It is also used in other organs if the specimen retrieved by the capillary technique is scant and if hypervascularity of the target is not expected or observed by imaging or previous needle passes.

In both techniques the needle should not be moved outside the target once the needle tip is inserted, since tissue mainly from the lesion should be obtained for cytological analysis and since damage to adjacent organs or structures as well as bleeding and potential risk for seeding of malignant tumor cells should be minimized. To maximize the diagnostic yield and to obtain the most representative cell type from the lesion of interest, the needle should be directed in a fan-shaped fashion in various directions inside the lesion within the imaging plane if a real-time guidance method is used. Rotating the needle with or without aspiration within the target is also used by some operators, but no statistically significant superiority of one method over the other has been reported so far, with the exception of inferiority of the nonsuction method compared to aspiration technique [6].

16.2.1.2 Ultrasound Guided Procedures

If the procedure is performed under ultrasound guidance, several points have to be considered. Fine needles, specifically smaller than 20G, are less conspicuous than thicker needles. Visualization also depends on background echogenicity of the tissues and angle with which the needle is inserted in relation to the scanning direction. The closer the angle is to 90° from the scan plane, the stronger the reflected ultrasound acoustic signal from the needle. Needle conspicuity is best at 90° and worst at 0° (Figures 16.3 and 16.4).

Needle visualization also depends on acoustic penetration and accurate position of the focal zone of the acoustic beam. Consequently, deeply located lesions such as paraaortic lymph nodes or other small retroperitoneal targets are not generally accessible for ultrasound guidance. Bowel gas and overlying organs may also limit the utility of ultrasound. However, challenging locations in the hands of an experienced interventionalist may still be accessed by ultrasound guidance [10]. CT guidance is the most commonly used alternative in these instances.

Because of the smaller field of view using ultrasound guidance compared to CT or MR, it is technically more demanding on the user to keep the needle in the imaging plane. To keep the needle in the scanning field, two basic techniques are commonly used: free-hand and guided technique. For the free-hand technique the operator fully controls the angle of the needle in two dimensions relative to the

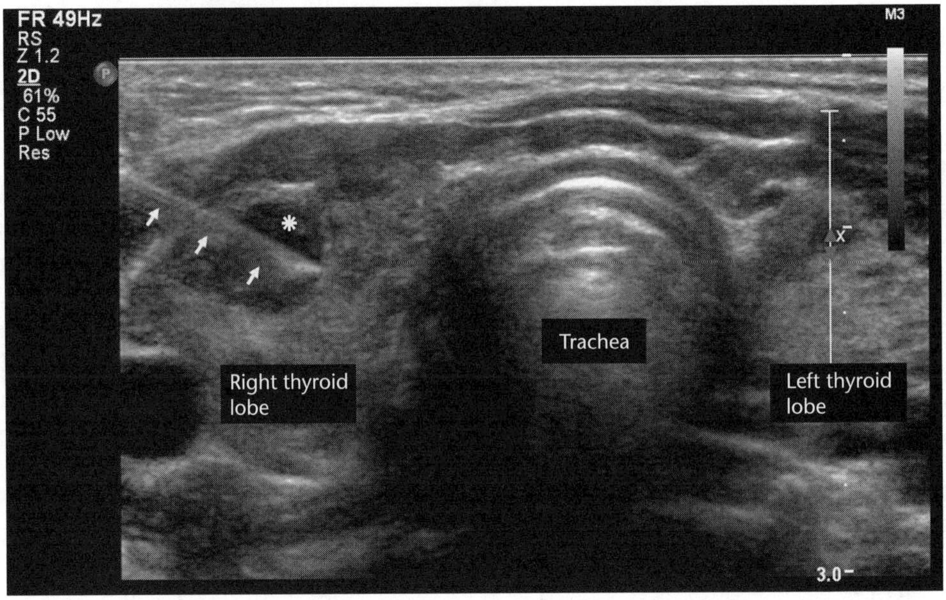

Figure 16.3 Sonographic axial view of the thyroid gland: the 25G spinal needle (arrows) in the small hypoechoic round mass (✱) is easily seen, with a relatively shallow angle of the needle to the scanning direction. Cytological evaluation revealed benign adenoma.

transducer. Alternatively, physical guides are available that determine the angle of the needle to the scanning plane (Figure 16.5). Once inserted into the guide, the needle follows the given angle until it reaches the target. At any time the guide can be removed to convert to a free-hand technique.

The angle that the needle would be following using the guide is represented on the display by a line or a sector segment that can be activated to better plan the procedure (Figure 16.12). However, feasibility of utilizing the displayed needle path on the image depends on anatomic and logistical obstacles such as ribs, gas, and interposed organs at risk or external dressings, wounds, and nonfeasible patient positioning.

Two major types of physical needle guides are available: side and end applicators. End applicators have generally replaced side applicators since they can be added to almost any transducer without modifying the transducer array design. In-plane side applicators have been designed to allow the shortest possible path from skin to target through the mid portion of the imaging plane; however, they require specific array designs with a notch in the center of the array to accommodate the needle. This decreases the cost efficacy, since these transducers would be used for guidance purposes only. Another disadvantage of this design is the inferior conspicuity of the needle, as this is a function of the angle of the needle in relation to the scanning direction—needle conspicuity is best at 90° and worst at 0° because of the basic cosinus dependence of the received echo pulse. Organs where an ideal 90° or almost 90° needle angle in relation to the imaging plane can be achieved are the thyroid gland, the breast, and other superficially located lesions (Figures 16.3 and 16.11). Steeper angles have to be used for peritoneal targets such as the liver,

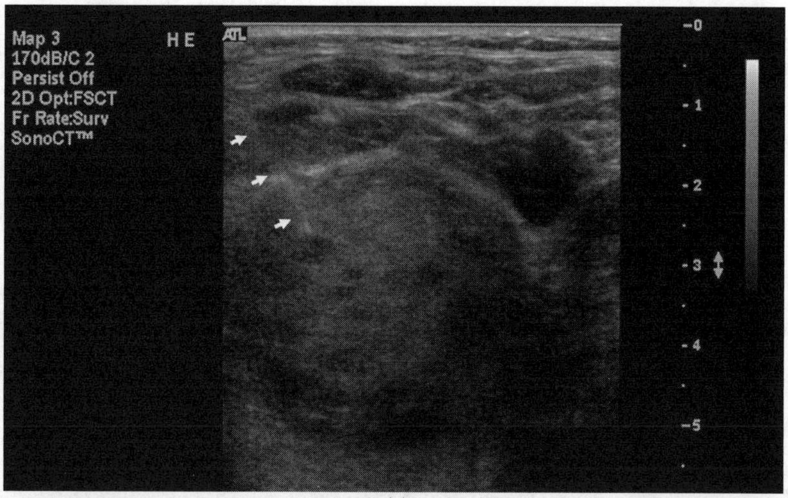

(a)

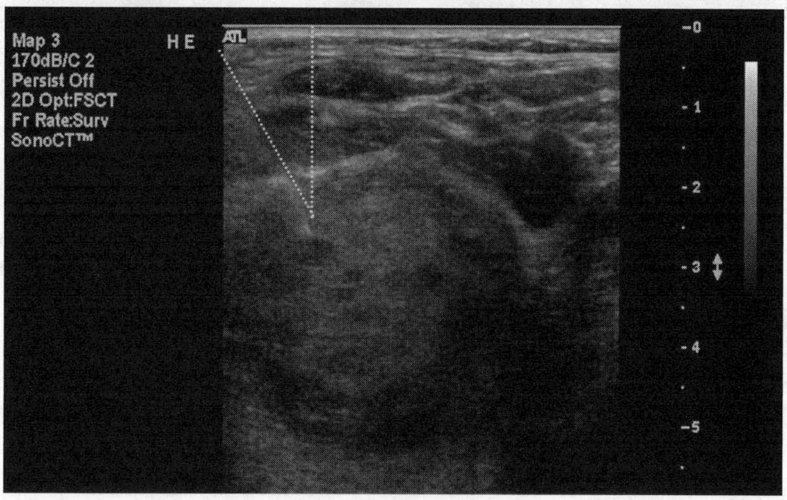

(b)

Figure 16.4 Free-hand ultrasound guided fine needle aspiration of thyroid mass. (a) Axial ultrasound image of a large thyroid mass with 25G fine needle poorly visualized (arrows). (b) Angle of the needle to the scanning direction is clearly less than on Figure 16.3, contributing to poor visualization of the needle.

kidney, and intraperitioneal masses and fluid collections. Newer guides allow more than one needle angle.

16.2.1.3 CT Guided Procedures

CT guidance is used for locations that are not visualized by ultrasound such as biopsies of masses in the lung that are completely surrounded by air containing lung parenchyma, lesions in the retroperitoneum, where an acoustic window might be impossible to get due to the surrounding bowel gas, or in the pelvis, where bowel gas and bony structures may obscure the target. CT is also used to visualize structures at risk that are not sufficiently well seen sonographically for guidance, even if the target can be visualized sonographically. Structures at risk include vessels,

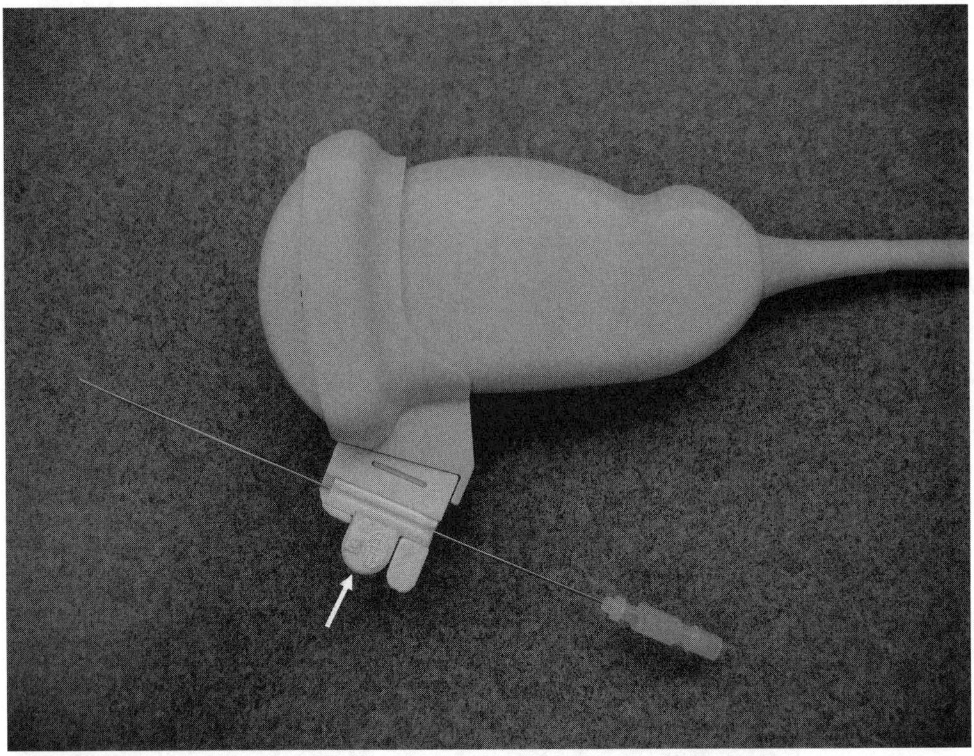

Figure 16.5 End applicator mounted on a curved array transducer. Note the snap-in insert that can be chosen according to the required needle diameter (arrow). The angle of the guide corresponds to electronic guide on the ultrasound display [compare with Figure 16.12(b)].

ureters, bowel, and lung. Other applications for CT guided interventions include drainage of fluid collections or therapeutic nerve blocks in locations that are not seen by ultrasound secondary to poor sonographic soft tissue contrast or due to the limited acoustic penetration of ultrasound such as the pudendal nerve. Indications for nerve blocks are pain of unknown (idiopathic) or known etiology such following trauma, inflammatory processes, surgery, or radiation. For example pelvic pain refractory to pain medication can be treated by pudendal nerve blocks using incremental or real-time fluoroscopic CT guidance. Once a 22G spine needle is inserted into the appropriate location of the pelvis, a mix of local numbing medication, long acting anti-inflammatory medication, and radio-opaque contrast is injected (Figure 16.6). The contrast agent demonstrates the distribution of the medication along the neural anatomic compartments and allows distinction between technical error and methodical failure in case the expected relief from the pain, is not seen. The local anesthetic serves as immediate feedback if the treatment is successful, since it causes numbness of the corresponding anatomic compartment minutes after the intervention.

Other indications for CT guided nerve blocks are painful conditions of the nerve roots (radiculopathies) resulting from impingement of a spinal nerve or celiac nerve blocks for upper abdominal and back pain resulting from tumor encasement, radiation, port operative scarring or inflammation of the solar plexus in the upper retroperitoneum. These areas may be accessed with CT guidance; however, fluoro-

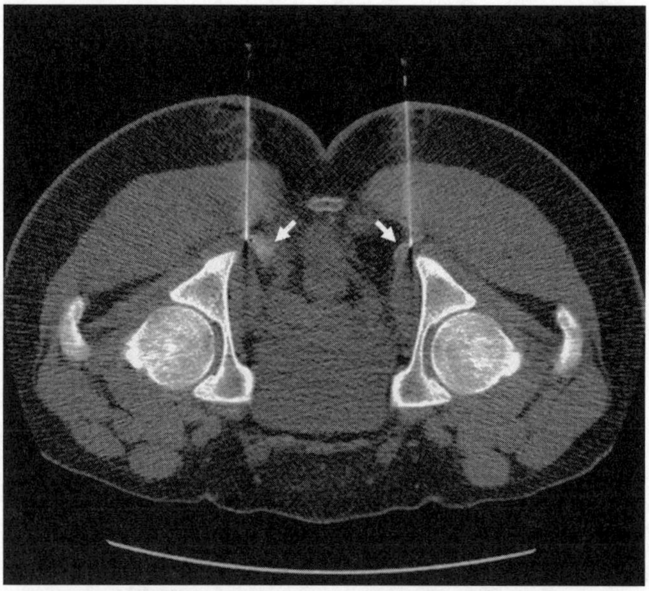

(a)

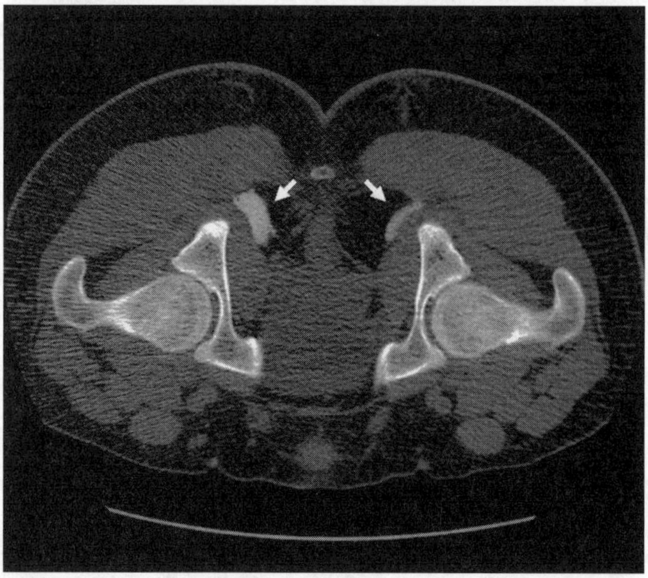

(b)

Figure 16.6 CT guided bilateral pudendal nerve block in prone position. (a) Two 22G spinal needles are inserted through the gluteal musculature immediately posterior to the pudendal nerves. Test injection of 2cc diluted iodine contrast of both pudendal nerves verifies correct location of the needle tips within the canal of the pudendal nerves (arrows). (b) Subsequently a mixture of local anesthetic, long acting anti-inflammatory drug, and iodine contrast is injected for treatment—image showing adequate distribution of medication within the neural anatomic compartment (Alcocks' canal). The patient experienced immediate superficial numbness in the perineum and both inner thighs, as expected, proving technically successful nerve block.

scopically, sonographically, or endo-sonographically guided approaches may be an alternative depending on the anatomic location and on the operators' expertise and preference.

16.2.2 Core Needle Devices and Techniques

If histological evaluation is the goal of the biopsy, a mostly automated core needle system is used. End-core and side-notch devices are available for this purpose. Both types of systems are available as hand-held devices with manual advancement of the retrieval component or with an automated high-speed spring mechanism that allows rapid acceleration of the cutting component of the device through the target tissue. The result is a tissue core that can be retrieved for microscopic evaluation, ideally of sufficient length and diameter to allow preparation of various histological and immuno-histochemical stains from one submitted block tissue (Figure 16.7).

End-core systems allow larger tissue volume samples than side-notch systems of comparable caliber.

The needle shafts are often equipped with centimeter markings and the handle has an incrementally adjustable throw length. Once the needle with the exposed stylet tip is positioned within the target, the cutting component is released by the push of the trigger. The sharp core needle tip, comparable to the Franseen fine needle, cuts through the tissue at the set throw length. The high velocity with which the cutting needle is advanced through the tissues and the end-notch design result in larger cores and minimize crush artifacts of the specimen. With actuation of the device on some systems such as the triaxial BioPince full core device (Angiotech Interventional, Gainesville, Florida), a cutter is advanced within the cannula which cuts the retrieved tissue cylinder at its distal margin and keeps it secured within the cannula (Figure 16.8).

This is an advantage compared to earlier end-core designs without specimen cutter, where "empty" biopsies were a serious problem with some end-core systems. The specimen gets expelled from the cannula by recocking the device again outside

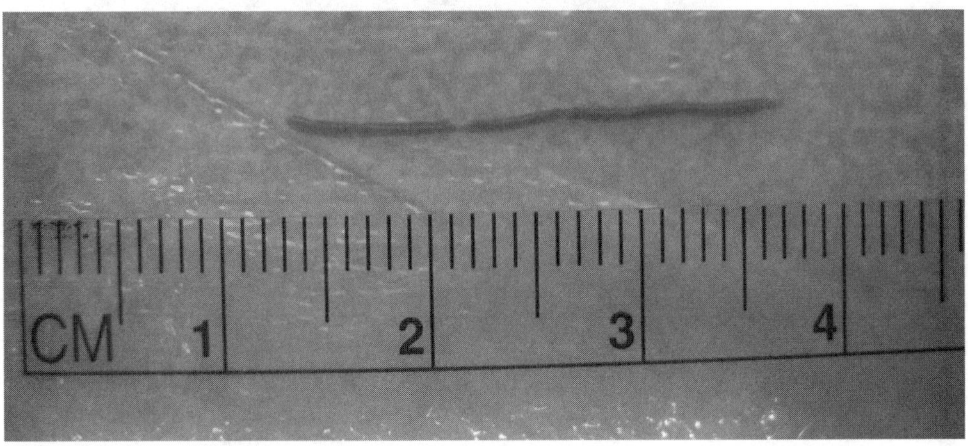

Figure 16.7 A 2.3-cm core biopsy specimen of the liver obtained with 17/18G full core coaxial system.

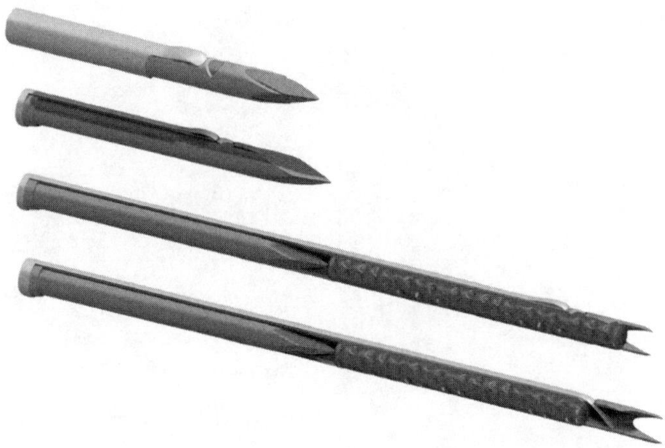

Figure 16.8 Triaxial core needle biopsy device. (Biopince, courtesy Angiotech Interventional, Gainesville, Florida, USA. © 2008 Medical Device Technologies, Inc. © 2008 Angiotech Pharmaceuticals, Inc. All Rights Reserved, with permission.)

the body, which simultaneously sets it up for the next biopsy pass if desired. Caution must be used in these systems when small lesions are targeted, since the throw cannot be influenced once the cutting cannula is released and possible tissue damage of structures distal to the target may occur. Careful measurement from the end of the inserted tip to the calculated throw length on the imaging display is sometimes necessary to ensure a safe biopsy pass.

Side-notch systems have adjustable or nonadjustable throw lengths. They have an inner side-notch needle, the so-called trough (Figure 16.9).

However the volume of the specimen is smaller since one part of the full core diameter is used up by the trough that is necessary to accommodate the specimen (Figure 16.10).

The throw length of some of the adjustable models can be modified nonincrementally or in increments with set throw lengths. The advantage over the end-core systems is that they have a tactile plunger allowing controlled advancement of the

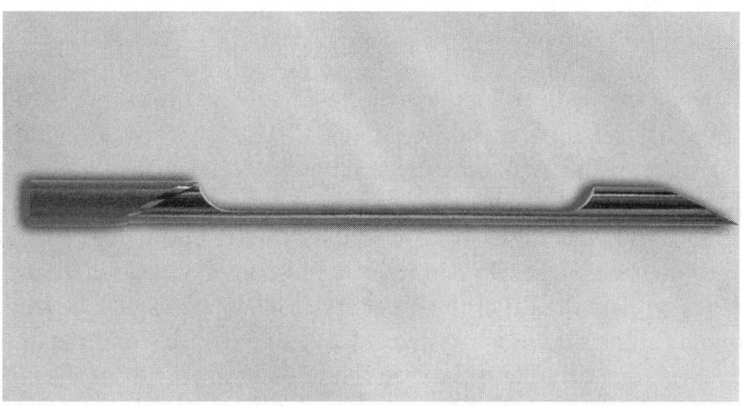

Figure 16.9 Side-notch core needle with a sample notch of 19-mm length. (Tru-Core, courtesy Angiotech Interventional, Gainesville, Florida, USA. © 2008 Medical Device Technologies, Inc. © 2008 Angiotech Pharmaceuticals, Inc. All Rights Reserved, with permission.)

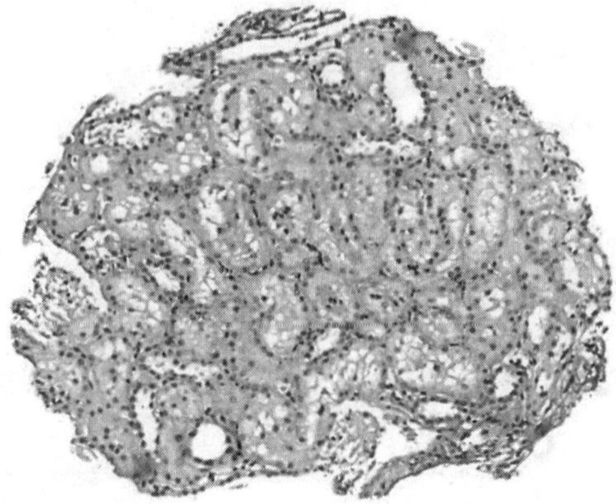

(a)

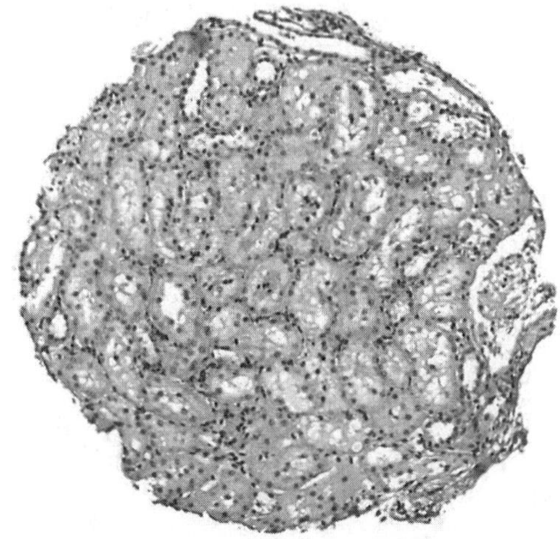

(b)

Figure 16.10 Two histological specimens in axial section. (a) Specimen obtained with side-notch system, showing slightly smaller tissue than (b) full core specimen harvested with end-core system. (Courtesy Angiotech, Inc., Gainesville, Florida, USA. © 2008 Medical Device Technologies, Inc. © 2008 Angiotech Pharmaceuticals, Inc. All Rights Reserved, with permission.)

tip, which can help to increase the safety of the procedure in small targets or in lesions that are surrounded by organs at risk. If ultrasound guidance is used, this inner stylet, which will carry the specimen, can be pushed out gradually under real guidance (Figure 16.11).

Once the inner stylet is advanced, the outer cutting cannula is spring-released by pushing the trigger. In contrast to end-core devices, where the cutting cannula extends beyond the tip of the inner stylet when activated, the length of the cutting cannula on the side-notch systems does not extent beyond the inner stylet. Instead the sharp outer cannula slides over the side-notch portion of the inner stylet, thereby enclosing the specimen cylinder. A cutter at the end of the cutting needle is obsolete, since a metal block at the end of the inner stylet prevents the specimen from being pulled out of the cannula when the needle is removed.

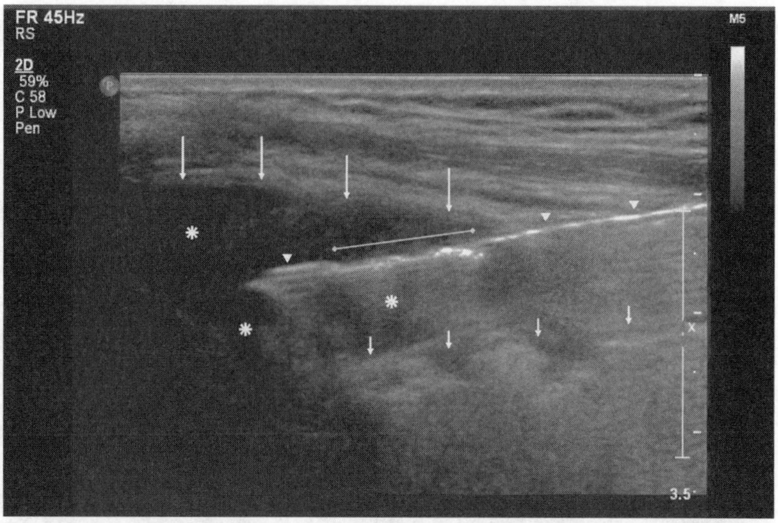

(a)

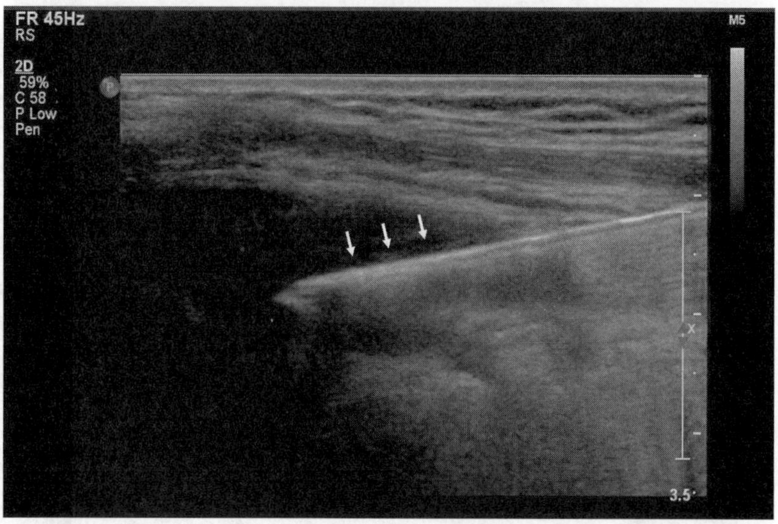

(b)

Figure 16.11 Intercostal ultrasound guided free-hand biopsy of solid 1-cm thickening of the pleura using a coaxial core side notch system. (a) The trough of the needle (arrowheads) is well seen in the pleural space (✱). Note pleura (long arrows) and lung (short arrows) delineating the small pleural space. Ultrasound provided real-time guidance in this challenging location close to the lung, which had to be avoided for biopsy. (b) After firing the cutting cannula the side-notch is covered (arrows), entrapping the specimen. Note that the absolute length of the needle tip does not change after the cutting cannula is advanced. Histological evaluation showed benign fibrous tissue.

16.2.3 Coaxial Needle Techniques

Both fine and core needle biopsies can be performed by coaxial technique. In this case a larger caliber introducer is inserted into the target tissue first, functioning as a sheath for the biopsy device. Whereas the introducer is placed through the normal tissues only once before its tip is positioned in or close to the target, the

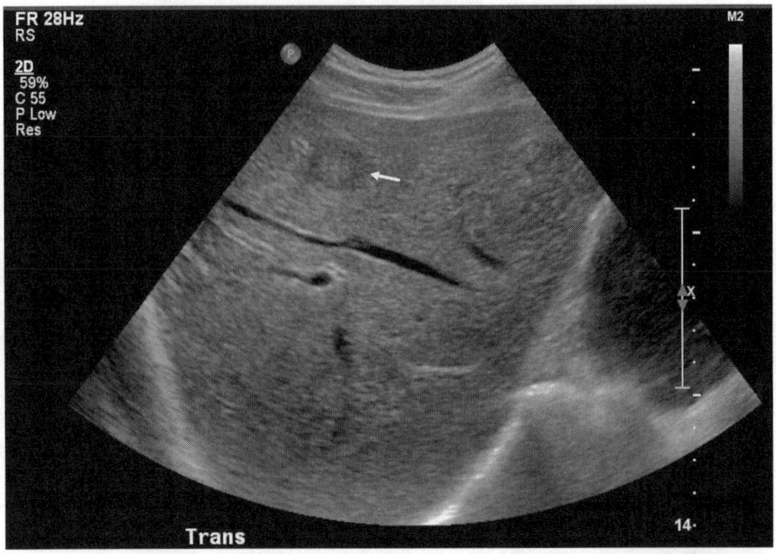

(a)

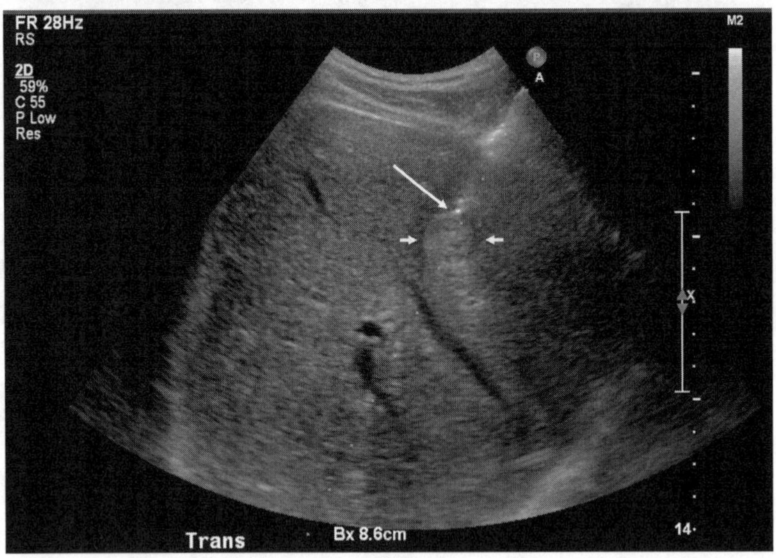

(b)

Figure 16.12 Ultrasound guided coaxial core needle biopsy of new small liver mass in a patient with history of rectal melanoma performed with an attached needle guide. (a) Target sign lesion with echogenic center and hypoechoic rim, suspicious for metastasis (arrow). (b) Tip of the inserted 17G introducer (long arrow) abutting the proximal margin of the mass (short arrows). Dotted lines represent electronic needle guide measuring the distance from the top of the attached needle guide to the proximal margin of the mass. (c) Fired 18G end-notch needle (long arrow) within the mass terminating intentionally beyond the distal margin of the mass (short arrow) in order to include adjacent liver tissue as a reference. The projected electronic path predicted quite accurately the actual biopsy trajectory thanks to no deflection of the relatively stiff 17/18G coaxial needle system. Histology showed unexpected metastasis of neuroendocrine tumor, not related to primary rectal melanoma.

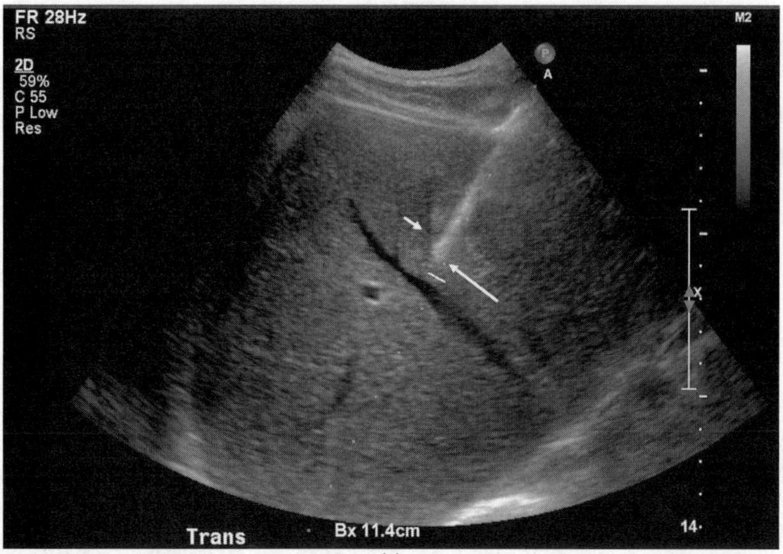

(c)

Figure 16.12 (*continued*)

actual biopsy device can be inserted through this sheath and into the lesion multiple times without transgressing other tissues. This option reduces the number of passes through normal tissues ideally to a single pass if no adjustment of positioning is required. This is chosen in the following scenarios:

- Multiple passes through the same target are planned and the target organ poses a relative risk for post-interventional bleeding, since it is well perfused or the lesion is hypervascular or both. Examples are all abdominal organs such as the liver, kidney, spleen, or vascular abdominal masses (Figure 16.12). However, no significant difference in complications could be found in a recent retrospective review of the coaxial versus the noncoaxial technique on liver and kidney biopsies [11].
- A fine needle aspiration biopsy of a lung lesion is planned with a cytologist in the procedure room. Since the introducer provides access to the lesion, repeated passes through the introducer can be performed if the first pass in inadequate without adding another pass through lung tissue. This technique is used to decrease the risk for a pneumothorax and bleeding. It is also being used for core biopsies of lung lesions.
- The risk of seeding malignant tumors cells from a potentially cancerous target. The idea behind this approach is that with coaxial technique the introducer functions as a sheath shielding the normal tissue from the biopsy device, which may also carry malignant cells at its end. In the noncoaxial technique with more than one pass the same needle is inserted into and removed from the target multiple times, so that the risk for seeding may increase with the

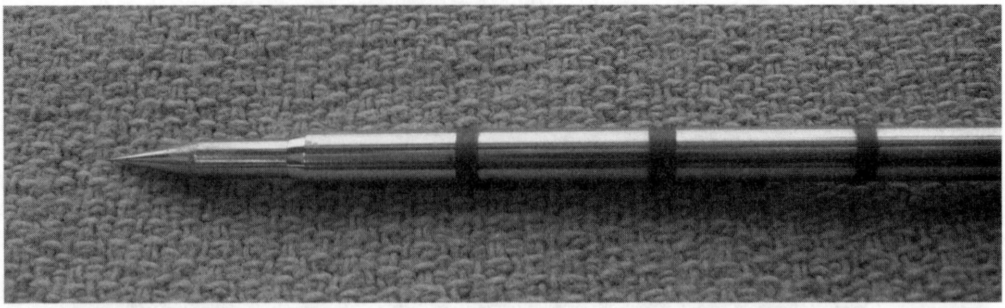

(a)

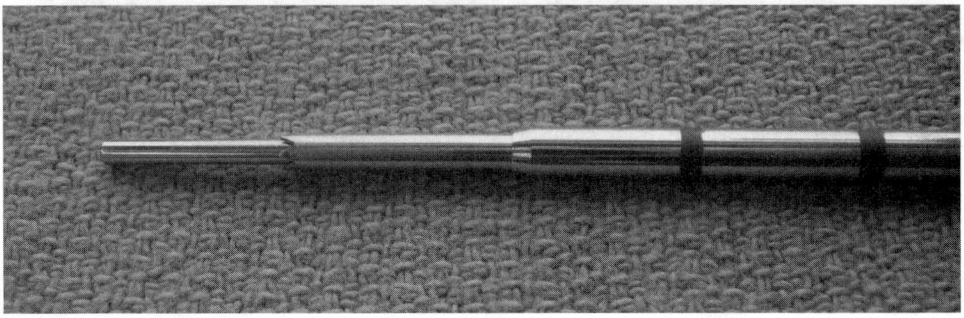

(b)

Figure 16.13 Reusable Ackermann needle for coaxial core biopsies of the bone: (a) introducer with inner stylet is advanced to cortex of bone; and (b) drill is advanced through the cortex and into the marrow; specimen expelled with pusher.

number of passes. With the coaxial technique the introducer is inserted and removed only once, allowing multiple coaxial biopsy passes while protecting the surrounding tissue from contamination with malignant cells [12].

- Administration of an injectable sealant is planned after only one pass in a patient at increased risk for postprocedural bleeding or pneumothorax. Indications may be reduction of pneumothorax risk after lung biopsies, various blood disorders, bleeding disorders, treatment-induced abnormalities of the coagulation system, and organs at increased risk for bleeding such as the spleen [13, 14].

It should be noted that when a coaxial approach is used, the introducer has to be at least one diameter size larger than the outer caliber of the biopsy device. This ratio of outer caliber of the introducer to the outer diameter of the biopsy device is variable.

Most introducers are equipped with a roughened or coated segment of the surface at the tip in order to increase acoustic reflection. This is designed to increase needle conspicuity when an ultrasound guided procedure is performed.

For biopsies of osseous structures with an intact bone cortex, a coaxial or triaxial technique with a special bone cutting introducer is required. Either the cutting cannula itself is designed to penetrate through the bone and obtain the specimen (Figure 16.13) or the cutting device can be used to drill a hole through the cortex in order to allow a conventional end-core or side-notch device to obtain the softer target tissue within the bone marrow.

For biopsies of the breast, where a large sample volume has shown to provide additional information for further management of the patient rather than 16G to 18G core biopsies, vacuum assisted biopsy devices are used [15]. Like spring-loaded core needle biopsy systems, vacuum biopsy devices can be used for stereotactic plain film or MR guided biopsy procedures. They are usually among the largest biopsy devices, in the range of 9G to 10G.

16.2.4 Drainage Devices Without a Guide Wire

For temporary therapeutic removal of larger volumes of fluid, a catheter-based approach may be preferred. The catheter may be inserted for the duration of the procedure only and removed immediately afterward. Alternatively, larger caliber catheters may be placed with the intention of being left for a longer time period, in the range of days to a few weeks if the collection is known to reaccumulate or if the fluid is of more viscous nature. These drainage techniques will not be discussed in this chapter.

Two main cavities in the body appropriate for catheter-based aspirations are the pleural cavity in the chest and the peritoneal cavity in the abdomen and pelvis. Besides these two physiologic cavities, fluid collections may occur elsewhere in the body including within the calvaria, an organ, or the muscles or soft tissues.

All larger fluid collections with exception of the intracranial ones may be drained with a simple small 19G pigtail catheter (Yueh needle, Cook Medical, Bloomington, Indiana), which is removed after the procedure (Figure 16.14).

The catheter has a curled ("pigtail") configuration (Figure 16.15); four side ports located along the inner curvature of the curled tip are designed to prevent occlusion by adjacent lung or bowel loops. The catheter has a thin outer sheath, allowing it to be straightened and advanced over the introducing needle before the needle is inserted. The blunt inner stylet can only be used after the needle has been advanced through the tissues into the fluid compartment, and requires some experience in its use. Other devices such as certain thoracentesis devices are designed with a blunt spring activated inner stylet for protection of the lungs (see below). Once the entire straightened device including the introducing needle and stylet is positioned in the fluid collection, the needle and stylet are removed and the catheter tip follows its preformed curled configuration (Figure 16.15). After evacuation of the collection the catheter can be removed.

Abdominal fluid collections and pleural effusions can also be accessed with dedicated systems such as the Turkel safety device (Kendall, Covidien, Mansfield, Massachusetts) designed to minimize the risk for organ perforation or pneumothorax. These systems are available as a prepared set along with the drainage device (Figure 16.16).

The set includes items such as a scalpel, glass slides for cytological evaluation, local anesthetic, syringes and smaller needles for the numbing part of the

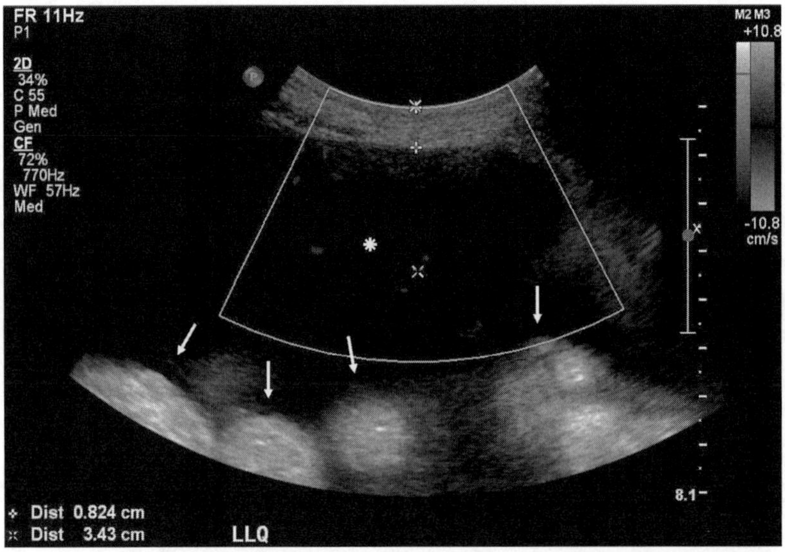

(a)

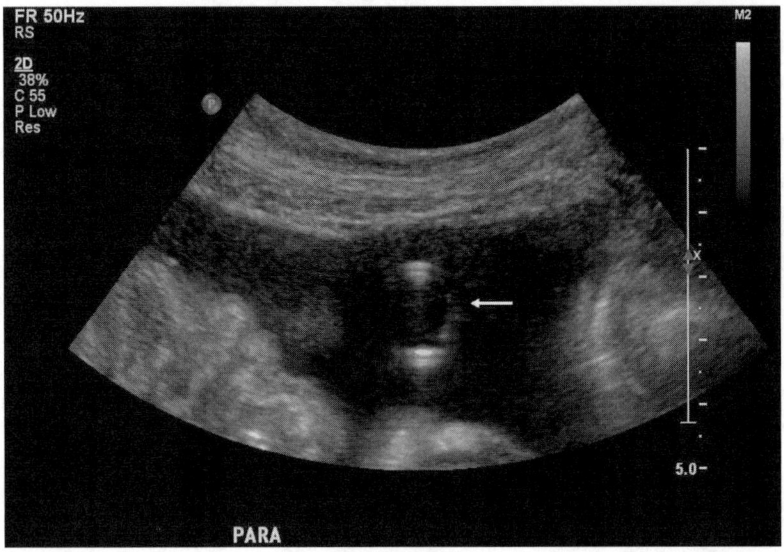

(b)

Figure 16.14 Therapeutic ultrasound guided paracentesis on a patient with metastatic gastric cancer causing malignant ascites. (a) Large volume of ascites (✱). Distance from the skin to the mid-depth of the fluid is measured to avoid contact of needle with the underlying small bowel loops (arrows). Color Doppler excludes significant vessels in the trajectory of the catheter within the abdominal wall. (b) Curled portion of Yueh catheter (Cook Medical, Bloomington, Indiana, USA) is visualized within the fluid (arrows). (c) With progressive removal of ascites the catheter comes in contact with the bowel loops without causing damage (arrow). (d) 3.5 liters of ascites are drained thanks to the inner side ports of the curled catheter tip, in spite of the catheter being surrounded and abutted by bowel loops. Arrow indicates incompletely visualized loop of the catheter.

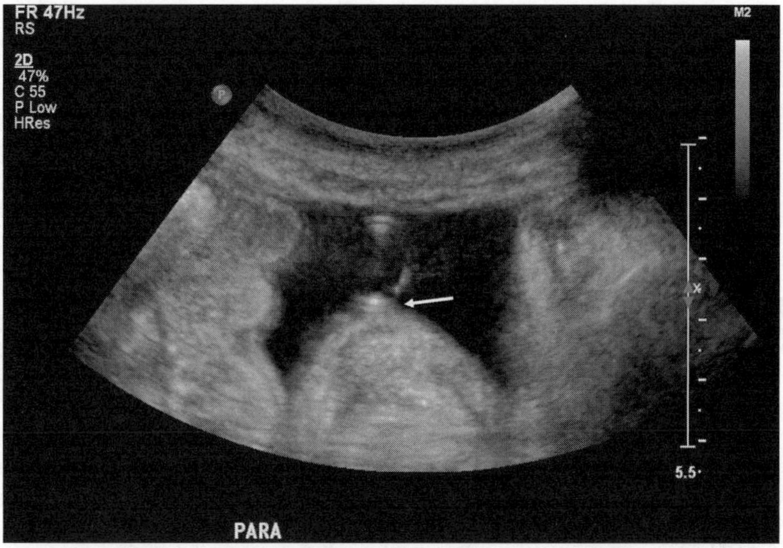

(c)

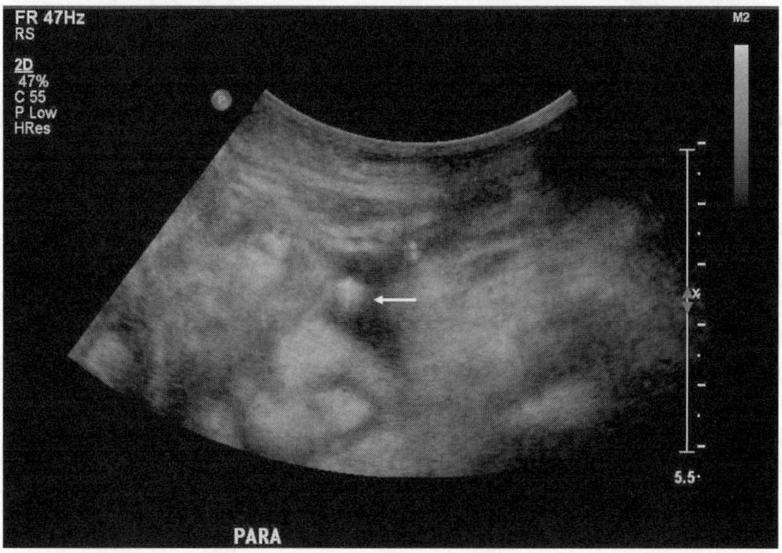

(d)

Figure 16.14 (*continued*)

procedures, gauzes and more. The device itself has the same basic configuration as other pigtail catheters consisting of an introducing needle and a catheter. One main difference with the Yueh needle is a built-in valve that allows the introducing needle to be inserted and removed without allowing air to enter the pleural cavity through the end of the catheter. Another feature is a spring-activated inner stylet with a blunt tip, which is longer than the introducing needle. The spring allows the blunt tip to be pushed back so that the cutting introducing needle is exposed while it passes through solid tissues of skin, subcutaneous fat, and intercostal musculature. Once the sharp needle tip reaches the pleural effusion, the lack of solid tissue

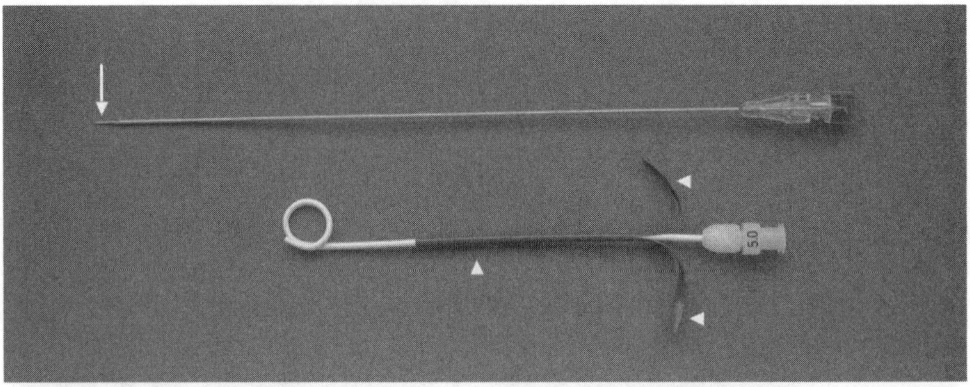

Figure 16.15 Yueh needle and catheter device. 19G introducing needle (upper) with blunt tip (arrow) longer than the sharp introducer needle to protect sensitive organs. 5 French catheter (lower) with curled tip and sheath (arrow heads), which allows straightening of the curled tip when slipped over the introducer.

resistance allows the blunt inner stylet to be immediately advanced beyond the end of the sharp introducing needle, shielding potentially adjacent lung from the sharp needle. While the blunt stylet is pushed into the introducing needle a red marker at the end of the device indicates that the sharp needle tip is exposed. Once the blunt stylet reaches the fluid collection, the marker turns green indicating exposure of the blunted and safer tip. At this point an attached syringe at the straight end of the introducing needle allows immediate retrieval of fluid for diagnostic purposes. Once the introducing needle is fully withdrawn, the introducer cannot be reinserted into the catheter, since the valve prevents air and the needle from entering the pleural cavity. A side hole at the hub end of the drain allows connection to larger syringes or vacuum bottles for aspiration. Immediately after the procedure the catheter can be withdrawn.

Permanent catheters of larger calibers are inserted with help of a guide wire and dilators, which is not described in detail in this chapter.

16.3 Complications

Complications of percutaneous minimally invasive procedures include general risks such as pain, hemorrhage, and infection (Figure 16.17). Complications specific to the anatomic regions exist in addition, such as pneumothorax and hemoptysis (coughing up blood) for lung related interventions and damage to other organs such as stomach, bowel, and urinary system for abdominal and pelvic procedures (Figure 16.18).

Overall, image-guided minimally invasive needle-based interventions have gained significant popularity over the last two decades thanks to their high level of accuracy, reproducibility, safety, and ease of use. The choice of which imaging modality is best for the specific patient depends on various parameters such as the purpose of the procedure, anatomy of the patient, availability of the modality, and the operator's expertise and preference.

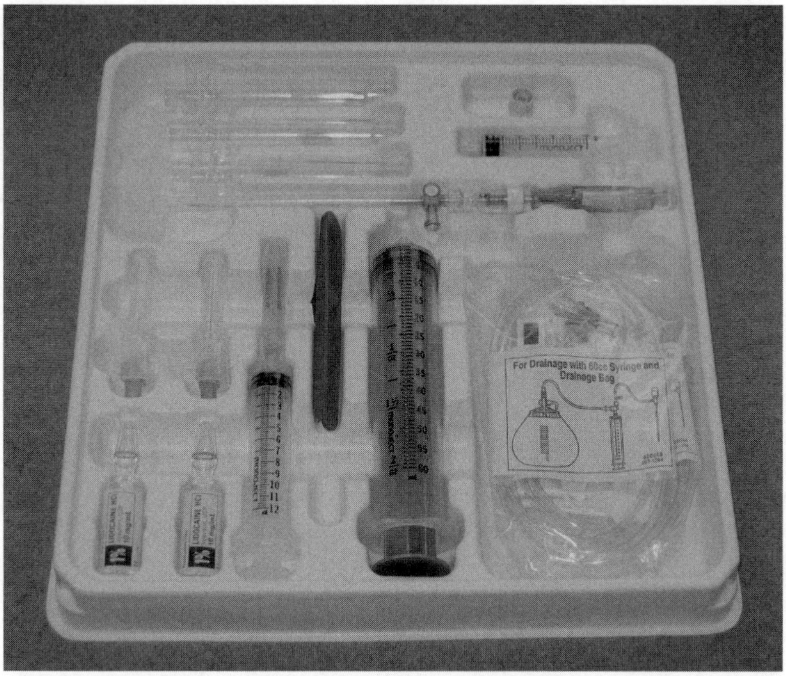

(a)

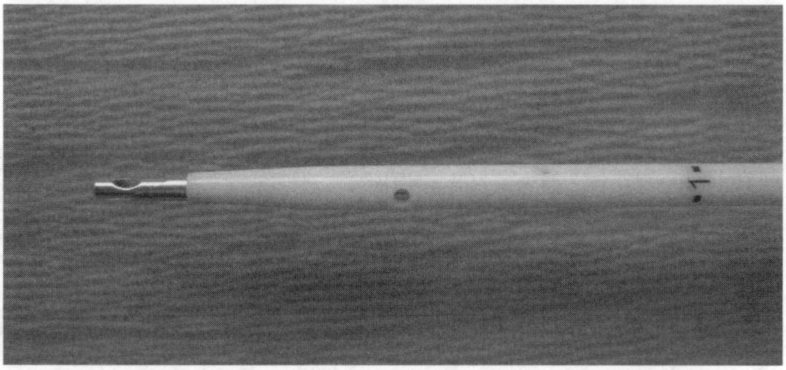

(b)

Figure 16.16 (a) Tray with safety needle and mounted straight catheter as well as multiple syringes, needles, local anesthetic, specimen bag, containers, and scalpel. (b) Tip with blunt spring-activated inner stylet for protection of sensitive organs. (c) Hub with bicolored indicator (white arrow) changes from green to red when the blunt stylet is pushed back by tissues exposing the sharp needle, indicating organs are at risk of being damaged by the needle. Once the needle enters the peritoneal or pleural cavity, the blunt tip is automatically advanced protecting organs from the sharp needle. A ball valve (black arrow) prevents air from entering the device. The dotted arrow indicates the side-port with three-way stop cock for connection to specimen retrieval bag or container.

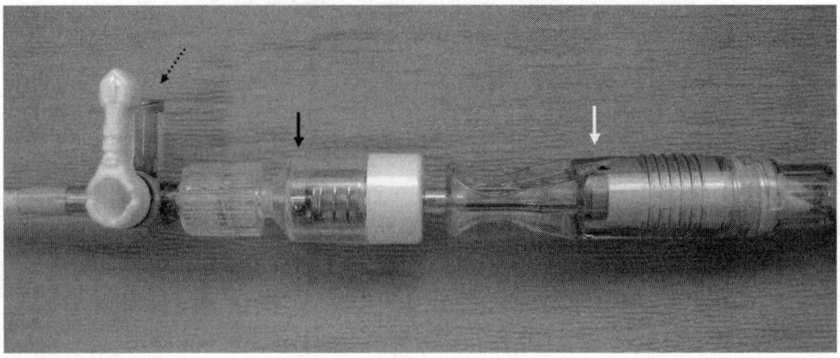

(c)

Figure 16.16 (*continued*)

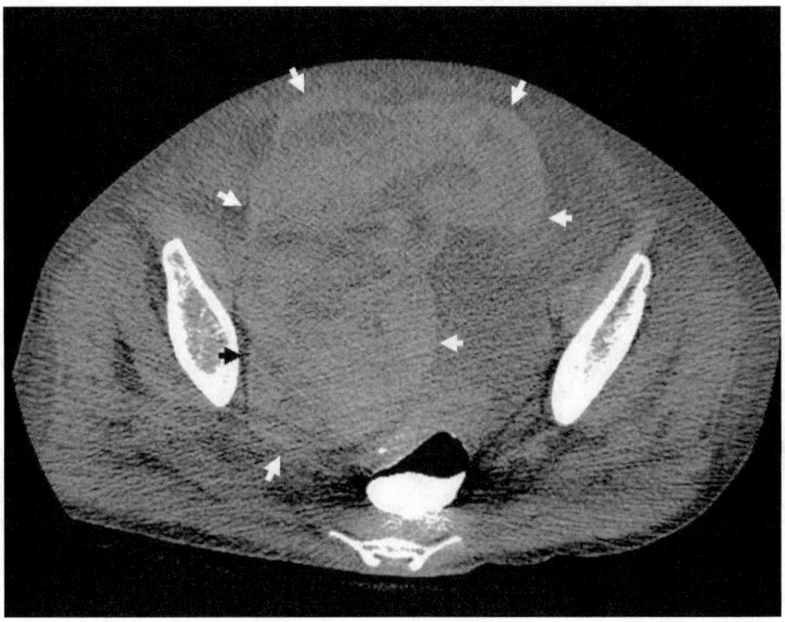

Figure 16.17 Large retroperitioneal hematoma in the pelvis at the puncture site 1 day after ultrasound guided paracentesis for malignant ascites in a patient with metastatic lung cancer.

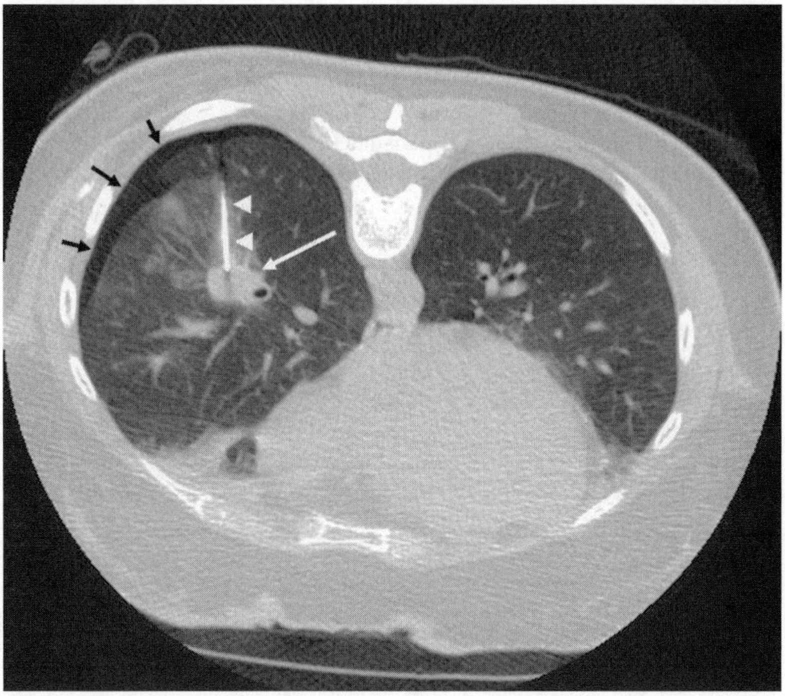

Figure 16.18 CT guided coaxial fine needle aspiration of right small nodule in prone position. 22G Chiba needle (arrowheads) is inserted into the mass (long white arrow) with immediate development of small pneumothorax (black arrows) that resolved spontaneously over the next hours. Histology showed metastasis of malignant liver tumor.

References

[1] Geraghty, P. R., et al., "CT-Guided Transthoracic Needle Aspiration Biopsy of Pulmonary Nodules: Needle Size and Pneumothorax Rate," *Radiology*, Vol. 229, 2003, pp. 475–481.

[2] Matsubara, J., et al., "Ultrasound-Guided Percutaneous Pancreatic Tumor Biopsy in Pancreatic Cancer: A Comparison with Metastatic Liver Tumor Biopsy, Including Sensitivity, Specificity, and Complications," *J. Gastroenterol.*, Vol. 43, 2008, pp. 225–232.

[3] Schmidbauer, J., et al., "Diagnostic Accuracy of Computed Tomography-Guided Percutaneous Biopsy of Renal Masses," *European Urology*, Vol. 53, 2008, pp. 1003–1012.

[4] Ng, Y. L., et al., "CT-Guided Percutaneous Fine-Needle Aspiration Biopsy of Pulmonary Nodules Measuring 10 mm or Less," *Clinical Radiology*, Vol. 63, 2008, pp. 272–277.

[5] Savage, C. A., et al., "Fine-Needle Aspiration Biopsy Versus Fine-Needle Capillary (Nonaspiration) Biopsy: In Vivo Comparison," *Radiology*, Vol. 195, 1995, pp. 815–819.

[6] Hopper, K. D., et al., "Fine-Needle Aspiration Biopsy for Cytopathologic Analysis: Utility of Syringe Handles, Automated Guns, and the Nonsuction Method," *Radiology*, Vol. 185, 1992, pp. 819–824.

[7] Fagelman, D., and Q. Chess, "Nonaspiration Fine-Needle Cytology of the Liver: A New Technique for Obtaining Diagnostic Samples," *Am. J. Roentgenol.*, Vol. 155, 1990, pp. 1217–1219.

[8] Hueftle, M. G., and J. R. Haaga, "Effect of Suction on Biopsy Sample Size," *Am. J. Roentgenol.*, Vol. 147, 1986, pp. 1014–1016.

[9] Kinney, T. B., et al., "Fine-Needle Biopsy: Prospective Comparison of Aspiration Versus Nonaspiration Techniques in the Abdomen," *Radiology*, Vol. 186, 1993, pp. 549–552.

[10] Winter, T. C., F. T. J. Lee, and J. L. Hinshaw, "Ultrasound-Guided Biopsies in the Abdomen and Pelvis [Review]," *Ultrasound Quarterly*, Vol. 24, 2008, pp. 45–68.

[11] Hatfield, M. K., et al., "Percutaneous Imaging-Guided Solid Organ Core Needle Biopsy: Coaxial Versus Noncoaxial Method," *Am. J. Roentgenol.*, Vol. 190, 2008, pp. 413–417.

[12] Maturen, K. E., et al., "Lack of Tumor Seeding of Hepatocellular Carcinoma After Percutaneous Needle Biopsy Using Coaxial Cutting Needle Technique," *Am. J. Roentgenol.*, Vol. 187, 2006, pp. 1184–1187.

[13] Billich, C., et al., "CT-Guided Lung Biopsy: Incidence of Pneumothorax After Instillation of NaCl into the Biopsy Track," *European Radiology*, Vol. 18, No. 6, June 2008, pp. 1146–1152.

[14] Herman, S. J., and G. L. Weisbrod, "Usefulness of the Blood Patch Technique After Transthoracic Needle Aspiration Biopsy," *Radiology*, Vol. 176, 1990, pp. 395–397.

[15] Liberman, L., et al., "Calcifications Highly Suggestive of Malignancy: Comparison of Breast Biopsy Methods," *Am. J. Roentgenol.*, Vol. 177, 2001, pp. 165–172.

CHAPTER 17

Robotic Radical Prostatectomy: History, Present, and Future

Fernando J. Bianco, Jr.

The last years of the 1990s witnessed through the eye of the laparoscope an unprecedented evolution regarding the surgical removal of the prostate gland. Laparoscopic radical prostatectomy started to generate great expectations. However, the required laparoscopic technical skills and the complex prostate location in the pelvis made it very difficult to teach and reproduce. The introduction of the DaVinci robot—master-slave system—cleared most of these hurdles for the surgeon. Today, robotic assisted laparoscopic prostatectomy is the most used surgical approach to remove the prostate gland. Consistent advantages of this technique are: a shorter convalescent state and a very marked decrease in the amount of blood loss during and after surgery without compromising the cancer control rates. The long-term functional and oncologic results are not mature at this moment. The postoperative morbidity and mortality results are at least as good or better as the ones obtained with traditional prostatectomy. However, the major challenge for robotic surgeons is not different than for its predecessors. To establish a paradigm that breaks with the tradition and prevents biased reporting due to technology enthusiasm, but rather takes a critical approach based in prospective, controlled, randomized clinical trials. If the latter objective is reached, the robotic surgeon movement will represent a new generation of surgeons with the ability to offer excellent clinical evidence to their patients.

17.1 Historical Background of the Robotic Technology

Several approaches have been mixed in order to get to the robotic surgery as it is known today. Robotic systems are considered according with the movement commands, as follows: (1) master-slave systems, movements are done under a device (arms in a console) and the robotic instruments reproduce them; (2) precise trajectory systems, where movements are preprogrammed under a series of parameters but there is no an external control; and (3) internal substitution devices, which execute precise actions under voice commands or they are positioned and their work is passive.

The antecedent of the technology best known by the urologic community is based in the prototype master-slave system, in which the surgeon make the movements in the console and the robotic instrument reproduce them in the patient. Examples of this technology are the DaVinci Surgical System (Intuitive Surgical, Sunnyvale, California). The second type of robots with surgical applications performs preprogrammed movements over a series of patient's parameters, but there are no external controls. These are known as precise trajectory systems. Examples of those are: the ROBODOC (Integrated Surgical Systems, Davis, California), used to implant joint prosthesis (the procedure called "Surgeon Robot for Prostatectomies" developed by Wickham [1]), and the PAKY developed for the renal percutaneous access in the Johns Hopkins Medical Center. There is another type of surgical robot known as internal substitution devices, like the recently discontinued AESOP (Intuitive Surgical, Sunnyvale, California) which provides computerized support for the camera and it is controlled by the surgeon's voice. Another system is named navigation-position system and one of its applications is called Neubluntte (Integrated Surgical Systems, Davis, California) and it is used in neurosurgery.

The master-slave technology can be defined as computer assisted due to the fact that the instruments do not work autonomously; rather they reproduce with precision the movements that the surgeon does in the console. The precise trajectory systems are the ones that best suit the concept of robotic surgery due to their semi-autonomous movements. It is obvious that there are semantic differences, but in this chapter we are going to use the term robotic surgery to talk about the master-slave systems.

The master-slave systems in which the surgeon directly starts the movements of the surgical technique were developed initially at the end of the 1980s through a joint research initiative: researchers from the National Aeronautics and Space Administration Ames Research Center (California) working in virtual reality systems collaborated with a group of mechanical engineers from the Stanford Research Institute (SRI, Menlo Park, California) interested in robotic techniques. The first outcome of this cooperative project was the development of one tele-assisted surgical system to increase the precision in microsurgery. The demonstration of its efficacy was done by practicing termino-terminal anastomosis of the femoral artery in 10 rats, achieving permeability in 100% of the cases [2].

The next step from the initial conception of the SRI system to help with microsurgical techniques was the study of the general applications in macroscopic surgery. The first laparoscopic cholecystectomy was done in 1989 by Perissat et al. [3] and was presented in the American Society of Gastrointestinal Surgeons Meeting in Atlanta, representing a historic point in the development of the laparoscopic surgery. The demonstration of this technique led the programmers of the SRI system to the consideration that their devices for robotic tele-manipulation could have ideal applications in the field of laparoscopic surgery in addition to their initial applications in microsurgery [4]. Based on these experiences, a tele-assisted system was developed with the financial support from the U.S. Department of Defense that included a control console for the surgeon and a remote control working device. However, the initial application of this system was for open surgery rather that laparoscopic surgery. The system was called SRI Green Telepresence Surgery System, recognizing Phil Green, SRI investigator. This system was developed as a surgical device to facilitate performing surgical procedures at a distance—surgery at war. It would include a mobile and armored operating room vehicle, equipped with the surgical robotic devices to be controlled by a surgeon located in a hospital. It was designed in order to control potentially lethal injuries, such as vascular trauma. Initial studies showed that the outcomes were adequate for trauma surgery, but the surgical times were 2.7 times greater compared with the open surgery [5]. Even though the technology of the tele-presence has not been used for its initial application, it has given a place for the development and commercialization of the DaVinci Surgical System.

In its initial phases, the SRI Green System was tried in urologic procedures. Bowersox and Cornum [6] used the system to practice open surgeries such as nephrectomies, closure of cystostomies, and uretheral anastomosis in pigs. The first systems only had 4 degrees of freedom (the same as the conventional laparoscopic instruments) and they presented marked functioning problems, leading to an initial stop to their clinical development. Simultaneously in Europe, Schurr et al. [7] developed in Germany another master-slave system called ARTEMIS (Advanced Robotic Telemanipulator for Minimally-Invasive Surgery). It included remote telecontrols, 6 degrees of freedom of its instruments, and a tridimensional visual system. Even though this was the first system that reached 6 degrees of freedom, it was not possible to find the needed financial support for the project, and commercial development never took place.

17.2 System Development and Commercialization

The device for hip arthoplasty known as ROBODOC was the first commercialized robotic surgical system (Integrated Medical System, Birmingham, Alabama, 1992). After that, it was commercialized as the Automated Endoscopic System for Optimal Positioning (AESOP) developed by Computer Motion (Santa Barbara, California) and introduced in 1993. This system, previously described, allowed several surgeons to become familiar with the robotic application in the laparoscopic surgery.

At the same time, Fredrick Moll obtained the commercialization rights from the SRI Greene Telepresence Surgery System and funded Intuitive Surgical System (Sunnyvale, California) in 1995. After several modifications, in April 1997, the system was presented as a renewed master-slave system, the prototype for the DaVinci Surgical System. This system was approved by the FDA in July 2000. The basic difference with its predecessor was the fact it was designed for laparoscopic surgery not for open surgery.

A year later, Computer Motion introduced its own master-slave system, ZEUS Surgical System, which was approved by the FDA in October 2001. Starting with the application of their own technology, AESOP, Computer Motion added two robotic telecontrolers under control of the surgeon to complete the system. Finally, in June 2003, Intuitive Surgical merged with Computer Motion, combining the patents and commercial efforts to promote the DaVinci Master-Slave Robot.

17.3 Clinical Evolution of the Robotic Radical Prostatectomy: Historical Perspective

Prostate cancer, the most common solid malignancy in men, represents a unique oncologic entity that for more than a century has fascinated surgeons trying to cure their patients with the "surgical extirpation of the disease." There is evidence that the first radical prostatectomy was done by Billroth in the 1860s. The initial approach is to perform the surgery via perineum. The success of this procedure in 40 patients was initially described by Young more the 100 years ago and it represents a starting point in the history of the oncologic surgery [8]. The retropubic approach introduced by Millin in 1948 became popular due to the advantages of having an ample surgical field that provides the flexibility to adapt the surgical procedure to the specific anatomy of the patient, a better control of the hemorrhage and the possibility to completely remove cancer in the majority of patients [9]. Better comprehension of the pelvis anatomy as a result of the work performed by Walsh opened the field for these procedures, and in 1982 (with the technical modifications proposed by Walsh and Donker for the neurovascular preservation) the procedures were done in selected patients, without significant risk regarding the oncologic control and preserving the sexual function and urinary continence [10]. All these principles represented a challenge for any prostatic dissection; besides that, the new laparoscopic approach for the radical prostatectomy (LRP)—Montsouris' technique—was very successful, judging for the satisfactory report in the series of patients described by Guillonneau and Vallancien [11, 12].

The established surgical perception of a radical prostatectomy was moved by the clinical evidence generated at the Montsouris Institute of Paris [12, 13]. The first LRP in that institute was performed in January 1998, and the technical viability and satisfactory results on the treated patients lead to establishing the first Urologic Services with focus on LRP. The LRP technique was validated by surgeons in several countries. It became incrementally clear that this technique was quite challenging. It required a important set of skills from the surgeon, and this hindered the procedure's reproducibility. Robotic techniques laboratories provided great help with resolving this problem.

Henry Ford Health System Urology Department in the United States (Detroit, Michigan), led by Dr. Menon, started its laparoscopic/robotic program in 2001. Initially, they tried the development of a pure LPR program under the tutelage of Drs. Guillonneau and Vallancien, but after a year, it was clear that Dr. Menon was not able to master the technique, as he colloquially refers to it. The advance of the DaVinci robot proved pivotal. Thus, during 2001, the Henry Ford team developed an anatomic approach for the radical prostatectomy with robotic support following open and laparoscopic principles plus pivot robotic procedures [14–18].

17.4 DaVinci Surgical System Description

The DaVinci Surgical System is composed of three parts (Figure 17.1). The device has a surgical console, in which the surgeon is located. The surgeon receives tridimensional images of the surgical field while using a binocular device. The DaVinci system uses a laparoscopic device, which has double optics with tridimensional binocular vision. It is composed of two parallel cameras with lenses of 0° or 30° that capture the image and convert it to a 3D digital image. The surgeon interacts with the system through a device known as "master gloves." These master gloves allow free movement of the surgeon's hands, and these movements are intuitively reproduced by the robotic instruments with 7 degrees of freedom. The surgical

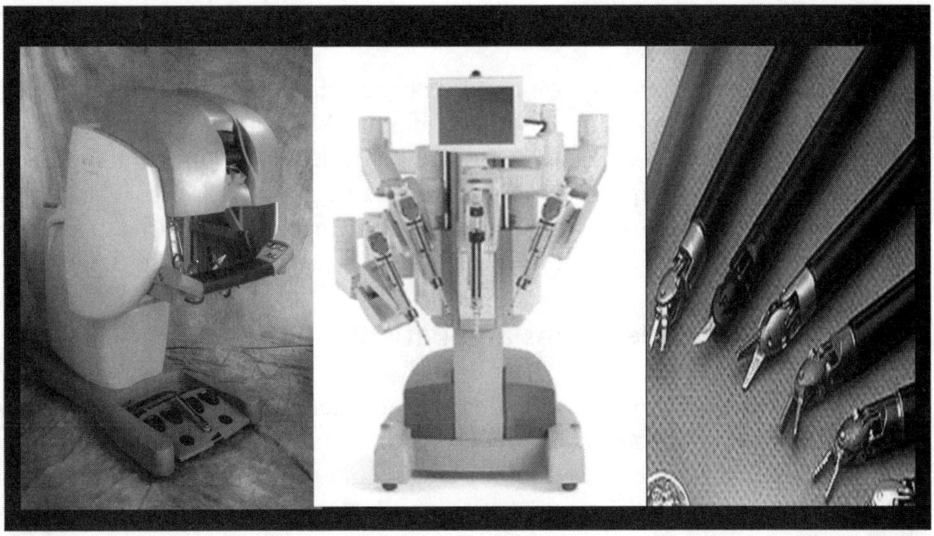

(a) (b) (c)

Figure 17.1 (a) Console—surgeon module. (b) Surgical robot (s-HD Model). (c) Instrumentation.

car can be composed of three or four arms, depending on the model. The camera is located in one of the arms. The technical tower is where all the audiovisual and illumination equipment is located. In the other arms, the robotic surgical instruments are adapted. These instruments include scissors, graspers, and so on. The end of the instruments can articulate in several planes similar to the human wrist (ENDOWRIST Intuitive Surgical). The DaVinci Surgical System allows the surgeon to practice manual movements in the surgical console; those are digitalized and modified by the informatics system that controls the robot in real time, applying the movements in the patient.

This system offers several advantages over the conventional laparoscopy:

1. The surgical console has adequate ergonomic characteristics for the practice of a surgical procedure in optimum conditions. The surgeon can make manual and natural movements, instead of the contra-intuitive movements and the uncomfortable positions that the conventional laparoscopy involves.
2. Due to the digitalization of the movements of the surgeon's hand, the robotic system eliminates the tremor and step movements, such that an ample hand movement in the console is translated into a fine and precise movement in the surgical field.
3. The robotic arms can provide additional degrees of freedom inside the patient, in order to increase the precision and the agility. When compared to conventional laparoscopic instruments, the robotic arms have articulated instruments that reproduce with greater fidelity the movements of the human wrist.
4. The possibility of tridimensional images improves the surgeon's depth perception of the surgical field.

17.5 Robotic and Laparoscopic Instrumentation

The robotic instruments are expensive; hence, their use should be cost effective. The minimal equipment is composed by a bipolar Maryland type grasper, a monopolar scissors, and two needle handlers (Figure 17.1). At the same time it is necessary to use conventional laparoscopic instruments as graspers, scissors, metallic clips (5 and 10 mm), Hem-o-lock type clips, surgical bags, and irrigator/suction devices.

17.6 General Considerations and Patient's Position

The procedure is done under endotracheal general anesthesia, in general with halogenated gases. Nitrous oxide is avoided since it can produce abdominal distension. The IV liquids are restricted to 600 to 800 ml until the urethro-vesical anastomosis is completed. This recommendation avoids the excessive urine production, reducing the needed suction to keep a clean surgical field. The antibiotic prophylaxis is done according to the respective hospital protocol. Also, it is recommended to use perioperative tromboembolic prophylaxis and pneumatic hoses during the surgical procedure.

The patient should be supine decubitus with both arms along the body, in order to avoid lesion of the braquial plexus. It is recommended to use a thoracic pillow fixed with tape. The legs should be positioned in low lithotomy, legs are separated and in abduction, with a pillow or sand bag below buttocks. The legs' position facilitates the location of the surgical car between them. It is very important to pad, and protect well all pressure areas. The surgical table should be placed in extreme Tredelemburg position and as low as possible.

17.7 Robotic Assisted Radical Prostatectomy: Surgical Technique

17.7.1 Transperitoneal Approach

17.7.1.1 Creating the Pneumoperitoneum and Insertion of the Entry Ports

The majority of groups use the transperitoneal approach, but an extraperitoneal approach is also possible. After the insertion of the Veress' needle trough a supra or infra umbilical incision, CO_2 is insufflated until a pressure of 15 mm Hg is obtained. The Veress' needle is replaced by a 12-mm trocar, where the tridimensional laparoscope is introduced. The abdominal cavity is explored, four other trocars are introduced under direct vision; if necessary, adhesions are taken down. Two DaVinci 8-mm trocars are inserted approximately 2.5 cm under the umbilicus and 10 cm lateral than the camera port. A hand breath lateral to each lateral port and close to the anterior ileac spite another robotic 8-mm and standard 12-mm ports are inserted. Optionally, a 5-mm trocar may be inserted between the umbilicus and the 8-mm trocars, according to the assistant preference side (Figures 17.2 and 17.3). Some considerations must be taken in tall patients where distance between the umbilicus and the pubic symphisis is greater than average; the best disposition may be the inverted U somewhat caudal, in order to achieve the correct angulation

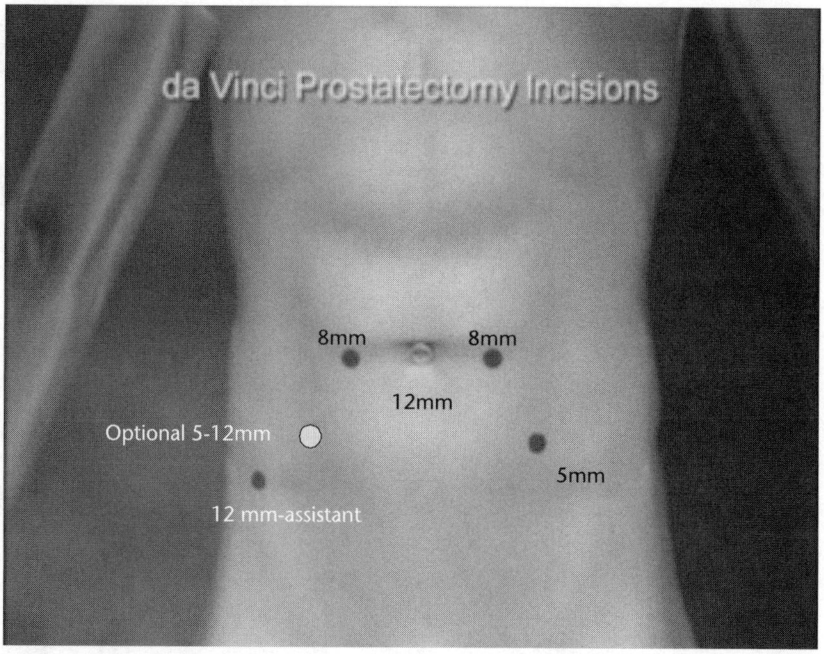

Figure 17.2 Schematic of port placement.

and triangulation over the pelvis. For obese patients, the best disposition should be an inverted U vertex located above the umbilicus, in order to achieve the correct positioning of the instruments. In general, the procedure is carried out with a 30° angle lens. Occasionally for challenging anatomical configurations, a 30° lens is used to facilitate visualization.

17.7.1.2 Creating the Retzius Space

The Retzius space is a virtual cavity occupied by loose connective tissue and fat between the pubic symphisis and the anterior wall of the bladder. The space is accessed by dissecting the umbilical structures through an inverted V incision of the parietal peritoneum, just lateral to each medial umbilical ligament (Figure 17.4). At the level of the pelvis, the lateral landmark is represented by the medial aspect of the vas deferent as it travels caudally toward the seminal vesicles. As fat and connective tissue is released the pelvic bowl is exposed and the bladder drops cranially. Once the anterior surface of the bladder is exposed the adipose tissue above the anterior face of the prostate is retired. The superficial dorsal vein should be exposed so is coagulated and cut. Similarly as the open technique, the endopelvic fascia is opened laterally (Figure 17.5). Little perforator veins are easily visible; they should be coagulated and cut. A complete release of the prostate and levator anni muscle fascia is performed. The pubovesical ligaments represent the distal boundary as they are preserved. Next, the dorsal venous complex is recognized laterally and ligated with a mattress suture (Vicryl 0 needle CT-1) (Figure 17.6). This suture is introduced horizontally in the groove between the urethra and the dorsal venous complex and it is directed back and below the more superficial fibers of the puboprostatic

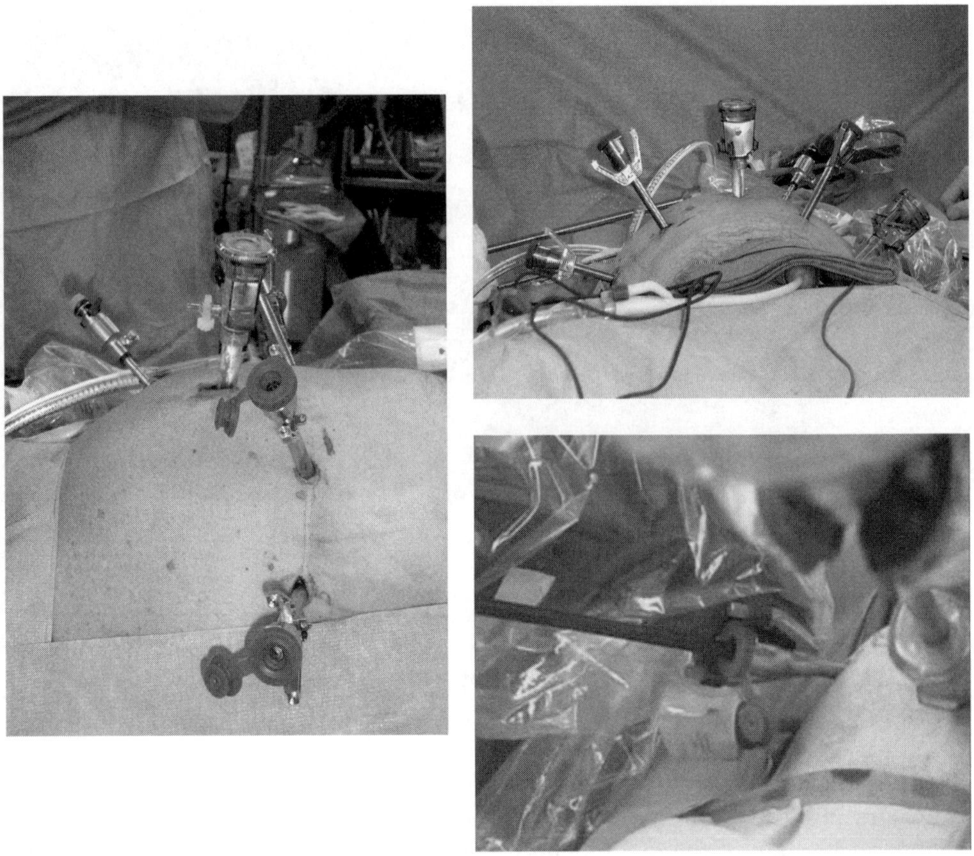

Figure 17.3 Pictures after port placement.

ligament. A second suture is done on the anterior surface of the prostate. The legs of the sutures are cut 1 cm long, in that way the assistant for the fourth arm can pull them during the dissection of the bladder neck and the prostatic apex (Figure 17.7).

17.7.1.3 Disection of the Vesical Neck

The dissection and cutting of the vesical neck is a paramount and potential pitfall of this surgical procedure. Delicate maneuvers can be done to facilitate its identification. In the middle line, detrusor muscle and the prostate are in close contact due to the continuity of the bladder neck urothelial mucosa to the prostatic urethral mucosa. The initial goal is to establish a well-defined dissection plane between the bladder and the prostate on the external side, where the fibroadipose tissue can be identified between the prostate and bladder. Under traction this distance can be almost 2 cm. We prefer to start the dissection of the vesical neck laterally, at the convergence of the posterior prostate and the anterior detrussor muscle. We then take down the anterior aspect of the bladder until we mucosa is entered. The Foley catheter is secured via superior traction by the fourth arm or an assistant. The posterior mucosa is identified, incised, and merged with the lateral plane. Inferiorly, the muscle of the seminal vesicles is identified and evenly divided with cautery exposing

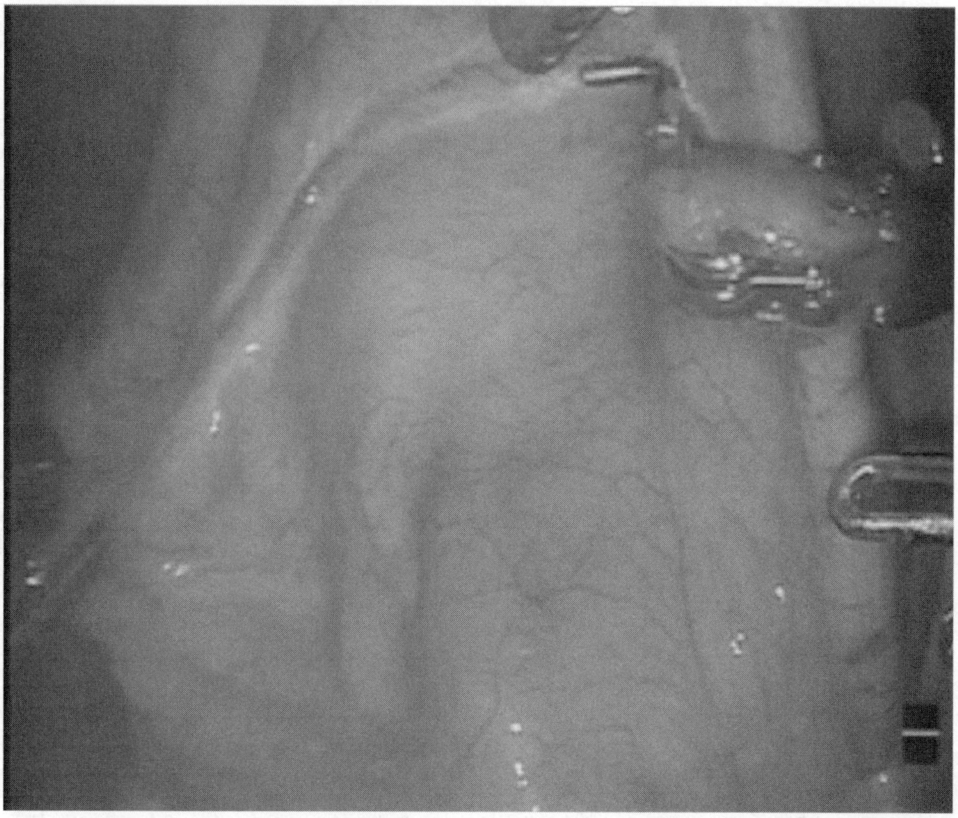

Figure 17.4 Incision of peritoneum providing access to the extra-pre-peritoneal space to drop the bladder.

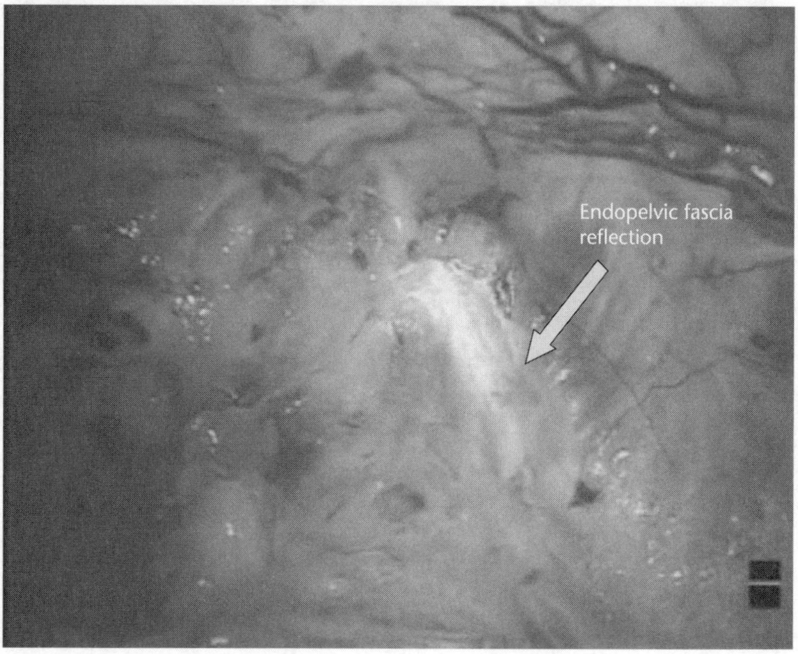

Figure 17.5 Anterior vision of the prostate covered by endopelvic fascia.

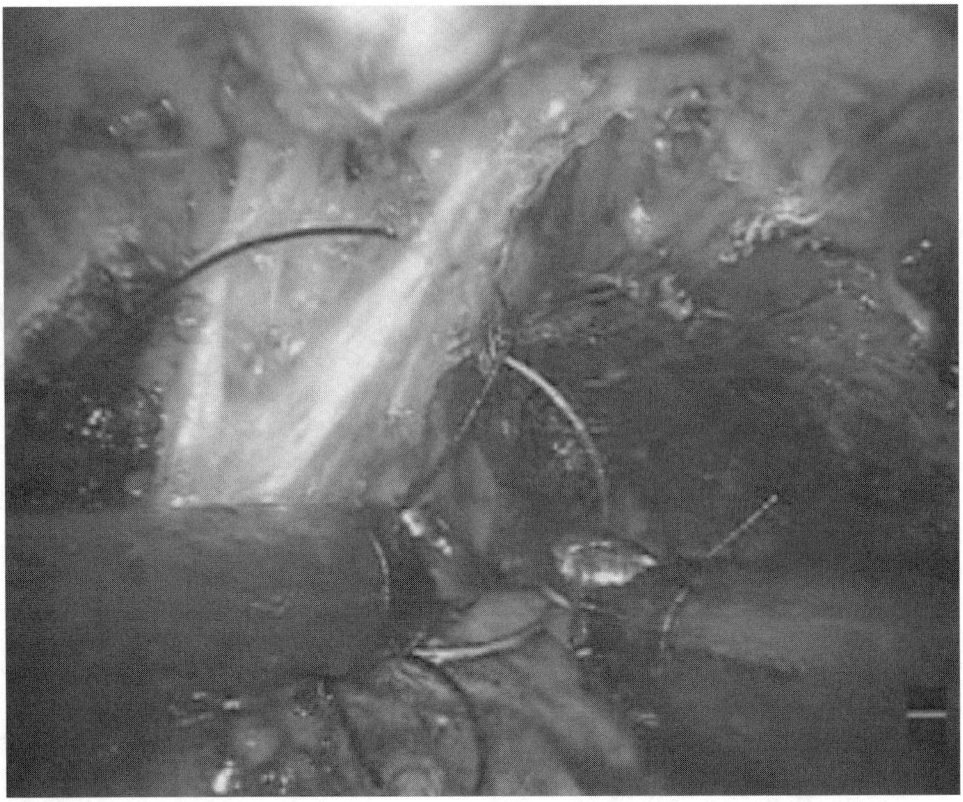

Figure 17.6 Dorsal vein complex (DVC) carefully ligated using endo-wrist needle holders.

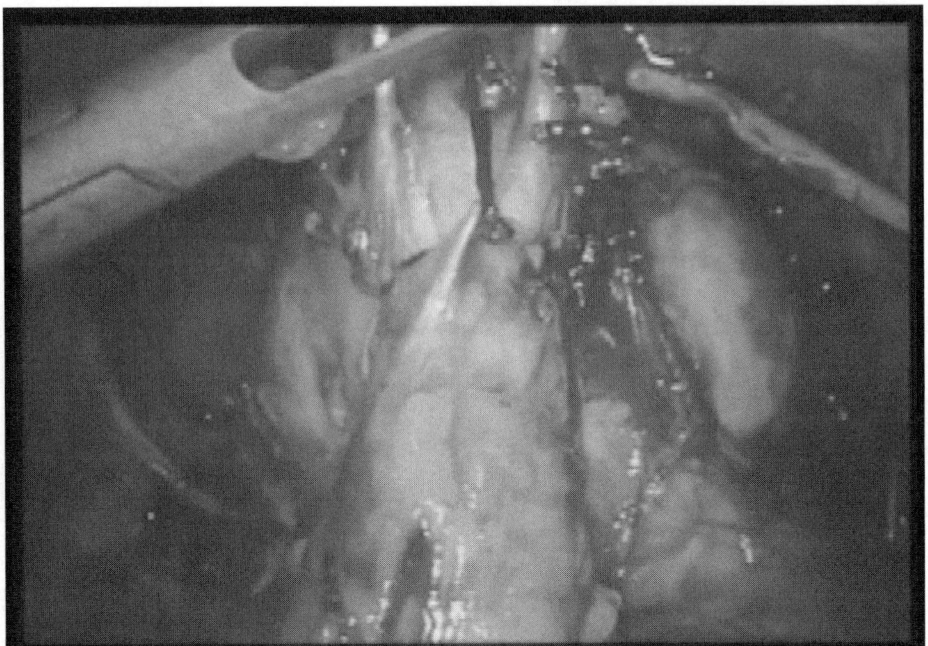

Figure 17.7 Exposure of bladder neck by pulling on fourth arm of robot.

the seminal vesicles and vas deferens (Figure 17.8). The size of the incision of the vesical neck changes according to the presence of cancer on base of the prostate, presence or absence of middle prostatic lobe, the size of the lateral lobules, and the intravesical extension of the lobules (Figure 17.9).

17.7.1.4 Disection of the Seminal Vesicles, Vas Deferens, Prostatic Pedicles, and Incision of the Denonvillier Fascia

The fourth arm or an assistant will grasp the distal aspect of the seminal vesicle muscle and pull upward. Countertraction in the bladder neck is exerted with the Maryland grasper as the vas is dissected, coagulated, and divided. At this time, the fourth arm is adjusted to grasp the distal cutted vas. The arteries of the vas deferent and those supplying the seminal vesicles are recognized and clip ligated. Bipolar cautery is used with caution and monopolar cautery is avoided. Both seminal vesicles and vas are released and secured with fourth arm, which exposes Denonvillier's fascia. The fascia is cut sharply and the dissection is continued caudally separating the prostate from the rectum (Figures 17.10 to 17.12).

17.7.1.5 Preserving the Nervous Structures

Clinical and experimental trials have demonstrated that the cavernous nerves can be found below the prostatic fascia in the anterolateral surface of the gland. These nerves are relevant in the physiology of the erectile function [10, 14, 19]. To facilitate the rapid recovery of the erection, the authors try to preserve the cavernous nerves in selected patients.

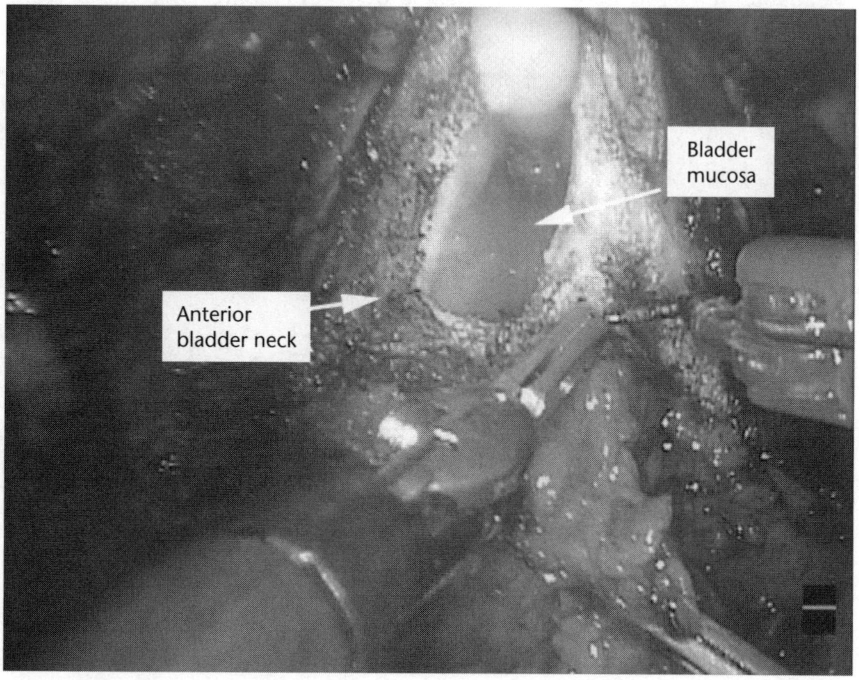

Figure 17.8 Bladder neck opening.

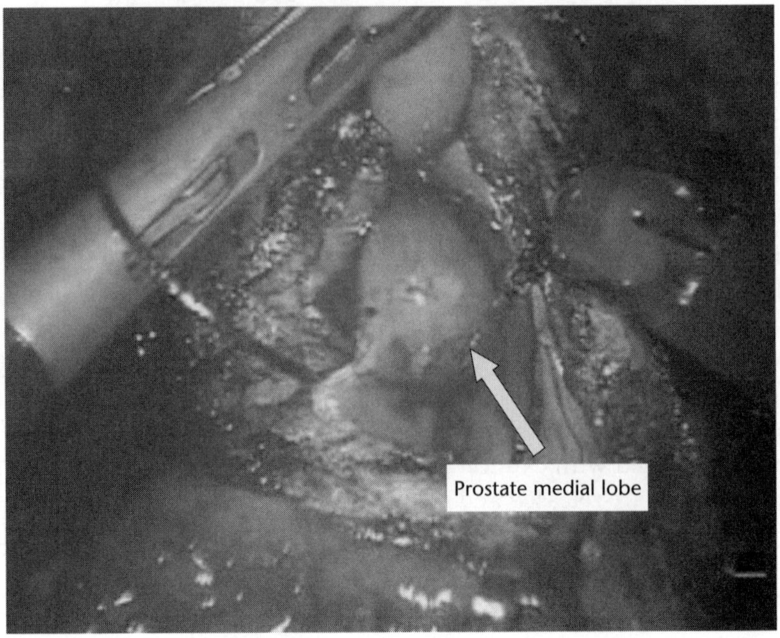

Figure 17.9 Dissection of posterior plate of bladder neck in the presence of a medial lobe of the prostate.

The dissection of the tissue that contains the neurovascular packet is done with the help of the robotic scissors, starting with incision of the lateral pelvic fascia and following in antegrade (cranial to caudal) or retrograde (caudal to cranial) direction releasing the neurovascular packet between the venous plexus and the prostatic capsule. The postero-lateral surface of the prostate is released from the base to

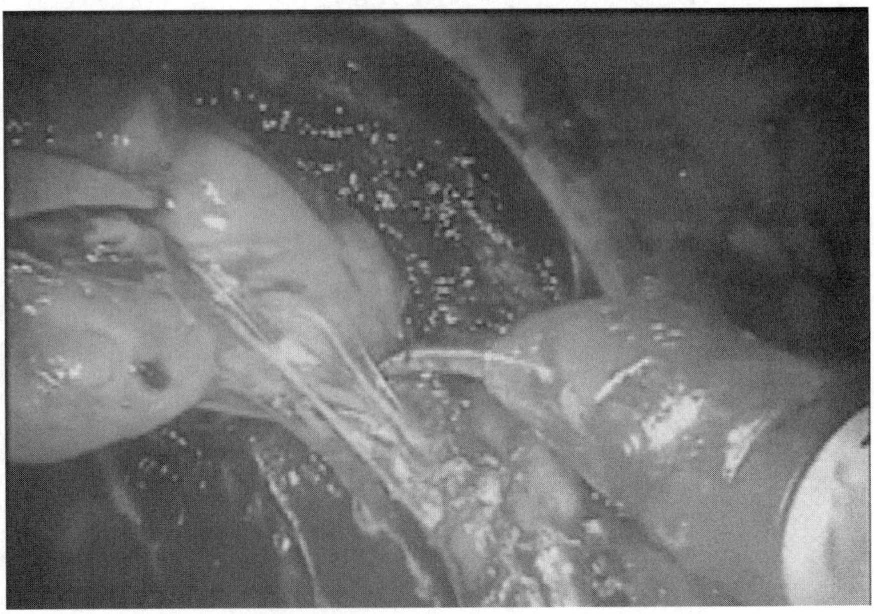

Figure 17.10 Seminal vesicle and vas deferent dissection.

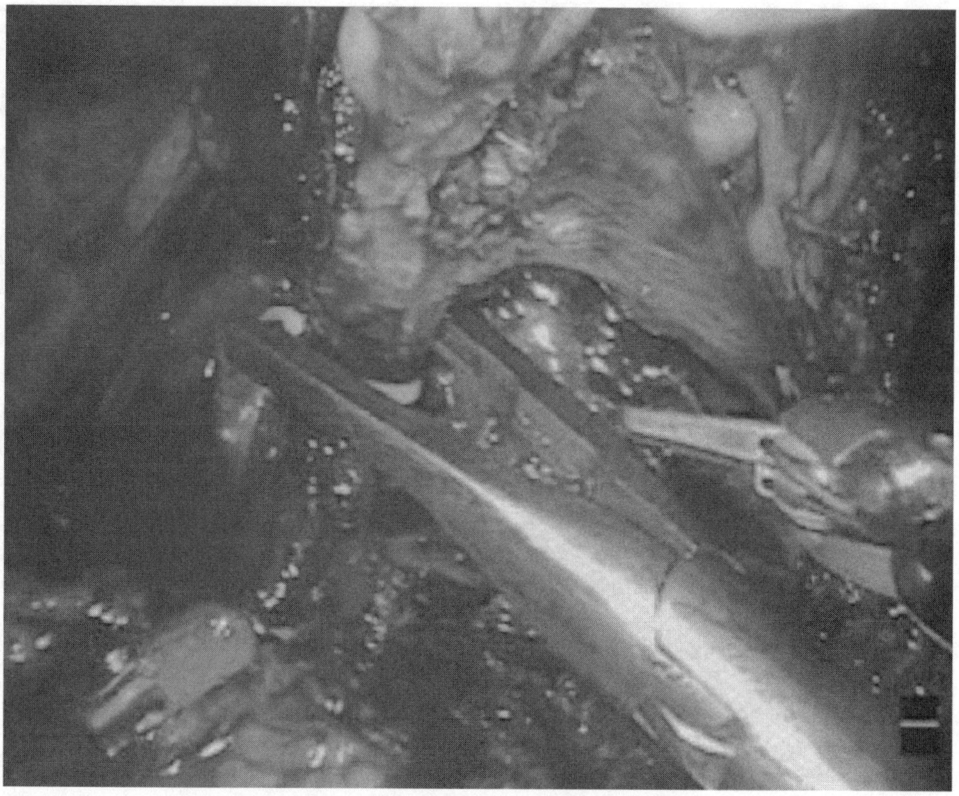

Figure 17.11 Control with hemoclips of the left vascular pedicle feeding the prostate.

the apex. The correct plane is the one located between the venous plexus and the prostatic surface, once there, the dissection is done under a plane almost avascular and it is possible to separate the prostate from the neurovascular packets (Figures 17.13 to 17.15). The vascular pedicles at the base are controlled with clips and cut with scissors.

17.7.1.6 Apical Disection and Urethral Section

Tissues distal to the DVC stitch are cut and dissection continues caudally towards the urethra. The urethra is cut distal to the apical prostate. The intent is to have as long and thick urethra as technically safe. Once the urethra has been severed, frozen sections samples may be obtained from the urethral stump or parietal apical borders, the prostate apex and/or base and from any suspicious area where the neurovascular bundles were released with the help of the articulated scissors. The magnification that the tridimensional optics provides allows obtaining of very precise periurethral samples, without damaging the urethra. In some cases, the authors also obtain samples for biopsy from the base and from the vesical neck. If one of the samples comes back positive, additional biopsies are obtained from the appropriate area; these procedures may reduce the incidence of positive surgical margins.

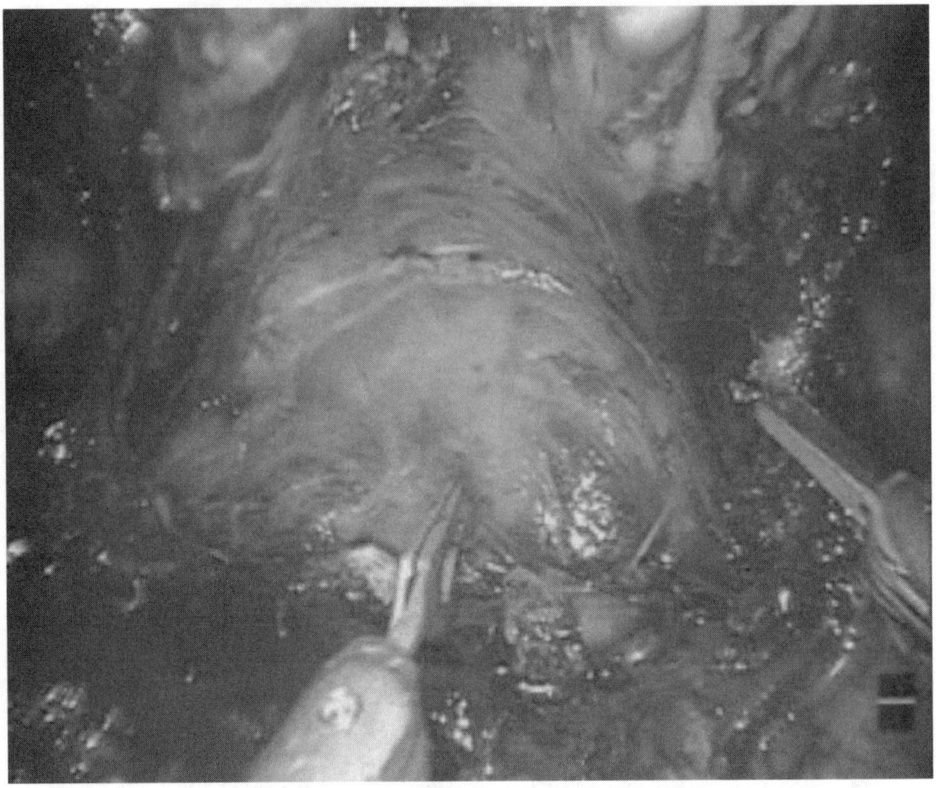

Figure 17.12 Opening of Denonvillier's fascia.

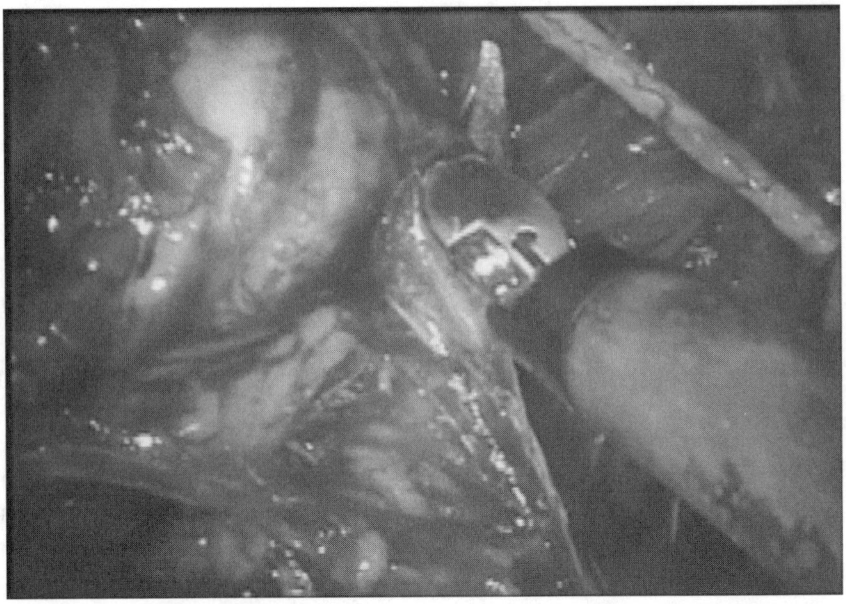

Figure 17.13 Dissection of the periprostatic fascia with preservation of the neurovascular bundles responsible for male erections.

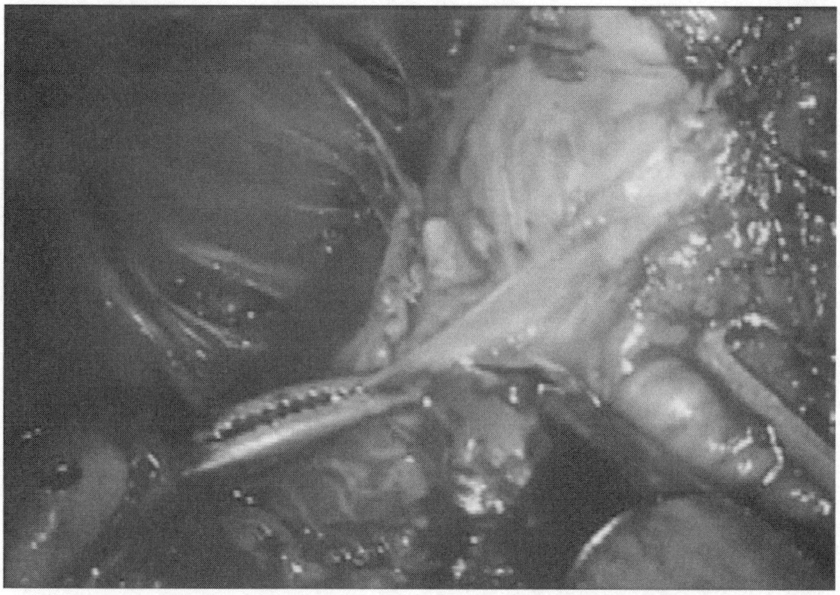

Figure 17.14 Example showing periprostatic fascia dissection on the left side.

17.7.1.7 Vesico-Urethral Anastomosis

The anastomosis is done with a modification of the technique proposed by Van Velthoben [20]. The procedure starts with a knot between the distal legs of two 3-0 Monocryl sutures (different colors and 15 to 20 cm long and needle type RB-1 17 mm). This way a suture of 30 to 40 cm is obtained. The vesico-uretral anastomosis is started by placing the needle of one of the legs at the 5 o'clock position in the

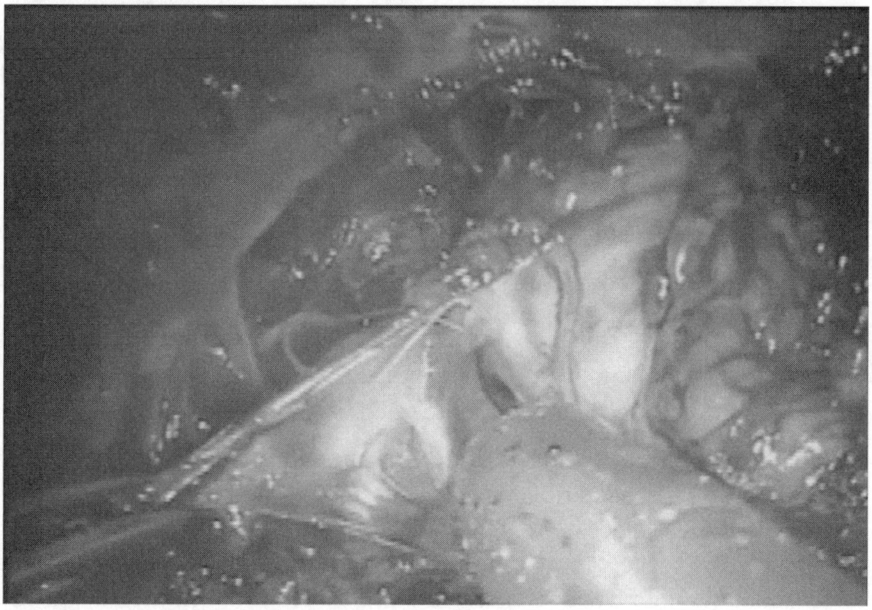

Figure 17.15 Intrafascial dissection of the neurovascular bundles.

vesical neck and from the inside out in the correspondent area or the urethra. The authors make a continuing suture clockwise with three passes of the needle in the bladder and two in the urethra. After completing the posterior wall, a knot is done. After that, the suture is continued until the 9 o'clock position, where the direction changes towards the bladder (Connell) until achieving the 12 o'clock position. The anastomosis is continued with the other leg of the suture in the 4 o'clock position from outside to inside in the urethra and from the inside to outside in the vesical neck. The suture continucs anticlockwise until it gets the other leg. This approach has allowed the authors to complete the urethrovesical anastomosis with only one intracorporeal knot. Finally an 18 F Foley catheter is introduced to assure permeability and a Jackson-Pratt drain in located in the Retzius space.

17.7.1.8 Bilateral Pelvic Lymphadenectomy

This part of the procedure can be done before or after the prostatectomy. The author prefers to do it at the beginning of the procedure. The dissection is done with a 30° lens, up first and then flips downward. The first step is the removal of the retroperitoneal adipose tissue over the iliac vein, circumvent and go to the pelvic sidewall. As the dissection progresses downwards, the obturator nerve and vessels are identified and spared. The lymphatic tissue may be split and rolled to achieve this objective. The external ileac, obturator, and hypogastrics nodes are meticulously dissected out. The dissection is continued cranially until the bifurcation of the external iliac vein.

17.7.2 Retroperitoneal Technique

This technique uses a hybrid approach to develop a big retroperitoneal space for neumoinsuflation. The port insertion and the gas suction are performed during the procedure. With the exception of the bladder descend step, the rest of the procedure is done in the extraperitoneal space. The procedure can be done with a complete extraperitoneal approach. Both are similar in the surgical steps, with the difference in the port insertion and the creation of the work space. Importantly, access to lymph node dissection is limited with this approach.

17.7.2.1 Patients Position Considerations

The position of the patient is similar to the classic technique, but the Tredelemburg is fixed at 15 degrees.

17.17.2.2 Creating the Extraperitoneal Space (Retzius)

An infraumbilical incision is done 2.5 cm below umbilicus; the dissection is done until getting the posterior fascia of the rectum muscles. With blunt dissection an extraperitoneal space is created in order to introduce the balloon of the insufflation device. This space can also be produced with the laparoscopy. After the space is created, a 12-mm trocar is inserted and through it the camera is introduced. Under direct vision the two 8-mm robotic ports are inserted, 2 cm above the camera's port in each side of the rectum muscles, forming a 90-degree angle. For the assistant two extra posts are introduced (5 and 12 mm). This approach has been used with good results by other groups for the radical laparoscopic prostatectomy, in some instances with robotic assistance [22, 23]. According to the authors' experience, the main problem of this approach is the lack of space to practice an appropriate bilateral pelvic lymphadenectomy.

17.8 Series Results of the Radical Robotic Prostatectomy

It is clear that the Radical Robotic Prostatectomy (RRP) has the original advantages of the LPR, reducing the loss of blood and the postoperative pain when compared to the open approach [23]. This translates to a faster hospital discharge (24 hours) [18]. A possible explanation for this observation relates to several sanitary systems that do not encourage the rapid discharge and patients do not require it either. There are centers that do not discharge the patient until retiring the vesical catheter [24]. Table 17.1 shows the results of series performed by a center in which the learning curve has been overcome (in our opinion).

Maybe the challenge now is to demonstrate the utility of the magnification and the tridimensional vision that this technique provides to improve the results. In general, the oncologic results from the published series using the robotic technique (Table 17.2) seem equivalent to the ones for the classic series for open and laparoscopic surgeries.

The risk for incontinence after RRP varies from 5% to 10% when the surgeon is the evaluator to 20% to 30% when the patient answers individually to a questionnaire [25]. Several authors have communicated very promising results regarding this issue after the RRP (Table 17.3). However, we must demand more hard core evidence, desirably coming from randomized studies.

The conversion numbers for the LPR are less than 5%. Currently, the more recent series for RRP show a rate of conversion almost 0% (Table 17.1). The perioperative complications (Table 17.1) in general are the same as for those with the laparoscopic surgery, but the learning curve and the operatory time are clearly better for the robotic surgery.

Table 17.1 Robotic Assisted Laparoscopic Prostatectomy: Perioperative Results

Autor	*Yr*	*N*	*Operative Time (min)*	*Blood Loss (ml)*	*Transfusion Rate (%)*	*Conversions (%)*	*Complications (%)*	*Stay (days)*
Menon [26]	2003	200	160	153	0%	1%	8%	1.2
Wolfram [21]	2003	81	250	300	12%	SD	SD	SD
Bentas [24]	2003	41	498	570	32%	5%	41.7%	1.7
Ahlering [27]	2004	60	231	103	0%	0%	6.7%	1
Costello [28]	2005	122	SD	SD	3%	SD	16%	2
Patel [29]	2005	200	141	75	0%	0%	1.5%	1.1
Hu [30]	2006	322	186	250	1.6%	0.6%	17.2%	SD
Joseph [31]	2006	325	130	196	1%	0%	9.6%	1

Table 17.2 Pathological Results for Robotic Prostatectomies for Prostate Cancer

Author	*Year*	*N*	*Path Stage*			*Positive Margins (%)*	*PM (%) by Stage*		
			pT2	*pT3*	*pT3b*		*pT2*	*pT3a*	*pT3b*
Menon [26]*	2003	200	87%	7%	6%	15%*	11%*	40%*	40%*
Wolfram [21]	2003	81	69%	31%		22%	13%	42%	
Bentas [24]	2003	41	63%	22%	15%	30%	8%	67%	
Ahlering [27]	2004	60	75%	24%		17%	5%	44%	
Costello [28]	2005	122	80%	16%	4%	16%			
Patel [29]	2005	200	78%	14%	8%	11%	6%	26%	33%
Joseph [31]	2006	325	81%	14%	5%	13%	10%	37%	27%

*Margins based on the first 100 cases.

Table 17.3 Urinary Continence Results for Robotic Prostatectomies for Prostate Cancer

Author	*Year*	*N*	*Continence Definition*	*Methodology*	*Continence (%)*		
					3-mo	*6-mo*	*12-mo*
Menon [26]	2003	200	0-1 PADS	Interview		96%	
Bentas [24]	2003	41	0-1 PADS	Questionnaire			84%
Ahlering [27]	2004	60	No PADS	Questionnaire	76%		
Costello [28]	2005	122	0-1 PADS	Questionnaire	73%	82%	
Patel [29]	2005	200	No PADS	Questionnaire	82%	89%	98%
Joseph [31]	2006	325	No PADS	Questionnaire	93%	96%	

17.9 Conclusions and Future Vision

We have done a summary of the most important aspects of this very exciting intervention. We believe that the most important contribution of the RRP is its reproducibility. The optic magnification and the advance of the technology should make the teaching and learning of this approach easier. The magnified vision serves as a historic reference in the study of the surgical technique and the implications that its variations have. Ideally, it would possible to randomize the patients to study the effect of the surgeon preferences. The excision of the prostate is one of more demanding procedures for the urologist. The real goal, the control of the cancer preserving the continence and the sexual function, is a challenge achieved in more than 50% of the patients in the hands of experienced surgeons. We expect that the increased data and experience will improve this rate of success.

References

[1] Davies, B. L., et al., "The Development of a Surgeon Robot for Prostatectomies," *Proc. Inst. Mech. Eng.*, Vol. 205, 1991, pp. 35–38.

[2] Hill, J. W., et al., "Telepresence Interface with Applications to Microsurgery and Surgical Simulation," *Stud. Health Technol. Inform.*, Vol. 50, 1998, pp. 96–102.

[3] Perissat, J., D. R. Collet, and R. Belliard, "Gallstones: Laparoscopic Treatment, Intracorporeal Lithotripsy Followed by Cholecystostomy or Cholecystostomy—A Personal Technique," *Endoscopy*, Vol. 21, 1989, pp. 373–374.

[4] Satava, R. M., "Robotic Surgery: From Past to Future—A Personal Journey," *Surg. Clin. North Am.*, Vol. 83, 2003, pp. 1491–1500.

[5] Bowersox, J. C., P. R. Cordts, and A. J. LaPorta, "Use of an Intuitive Telemanipulator System for Remote Trauma Surgery: An Experimental Study," *J. Am. Coll. Surg.*, Vol. 186, 1998, p. 615.

[6] Bowersox, J. C., and R. L. Cornum, "Remote Operative Urology Using a Surgical Telemanipulator System: Preliminary Observations," *Urology*, Vol. 52, 1998, pp. 17–22.

[7] Schurr, M. O., et al., "Robotics and Telemanipulation Technologies for Endoscopic Surgery. A Review of the ARTEMIS Project. Advanced Robotic Telemanipulator for Minimally Invasive Surgery," *Surg. Endosc.*, Vol. 14, 2000, pp. 375–381.

[8] Young, H. H., "The Early Diagnosis and Radical Cure of Carcinoma of the Prostate. Being a Study of 40 Cases and Presentation of a Radical Operation Which Was Carried Out in Four Cases," *J. Urol.*, Vol. 168, 2002, pp. 914–921.

[9] Millin, T., "Retropubic Prostatectomy," *J. Urol.*, Vol. 60, 1948, pp. 267–280.

[10] Walsh, P. C., and P. J. Donker, "Impotence Following Radical Prostatectomy: Insight into Etiology and Prevention," *J. Urol.*, 1982; Vol. 128: 492–497.

[11] Guillonneau, B., et al., "Laparoscopic Radical Prostatectomy. Preliminary Evaluation After 28 Interventions," *Presse Med.*, Vol. 27, 1998, pp. 1570–1574.

[12] Guillonneau, B., and G. Vallancien, "Laparoscopic Radical Prostatectomy: The Montsouris Technique," *J. Urol.*, Vol. 163, 2000, pp. 1643–1649.

[13] Guillonneau, B., et al., "Laparoscopic Radical Prostatectomy: Oncological Evaluation After 1,000 Cases at Montsouris Institute," *J. Urol.*, Vol. 169, 2003, pp. 1261–1266.

[14] Walsh, P. C., "Radical Retropubic Prostatectomy with Reduced Morbidity: An Anatomic Approach," *NCI Monogr.*, Vol. 7, 1988, pp. 133–137.

[15] Pasticier, G., et al., "Robotically Assisted Laparoscopic Radical Prostatectomy: Feasibility Study in Men," *Eur. Urol.*, Vol. 40, 2001, pp. 70–74.

[16] Binder, J., and W. Kramer, "Robotically Assisted Laparoscopic Radical Prostatectomy," *BJU Int.*, Vol. 87, 2001, pp. 408–410.

[17] Abbou, C. C., et al., "Laparoscopic Radical Prostatectomy with a Remote Controlled Robot," *J. Urol.*, Vol. 165, 2001, pp. 1964–1966.

[18] Menon, M., "Robotic Radical Retropubic Prostatectomy," *BJU Int.*, Vol. 91, 2003, pp. 175–176.

[19] Takenaka, A., et al., "Anatomical Analysis of the Neurovascular Bundle Supplying Penile Cavernous Tissue to Ensure a Reliable Nerve Graft After Radical Prostatectomy," *J. Urol.*, Vol. 172, 2004, pp. 1032–1035.

[20] Van Velthoben, R. F., et al., "Technique for Laparoscopic Running Urethrovesical Anastomosis: The Single Knot Method," *Urology*, Vol. 61, 2003, pp. 699–702.

[21] Wolfram, M., et al., "Robotic-Assisted Laparoscopic Radical Prostatectomy: The Frankfurt Technique," *World J. Urol.*, Vol. 21, 2003, pp. 128–132.

[22] Gettman, M. T., et al. "Laparoscopic Radical Prostatectomy: Description of the Extraperitoneal Approach Using the Da Vinci Robotic System," *J. Urol.*, Vol. 170, 2003, pp. 416–419.

[23] Tewari, A., A. Srivastava, and M. Menon, "Members of the VIP Team. A Prospective Comparison of Radical Retropubic and Robot-Assisted Prostatectomy: Experience in One Institution," *BJU Int.*, Vol. 92, 2003, pp. 205–210.

[24] Bentas, W., et al., "Robotic Technology and the Translation of Open Radical Prostatectomy to Laparoscopy: The Early Frankfurt Experience with Robotic Radical Prostatectomy and One Year Follow-Up," *Eur. Urol.*, Vol. 44, 2003, pp. 175–218.

[25] Noldus, J., J. Palisaar, and H. Huland, "Treatment of Prostate Cancer: The Clinical Use of Radical Prostatectomy," *EAU Update Series*, Vol. 1, 2003, pp. 16–22.

[26] Menon, M., et al., "Robotic Radical Prostatectomy and the Vattikuti Urology Institute Technique: An Interim Analysis of Results and Technical Points," *Urology*, Vol. 61, 2003, pp. 15–20.

[27] Ahlering, T. E., et al., "Robot-Assisted Versus Open Radical Prostatectomy: A Comparison of One Surgeon's Outcomes," *Urology*, Vol. 63, 2004, pp. 819–822.

[28] Costello, A. J., et al., "Installation of Telerobotic Surgery and Initial Experience with Telerobotic Radical Prostatectomy," *BJU Int.*, Vol. 96, 2005, pp. 34–38.

[29] Patel, V. R., et al., "Robotic Radical Prostatectomy in the Community Setting—The Learning Curve and Beyond: Initial 200 Cases," *J. Urol.*, Vol. 174, 2005, pp. 269–272.

[30] Hu, J. C., et al., "Perioperative Complications of Laparoscopic and Robotic Assisted Laparoscopic Radical Prostatectomy," *J. Urol.*, Vol. 175, 2006, pp. 541–546.

[31] Joseph, J. V., et al. "Robotic Extraperitoneal Radical Prostatectomy: An Alternative Approach," *J. Urol.*, Vol. 175, 2006, pp. 945–950.

CHAPTER 18

Modeling of Image-Guided Therapy

Isaac A. Chang and T. Joshua Pfefer

18.1 Introduction

Image-guided therapy has historically involved the use of anatomical information for device navigation and treatment monitoring during medical procedures. While these techniques provide significant advantage in terms of localizing and delineating critical biological structures, medical procedures can also be enhanced through the application of established knowledge of biophysical processes. For interventions which involve directed energy modalities such as X-ray, radiofrequency, and optical radiation, computational modeling represents a powerful tool that enables clinicians to exploit patient-specific three-dimensional (3D) morphology in order to identify optimal treatment parameters.

The use of medical images in guiding therapeutic treatment modalities is not new. Since the discovery that X-rays could be used to image bone structures in the human anatomy by Röntgen in 1895, much interest has been placed on incorporating imaging into clinical treatment. Over the years, a variety of imaging modalities have been used to localize both normal and diseased anatomical and pathological structures. X-rays, ultrasound, computed tomography (CT), magnetic resonance imaging (MRI), and impedance imaging all generate images that are essential in optimizing approaches for defining and targeting treatment volumes for therapy. Imaging is as critical of a component for treatment planning as it is for monitoring interventions.

Modeling also plays an essential role in the process of guiding therapeutic treatment. Computational models provide a representation of the behavior of a complex system. The implementation of models in therapeutic treatment is as diverse as the use of imaging. Models range from empirical estimations of phenomena, to mechanistic behavior of a device component, to morphologically thorough (whether this be whole body or high-resolution of a limited volume) simulations of nonlinear device-tissue interactions. As the complexity of modeling increases, the time and resources needed to solve such problems increase as well.

This chapter focuses on the modeling of image guided therapies. While the topic elicits a connotation of applicability to only real-time image guided therapies, it actually represents a spectrum of solutions where imaging and modeling are balanced in different proportions. To illustrate this spectrum, consider two cases involving oncologic treatment of tumors: ultrasound guided radiofrequency ablation and radiation oncology.

Radiofrequency (RF) ablation is a clinical therapy in which diseased tissue is necrosed by raising the temperature of targeted tissues. A conductive electrode is inserted into the diseased tissue. Once positioned, high frequency alternating current (450 to 550 kHz) is delivered through the electrode into the surrounding tissues to a dispersive ground pad that is applied to the patient. The electromagnetic energy is converted to heat by resistive heating [1]. In ultrasound guided radiofrequency ablation studies [2–6], ultrasound imaging is used to provide real-time feedback regarding the location of probe placement. Frequently, the ultrasound images are also used to track the progression of tissue necrosis by monitoring RF ablation-induced changes. Since actual cell necrosis is not discernable from the ultrasound image, histopathologic evaluation of tissue specimens post-procedure is used to determine whether an adequate treatment margin is produced around the tumor. Computational studies have been performed on the tumor ablation probe geometry by a number of investigators [7, 8]. These studies provide insight into the heating pattern of the probes and attempt to correlate the histopathologic evidence with surrogate markers (i.e., temperature) to predict the progression of lesion growth over the course of treatment. The availability of the modeling results serves to enhance and optimize the treatment approach by identifying new imaging markers to guide therapeutic treatment in real time. The case of ultrasound-guided radiofrequency ablation demonstrates a situation in which imaging dominates modeling in shaping real-time imaging therapy. The modeling aspects contribute greatly to the optimization of the therapy and provide a more robust means of anticipating the behavior of the radiofrequency ablation device under a variety of conditions.

Radiation oncology is the medical use of ionizing radiation to manage the growth of malignant tumor cells [9]. Although it can be used for total body irradiation, which is typical of bone marrow transplant procedures, for the management of tumors the radiation beams are typically shaped to minimize exposure to healthy tissues [10]. Modern computing has brought major advances in computerized imaging, computational technique, and visualization. These tools have found wide utility in radiation oncology applications. Preoperative images of the entire three-dimensional anatomy are used to create anatomical models, which help to localize, visualize, and target intended tissues. The models are used to calculate radiation dosing and identify the angles in which radiation beams are placed to provide greater absorbed dose in the targeted tissue than in the surrounding healthy tissue. The case of radiation oncology demonstrates a situation in which modeling plays a substantial role in the guided therapy. While imaging forms the basis of the models, the model itself forms the basis of the optimized guided therapy. Real-time imaging plays a minimal role in radiation oncology.

18.2 Role of Imaging and Modeling for Image-Guided Therapies

The interdependency of imaging and modeling for image-guided therapies can be thought of as a continuum, where the relative emphasis of modeling and imaging are different for each kind of guided therapy, Whether the image modality is intended to provide surface or subsurface detail, a structural or a functional view of tissue, or provide details on a molecular scale, the optimization of the guided therapy involves some aspects of both imaging and modeling.

18.2.1 Progression of Imaging

Figure 18.1 illustrates the spectrum of image-based guided therapies that involve modeling. The progression applies to therapies with geometries ranging from micro-cellular structures to whole-body geometries. The most basic form of image guided therapy involves acquiring images to determine treatment location and interventional placement of medical devices. These "image-guided placement" therapies form the early experience for nearly all therapies that involve imaging. Real-time imaging approaches are the next logical development of image guided placements. They allow the practitioner to gain feedback for navigation and assessment of treatment progress. In many cases, therapy monitoring need not be performed by real-time imaging. For example, in gynecological, cardiac, and oncologic radiofrequency ablation procedures, it is frequently only necessary to identify the placement of the device. When X-ray and other ionizing radiation are involved in imaging, real-time approaches are used sparingly to reduce the level of radiation exposure to the patient. In such cases, a fundamental understanding of how the device functions through device modeling is helpful to ensure a successful clinical outcome.

In addition to gaining a structural view of tissues for guiding placement of devices, imaging plays an integral role in modeling. Medical images are simplified into representative geometries, in many cases, as a matter of practicality. The resources needed to model systems at a high degree of realism may be prohibitively expensive in terms of memory or computational effort. Thus, models that incorporate simpler geometries are used to determine the behavior of a medical device. Figure 18.2 shows an example of a computational modeling study of how radiofrequency ablation of liver is affected by flow from major arterial vessels [11]. The liver tissue was imaged using MRI in Figure 18.2(a). Geometric reconstruction techniques were used to form a simpler rendering of the actual arterial geometry. The fine detail

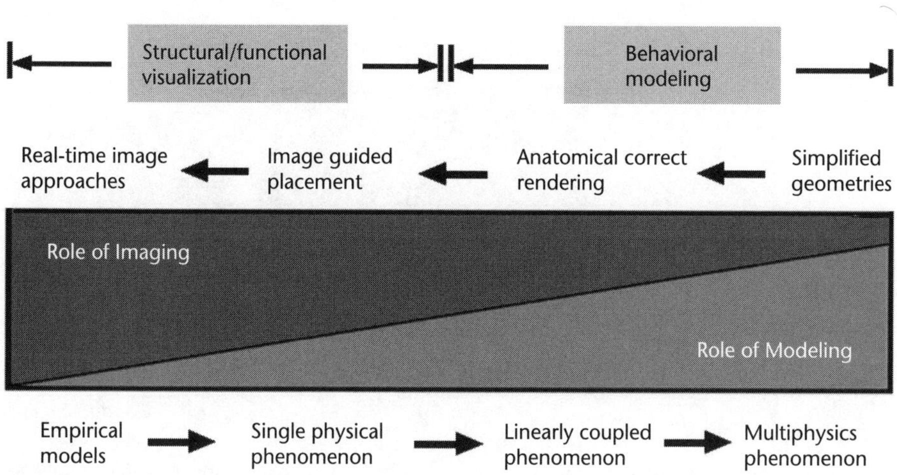

Figure 18.1 Spectrum of model and image-guided therapies.

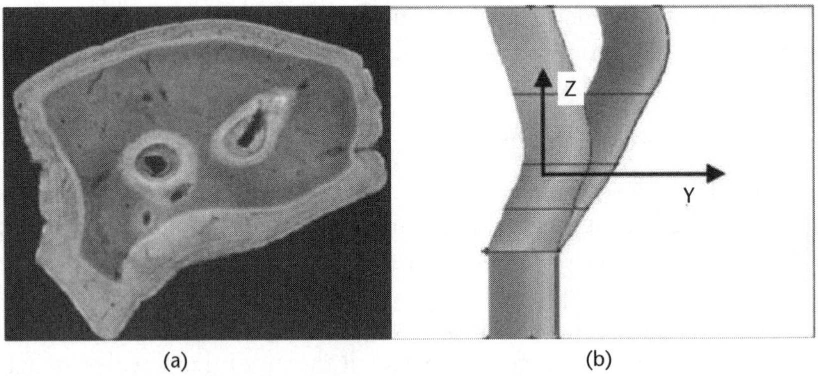

Figure 18.2 (a) Cross-sectional MRI image of excised porcine liver cross section. (b) Reconstructed bifurcated artery surrounded by hepatic tissue.

of microscopic structures are neglected completely in favor of a more manageable computational structure.

Frequently, geometric simplifications can be made by reducing the number of dimensions in a system, or by identifying axes or planes of symmetry [12–17]. For example, Figure 18.3 shows the geometry of a commercially available multiprong radiofrequency ablation probe used in the treatment of liver metastatic tumors. The figure identifies two planes of symmetry that can be used to reduce the scope of the model geometry. By simplifying the model in this manner, memory requirements are substantially decreased and computational speeds are increased dramatically. Localized geometries are often represented by idealized structures that represent layers of tissue of various dimensions with bulk intrinsic tissue properties of whole organ level tissues [18–20].

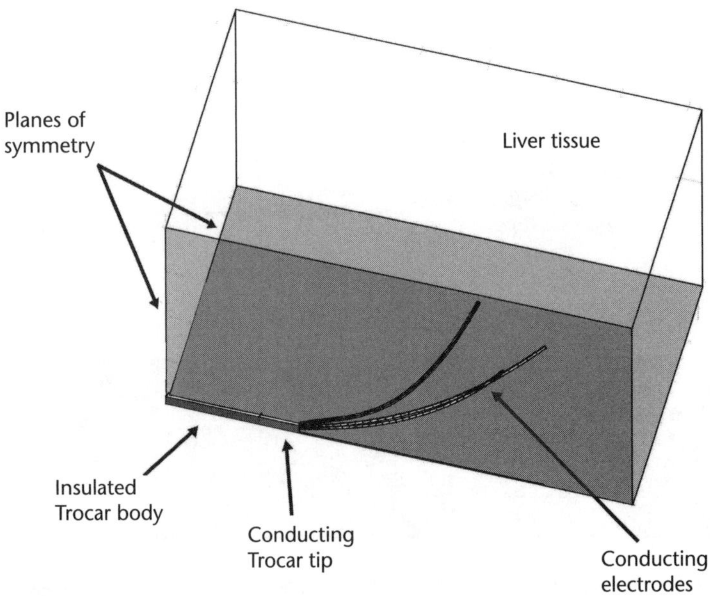

Figure 18.3 Example geometry of a complex multiprong oncologic radiofrequency ablation device showing planes of symmetry.

In recent years, an effort has been made to incorporate anatomically correct structures in computational modeling [21–25]. In these applications, the actual body geometry is frequently too complicated to be accurately depicted or modeled. Smoothing and rendering algorithms are used to simplify the geometry of body structures. Beard and Kainz [26], for example, have used anatomically correct renderings of the head to calculate the exposure from cell phones. In this study, the authors compared computational results of specific absorption rate (SAR) calculations between a standardized cell-phone head model and anatomically correct renderings of the human head. The anatomically correct data set of the human head was adapted from the Visible Human Male (Figure 18.4), which originated at the National Institutes of Health. Figure 18.4(a) shows a three-dimensional rendering of the human male model. The model is a geometrically correct rendering of a man subdivided into 5 × 5 × 5 mm volumes, for a total of 4.3 million cubes. Each cubic volume is assigned to one of 34 different types of body tissue. Figure 18.4(b, c) shows coronal projections of muscle tissue and bone. In other studies, Kainz et al. have calculated the internal fields and current densities induced in a pregnant women and her fetus when exposed to handheld metal detectors [27]. In these studies, geometrically reconstructed models of a pregnant woman and a fetus at

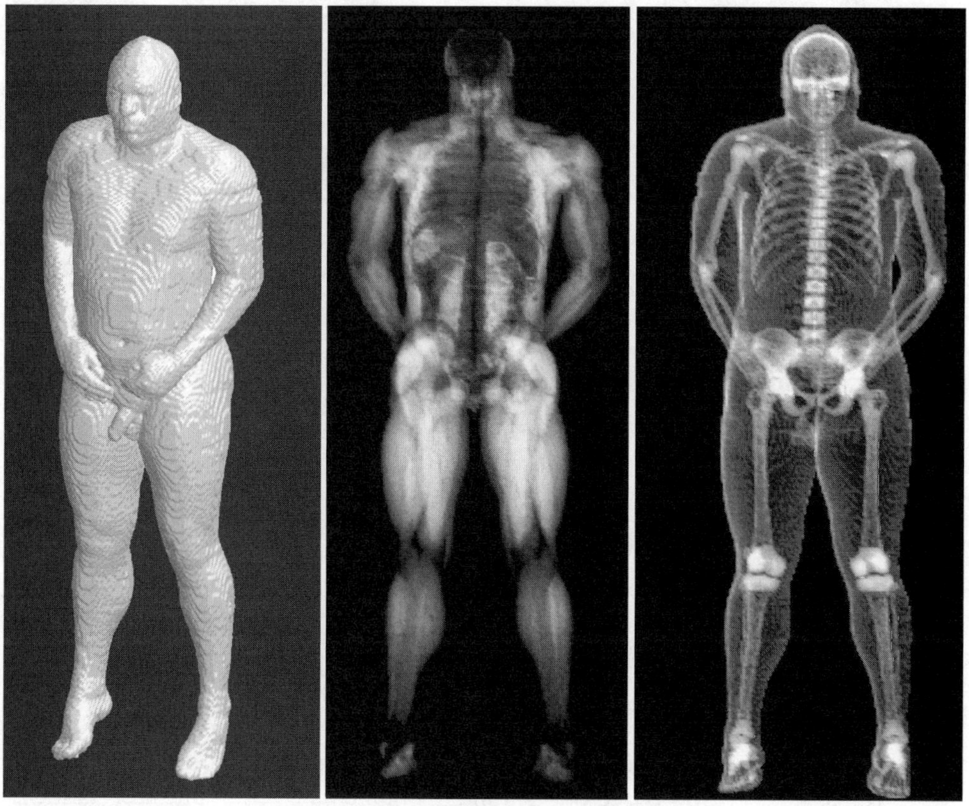

(a) (b) (c)

Figure 18.4 Anatomically correct rendering of an adult human: (a) 3D exterior view; (b) coronal projection of muscle tissue; and (c) coronal projection of bone.

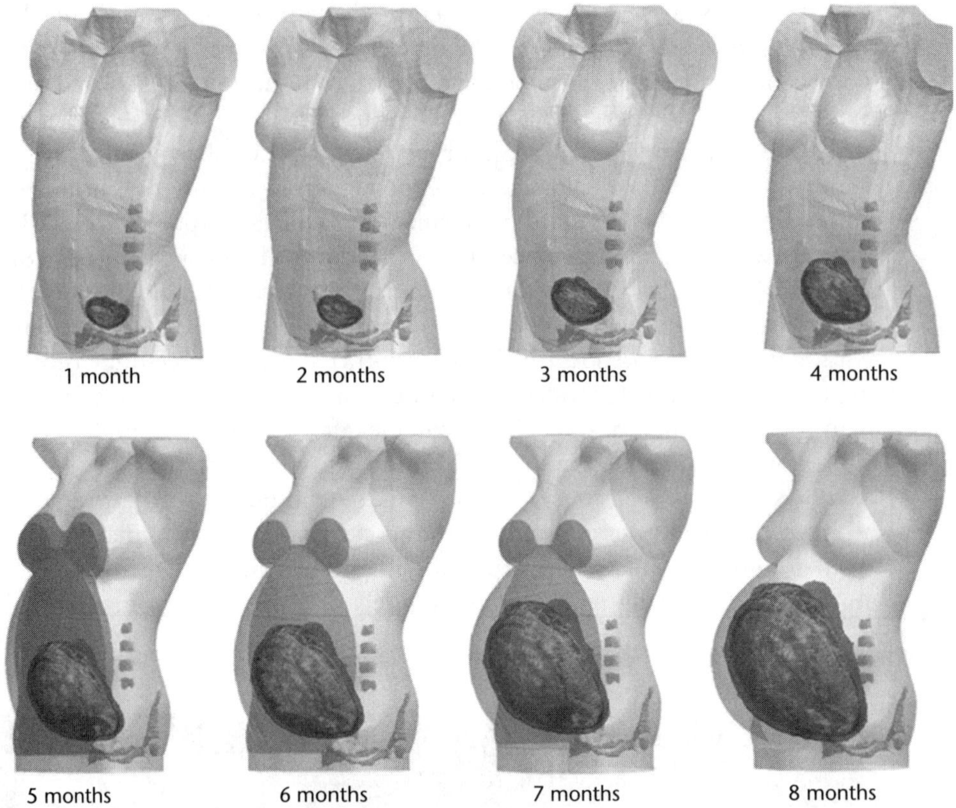

Figure 18.5 Geometric reconstruction of a pregnant woman and fetus model used for the evaluation of induced current densities and specific absorption rates for pregnant women exposed to hand-held metal detectors.

varying points in pregnancy were created. The model geometries were scaled from a scanned image of a woman in the 34th week of pregnancy (Figure 18.5). Most recently, CAD based anatomical models of two adults and two children have been developed by the U.S. Food and Drug Administration in collaboration with the ITIS foundation. These models are freely available for academic and scientific distribution through the ITIS Foundation (www.itis.ethz.ch).

18.2.2 Progression of Modeling

The complexity of computational models has varied widely. The simplest models are numerical approximations of observed clinical data. Empirical data can be represented numerically by the use of polynomial or other functional expressions. These simple models allow for interpolation between known clinical observations and are extremely useful in optimizing a specific procedure. While no less accurate than more complicated modeling schemes, empirical models have severe limitations. They are not based on the fundamental equations of physics. As such, a major assumption for empirical models is that the observable outcome is dependent on only a few measurable variables. A consequence of this assumption is that variations in any other parameter in the model are not allowed. For example, a model that predicts the behavior of a therapy on healthy tissues may behave completely different in the presence of diseased tissues.

The introduction of the fundamental equations of physics into modeling greatly improves the ability to predict system behavior and can be used to optimize guided therapies. Fundamental relations such as Maxwell's equations (electromagnetic), Pennes Bioheat equation (heat transfer), and the Navier-Stokes equation (fluid mechanics) can be used to predict the distribution of energy and forces throughout a body system. Models that account for the equations governing physical phenomena are useful in anticipating how the system behaves to changes in the applied sources as well as changes in the intrinsic characteristics. For example, the spatial distribution of temperature in body tissues is found by solving the Pennes Bioheat [28] equation:

$$\rho C\frac{dT}{dt} = \nabla \cdot (k\nabla T) - \rho_b C_b \omega (T - T_{ambient}) + Q_m \tag{18.1}$$

where ρ is the density; C is the heat capacity; k is the thermal conductivity; T is the temperature, ρ_b is the density of blood; C_b is the heat capacity of blood; ω is the tissue perfusion; $T_{ambient}$ is the ambient blood temperature, Q_m is the metabolic heat generation term; and ∇ is the gradient operator. Models based on this equation can predict the behavior of the system (i.e., temperature rise) as a result of changes to any one of these variables. This offers distinct advantages over empirical models, as the relationship between the parameters governing the behavior of the system are defined and can be changed, without compromising the inherent behavior of the model.

In describing more complex behavior, several sets of governing equations may be used. In these cases, one must consider the manner in which these equations are coupled to each other. Depending on how they are coupled, the system will behave in a simple linear manner or, alternatively, in a highly nonlinear and complex manner [29]. For example, in radiofrequency ablation problems, three sets of governing equations apply [1]. In addition to the Pennes Bioheat equation, Laplace's equation and the Arrhenius equation are often solved. The electric field is solved by using Laplace's equation,

$$\nabla \cdot [\sigma \nabla V] = 0 \tag{18.2}$$

where σ is the electrical conductivity and V is the electric potential. Temperature is then solved by using a modified Pennes Bioheat equation,

$$\rho C\frac{dT}{dt} = \nabla \cdot (k\nabla T) + \sigma |\nabla V|^2 - \rho_b C_b \omega (T - T_{ambient}) + Q_m \tag{18.3}$$

where the added term $\sigma |\nabla V|^2$ represents the electromagnetic source term. The Arrhenius equation is used to calculate the cumulative damage integral, which indicates the degree of tissue injury, $\Omega(t)$:

$$\Omega(t) = A \int_{0}^{t=\tau} \exp\left(-\frac{\Delta E}{RT(t)}\right) dt \tag{18.4}$$

where R is the universal gas constant, A is a "frequency" factor for the kinetic expression, and ΔE is the thermodynamic activation energy for the irreversible damage reaction. The kinetic parameters account for morphologic changes in tissue relating to the thermal degradation of proteins in tissue. In many models [7, 8, 12, 17, 30, 31], these equations are coupled sequentially. In such settings, (18.2) is solved to calculate the electric potential (V) at all points in the model. The potential is then used to calculate the electromagnetic source term in (18.3), where it is then used to calculate temperature (T) everywhere. The temperature is then used to solve the thermal injury integral Ω (18.4).

Since it is known that electrical [12, 15, 32–40] and thermal [13, 32, 33, 39, 41–43] conductivity are strong functions of temperature, and tissue perfusion is a function of thermal injury, (18.2) and (18.3) can be written more completely as:

$$\nabla \cdot [\sigma(T) \nabla V] = 0 \tag{18.5}$$

$$\rho C \frac{dT}{dt} = \nabla \cdot (k(T) \nabla T) + \sigma(T) |\nabla V|^2 - \rho_b C_b \alpha \omega (T - T_{ambient}) + Q_m \tag{18.6}$$

where

$$\alpha = \frac{1}{\exp(\Omega(t))} \tag{18.7}$$

This set of equations produces highly nonlinear results as the electrical and thermal equations are closely coupled. Likewise, the thermal and thermal injury equations are closely coupled. In this setting, sequential coupling of the equations will not account for the nonlinear behavior and the equations must be solved simultaneously. The first step in solving the system of equations is to solve the electrical potential and the temperature simultaneously at a time step. This is frequently best approached using an iterative method, such as a Gauss-Seidel approach [1]. Once convergence is achieved, the level of tissue injury is calculated using (18.4). The resulting thermal injury integral, Ω, is then used to calculate the tissue injury parameter (α). Since it is known that the tissue perfusion ceases when tissues are sufficiently coagulated, the thermal injury parameter represents the degree of tissue perfusion associated with corresponding levels of tissue injury. Figure 18.6 shows a modeling algorithm developed by Chang et al. for implementing simultaneous calculation of (18.4) through (18.7) [44].

Studies have shown that substantial calculation error can result when the governing equations are coupled in a sequential manner [44]. Models that use simultaneous calculations have been found to account for the nonlinear behavior of tissue injury when compared to actual experimental observation. However, these approaches are computationally more intensive and can take several orders of magnitude longer to calculate [1].

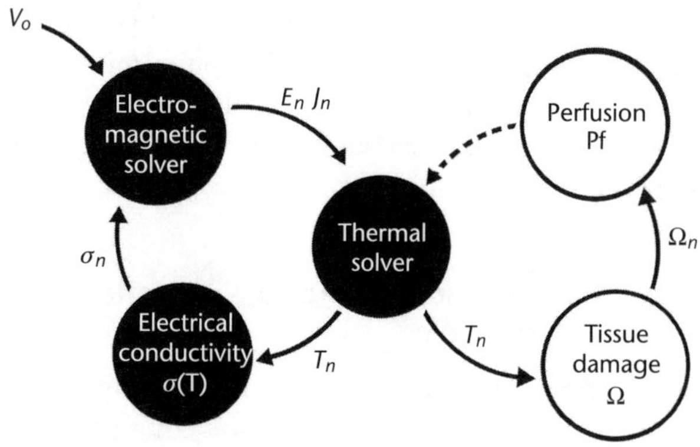

Figure 18.6 Algorithm for simultaneous calculation of thermal injury for radiofrequency ablation devices.

The complexity of calculation is also greatly influenced by the size of the model, resolution, and the number of degrees of freedom. While the full-body geometries in Figures 18.4 and 18.5 may require substantial computational resources for calculations, so too can small localized tissue regions that are modeled with high spatial resolution. Figure 18.7 shows an example of calculations of thermal injury resulting from laser irradiation of abnormal cutaneous vasculature. The volumetric tissue reconstruction was generated by imaging and labeling serial optical microscopy images. On the left is a high-resolution reconstruction of a human port wine stain biopsy specimen. While the physical dimensions of the model are small (268 × 312 × 460 μm), the resolution of the model is quite high (2 × 6 × 2 μm) resulting in a computational model containing more than 1.6 million voxels. Figure 18.7 illustrates the sequential modeling methodology used, including calculation of the

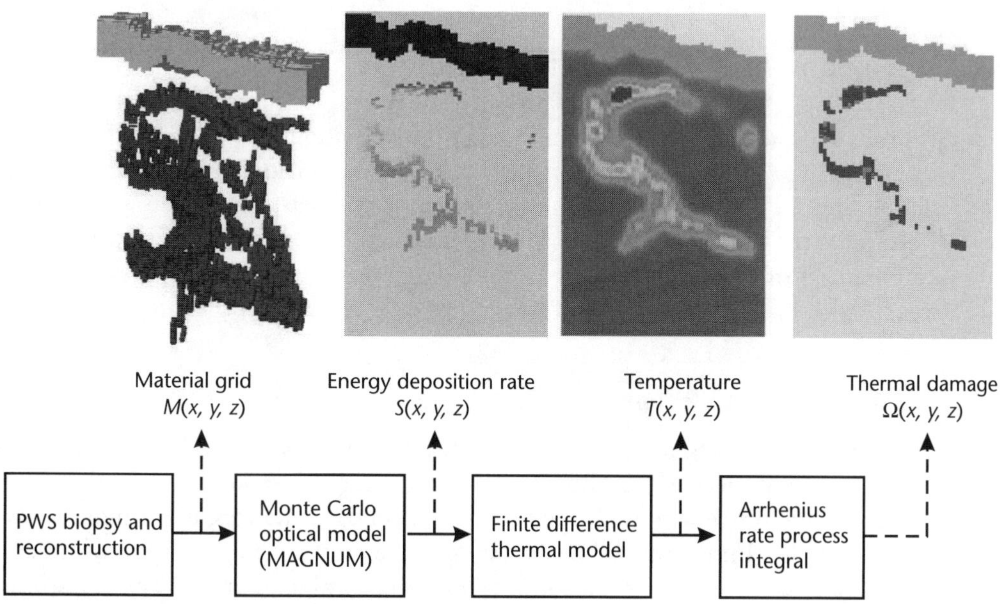

Figure 18.7 Optical-thermal simulation of laser irradiation using a human port wine stain biopsy model.

energy deposition rate, transient temperature distribution, and thermal damage generation. This calculation scheme limits the number of degrees of freedom as at any given time, only one of the three variables (S, T, or Ω) is calculated. Conversely, by employing a simultaneous calculation scheme, the number of degrees of freedom greatly increases, requiring additional memory and computational resources.

18.2.3 General Observations of the Role of Models and Imaging for Guided Therapies

Several general statements can be made with regards to the balance of imaging and modeling in guided therapies. In many ways, imaging and modeling play complimentary roles. Imaging provides qualitative and quantitative data on tissue structure and function as well as treatment monitoring. While imaging provides limited understanding with regards to underlying physical processes, modeling provides a complementary knowledge of the system's behavior. By describing the mechanistic behavior of the system more robustly, modeling provides valuable insight with direct benefit to guided therapy.

In terms of the spectrum of image guided modeling (Figure 18.1), we observe that as we move to the right, models become increasingly complex and can account for greater nonlinearity in describing the physical behavior of the system. By necessity, model geometries become more simplified renditions of the medical images that they simulate. As a therapy, image guided therapies on the right rely on a greater understanding of system behavior and are wholly appropriate for situations in which images are difficult to acquire. As we move to the left, the ability to directly observe local phenomena increases. In these cases, modeling plays a more secondary role. However, as technological advances are made in computational speed, more complex modeling schemes will find their way into image guided therapies to enhance the overall availability of information to the clinical practitioner.

18.3 Development of Computational Models

In principle, the development of all image derived computational models involves four steps: (1) image acquisition, (2) image segmentation, (3) meshing, and (4) computational methodology. While several review articles have been written about each topic, the larger structure of all four steps is often skipped in lieu of a greater examination of each area. In this section, we present an overview of each of these areas.

18.3.1 Image Acquisition

Modern medical imaging techniques employ a variety of methods that are used to create representations of the human body. While we customarily associate imaging and image processing with the determination of structures, at a fundamentally mechanistic level imaging is the process of producing a representation of function or structure that captures variations in some measurable quantity. The variation of these measurable quantities is referred to as image contrast. Each image modality measures a different intrinsic tissue characteristic. For example, ultrasound imaging techniques measure the propagation of ultrasonic pressure waves in tissues. X-ray radiography measures the absorption of X-ray radiation in tissue. The contrast in the image results from different rates of absorption or propagation in different types of tissues.

Imaging modalities are classified into three categories: (1) projection imaging, (2) tomographic imaging, and (3) optical imaging.

18.3.1.1 Projection Imaging

Projection imaging encompasses the variety of techniques where images are acquired primarily by the absorption or propagation of a source through different types of tissue along a linear pathway. They include methods such as projection radiography, fluoroscopy, and nuclear medicine, as well as photoacoustic imaging [45].

Projection radiographs, more commonly referred to as X-rays, produce a two-dimensional X-ray image by measuring X-ray absorption in tissues. Radiographs are generated by exposing tissues to an X-ray beam. As the X-rays pass, they are absorbed by the tissue. Hard tissues, such as bone or teeth, tend to absorb more X-rays than softer tissues such as muscle and skin. The resulting images are captured from the remnant beam that is captured on a photographic film. X-rays are commonly used for imaging fractures in bones and teeth and in looking for pathologic anomalies in the lungs. Soft tissues can also be imaged by the use of radio-opaque contrast medium, such as barium sulfate or iodine-containing radiocontrast agents (diatrizoic acid).

In principle, fluoroscopy produces two-dimensional images similar to projection radiography, but employs a constant stream of X-rays. While projection radiographs are usually captured on photographic film, fluoroscopy images are projected on to fluorescent screens. This allows the physician to acquire real-time information during clinical procedures. While more sophisticated and higher-resolution imaging schemes exist, fluoroscopy remains a mainstay in minimally invasive clinical procedures owing to its real-time capability.

While projection radiographs and fluoroscopy use an external source to generate structural images, nuclear medicine uses short lived isotopes that are readily absorbed into biological active areas (such as tumors and fractured bone regions) to form images. Isotopes such as iodine-131, phosphorus-32 and other radio-labeled drugs are administered to the patient. The radiation emitted by the tissues is collected using a gamma camera. Nuclear medicine differs from most imaging processes as the images produced reflect biological activity at the cellular and sub-cellular level. In practice, nuclear medicine images are superimposed on to data acquired by other imaging techniques [45].

18.3.1.2 Tomographic Imaging

Tomography is the method of producing single plane images of the internal structures of the human body by the observation and recording of signals from multiple locations. Unlike projected images, tomographic images are two-dimensional slices of a three-dimensional reconstruction of the body. Tomographic imaging methods include computed tomography (CT), positron emission tomography (PET), magnetic resonance imaging (MRI), ultrasound imaging, and electrical impedance tomography (EIT).

Computed tomography is an extension of fluoroscopy. An X-ray source and an X-ray detector are positioned on opposite sides of a circle, through which a patient is placed (Figure 18.8). Several X-ray projections are acquired by rotating the X-ray source and detector around the circle. Each projection represents a line integral of X-ray attenuation though the object. Johann Radon first described the mathematical basis for the projections as

$$p(r,\theta) = \int_{-\infty}^{\infty}\int_{-\infty}^{\infty} f(x,y)\,\delta\,(x\cos\theta + y\sin\theta)\,dxdy \tag{18.8}$$

where $p(r, \theta)$ is the projected line integral through the object $f(x, y)$, δ is the Dirac delta, which is infinite at $(x{\cdot}\cos\theta + y{\cdot}\sin\theta)$ and zero for all other arguments. (Note the integral if δ is one.) In CT, the objective is to solve for the inverse function $f(x, y)$ given a measured set of projections. A number of techniques, such as the inverse Radon transformation, or the filtered back projection algorithm are used to compute the reconstructed image [46].

In principle, positron emission tomography bears many similarities to nuclear medicine. Radionuclides that emit positrons are used as a short half-life radiation source to generate a pair of gamma rays. Isotopes such as carbon-11 (~ 20-minute half life), nitrogen-13 (~10 minutes), oxygen-15 (~2 minutes), and Flourine-18 (~110 minutes) are incorporated into compounds normally present in the body

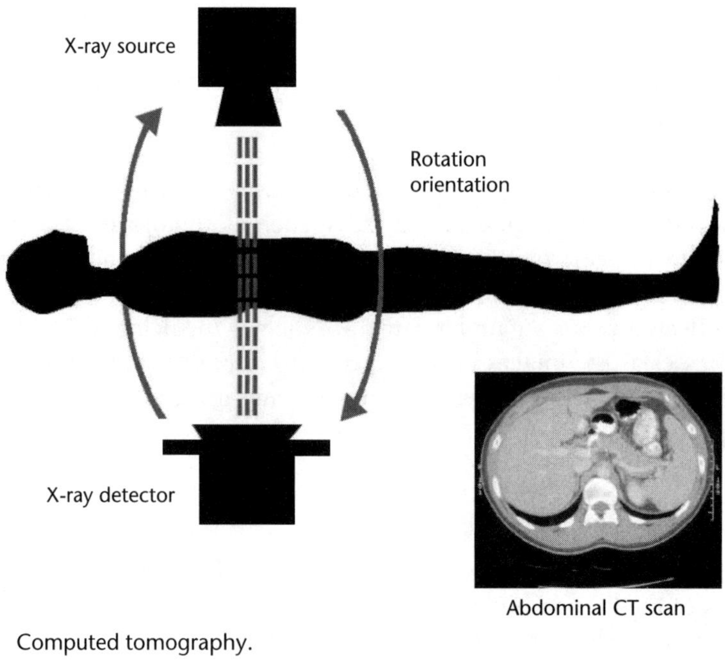

Figure 18.8 Computed tomography.

(such as water, ammonia, and glucose) to track metabolic processes. The most common molecule used for PET is fluorodeoxyglucose, a sugar. The radioisotope decays and emits a positron which annihilates with an electron, producing a pair of gamma rays that move in opposite directions. These gamma rays are then absorbed by scintillator material (high energy absorbers) creating bursts of light that are sensed by multiple detector blocks that are arranged in a ring surrounding the patient. A tomographic reconstruction similar to that used in CT is used to generate a functional image of metabolic processes [47].

Magnetic resonance imaging is a tomographic technique that produces images by using powerful magnets to polarize and excite hydrogen nuclei in water molecules in body tissues. Unlike CT and PET, MRI uses no ionizing radiation. Instead, three kinds of electromagnetic fields are used. A strong static magnetic field is used to polarize the hydrogen nuclei. The static magnetic field is generated by using a superconducting electromagnet made of a niobium-titanium alloy which is cooled by liquid helium. A weaker time-varying magnetic field is generated by a gradient coil. By tuning this gradient coil, hydrogen protons in one slice can be manipulated to create a perturbation that can be used to spatially identify (encode) the plane. A weak radiofrequency (RF) field is used to manipulate the hydrogen nuclei to produce a measurable signal. Radio waves at a specific frequency are absorbed by the protons which pushes some of them out of alignment. When the protons "snap" back into alignment, they produce a rotating magnetic field, which is detected. Each type of tissue realigns these protons at different speeds, which allows reconstruction of the various body structures. Spectroscopic methods have been adapted to MRI, which allow for measurement of different metabolite levels in body tissues. Such methods have been termed magnetic resonance spectroscopy (MRS) or magnetic resonance spectroscopy imaging (MRSI). MRI is particularly effective for imaging soft tissues, such as muscle and fat, due to the generally higher water content in these tissues [47].

Ultrasound imaging uses high-frequency sound waves between 2 and 10 MHz to produce 2D slice images in body tissues. A piezoelectric transducer is used to create mechanical pressure waves in tissues. Density changes and differences in the acoustical properties of tissues cause the sound waves to reflect and change directions. The sound waves return to the transducer and are converted to electrical pulses. The intensity of the reflection and the amount of time needed for the echo to be received are analyzed to reconstruct the image. As an imaging modality, ultrasound produces less detail than other tomographic techniques such as MRI or CT. Ultrasound modalities do not readily lend themselves as image source for computational modeling. However, they are commonly used clinically for treatment planning. Ultrasound's portability and nondestructive means of assessing body structures in real time make it an affordable and convenient imaging modality for guided therapies [45].

Although it has not been applied widely, electrical impedance tomography represents a form of tomographic imaging that has found specific uses in the clinical diagnostics of lung functioning, breast tumor detection, and monitoring bowel function [48]. Electrical impedance tomography is an image modality that is sensitive to changes in the electrical conductivity and permittivity of body tissues. Conducting electrodes are attached to the skin of the patient and small alternating currents are applied between electrodes pairs. The induced electrical potentials are measured from the electrodes using one of several measurement algorithms. Computational techniques are used to iteratively solve for the inverse solution, which produces a structural map of electrical impedance [49]. To date, this is the only tomographic imaging modality that is sensitive to changes in the electrical properties of tissues. EIT, however, generally produces low-resolution images, as the methodology is greatly dependent on the number of electrodes and produces highly variable results resulting from difference in skin impedance. Despite these limitations, EIT is used successfully in applications of bowel and lung imaging and is considered the standard of care for these clinical applications (see Figure 18.9).

18.3.1.3 Optical Imaging

Optical imaging typically infers the structural and biochemical properties of tissue by examining spectral and spatial variations in light due to elastic scattering and absorption by tissue, or by inelastic scattering (e.g., the generation of fluorescence). Optical imaging systems are typically designed to either provide two-dimensional images of a tissue surface or depth-resolved images which provide two-dimensional cross-sections or three-dimensional data volumes.

Surface imaging techniques based on optical spectroscopy have been incorporated into clinical use for a variety of applications, such as detection of cancers and precancers arising in epithelial tissues lining the bronchi, gastrointestinal tract, and cervix. While these techniques can provide real-time information for localization and monitoring of therapy, they are not well suited to provide the volumetric data that is most useful for incorporation into three-dimensional computational models.

Subsurface optical imaging techniques can be divided into three main categories: ballistic, diffuse, and photoacoustic. Techniques which fall into the ballistic category produce high spatial resolution images (on the order of microns or less) of tissues that are a few millimeters thick [50–52]. Ballistic optical imaging considers only the photons that travel through tissue and essentially undergo a single 180° backscatter event with minimal other deflections due to scattering. These singly scattered photons are used in high-resolution imaging techniques such as confocal microscopy and optical coherence tomography (OCT). The latter approach measures backscattered light in a manner analogous to ultrasound and achieves a spatial resolution of 1 to 20 μm and imaging depths of several millimeters in turbid tissues. While time-domain OCT systems use a moving mirror to collect interference patterns and quantify backscatter intensity as a function of depth, Fourier-domain systems now employ a static reference arm and spectrally resolved detection system to achieve the same information. A depth-resolved map of reflectance is then attained by scanning across the tissue. While detected OCT signals are primarily determined by changes in index of refraction and scattering levels, they can also be affected by absorption, flow, and birefringence. The high resolution and short penetration depth of ballistic techniques cause the resulting images to be useful primarily for defining microstructures such as capillaries and small tumors for modeling of highly localized treatments. For example, OCT has been used to define tissue morphology for numerical models of selective photothermal coagulation of cutaneous vasculature [53].

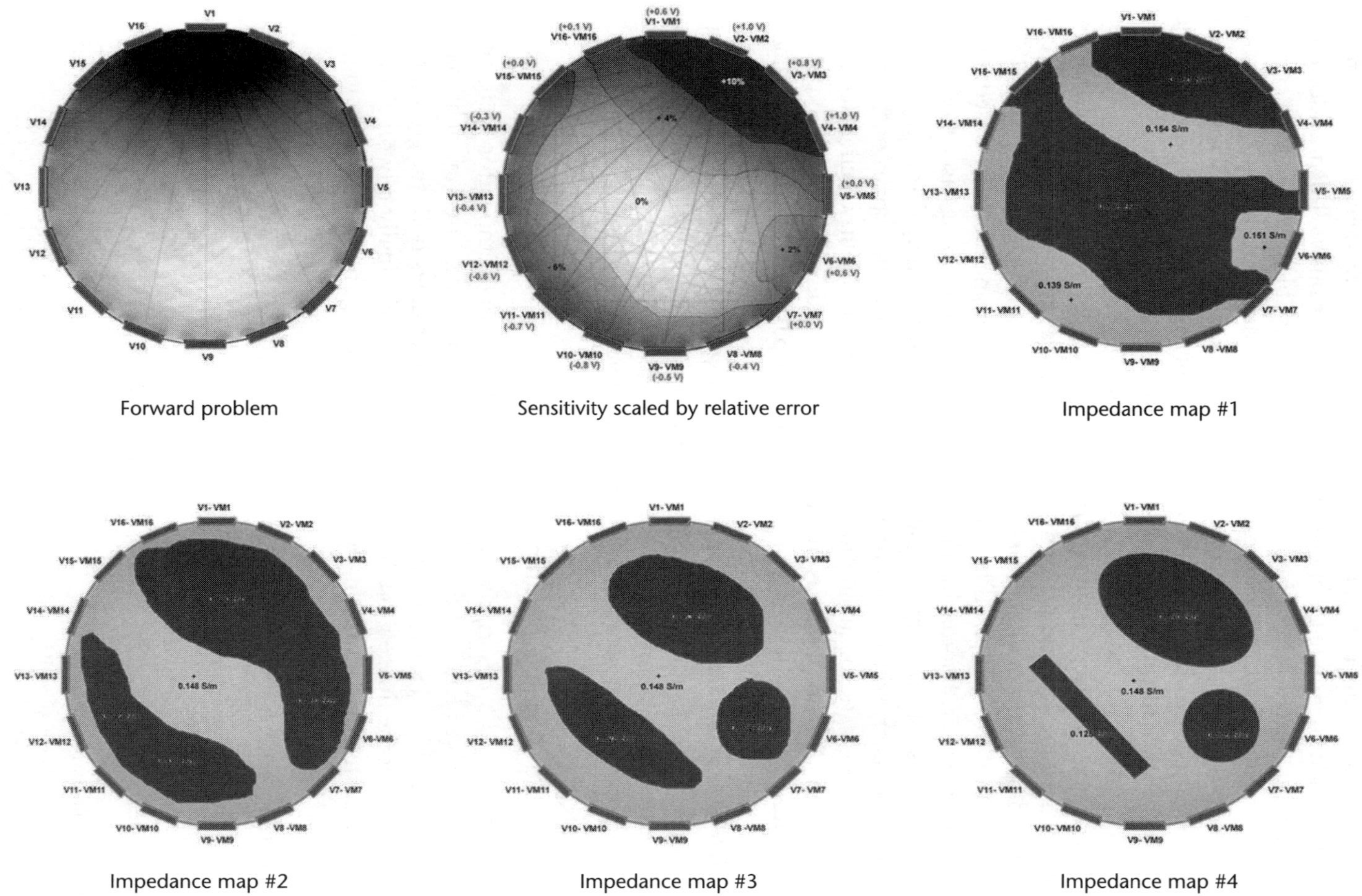

Figure 18.9 Electrical Impedance Tomography Algorithm. The conductivity from inside the body is mapped by applying currents through electrodes attached to the surface of the body. The forward problem is solved with an estimated conductivity for a homogenous case at first to obtain the initial sensitivity map. The difference between the measured voltages and estimated voltages is then used to scale the sensitivity map and calculate the impedance map. Steps 1–3 are repeated until the image converges.

Nonballistic imaging approaches, such as diffuse optical tomography, exploit established techniques for simulating the random walk behavior of photons that propagate through turbid media to generate two- and three-dimensional reconstruction of absorption and scattering distributions [54]. By delivering light to the surface of a tissue region (e.g., breast, head, wrist) at various well-defined locations and detecting remitted light at other locations, it is possible to reconstruct the spatial distribution of absorbers and scatterers (and fluorophores) using computationally intensive tomographic reconstruction algorithms. While the resolution of these approaches is on the order of millimeters to centimeters, they provide much deeper penetration than ballistic approaches and more thorough information regarding optical properties and biochemistry. Diffuse optical imaging techniques are effective for imaging variations in near-infrared absorbers such as oxyhemoglobin and water, and have shown promise for applications such as monitoring of brain trauma patients and detection of angiogenesis.

Related to diffusive optical imaging is a hybrid imaging modality based on the photoacoustic effect. Photoacoustic imaging uses a nonionizing laser to deliver a pulse of photons into biological tissues. A portion of the energy from this pulse is converted into heat, which leads to a localized thermoelastic expansion of the tissue. The thermoelastic expansion induces an acoustic transient which is detectable by ultrasound. This technique is highly effective for imaging hemoglobin concentrations and oxygen saturation in tissue, making it particularly useful for imaging vascular and tumor tissues [55].

While we are not aware of diffuse optical tomography or photoacoustic images having been used to simulate therapeutic techniques, as the quality of reconstructions improve, these approaches have the potential to provide volumetric data for simulating optical treatments such as photodynamic therapy.

18.3.1.4 Image Acquisition Summary

We have presented a descriptive summary of the major methods for imaging. In each case, we have identified the principle metric that is measured in each imaging modality. (See Table 18.1.) The principle metric determines both the strength and the weakness of the image modality. Techniques that principally rely on X-ray absorption are effective for imaging hard structures, but are not effective for imaging

Table 18.1 Principle Metrics for Various Imaging Modalities

Imaging Modality	*Principle Metric*
Projection radiographs	X-ray absorption
Fluoroscopy	X-ray absorption
Nuclear medicine	Gamma emission
Computed tomography	X-ray absorption
Positron emission tomography	Gamma emission
Magnetic resonance imaging	Hydrogen magnetic field
Ultrasound imaging	Density changes
Electrical impedance tomography	Changes in electrical properties
Diffusive optical imaging	Light scattering and absorption
Photoacoustic imaging	Thermoelastic expansion / Ultrasonic emissions
Optical Coherence Tomography	Light Scattering and Absorption

soft tissues. Ultrasound imaging, which is effective for detecting density changes, may not detect adjacent tissues with large variations in electrical conductivity. The choice of the metric may inherently have limitations. For example, in electrical impedance tomography, the choice of the frequency of measurements will determine the kinds of structures that are potentially imaged. At low frequencies (< 1 kHz), for example, current passes through the extracellular space of cells causing the electrical conductivity to be low and the dielectric permittivity to be high. At higher frequencies (> 10 MHz), tissue membranes are shorted causing current to flow in both the extracellular and intracellular spaces of cells. The electrical conductivity increases and the dielectric permittivity decrease substantially. At higher frequencies, it is much more difficult to distinguish between tissue types, since the electrical properties of tissues at higher frequencies tend to be very similar [18]. Another example of inherent limitations in metric selection is optical coherence tomography, which is highly effective at measuring microscopic tissue structures that are a few millimeters wide but terribly ineffective for structures beyond this distance.

18.3.2 Image Segmentation

Image segmentation is the process of separating an image into multiple regions to simplify the representation of the image and/or add meaning to substructures within the image. A body, for example can be represented in several ways according to body structure. It can be segmented into smaller body parts that represent the extremities (i.e., head, arms, legs, torso). Alternatively, it can be subdivided according to anatomical structures (i.e., heart, liver, skin, muscle, fat). The body can also be segmented by nonstructural means. For example, X-ray images represent a grayscale of intensities which, by themselves, can be used to separate tissues by the amount of X-rays absorbed. In this case, soft tissues are not distinguishable from one another. Positron emission tomography, for example, represents only the *locations* with greatest gamma emission, but does not inherently identify the *structures* where the gamma emissions originate.

Fundamentally, all image segmentation involves two properties: a *location* and an *attribute*. In the case of representing body structures by the extremities, the location is the geometric position of the appendage; the attribute is the name (e.g., Location – area located between the left elbow and the left hand; Attribute – classified as "Left Forearm") When representing the body by anatomical structures, several attributes can be "tagged" to the location. For example, Location: the liver is an organ in the upper abdomen; Attribute 1: organ that aids in digestion and removal of waste products in the blood; Attribute 2: Liver has electrical conductivity of 0.147 S/m at 500 kHz [18]; Attribute 3: Liver has a density of 1,060 kg/m^3 [20].

While some segmentation methods involve more attributes than others, this does not make them any more useful than segmentations that involve fewer attributes. For example, knowing that muscle has an electrical conductivity of 0.4459 S/m at 500 kHz [18] does not help one to identify what limb the muscle belongs to. Adding to the complication is the fact that sometimes segmentation does not produce mutually exclusive classifications. The ball and socket of a femur may belong to the pelvis or may constitute part of the upper leg. Worse still, classifications are sometimes ambiguous. A debate by the cellular phone community, for example, raged for several years over whether the pinna (external ear) was technically part of the human head. According to the guidelines of the Institute of Electrical and Electronics Engineers (IEEE) and the International Commission on Non-Ionizing Radiation Protection (ICNIRP), the pinna is part of the head and is not considered an extremity. Other investigators considered the pinna to be an extremity and ignored it in calculating radiofrequency dosimetry in the head as calculations within the pinna were characteristically higher than any other location within the human head [56] (see Figure 18.10).

There are many approaches to segmentation. Objects within an image can be separated into regions defined by surfaces (volumes) and boundaries (surfaces). The segmentation algorithm relies on identifying similarities in some characteristic, such as image intensity, coloration, or some other computed property. The end result of segmentation is a set of defined regions whose attributes are distinctly different from each neighboring region, and whose collective area covers the entire image. In general, there is no single technique used to segment images. However, there have been a number of common approaches.

18.3.2.1 Clustering Methodologies

The clustering methodology (K-means algorithm) is an iterative approach to segmenting images that separates areas of an image according to its proximity to predefined cluster centers. These centers technically can be chosen at random or by using some other methodical method. Each pixel in the image is assigned to the closest cluster center by minimizing the distance between the pixel and the cluster center. For each subsequent iteration, the cluster center is recomputed by averaging all of the pixels in the cluster; and all of the pixels are again assigned to the closest cluster center. Final assignment of each pixel to a cluster is attained when none of the pixels change clusters. For medical imaging, this approach is highly useful for defining structures that, when deformed, may have a loose association with a specific attribute. For example, the body torso consists of two areas, the abdomen and

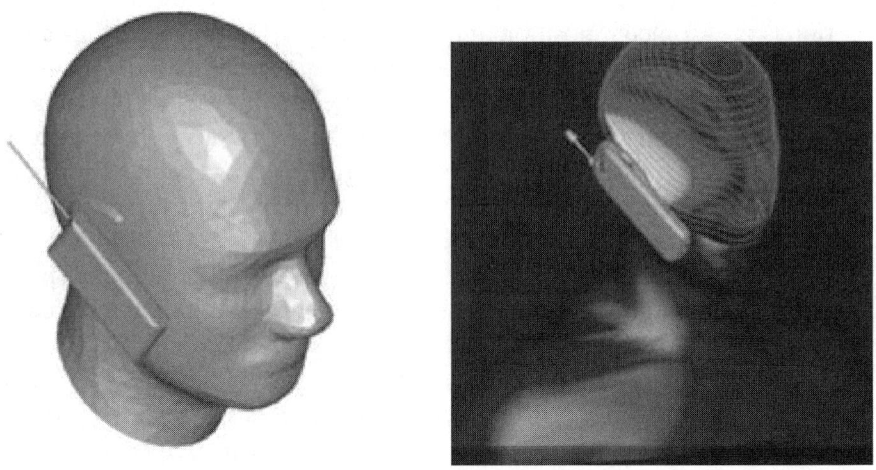

Figure 18.10 Radiofrequency dosimetry calculations from cell phones in the standardized anthropomorphic mannequin (SAM) of the human head.

the thorax. When assigning body organs in the torso under a variety of postures, clustering methodology can be used to identify which body organs belong to the abdomen and thorax. In this example, all pixels in a body geometry are partitioned into two group clusters. The clustering method creates regions that are weighted by proximity to the cluster centers and conform to the geometry of the torso. Once the cluster regions are finalized, the resulting partition between the clustering region is the plane defining the abdomen and the thorax. When the torso undergoes significant deformation, body organs may switch cluster regions.

A variant of the clustering methodology uses histograms. This variant uses a histogram of some parameter (e.g., intensity) to help preseed the cluster centers. Clusters can also be subdivided efficiently using histogram-based methodologies, which allows for greater refinement of boundary regions (see Figure 18.11).

18.3.2.2 Edge Detection Methods

Edge detection methodologies seek to define a region by locating edges which define the borders between adjacent regions. In some cases, these edges are well defined by

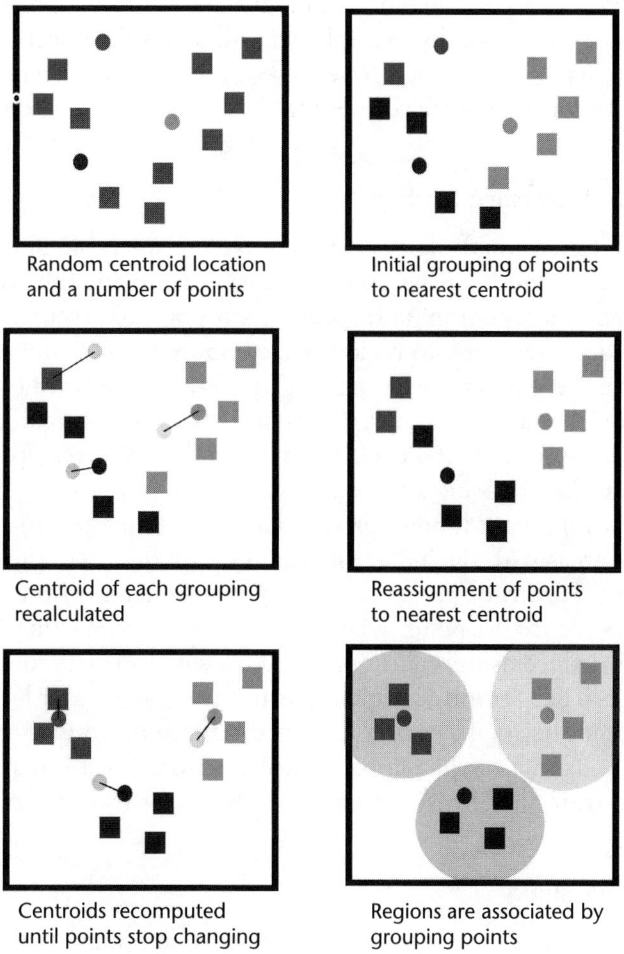

Figure 18.11 Clustering segmentation algorithm.

abrupt changes in the intensity of an image. In other cases, edges are defined only by a border of boundaries with no associated intensity changes. A wealth of image processing techniques have been developed to detect and enhance edges, contributing to wide use as the basis for more complicated segmentation techniques. An important consideration in applying edge detection methods is the difficulty in defining regions (which are closed structures) from boundaries that are often disconnected. In many cases, these discontinuities can be closed by bridging the gaps between segments when the proximity is below a predefined threshold.

18.3.2.3 Region Growing Methods

At first glance, region growing methods appear to closely resemble clustering methods with the notable exception that there are no cluster centers. In this methodology, a seed is used to mark every object to be segmented in the image. Each seed is allowed to expand in size, stopping only when it encounters a geometric boundary or the border of another seed region. For example, one wishing to identify the left and right side of a body can place two seeds that are equidistant from the centerline of the body image. The regions will grow until the entire body is identified as being left and right.

As with the clustering methodology, region growing methods are iterative and quite slow. One difficulty in implementing this is the selection of the starting point for the seeds. If, for example, one seed starts in the left forefinger and the other seed starts within the chest, the centerline of the body will be skewed significantly.

18.3.2.4 Watershed Method

For two-dimensional images that involve considerable gradients in intensity, the watershed method can be used to classify an image into regions by considering the image as a topographic surface. In a topographic sense, a watershed is a ridge that divides a terrain into regions based upon where water is likely to flow. Water placed on the gradient slope leading up to the ridge will flow in the direction that minimizes the slope, resulting in a pooling reservoir (catchment basin) when water is allowed to accumulate. Each reservoir, in this context, represents a region. Water placed on the opposing side of the watershed will flow in the other direction and will form a different topographic region. Translating this to an image segmentation strategy, areas with the highest image intensity represent the watershed. Water will move in the locus of points defined by the direction of the steepest gradient until it reaches the lowest point, where the slope is zero. Starting from this location, the region is defined as the collection of pixels with intensity that fall within a specified tolerance. The tolerance is analogous to raising the water level to define the size of a catchment basin. The watershed method differs from normal thresholding algorithms in that the catchment basins are used to define the distinct regions. Thus, the resulting watershed lines may have variable intensity thresholds (see Figure 18.12).

18.3.3 Meshing

The governing equations that are modeled by computational models are rarely solvable using analytical solutions, except for the most simplest of geometries. To ana-

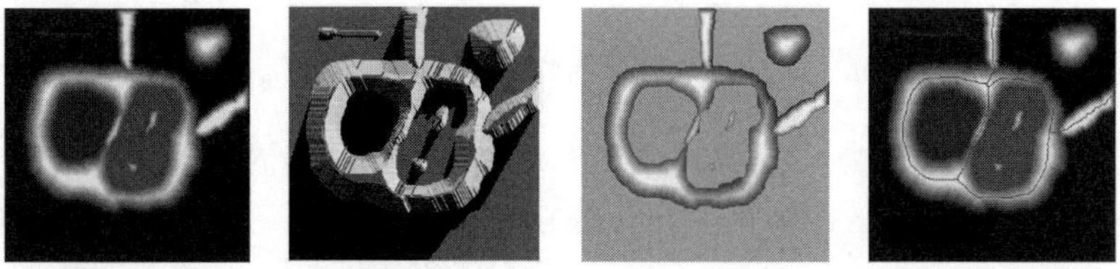

Figure 18.12 Watershed segmentation method.

lyze these problems, requires the subdivision of a problem into smaller subdomains that are made up of simpler geometries, where analytical solutions are possible. Triangular (tetrahedral) and rectangular (block) geometries, referred to as elements, can be combined to approximate the geometry of more complicated structures. The governing equation is solved for each element such that the solution at the boundary of each element is piecewise continuous to the elements that share its border. By dividing up a complex geometry into increasingly smaller pieces, a highly nonlinear solution can be computationally calculated using piecewise analytic solutions. Representing a geometry with too few elements results in a highly linearized solution. Representing a geometry with too many elements creates complications in solution convergence and requires increased time and computational resources.

A key concept in meshing is geometric simplification of structures. While the geometry of structures can be readily simplified by reducing the overall image resolution, meshing takes a more selective approach to simplifying geometries. Through the image acquisition process, we attain data representing an area of interest. Through the segmentation process, we are able to identify structures within the volume. Once a complex shape has been identified, the meshing process allows one to subdivide the structure (not the entire volume) into simpler elements. Meshes can be classified either by the type of elements that are used or by the manner in which the elements are connected.

18.3.3.1 Element-Based Classification Schemes

The simplest representation of a two-dimensional plane is a triangular element. While square elements are easier to obtain (often directly from imaging), triangular elements are often easier to solve, since the solution of the element is constrained by fewer equations describing the behavior at each point (i.e., node). All 2D meshes have mesh nodes that lie within a plane. The majority of 2D solvers use triangular or quadrilateral elements.

In three-dimensional problems, the simplest representation is the tetrahedral. Hexahedral (or brick), pyramidal, and wedge elements are also used. Since all 3D elements are bounded by 2D surfaces, all 3D meshes produce 2D surfaces which conform to the geometry of the surface, but may have elements that do not lie within a plane. These 2D surface surfaces, or surface meshes are extremely important in meshing 3D objects, as they heavily influence how coarse or fine the 3D mesh will need to be to define a continuous domain for the entire object geometry (see Figure 18.13).

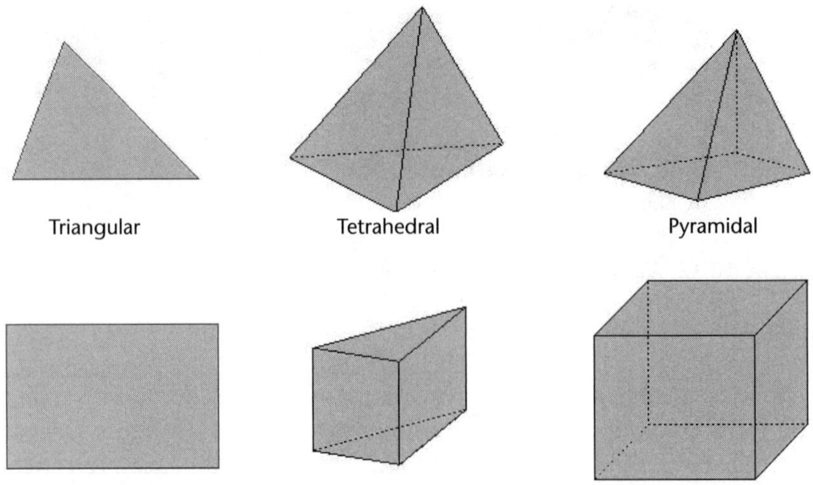

Figure 18.13 Element shapes used in meshing.

18.3.3.2 Connectivity-Based Classification Schemes

The connectivity of elements can have a structured mesh, an unstructured mesh, or be some hybrid combination of the two. Structured meshes are meshes that have a regularized connectivity. An $n \times m$ array, for example, is a regularized structured mesh. In most cases, the connectivity of a structured mesh consists of only one type of element, which greatly simplifies the description of how elements are connected. Unstructured meshes, on the other hand, are flexible in that all of the different element shape types can be used. However, the connectivity is more difficult to describe and must be explicitly stored, which may require substantially larger storage requirements. Hybrid meshes are meshes that contain both structured and unstructured portions. Depending on the complexity of problems, more than one meshing scheme may be used. For example, in the calculation of electromagnetic field problems, the time-domain technique known as finite difference time domain (FDTD) uses one mesh to calculate electric field components, and a second mesh (that is offset by 1/2 the regularized spacing) to calculate magnetic field quantities. Another example is in multiphysics modeling of thermal injury from electromagnetic sources where it is sometimes advantageous to use overlapping unstructured mesh (electromagnetic/thermal) and structured mesh schemes (thermal injury) to model different governing equations [1].

18.3.3.3 Grid Generation

While elegant algorithms for automatic grid generation are increasingly more common today, the development of gridding techniques remains an active area of research. Meshing is the most time-consuming and the least optimized of the four steps for computational modeling. A major issue in developing three-dimensional meshes arises from the generation of "water-tight" surface meshes. Since surface meshes are not planar, gaps sometimes occur in the surface mesh, making it impossible to define the three-dimensional volume. Special care is taken to "heal" the surface meshes using interpolation techniques (i.e., cubic spline, Bezeir curves, nonuniform rational β-splines) so that a continuous boundary can be defined for volumetric meshing.

18.3.4 Computational Methodologies

Computational models are designed according to the questions that need to be answered. In many situations, several approaches can be used. For example, in the study of drug-eluting stents, one examines the kinematics of drug delivery. This can be done by modeling the distribution of the drug everywhere throughout the polymer matrix. One can also model the drug dissolution by assuming a bulk rate constant. Both of these approaches are useful in describing how the drug is released from the stent. However, one may also wish to examine the uptake and metabolism of the drug in the body. Locally, this may involve an anatomically based model in which the distribution of the drug diffuses into the various body tissues. These local models may be helpful in modeling tissue restenosis and cell proliferation. Alternatively, a compartmental model involving known tissue organ uptake may be used to look at whole-body distribution of the drugs. This approach may provide insight into how the body metabolizes the drug. The approach to modeling varies considerably. However, every method involves imaging in some capacity. Computational models can be classified into three categories: compartmental models, statistical models, and field models.

18.3.4.1 Compartmental Models

The simplest compartmental models involve two compartments. One compartment represents a region in which the behavior of an object within a system is describable using a set of rules or equations. The other compartment represents the rest of the system. The object of compartmental models is to examine the interaction between compartments. One common use of compartmental models is in the modeling of drug absorption and metabolism in the body. Physiologically based pharmacokinetics modeling (PBPK) is widely used to predict the absorption, distribution, metabolism, and excretion of drugs and other chemical substances by the human body. Figure 18.14 shows a system in which drugs are introduced intravenously. The behavior of each component is governed by the compartment's binding kinetics, the flow rate, and the mass of the organ. In general, this kind of modeling does not directly involve imaging. However, imaging is used to define the connection between compartments as well as define the size of the compartments relative to each other [57].

The differential equations of a PBPK model are derived through mass balance across various components. For each compartment of the cell, the mass of drug entering, leaving, and binding to the compartment is calculated. For example, if we examine the liver compartment in Figure 18.14, the differential equation governing the mass of drug in the compartment can be written as

$$\frac{dC_L}{dt} = -\frac{Q_L}{V_L \cdot K_p} \cdot C_L + \frac{Q_L}{V_L} \cdot C_{arterial} \tag{18.9}$$

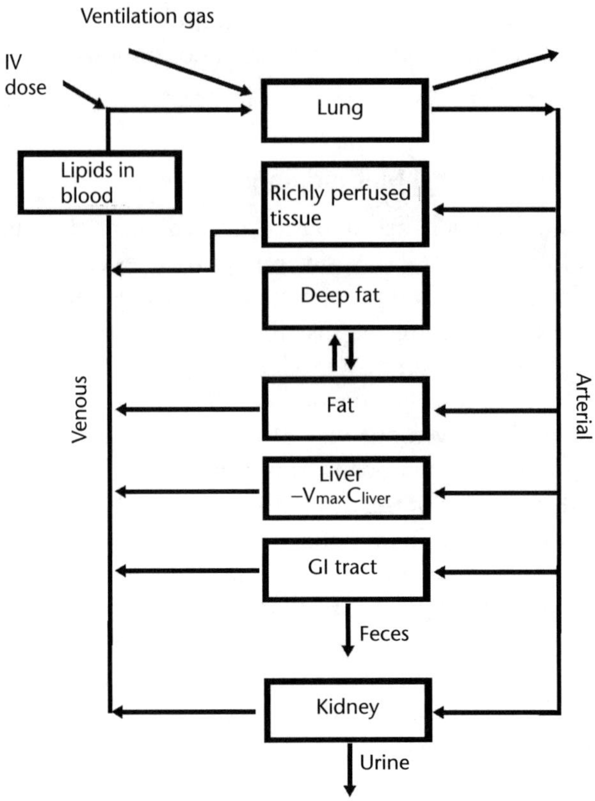

Figure 18.14 Physiological based pharmacokinetics (PBPK) model.

where C_L is the concentration of a drug in the liver, Q_L represents the net flow rate, V_L is the volume of the liver, K_p is the tissue: plasma distribution coefficient, and $C_{arterial}$ is the concentration in the arterial blood supply. Governing equations are generated for each compartment in the model and solved simultaneously at each time step. Each parameter used in the model is experimentally measured. The result of this kind of modeling gives a time course of drug concentration in each organ.

18.3.4.2 Statistical Models

Statistical models encompass a variety of techniques in which the parameters of an established model are repetitively calculated using parameters that vary according to some kind of distribution. This variation may be the result of variations in the input characteristics of a model (source variation), in the intrinsic properties of an object's characteristics (parameter variation), or in the relationship between one object in the model and another (process variation). In many cases, the end goal of these models is to characterize the robustness of the behavior of a system to changes. In other cases, the added value of statistical modeling is to characterize the behavior of a process in a population. In the field of biomedical optics, for example, statistical simulation is essential for characterizing what are essentially random light scattering processes in tissue.

Light transport in tissue where multiple scattering processes predominate can be described by Maxwell's equations. However, these kinds of solutions are not practical for use in evaluating light propagation in tissue, due to the unmanageable number of potential reflections. Instead of considering the wave-like behavior of light, a more practical approach is to consider light as consisting of a large quantity of individual photons which can be scattered or absorbed, otherwise known as radiative transfer theory. This is governed by the equation,

$$\frac{dL(\vec{r},\hat{s})}{ds} = -\mu_a L(\vec{r},\hat{s}) - \mu_s L(\vec{r},\hat{s}) + \mu_s \int_{4\pi} p(\hat{s},\hat{s}')L(\vec{r},\hat{s})d\omega + S(\vec{r},\hat{s}) \tag{18.10}$$

where $L(\vec{r},\hat{s})$ is the radiance (w/m^2/Steradian) at position $\vec{r}$ in the direction of the unit vector $\hat{s}$. The left-hand-side term represents the gradient of the radiance. The first two terms on the right-hand side represent losses due to absorption and scattering, respectively. The integral term is the gain due to scattering and the final term is a source term. Variables μ_a (cm^{-1}) and μ_s (cm^{-1}) represent the material properties known as the absorption and scattering coefficients, respectively. The probability of a photon being absorbed within a length *ds* is represented by the quantity $\mu_a ds$. Similarly, $\mu_s ds$ represents the probability of a photon being scattered within *ds*.

Since (18.10) cannot be solved analytically for realistic conditions, various numerical methods and approximations have been developed. Some methods, such as the diffusion approximation of radiative transfer equation are useful only for light transport across larger distances (i.e., centimeters) in homogenous media. However, body tissues are highly heterogeneous and the photon pathways of interest are often far shorter. In these circumstances, the best option is often a Monte Carlo statistical approach, which simulates the random walk of photons. Monte Carlo methods do not involve solutions of governing equations across the region of interest, rather they apply fundamental laws and stochastic relations to determine the movement and interaction of individual particles with tissue. As the number of simulated photon paths increases, the more robust the final distribution of light absorption becomes. The process is highly flexible, yet rigorous. It is particularly useful for evaluating a variety of illumination geometries including collimated, diverging, and converging beams or for fiber optic delivery. Furthermore, realistic morphology—implemented as spatial variations in optical properties—can be readily implemented into Monte Carlo models. In fact, volumetric reconstructions of the brain acquired by MRI [58] and high-resolution images of trabecular bone acquired by micro-CT [59] have been implemented in Monte Carlo models.

18.3.4.3 Field Models

In some cases, it is necessary to know the distribution of energy or dose everywhere in the model volume. The goal of electromagnetic dosimetry is to calculate the electric field distribution from an antenna. In this case, the governing equations must be solved at every point in the model. There are many methods to accomplish this. The two most common approaches are the finite difference and the finite element method.

Finite Difference

Finite difference calculations are derived from the fundamental definition of the derivative f at a point x.

$$\frac{df}{dx} = \lim_{\Delta x \to 0} \frac{f(x + \Delta x) - f(x)}{\Delta x} \tag{18.11}$$

In situations where the limit is not applied, Δx approaches a nonzero fixed value and the quotient is called a finite difference.

$$\left.\frac{\Delta f}{\Delta x}\right|_R = \frac{f(x + \Delta x) - f(x)}{\Delta x} \tag{18.12}$$

$$\left.\frac{\Delta f}{\Delta x}\right|_L = \frac{f(x) - f(x - \Delta x)}{\Delta x} \tag{18.13}$$

Since Δx is a finite quantity, the center of the derivative is shifted $\Delta x/2$ to the right of center (18.12) or to the left (18.13). Equations (18.12) and (18.13) are referred to as the "right shifted" and "left shifted" derivative expressions, respectively. Alternatively the derivative by calculated by a half shift to the right and left such that

$$\left.\frac{\Delta f}{\Delta x}\right|_R = \frac{f\left(x + \frac{\Delta x}{2}\right) - f\left(x - \frac{\Delta x}{2}\right)}{\Delta x} = \frac{f(x+1) - f(x-1)}{2} \tag{18.14}$$

An analogous second derivative expression can be found by first right shifting, than left shifting:

$$\frac{\Delta^2 f}{\Delta x^2} = \left.\frac{\Delta}{\Delta x}\right|_R \left.\frac{\Delta f}{\Delta x}\right|_L = \frac{f(x+1) - 2f(x) + f(x-1)}{\Delta x^2} \tag{18.15}$$

Similar expressions can be determined for time dependent derivatives. As an example of how these finite element expressions are used to solve field problems, consider the example of solving the heat equation in one dimension with homogenous Direchelet boundary conditions:

$$\frac{dT}{dt} = \frac{d^2T}{dt^2}; U(0,t) = U(1,t) = 0; U(x,0) = U_0(x) \tag{18.16}$$

Adopting the convention that the evaluation of a function at time t and position x is

$$f(x,t) = f_x^t$$

we can apply the derivative expressions directly to solve the heat equation:

$$\frac{f_x^{t+1} - f_x^t}{\Delta t} = \frac{f_{x+1}^t - 2f_x^t + f_{x-1}^t}{\Delta x^2} \tag{18.17}$$

Equation (18.17) uses a forward difference at time t and a second-order central difference in x. Rearranging (18.17), we arrive at the evaluation of f_x^{t+1} to be

$$\begin{aligned} f_x^{t+1} &= (1 - 2\beta)f_x^t + \beta f_{x+1}^t + \beta f_{x-1}^t \\ \beta &= \Delta t / (\Delta x)^2 \end{aligned} \tag{18.18}$$

which can be solved everywhere in the one-dimensional domain using a regularized mesh. This method of solving finite the heat equation on a regularized mesh is referred to as the "explicit" method as all the terms on the right side of (18.18) are defined for the previous time step. The explicit method is the simple to implement, and converges when $\beta \leq 0.5$. While it is not always the most numerically stable method and can contribute to large errors, it is suitable for problems that involve small time-step solutions.

The heat equation can also be solved using a backward difference at time t and a second-order central difference in x. This is known as the implicit method:

$$\frac{f_x^{t+1} - f_x^t}{\Delta t} = \frac{f_{x+1}^{t+1} - 2f_x^{t+1} + f_{x-1}^{t+1}}{\Delta x^2} \tag{18.19}$$

Rearranging (18.19), we can solve f_x^{t+1} such that

$$(1 + 2\beta)f_x^{t+1} - \beta f_{x+1}^{t+1} + \beta f_{x-1}^{t+1} = f_x^t \tag{18.20}$$

which, although is more difficult to solve since a system of numerical equations is solved at each time step, is always numerically stable and converges. The implicit method, though difficult, is the most accurate method for addressing large time-step solutions.

To improve the accuracy of short time-step solutions, we can combine the explicit and implicit approaches by taking their average. This gives rise to the Crank-Nicolson method for solving finite-difference problems, which is considered to be the most accurate and widely used method for solving small time step problems:

$$\frac{f_x^{t+1} - f_x^t}{\Delta t} = \frac{\frac{f_{x+1}^t - 2f_x^t + f_{x-1}^t}{\Delta x^2} + \frac{f_{x+1}^{t+1} - 2f_x^{t+1} + f_{x-1}^{t+1}}{\Delta x^2}}{2} \tag{18.21}$$

$$2(1+\beta)f_x^{t+1} - \beta f_{x+1}^{t+1} + \beta f_{x-1}^{t+1} = 2(1-\beta)f_x^t - \beta f_{x+1}^t + \beta f_{x-1}^t \tag{18.22}$$

The expression f_x^{t+1} is solved using the Crank-Nicholson expression by simultaneous calculation of the system and is always convergent and numerically stable. For each expression, the values at the boundaries are replaced with the appropriate boundary conditions. The explicit (18.17), implicit (18.19), and Crank-Nicholson (18.21) expressions can be generalized to multiple dimensions (i.e., x, y, z). The descretization algorithm presented here is applicable for the development of any governing expression that is called for when using finite-difference modeling schemes.

In solving problems involving complicated geometries, such as those encountered in whole-body simulation models, the finite difference method is the preferred approach for developing computational simulations. Accuracy in the finite difference solutions is governed by the size of elements and the time-step size used in the calculation. Finite difference methodology is most suitable for problems involving regularized meshing schemes.

Finite Element

The finite element method is fundamentally different from the finite difference method. Whereas the finite difference method is an approximation of the governing differential equation, the finite element method is an approximation of the *solution* of the governing differential equation. In this sense, finite element expressions may or may not actually satisfy the finite element equations at every point. Finite element problems are particular effective for problems that do not have a regularized meshing structure, and thus the method is extremely effective for handling objects with complex geometries. Meshing is accomplished by dividing a domain into a series of nonoverlapping discrete elements (see Figure 18.15).

The behavior of each element is first analyzed to relate the response at node points to changes in loading characteristics at these nodes. In the case of structural mechanics, for example, changes in the forces applied to the corners of a triangular truss result in linear displacement changes at each corner (nodes). As a triangle represents a two-dimensional object, the applied forces exert deformation changes in both the x and y directions at each node. The forces (f) and displacements (u) can

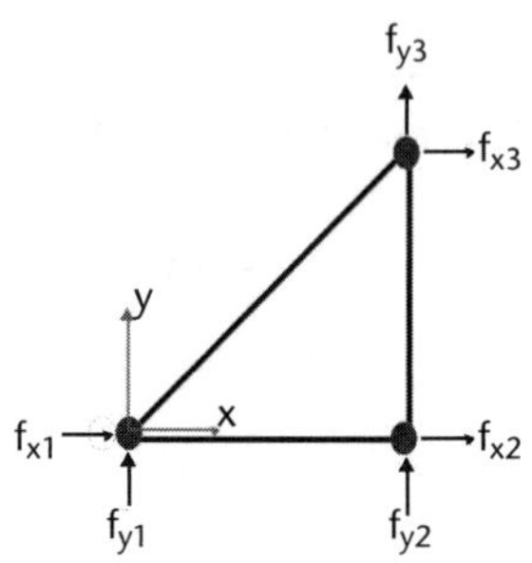

Figure 18.15 Idealized structural truss.

be written in vector form. The relationship between the forces and the displacement forms a matrix (stiffness matrix) such that

$$f=\begin{bmatrix} f_{x1} \\ f_{y1} \\ f_{x2} \\ f_{y2} \\ f_{x3} \\ f_{y3} \end{bmatrix};\ u=\begin{bmatrix} u_{x1} \\ u_{y1} \\ u_{x2} \\ u_{y2} \\ u_{x3} \\ u_{y3} \end{bmatrix};\ K=\begin{bmatrix} K_{x1x1} & K_{x1y1} & K_{x1x2} & K_{x1y2} & K_{x1x3} & K_{x1y3} \\ K_{y1x1} & K_{y1y1} & K_{y1x2} & K_{y1y2} & K_{y1x3} & K_{y1y3} \\ K_{x2x1} & K_{x2y1} & K_{x2x2} & K_{x2y2} & K_{x2x3} & K_{x2y3} \\ K_{y2x1} & K_{y2y1} & K_{y2x2} & K_{y2y2} & K_{y2x3} & K_{y2y3} \\ K_{x3x1} & K_{x3y1} & K_{x3x2} & K_{x3y2} & K_{x3x3} & K_{x3y3} \\ K_{y3y1} & K_{y3y} & K_{y3x2} & K_{y3y2} & K_{y3x3} & K_{y3y3} \end{bmatrix} \tag{18.23}$$

Given that the forces and displacements have a linear relationship, the resulting expression has the form,

$$\begin{bmatrix} K_{x1x1} & K_{x1y1} & K_{x1x2} & K_{x1y2} & K_{x1x3} & K_{x1y3} \\ K_{y1x1} & K_{y1y1} & K_{y1x2} & K_{y1y2} & K_{y1x3} & K_{y1y3} \\ K_{x2x1} & K_{x2y1} & K_{x2x2} & K_{x2y2} & K_{x2x3} & K_{x2y3} \\ K_{y2x1} & K_{y2y1} & K_{y2x2} & K_{y2y2} & K_{y2x3} & K_{y2y3} \\ K_{x3x1} & K_{x3y1} & K_{x3x2} & K_{x3y2} & K_{x3x3} & K_{x3y3} \\ K_{y3y1} & K_{y3y} & K_{y3x2} & K_{y3y2} & K_{y3x3} & K_{y3y3} \end{bmatrix} \begin{bmatrix} u_{x1} \\ u_{y1} \\ u_{x2} \\ u_{y2} \\ u_{x3} \\ u_{y3} \end{bmatrix} = \begin{bmatrix} f_{x1} \\ f_{y1} \\ f_{x2} \\ f_{y2} \\ f_{x3} \\ f_{y3} \end{bmatrix} \tag{18.24}$$

which can be rewritten in matrix notation as: $[K]u = f$. Each element in the stiffness matrix establishes a relationship between the load force and displacement. Each element K represents an intrinsic material property. For example, in structural mechanics, $K = EA/L$ where E is the elastic modulus, A is the cross-sectional area of the truss beams, and L is the initial length of the beam. Forces can be easily solved if the relationships in K and the displacement vectors u are known.

The finite element problem can be stated concisely using the above example: Given a known relationship (K) between forces and displacement, what are the displacements at the nodes when forces are exerted on the system. Mathematically, the problem can be stated as: Given: $[K]u = f$, where f and $[K]$ are known, find u. The solution to this equation ultimately involves finding an inverse for the matrix $[K]$ such that

$$u = [K]^{-1}f \tag{18.25}$$

A number of direct methods and iterative methods have been developed that efficiently tackle this problem. Direct methods obtain an exact solution for (18.24). The most widely known method is Gaussian elimination, in which the matrix expression is rearranged algebraically to eliminate all entries in the lower triangle of the matrix. Back-substitution is then used to solve for u in every row entry. LU decomposition is another method in which the matrix K is first divided into an upper and lower triangle. Since the matrix $[K] = [L][U]$, the matrix $[K]u = [L][U]u = f$. LU decomposition proceeds by first solving the forward expression $[L]y = f$, where $y = [U]u$ is substituted to transform the equation. Once $[L]y = f$ is solved, a backward substation is then solved where $[U]y = f$ to get the original matrix $[K]$.

Iterative methods generate a sequence of approximate solutions that (like the finite difference method) converges to the exact solution. The object in the iterative method is to minimize a residual. After n iterations, we obtain an approximate solution for $[K]u = f$:

$$[K]u^{(n)} = f - r^{(n)} \tag{18.26}$$

Defining the error in u as

$$\varepsilon^{(n)} = u - u^{(n)} \tag{18.27}$$

the iterative process is solved until the error is minimized. There are numerous iterative methods for solving finite element problems [i.e., Gauss-Seidel, successive overrelaxation methods (SOR), quasi-minimal residuals, and conjugate gradient method]. A more complete discussion on specific methodologies is described in the literature [60–62].

18.4 Summary

In this chapter, we surveyed a number of topics regarding the modeling of image guided systems. We discussed the role of imaging and modeling for image guided therapies. Both imaging and modeling play important roles in optimizing guided therapies—each enhances the other. As image modalities improve, the breadth of geometries that can be modeled increases. As modeling improves, our understanding of what happens in tissues increases. Ultimately, the development of all computational models requires four steps: image acquisition, segmentation, meshing, and computational methods. While the relative importance of each step is dependent on the specific modeling situation, each step is represented. As computer technology evolves, the speed in which the various steps can be accomplished improves significantly. The effect is that increasingly more complex modeling can be integrated into image guided therapies.

References

[1] Chang, I. A., and U. D. Nguyen, "Thermal Modeling of Lesion Growth with Radiofrequency Ablation," *Biomedical Engineering Online*, Vol. 3, 2004, p. 27.

[2] Hynynen, K., et al., "MR Imaging-Guided Focused Ultrasound Surgery of Fibroadenomas in the Breast: A Feasibility Study," *Radiology*, Vol. 219, 2001, pp. 176–185.

[3] Kopelman, D., and M. Papa, "Magnetic Resonance-Guided Focused Ultrasound Surgery for the Noninvasive Curative Ablation of Tumors and Palliative Treatments: A Review," *Annuals of Surgical Oncology*, Vol. 14, No. 5, 2007, pp. 1540–1550.

[4] Marcy, P. Y., et al., "Ultrasound-Guided Percutaneous Radiofrequency Ablation in Elderly Breast Cancer Patients: Preliminary Institutional Experience," *Br. J. Radiol.*, Vol. 80, No. 952, 2007, pp. 267–273.

[5] Goldberg, S. N., "Comparison of Techniques for Image-Guided Ablation of Focal Liver Tumors," *Radiology*, Vol. 223, No. 2, 2002, pp. 304–307.

[6] Fornage, B. D., et al., "Small (<2-cm) Breast Cancer Treated with US-Guided Radiofrequency Ablation: Feasibility Study," *Radiology*, Vol. 231, 2004, pp. 215–224.

[7] Tungjitkusolmun, S., et al., "Three-Dimensional Finite Element Analyses for Radio-Frequency Hepatic Tumor Ablation," *IEEE Transactions on Biomedical Engineering*, Vol. 49, 2002, pp. 3–9.

[8] Haemmerich, D., et al., "Finite-Element Analysis of Hepatic Multiple Probe Radio-Frequency Ablation," *IEEE Transactions on Biomedical Engineering*, Vol. 49, 2002, pp. 836–842.

[9] Weber, D. C., et al., "Radiation Therapy Planning with Photons and Protons for Early and Advanced Breast Cancer: An Overview," *Radiation Oncology*, Vol. 1, 2006, p. 22.

[10] Menkarios, C., et al., "Optimal Organ-Sparing Intensity-Modulated Radiation Therapy (IMRT) Regimen for the Treatment of Locally Advanced Anal Canal Carcinoma: A Comparison of Conventional and IMRT Plans," *Radiation Oncology*, Vol. 2, 2007, p. 41, http://www.ro-journal.com/content/2/1/41.

[11] Hariharan, P., et al., "Radio-Frequency Ablation in a Realistic Reconstructed Hepatic Tissue," *Journal of Biomechanical Engineering*, Vol. 6, 2007, pp. 129, 354–364.

[12] Tungjitkusolmun, S., et al., "Thermal–Electrical Finite Element Modelling for Radio Frequency Cardiac Ablation: Effects of Changes in Myocardial Properties," *Med. Biol. Eng. Comput.*, Vol. 38, 2000, pp. 562–568.

[13] Berjano, E. J., J. L. Alio, and J. Saiz, "Modeling for Radio-Frequency Conductive Keratoplasty: Implications for the Maximum Temperature Reached in the Cornea," *Physiol. Meas.*, Vol. 26, 2005, pp. 157–172.

[14] Haines, D. E., and D. D. Watson, "Tissue Heating During Radiofrequency Catheter Ablation: A Thermodynamic Model and Observations in Isolated Perfused and Superfused Canine Right Ventricular Free Wall," *Pacing Clin. Electrophysiol.*, Vol. 12, 1989, pp. 962–976.

[15] Labonte, S., "A Computer Simulation of Radio-Frequency Ablation of the Endocardium," *IEEE Transactions on Biomedical Engineering*, Vol. 41, 1994, pp. 883–890.

[16] Cao, H., et al., "FEM Analysis of Predicting Electrode-Myocardium Contact from RF Cardiac Catheter Ablation System Impedance," *IEEE Transactions on Biomedical Engineering*, Vol. 49, 2002, pp. 520–526.

[17] Haemmerich, D., et al., "Hepatic Bipolar Radio-Frequency Ablation Between Separated Multiprong Electrodes," *IEEE Transactions on Biomedical Engineering*, Vol. 48, 2001, pp. 1145–1152.

[18] Gabriel, S., R. W. Lau, and C. Gabriel, "The Dielectric Properties of Biological Tissues: II. Measurements in the Frequency Range 10 Hz to 20 GHz," *Phys. Med. Biol.*, Vol. 41, 1996, pp. 2251–2269.

[19] Stoy, R. D., K. R. Foster, and H. P. Schwan, "Dielectric Properties of Mammalian Tissues from 0.1 to 100 MHz: A Summary of Recent Data," *Phys. Med. Biol.*, Vol. 27, 1982, pp. 501–513.

[20] Duck, F., *Physical Properties of Tissue: A Comprehensive Reference Book*, New York: Academic Press, 1990, pp. 167–223.

[21] Wu, D., et al., "Possible Overexposure of Pregnant Women in the Third Trimester Due to Scanning in One Model of Walk Through Metal Detector," *Phys. Med. Biol.*, 2007, Vol. 52, pp. 5735–5748.

[22] Wu, D., et al., "Safety Evaluation of Walk-Through Metal Detectors," *IEEE EMC Society Newsletter*, Summer 2007, No. 214, pp. 60–65.

[23] Badano, A., and J. Sempau, "MANTIS: Combined X-Ray, Electron and Optical Monte Carlo Simulations of Indirect Radiation Imaging Systems," *Phys. Med. Biol.*, Vol. 51, 2006, pp. 1545–1561.

[24] Siegel, E., et al., "Digital Mammography Image Quality: Image Display," *Journal of the American College of Radiology*, Vol. 3, 2006, pp. 8, 615–627.

[25] Pfefer, T. J., et al., "Bioheat Transfer Analysis of Cryogen Spray Cooling During Laser Treatment of Port Wine Stains," *Lasers Surg Med.*, Vol. 26, No. 2, 2000, pp. 145–157.

[26] Beard, B. B., and W. Kainz, "Review and Standardization of Cell Phone Exposure Calculations Using the SAM Phantom and Anatomically Correct Head Models," *Biomed. Eng. Online*, Vol. 3, 2004, p. 34.

[27] Kainz, W., et al., "Calculation of Induced Current Densities and Specific Absorption Rates (SAR) for Pregnant Women Exposed to Hand-Held Metal Detectors," *Phys. Med. Biol.*, Vol. 48, 2003, pp. 2551–2560.

[28] Pennes, H. H., "Analysis of Tissue and Arterial Blood Temperature in the Resting Human Forearm," *J. Appl. Physiol.*, Vol. 1, 1948, pp. 93–122.

[29] Chang, I., "Finite Element Analysis of Hepatic Radiofrequency Ablation Probes Using Temperature-Dependent Electrical Conductivity," *Biomed. Engineering Online*, Vol. 2, 2003, p. 12.

[30] Curley, M. G., and P. S. Hamilton, "Creation of Large Thermal Lesions in Liver Using Saline-Enhanced RF Ablation," *Engineering in Medicine and Biology Society Proceedings of the 19th Annual International Conference of the IEEE*, 1997, pp. 2516–2519.

[31] Panescu, D., et al., "Three-Dimensional Finite Element Analysis of Current Density and Temperature Distributions During Radio-Frequency Ablation," *IEEE Transactions on Biomedical Engineering*, Vol. 42, 1995, pp. 879–890.

[32] Shahidi, A. V., and P. Savard, "A Finite Element Model for Radiofrequency Ablation of the Myocardium," *IEEE Transactions on Biomedical Engineering*, Vol. 41, 1994, pp. 963–968.

[33] Tungjitkusolmun, S., et al., "Finite Element Analyses of Uniform Current Density Electrodes for Radio-Frequency Cardiac Ablation," *IEEE Transactions on Biomedical Engineering*, Vol. 47, 2000, pp. 32–40.

[34] Lai, Y. C., et al., "Lesion Size Estimator of Cardiac Radiofrequency Ablation at Different Common Locations with Different Tip Temperatures," *IEEE Transactions on Biomedical Engineering*, Vol. 51, 2004, pp. 1859–1864.

[35] Jain, M. K., and P. D. Wolf, "Temperature-Controlled and Constant Power Radio-Frequency Ablation: What Affects Lesion Growth?" *IEEE Transactions on Biomedical Engineering*, Vol. 46, 1999, pp. 1405–1412.

[36] Jain, M. K., et al., "Effect of Skin Electrode Location on Radiofrequency Ablation Lesions: An In Vivo and a Three-Dimensional Finite Element Study," *J. Cardiovasc. Electrophysiol.*, Vol. 9, 1998, pp. 1325–1335.

[37] Berjano, E. J., and F. Hornero, "Thermal-Electrical Modeling for Epicardial Atrial Radiofrequency Ablation," *IEEE Transactions on Biomedical Engineering*, Vol. 51, 2004, pp. 1348–1357.

[38] Ekstrand, V., et al., "Influence of Electrical and Thermal Properties on RF Ablation of Breast Cancer: Is the Tumour Preferentially Heated?" *Biomed. Eng. Online*, Vol. 4, 2005, p. 41.

[39] Tungjitkusolmun, S., et al., "Using ANSYS for Three-Dimensional Electrical-Thermal Models for Radio-Frequency Catheter Ablation," *Engineering in Medicine and Biology Society Proceedings of the 19th Annual International Conference of the IEEE*, 1997, pp. 161–164.

[40] Tungjitkusolmun, S., et al., "Modeling Bipolar Phase-Shifted Multielectrode Catheter Ablation," *IEEE Transactions on Biomedical Engineering*, Vol. 49, 2002, pp. 10–17.

[41] Berjano, E. J., and F. Hornero, "A Cooled Intraesophageal Balloon to Prevent Thermal Injury During Endocardial Surgical Radiofrequency Ablation of the Left Atrium: A Finite Element Study," *Phys. Med. Biol.*, Vol. 50, 2005, pp. N269–N279.

[42] Berjano, E. J., and F. Hornero, "What Affects Esophageal Injury During Radiofrequency Ablation of the Left Atrium? An Engineering Study Based on Finite-Element Analysis," *Physiol. Meas.*, Vol. 26, 2005, pp. 837–848.

[43] Hornero, F., and E. J. Berjano, "Esophageal Temperature During Radiofrequency Catheter Ablation of Left Atrium: A Three-Dimensional Computer Modeling Study," *J. Cardiovasc. Electrophysiol.*, Vol. 17, 2006, pp. 405–410.

[44] Chang, I., F. Razjouyan, and U. Nguyen, "Analysis Considerations for Modeling Thermal Injury Using RF Ablation Devices," *2nd Young Vietnamese Scientists Meeting*, Hanoi, Vietnam, July 25–28, 2007.

[45] Yoo, T., *Insights into Images*, Wellesley, MA: A.K. Peters, 2004.

[46] Manzke, R. M., "Cardiac Cone Beam CT," Dissertation, Division of Imaging Science, Kings College, London, U.K., September 2004.

[47] Phelps, M. E., et al., "Application of Annihilation Coincidence Detection to Transaxial Reconstruction Tomography," *Journal of Nuclear Medicine*, Vol. 16, 1875, No. 3, pp. 210–224.

[48] Holder, D. S., *Electrical Impedance Tomography: Methods, History and Application*, London, U.K.: Institute of Physics, 2004.

[49] Beck, M. S., and R. Williams, *Process Tomography: Principles, Techniques and Applications*, Boston, MA: Butterworth-Heinemann, 1995.

[50] Boppart, S. A., "Optical Coherence Tomography: Technology and Applications for Neuroimaging," *Psychophysiology*, Vol. 40, 2003, pp. 529–541.

[51] Fercher, A. F., et al., "Optical Coherence Tomography—Principles and Applications," *Rep. Prog. Phys.*, Vol. 66, 2003, pp. 239–303.

[52] Fujimoto, J. G., "Optical Coherence Tomography for Ultrahigh Resolution In Vivo Imaging," *Nature Biotechnology*, Vol. 21, No. 11, 2003, pp. 1361–1367.

[53] Barton, J. K., et al., "Optical Low Coherence Reflectometry to Enhance Monte Carlo Modeling of Skin," *Journal of Biomedical Optics*, Vol. 2, No. 2, 1997, pp. 226–234.

[54] Gibson, A., J. Hebden, and S. Arridge, "Recent Advances in Diffuse Optical Imaging," *Phys. Med. Biol.*, Vol. 50, 2005, pp. R1–R43.

[55] Zhang, H. F., et al., "Functional Photoacoustic Microscopy for High-Resolution and Noninvasive In Vivo Imaging," *Nature Biotechnology*, Vol. 24, No. 7, 2006, pp. 848–851.

[56] Beard, B. B., and W. Kainz, "Review and Standardization of Cell Phone Exposure Calculations Using the SAM Phantom and Anatomically Correct Head Models," *Biomedical Engineering Online*, Vol. 3, 2004, p. 34.

[57] Hutter, J. C., H. D. Luu, and C. S. Kim, "A Dynamic Simulation of Bisphenol A Dosimetry in Neuroendocrine Organs," *Toxicology and Industrial Health*, Vol. 20, 2004, pp. 29–40.

[58] Boas, D. A., et al., "Three Dimensional Monte Carlo Code for Photon Migration Through Complex Heterogeneous Media Including the Adult Human Head," *Optics Express*, Vol. 10, No. 3, 2002, pp. 159–170.

[59] Margallo-Balbás, E., P. J. French, "Micro-CT Defined Geometry Shape Based Monte Carlo Code for Light Transport in Complex Heterogeneous Tissues," *Optics Express*, Vol. 15, No. 21, 2007, pp. 14086–14098.

[60] Grandin, H., *Fundamentals of the Finite Element Method*, New York: Macmillan, 1986.

[61] Logan, D. L., *A First Course in the Finite Element Method*, New York: CENGAGE-Engineering, 2005.

[62] Comini, G., *Finite Element Analysis in Heat Transfer: Basic Formulation & Linear Problems*, Series in Computational and Physical Processes in Mechanics and Thermal Sciences, Oxford, U.K.: Taylor & Francis, 1994.

CHAPTER 19

The Socioeconomic Benefits of Image-Guided Therapies

Arthur H. Chan

When planning a road trip and navigating a new city, we used to rely on paper maps. However, nowadays we use 3D satellite imagery to look at where we are traveling to before even getting in the car. Once on the road, a GPS navigation system shows the precise location of where we are and accurately directs us to our destination, informing us of traffic problems and road closures that we should avoid.

This analogy portrays the recent advances in image-guided therapy, which has revolutionized traditional surgical procedures by providing physicians 3D images to navigate through the body with great precision. An exact surgical plan, the optimal path to the lesion, obstacles to treatment and the surrounding tissues can be accurately mapped out before surgery and during the surgery. As such, image-guided surgery systems provide much benefit to patients in terms of improved efficiency, accuracy, and safety.

However, similar to a GPS navigator, these image-guided procedures will be accepted and adopted only if the electronics and software are reliable, and if the procedures are physician and operating room friendly. Accuracy and simplicity are important, and long-term durability data need to show that the image-guided procedure is as good as the traditional open surgery approach.

The clinical benefits and breakthrough technology associated with image-guided treatments continue to drive their acceptance and growth worldwide. Equally important in ensuring the viability and growth of image-guided therapies are the socioeconomic benefits associated with these treatments. Although socioeconomic benefits are important to the adoption and implementation of new medical technologies, it is also equally important to realize that the fundamental reason for them is due to patient benefit. Image-guided therapies are developed to be minimally or noninvasive alternatives to surgery. Less sedation, smaller incisions, less hospitalization, reduced follow-up care, and faster recovery are all associated with significant cost savings. These savings make image-guided therapies attractive to not just patients but physicians, hospitals, and healthcare insurance providers.

This chapter discusses concepts, dilemmas, and scenarios related to the socioeconomics of image-guided therapies. Although specific examples are used to illustrate each concept, the ideas and predicaments presented in each case can be applied to any image-guided therapy. When reading this chapter, imagine how these benefits can be realized for various treatments and think about how some of the challenges presented here can be overcome.

19.1 Infrastructure Changes

The advancement of multimodality image-guided therapy will necessitate changes in hospital design and infrastructure. Imagine the treatment of a prostate cancer patient who chooses focused ultrasound therapy for his tumor. His intentions are to avoid a prostatectomy and have a minimally invasive procedure to maintain potency and continence. However, his oncologist believes a low dose of radiation for the entire prostate to accompany focused ultrasound for the tumor would result in a greater chance that the entire prostate would be free of cancer while also minimizing toxicity. One could envision the patient moving to different treatment rooms within a hospital, or even traveling to different treatment centers to complete the prescribed treatment regimen. However, patients would prefer to have a complete set of treatment options available to them at one location. This desire would not just be for convenience but as reassurance that there will be no bias in the treatments recommended to them. As multimodality image-guided therapies become more prevalent, hospitals are planning image-guided surgical suites.

At the National Center for Image Guided Therapy, physicians and researchers at the Brigham and Women's Hospital and Harvard Medical School in Boston have combined a MRI, PET/CT scanner, an X-ray, and a surgical microscope all in one room. In this room, known as the AMIGO or the Advanced Multimodality Image Guided Operating suite, the patient is transported between imaging modalities on a special surgical table and a tracking and navigation system integrates treatment locations with anatomical and physiological information provided by the imaging technologies. Equipment, instruments, and supplies for minimally invasive surgery would all be in this room with the imaging modalities. Similarly, the image-guided surgery suite at University of Minnesota combines a 1.5 Tesla magnet with vascular X-ray.

Until recently, preoperative images have been used to aid surgeons in performing image-guided treatments. However, such preoperative images and the treatment plans based upon them need to be updated as the treatment progresses. Anatomical changes and physiological motion such as organ displacement and tissue deformation also need to be accounted for during image-guided procedures. Thus, having the imaging modalities able to capture and analyze images in real time during surgery is important and will be possible in the AMIGO suite.

Cancer centers are incorporating image-guided therapy into their facilities more than ever before. For example, the Holden Comprehensive Cancer Center at the University of Iowa added a Center of Excellence in Image Guided Radiation Therapy. This facility currently occupies 40,000 square feet and houses PET, CT, and MRI scanners, linear accelerators, and offers procedures such as intensity modulated 3D and 4D radiotherapy, ultrasound guided extracranial radiosurgery, and image-guided seed implantation into the prostate to name a few, according to the University of Iowa. In addition, cancer center chains such as US Oncology and the Cancer Treatment Centers of America offer an array of image-guided treatments for their patients. This illustrates the demand for, and acceptance of, image-guided procedures as standards of care due to the many benefits that image-guided therapies offer, namely minimal invasiveness and quick recovery time.

19.2 Patient Benefits

Image-guided therapies have allowed invasive surgical procedures to become minimally invasive. Minimally invasive procedures are less complex, shorter in duration, and safer for the patient. Endoscopy has reduced the need for exploratory surgery and has made the diagnosis and treatment of GI tumors simpler. Angioplasty is a lot less invasive, and carries a lot fewer risks, than open-heart surgeries. Image-guided therapy has certainly benefited patients seeking knee replacement surgeries. Aided by computers, surgeons are able to acquire and use a 3D image of the knee joint to align the leg and the implants during knee replacement procedures. Deformities are corrected, and the proper implant size can be modeled and selected prior to cutting the patient's bone. These techniques can also be applied to hip and pelvic surgeries as well. Even otolaryngologists (ear-nose-throat physicians) are performing image-guided endoscopic surgery to open up inflamed sinuses while minimizing risk to the optic nerve and carotic artery. This section explores how image-guided therapies have truly benefited patients in various specialties.

19.2.1 Image-Guided Neurosurgery

In 1908, an English neurosurgeon by the name of Sir Victor Horsley and a mathmetician named Robert Henry Clarke designed and developed a device that was used to guide an electrode into a monkey brain to study cerebral function [1]. A hundred years later, the work done by these pioneers would evolve into image-guided neurosurgery used by physicians today—to stay oriented in the cranium and minimize the amount of surgical exposure a patient would require.

In image-guided neurosurgery, computed tomography (CT) and functional magnetic resonance (fMR) imaging modalities are used to scan the patient's brain for anomalies. Rather than reconstructing a set of 2D images in their mind, surgeons can now have these images processed by a computer which creates a 3D rendering of the skull and brain. This dataset of images helps surgeons to see lesions, and provide a "map" of the brain to determine what surrounds the region they intend to operate on. The other important aspect of image-guided neurosurgery is to ensure that the surgical instruments used are continuously visualized relative to the preoperative diagnostic images. Being able to track the location of the instruments and surrounding structures to submillimeter accuracy, image-guided neurosurgery has allowed brain surgeons to access tumors and vascular abnormalities much more safely and less invasively. The Gamma Knife is a minimally invasive stereotactic radiosurgery procedure where a single high dose of ionizing radiation is delivered to specific targets in the brain. Lesions are targeted using 3D planning images and these images are used in treatment planning to precisely focus the radiation on the target tissue while minimizing radiation to surrounding brain tissues.

19.2.2 Image-Guided Drug Delivery

Chemotherapy works well in preventing cancer cells from reproducing and spreading, but chemotherapy affects normal cells as well. Chemotherapy, which is systemically administered, results in the entire body being affected when the intended target is a specific site. Tumor-targeting drugs have been developed which are used to specifically target and kill remaining cancer cells after a tumor has been removed. These drugs are injected to the tumor site via catheters in an image-guided procedure. The image guidance ensures that the drugs are delivered to the intended location—and to ensure that targeted drug delivery truly is targeted. As a result, patient side effects to chemotherapy can be diminished.

19.2.3 Reproductive Medicine

The less invasive a procedure, the less recovery time will be needed. Image-guided therapies offer patients a chance to be back to daily life sooner. An example of an indication that may benefit from having an image-guided therapy is male infertility. Male infertility may be caused by an enlarged and blocked varicose vein of the testicle, known as a varicocele. Open surgical ligation involves an incision above the scrotum to access and suture the testicular vein. Full anesthesia is required followed by a 2- to 3-week recovery period, with a quarter of all patients requiring an overnight hospital stay. An alternative to this option is varicocele embolization, which involves the insertion of a catheter through the femoral vein that is guided by fluoroscopy imaging into the testicular vein. The vein leading up to the varicocle is then occluded to reduce pressure and thus pain at the problem area. Patients take 1 to 2 days to recover and do not require anesthesia nor a hospital stay. In terms of efficacy, sperm concentration improvements have been similar or better with patients undergoing embolization compared with surgery, according to the Society of Interventional Radiology.

Once conception has been achieved a small number of fetuses will unfortunately require surgical intervention for developmental anomalies. Fetal intervention has remained a risky procedure for the child and the mother until recently. Traditionally, open fetal surgery involved opening up the abdomen, similar to a caesarian section, requiring the mother to be anesthetized and necessitating 3 to 7 days of recovery. A postprocedural epidural was needed for 2 to 3 days after the procedure for pain control and drugs were needed to prevent preterm labor. After this procedure, the only option for delivery was C-section, and a risk of preterm delivery was high.

Pioneers of fetal surgery at the University of California, San Francisco, have developed a method called Fetal Image Guided Surgery (FIGS), in which ultrasound imaging is used to guide fetal intervention. The mother is given local or regional sedation, and if an incision is required it is generally very small. FIGS can be done as an outpatient procedure, and an overnight stay to monitor for an unwanted side effect of preterm labor (still a risk) is generally all that is required. Comparing short-term morbidity with open surgery procedures, there are significantly fewer complications in the ultrasound guided procedures [2].

In weighing the above two options, most women would choose the latter lesser invasive procedure. However, image-guided minimally invasive options such as FIGS are often offered only in specialized centers with a few highly trained physician teams who can perform the procedures. Mention that a wait time for such procedures may end up being long and that these procedures may not be covered by insurance. As such, it is reasonable to believe that such procedures may not be presented as options during patient-physician consultations. So how do the approximately 3% of mothers whose fetuses need intervention discover image-guided treatment alternatives to open surgery? Women today are more than ever using the Internet as a resource during their pregnancy, to seek answers about fetal development, medical treatments, and seek support from other expectant mothers.

19.2.4 Spine Surgery

The benefits of image-guided therapy, as it pertains to patient safety, are illustrated in image-guided spine surgery. This procedure uses X-ray images reconstructed into 3D computer models that are used in real time to allow surgeons performing spinal surgery to be able to be more efficient and safe. Not only does the image-guided therapy show a 3D model of the patient's spine, it also shows virtual images of the surgeon's tools and instruments. According to Seattle's Orthopedics' International [3], image-guided spine surgery offers their surgeons the following benefits:

- It enhances the ability to navigate complex spinal anatomy in real time.
- It provides accurate measurements such as screw diameter and length.
- It allows us to more precisely implant instrumentation.
- It can pinpoint exactly where the tip of a surgeon's instrument is in relation to a patient's anatomy, providing invaluable information in case unexpected or unusual anatomy is encountered.
- It reduces operating time.
- It minimizes (and in some cases, eliminates) radiation exposure previously experienced with traditional X-rays.

19.3 Patient Education Drives Demand for Image-Guided Therapy

Patients are becoming more educated on healthcare options by going online. A 2002 study estimated that 62% of Americans (72% of women) with access to the Internet have used it to search for medical information and used it to supplement information provided by their physicians [4]. The study further reported that 68% reported that the information found on the Internet was influential in the treatment decision.

Since many patients are no longer solely relying on information provided by their physicians, it can be inferred that novel image-guided therapies are becoming discovered by patients as quickly as they are by their physicians. As patients seek low morbidity and quick recovery time associated with image-guided minimally invasive procedures, it would not be uncommon for a patient to have researched alternatives to surgery and demand certain procedures.

Patients seeking alternative therapies to surgery may also seek clinical studies related to their indication. A search of image-guided therapy on the U.S. government's Web site listing FDA clinical studies reveals more than a hundred studies involving image-guided therapies. From image-guided radiation therapy for prostates and pediatric brain tumors to MR guided focused ultrasound for the pain palliation of bone metastases, the Web site lists exclusion and inclusion criteria, the treatment regimen, participating sites and patient coordinator contact information. Although treatment outcomes are unknown and speculative, many patients are willing to attempt a minimally or noninvasive image-guided therapy prior to seeking surgical options.

However, patients need to be prudent in determining if they are a candidate for a novel image-guided treatment and if it truly is the best treatment for them in the long run. With that said, having physicians become educated in the latest image-guided treatments is equally critical in the widespread acceptance and offering of these procedures.

19.4 Physician Awareness and Training

As patient demand for minimally invasive image-guided therapies increases, researchers and physicians alike are spending more time discovering and performing these procedures. Founded in 1973 as the Society of Cardiovascular Radiology, the Society of Interventional Radiology (SIR) now comprises more than 4,000 members who specialize in image-guided procedures. At its annual meeting, many of its talks are about image-guided therapies, from angioplasty to kidney cancer tumor ablation.

When innovative image-guided therapies are first introduced, their availability is limited to large tertiary care medical centers (highly specialized in specific inpatient conditions and illnesses). Results from new procedures like image-guided ablation are often shared at society meetings like the SIR and the Radiological Society of North America (RSNA). Societies have even been formed within medical disciplines identifying physicians who practice image-guided minimally invasive procedures and providing them with a forum for discussion and training. An example is the American Association of Gynecological Laparoscopists (AAGL), comprised of gynecologists who perform image-guided procedures. At all medical meetings, there are a growing number of sessions, speakers, and round-table discussions on image-guided therapy. Physicians have a chance to learn about these procedures in scientific sessions, compare outcomes at roundtable discussions, and share best practices.

Due to the size and complexity of the computer systems and imaging modalities required, the teaching of most of these procedures are done via site visits and peer-to-peer training. Companies developing image-guided therapies often have workshops at medical society meetings or even dedicated training centers. These training centers may be a part of medical schools, or stand-alone facilities associated with corporate headquarters. Ethicon Endo-Surgery has three medical education facilities in Ohio, Germany, and Tokyo, which feature operating rooms and research labs designed to teach minimally invasive surgery. These "Endo-Surgery Institutes" have trained over 40,000 surgeons, operating room nurses, and other health care professionals worldwide. Companies who do not have dedicated training facilities have designated certain clinical sites as training centers, according to Ethicon Endo-Surgery.

Surgeons who are used to opening up the body and seeing actual organs and vessels are now relying on high-resolution pictures, image processing techniques, and computer equipment to guide them. The complexity and the learning curve of different image-guided therapies vary. A study published in the *New England Journal of Medicine* comparing open colectomy versus a laparoscopically assisted approach defined an experienced surgeon as one who has performed at least 20 laparoscopically assisted colorectal operations with knowledge of oncology [5]. However, it is often difficult to set a certain number of treatments as a determinant for physician proficiency. This is due to the varied backgrounds of physicians performing image-guided therapy and varied capabilities of these physicians.

It is important to have detailed requirements for training and certification, and defining what core competencies are needed for physicians performing image-guided treatments. A quantitative method of measuring proficiency and a consistent and objective training regimen should be implemented. Such a training program is often developed by the device manufacturer during the FDA approval process, and is based on physician training experience and physician input during the clinical study phases of a new image-guided treatment. Once the training program is developed, an approval or an endorsement of the training program by a medical society adds to its credibility.

A good example of a well-defined training document is one developed for credentialing physicians on carotid stenting [6]. Studies have shown improved patient outcomes with increasing operator experience which indicates a learning curve, and therefore ensuring that physicians who perform this procedure with an approved standard will generate better patient outcomes. This document details the cognitive, technical, and clinical requirements for a physician to perform carotid stenting. Here is an example of each: cognitive—understanding the pathophysiology of carotid artery disease; technical—having performed 25 stenting procedures with at least half of those as the primary operator; and clinical—determining patient risk/benefit and managing outpatient and inpatient responsibilities. This training guide also details the necessity for a hospital quality assurance program which includes case reviews, benchmark setting, outcomes measurement, and the tracking of physician treatments. These types of training standards are necessary for all image-guided minimally invasive and noninvasive procedures. Having all physicians well trained will lead to more success, adoption, and desire for these procedures.

The carotid stenting document also recommends the use of simulators, which have proven to be effective in physician training [7]. Simulators are computer systems that allow physicians to practice procedures, often with the actual surgical instruments used, with the aid of robotics or computer generated images, on phantoms. One of the unique aspects of image-guided therapy is that training can be done outside the surgical suite—on designated simulators, online, or even remotely. Although image-guided treatments may be more technologically involved and complex, getting trained may be easier as compared to traditional surgery trainings where cadaver and animal labs are required.

In a similar article that outlines credentialing for uterine artery embolization, the technical proficiency in terms of number of procedures is again stated. Also mentioned are standards for success and complications, with reported rates and suggested thresholds as goals for trainees and certified physicians to meet or exceed [8, 9]. It is documents like these that provide reassurance to patients and referring physicians that image-guided treatments will be consistent between credentialed physicians and will meet certain standards. It also allows patients to do consumer research as to whether or not physicians have met the society mandated requirements.

Once a physician is trained, it is important to foster continued education through medical conferences, physician training workshops which offer continuing medical education (CME) credits, or online courses. Not only is there new methodology to learn, but with the various software and graphical user interfaces involved with image-guided therapy, physicians are now more than ever in need to keep up with technology and system upgrades.

19.5 Physician Acceptance and Adoption

Just as important as physician awareness and education is physician willingness to adopt and include image-guided treatments as viable alternatives to surgery. Although there are many physicians who are early adopters of image-guided therapies, there are others who are more conservative and have less of a desire to be the first mover. These physicians would rather wait until a larger consensus has been reached on the long-term durability and safety profile of these treatments, especially as they compare to open surgery.

The early adopters are likely to be principal investigators in clinical studies to test out new image-guided therapies or advances in current technologies. Companies seeking to test new technologies may also seek influential key opinion leaders to be lead investigators. As clinical trial results are often presented at medical conferences, having key opinion leaders present these results may persuade and ease the acceptance of new image-guided therapies. It is also crucial for medical societies to be supportive of these treatments as many physicians who are members or affiliates of these organizations will look to their opinions as guidance for what to adopt in their practices. For adoption of novel image-guided therapies, the support of medical societies representing both the radiological side and the surgical side is equally important.

19.5.1 Barriers to Adoption

As many benefits as there may be with image-guided therapies, there are barriers to adoption as with all medical technologies. Two of the challenges to the adoption and widespread practice of new image-guided techniques are the learning curve involved and the time it takes to perform the procedure. With image-guided therapy, there may be a trade-off between reducing patient invasiveness and recovery time, and an increase in procedure time. The increase in procedure time is especially apparent when a physician first learns a novel image-guided procedure.

Take anterior lumbar spinal fusion, for example. In a multicenter study, Regan et al. compared 240 patients undergoing (image-guided) laparoscopic spinal fusion with 591 patients undergoing traditional surgical fusion with the same device. The laparoscopic group had shorter hospital stays and decreased blood loss but also had increased operating time due to a higher learning curve. Surgical complications were similar in both groups [10].

An increase in operating time may reduce the number of procedures that a physician can perform on a daily basis, or require more physicians to treat a certain number of patients. Thus, it is important for an image-guided therapy to not only meet or exceed the complication rate, but be as efficient as a current standard of treatment, both of which are part of the equation in a physician's decision to add image-guided therapy to their portfolio.

In considering whether or not an image-guided therapy should be used for a specific indication, and prior to a company investing millions of dollars in an FDA study, it is important to take into consideration the time it takes to currently treat the indication with available technology. For example, the fictitious procedure of MR guided cryo-vasectomy would probably not be a venture worth pursuing. First, a vasectomy currently takes minutes to complete. It is also already an outpatient procedure with a short recovery time, and reversal of the procedure is sometimes possible. It is doubtful that investing radiology and MRI time to perform such a procedure with cryo-ablation would make financial and practical sense.

The appeal of an image-guided technology may differ among and depend on the physicians and the indications that they treat. It takes a gynecologist approximately 2 hours of time to treat a 5-cm uterine fibroid with MR guided focused ultrasound (MRgFUS). If the same fibroid could be removed using a transcervical laparoscopic myomectomy, it might only take 30 minutes. Due to the high ultrasound absorption in bone, a radiation oncologist could use the same technology (MRgFUS) to potentially alleviate pain in a patient with a bone metastasis in less than an hour and a half [11]. This is not much different from the time takes to perform more invasive radiation therapy or RF ablation for the metastases. Thus, treatment for bone metastases may be adopted quicker.

The capital cost of the equipment used for image-guided therapies may also be a hindrance to adoption. Later on in this chapter, we will explore the increased demand for imaging due to image-guided therapies. This may require more CT, PET, or MRI scanners to be purchased, large capital expenses. However, this may actually have a positive financial impact as later explained. Image-guided therapy modalities may cost tens of thousands of dollars, or even up to a million dollars in the case of MRgFUS (not including the cost of an MRI). This results in the need for the equipment to be leased, and for physician groups to form partnerships as limited liability investors in such technology.

Finally, the willingness for healthcare insurance to cover image-guided therapy procedures determines the adoption rate. As obtaining insurance coverage is as challenging as obtaining FDA approval, a full discussion in healthcare reimbursement requires a book in itself. Here are some basics to consider whenever a new image-guided therapy is introduced.

The American Medical Association (AMA) classifies medical procedures into current procedural terminology (CPT) codes describing the procedure in terms of medical, surgical, and diagnostic services. A CPT I code is a permanent code for procedures and technologies with sufficient data and published literature. The CPT I code helps determine the amount payable for a procedure under the Medicare fee schedule for physicians. However, new image-guided therapies may fall under an emerging technology code, known as a CPT III code, are assigned to new technologies which may not have enough peer reviewed literature to classify it as a CPT I code. As such, since CPT III signifies that the procedure is still somewhat "experimental," insurance providers may be hesitant to pay for it.

In order to get a CPT I code, sufficient long-term data in peer-reviewed journals need to be available. For this to be possible, there needs to be a large population of patients treated. However, since these procedures require expensive technology and highly trained specialists, many patients cannot afford to pay for these procedures and would wait, if possible, until they are covered by insurance. This Catch-22 scenario may hinder the adoption of a new image-guided therapy.

Furthermore, insurers may be less likely to cover nondefinitive organ-sparing procedures, as most image-guided therapies are. The fear is that they do not want to cover additional procedures in the same patient for the same indication. For example, treating a prostate cancer tumor does not preclude another tumor from developing, whereas a radical prostatectomy (removal of the entire prostate) will.

Finally, insurance providers will have outlined certain criteria in which patients have to meet prior to receiving coverage. This ensures proper patient selection leading to durable and safe outcomes reducing the need for alternative treatments. Therefore, it is important in the development of a new image-guided therapy to specify a subset of a patient population for which the procedure is best suited.

19.5.2 Would Industry Cooperation Lead to Increased Adoption?

Another challenge with image-guided therapy is that there are multiple medical device companies developing imaging tools, software, and instruments for image-guided surgery. As one can imagine, compatibility becomes an issue. Images acquired with one manufacturer's software may have difficulty being read, processed, and rendered in another manufacturer's computer system. Collaboration between institutions to benefit a patient's care regimen may be hampered if they have competing manufacturers' systems. Physicians and technologists trained in one software may need to be retrained on a different software should they move hospitals. Surgical tools compatible with one image-guided therapy system may not be useable with another. Cooperation between device manufacturers or the idea of an open source development platform (similar to applications for the iPhone or Facebook) may lead to better tools and software. The use of a universal image format for MRI images, DICOM, has already resulted in many image processing tools capable of manipulating and optimizing these images for image-guided therapy.

19.6 Patient Selection: Image-Guided Therapy Is Not for Everyone

Proper patient selection is necessary to ensure optimal treatment outcomes. Renal cell carcinomas (RCCs) accounted for approximately 11,000 deaths in 2003. With advances in imaging technology, more renal cell carcinomas are being detected. These small asymptomatic nonaggressive tumors are good targets for a minimally invasive treatment approach with image-guided ablation. Results have shown high local control and low complication rates for image-guided RF and cryoablation [12]. Since RCCs are generally resistant to radiotherapy and chemotherapy, surgical resection or tumor destruction is often the only cure.

A kidney removal (radical nephrectomy) has been the standard of care for patients with RCCs until recently. Smaller tumors have been successfully treated with less invasive methods or removed laparoscopically, thus reducing morbidity [13]. Image-guided renal cryoablation and RF ablation have a complication rate of less than 10%, the majority of the complications being minor, compared to surgical complication rates of 14% with a 1% mortality [14]. Physicians at the Mayo Clinic performed cryo-ablation on solid renal tumors under ultrasound guidance and CT monitoring with a 95% success rate and an 8% complication rate [15]. In Japan, physicians using MR-guided cryo-ablation for RCCs also showed promising results [16]. These procedures have comparable efficacy to surgery but are safer, cost less, and can be performed as an outpatient procedure in patients who cannot tolerate or do not desire surgery.

To ensure good treatment results, one of the most crucial aspects to consider is patient selection. Although the risk of leaving viable cancer cells is minimal, it is still inherent in image-guided ablation. Therefore, resection is still the only definitive treatment option. While awaiting more long-term treatment durability data, physicians may advise only cancer patients who are not surgical candidates to undergo image-guided ablation. Patients who have metastatic disease would also most likely not choose a nonsurgical option.

An image-guided ablation requires the use of contrast-enhanced MR images for staging, planning, and treatment confirmation. There are patients who may be contraindicated for contrast, and in some cases unable to tolerate contrast agents such as gadolinium due to renal failure [17]. Patients also need to be able to fit in the imaging device—for example, the weight limit and bore dimensions of the MRI may exclude some patients from an MR guided procedure.

Equally important as choosing the right patients is tumor selection. The size of the tumor affects the procedure duration, energy delivered, and the risk of injury to the surrounding structures. As such, image-guided ablation is best suited for patients with tumors that are less than 5 cm in diameter [12]. By choosing appropriately sized tumors, technical success rates are improved and recurrence rates are lower. RCC recurrence rates after ablation are low (at 0% to 10%), but for tumors less than 4 cm, local recurrence rates are even less at (0% to 3%).

Tumor location also plays a role in as to whether or not the tumor can be successfully treated. First, the tumor has to be accessible. Second, the tumor should be in a location where treatment will not affect other sensitive structures. For image-guided ablation of RCCs, tumors on the periphery of the kidney are easier to treat than tumors located centrally. Treatment of central tumors may result in a higher risk of complications to the ureter. Tumors located anteriorly may be unsuitable for treatment due to potential risk to the bowel.

As exemplified with image-guided ablation of RCCs, minimally invasive image-guided therapies work best on patients and tumors that are suited for this procedure. It is important for patients to understand that just having a disease does not make the patient eligible for an image-guided treatment intended for that disease. One of the challenges for physicians will be to develop and optimize treatment guidelines defining what constitutes an ideal patient, and be able to define predictors of success to gauge whether or not a patient can benefit from a minimally invasive image-guided procedure. At the same time, reasons for patient ineligibility should be used to further improve the treatment devices so that a larger population of patients can become candidates for these sought after procedures.

19.7 The Economic Impact of Image-Guided Therapy

19.7.1 Spleens, Gallbladders, and Hernias All Benefit from Image-Guided Treatments

Image-guided therapies are generally considered minimally invasive or noninvasive. The perception of these procedures is that there is a tremendous healthcare cost savings associated with shorter recovery times, fewer complications, and shorter hospital stays. In an issue of the journal of *Surgical Laparoscopy, Endoscopy & Percutaneous Techniques*, three groups in Europe presented these benefits in separate studies.

Physicians in France examined medical records of patients to determine the benefits of image-guided minimally invasive surgery. They compared patients who had undergone laparoscopic splenectomy to those who underwent an open procedure. What they discovered was that mortality and morbidity of the open cases were 2.7% and 9% respectively, while there were no postprocedural complications associated with the laparoscopic splenectomy group. The time it took to perform the procedure was similar (approximately 75 minutes per case). Mean recovery time was shorter after laparoscopic splenectomy (3.95 ± 0.60 days) than after open splenectomy (7.0 ± 1.68 days) [18].

Another group of French doctors compared open versus laparoscopic cholecystectomy in elderly patients. The removal of the gallbladder is generally a last resort after attempts to break up gallstones with energy waves or treat them with medication proved unsuccessful. The patients in this study averaged 82 years of age. The length of the surgery (103.3 versus 149.7 minutes), postoperative length of stay (7.7 versus 12.7 days), and inpatient rehabilitation (15 versus 42 patients) were significantly shorter in the laparoscopic cholecystetcomy versus the open surgery group. The postoperative morbidity rate was not different between the groups [19].

Finally, a team in Italy compared the recovery of two groups of male patients requiring inguinal hernia repair. An inguinal hernia (the most common type of hernia) describes a part of the intestine that protrudes through a tear or weakened region in the lower abdominal wall causing pain. This study compared patients who had a laparoscopic hernia repair and those who had an open surgery for this condition. There was no difference in operating time between the two groups. The mean cost of laparoscopic hernioplasty was higher ($P < 0.001$). The intensity of postoperative pain was greater in the open hernia repair group which required a greater consumption of pain medication among these patients ($P < 0.05$). The median time to return to work was 30 days for the open hernia repair group and 16 days for the laparoscopic group ($P < 0.05$) [20].

19.7.2 Fibroids: An Example of How Image-Guided Treatments Could Save a Lot of Money

The economic impact of reducing the length of hospital stay, medications required, provider encounters, and time off work is huge. We can quantify this by looking at the costs of treating uterine fibroids, a benign growth in the uterus which may cause abnormal uterine bleeding, pelvic pain, urinary symptoms, and potentially hinder fertility. Although benign, the high prevalence of fibroids (approximately 25% of all women will have symptomatic fibroids) result in them being a huge problem. In 1997, the surgery and in-patient care costs for women with fibroids was over $2 billion per year according to the U.S. Center for Disease Control (CDC). Fibroids account for more than half of all hysterectomies (600,000 procedures per year), and cause women to spend 900,000 days in the hospital per year, more days than are spent in the hospital for either breast cancer or AIDS [21].

Surgery can be used to get rid of fibroids either through a hysterectomy (complete removal of the uterus) or a myomectomy (removal of a fibroid). However, image-guided therapies of uterine artery embolization and MR guided focused ultrasound (MRgFUS) have emerged as minimally and noninvasive outpatient uterine sparing procedures.

Uterine artery embolization, performed by interventional radiologists, involves guiding a catheter by fluoroscopy to deliver poly-vinyl alcohol particles that block blood flow in the uterine artery subsequently causing the fibroid to necrose and shrink. MRgFUS, performed by gynecologists and radiologists, involve focusing ultrasound waves into a small spot in the fibroid akin to how a magnifying glass focuses light. The focused ultrasound is able to heat the spot in the uterus to temperatures sufficient for cell death while sparing surrounding tissue.

19.7.3 Faster Recovery Achievable

One of the factors influencing the costs of fibroid procedures is the length of hospital stay required after the procedure (length of stay, LOS). Another factor to consider is the number of days it takes for patients to return to work after the procedure. When numbers reported in various studies were averaged, the LOS and lost work time for fibroid treatments were as shown in Table 19.1 [8, 22–27].

As expected, recovery from a surgical procedure takes longer than recovery from a minimally invasive procedure. Postoperative fever and pain were the reasons for hospital stays associated with UAE. In the case of MRgFUS, the patient receives intravenously infused conscious sedation, and the recovery time post procedure is 30 to 60 minutes [28]. In a study of 109 patients, only one required an overnight hospital stay for nausea [29].

The time away from work was also proportional to the invasiveness of the procedure. Patients from the United States, Canada, and Europe were averaged into the numbers, so there may be some cultural and workplace differences as to when it is required or appropriate for a patient to return to work.

Being able to return to work quickly after a procedure is equally important for employers, employees, and the self-employed. The costs associated with lost productivity, and the necessity for temporary workers, are certainly higher with surgical procedures versus UAE and MRgFUS. For many patients who cannot

Table 19.1 Length of Hospital Stay and Return to Work for Various Fibroid Treatments

Procedure	*Average Length of Stay (days)*	*Time Prior to Return to Work (days)*
Hysterectomy	3.0	47
Myomectomy	2.7	37
UAE	1.3	10.7
MRgFUS	0	0.8

afford to take a month or more off work, these minimally invasive and noninvasive procedures become their only option. Besides missed days from work, things like childcare and recovery care given by spouses, friends, and relatives need to be taken into account in the costs of recovery from surgery.

19.7.4 Overall Costs Are Less with Image-Guided Alternatives to Surgery

A cost analysis performed by the Ob/Gyn department at McGill University showed that the total inpatient cost (in Canadian dollars) of uterine artery embolization ($1,007.44 ± $60.65) was significantly lower than the cost of total abdominal hysterectomy ($1,933.37 ± $47.68), abdominal myomectomy ($1,781.73 ± $47.16), and vaginal hysterectomy ($1,515.39 ± $66.72) [25].

At the American Congress of Obstetrics and Gynecology's annual meeting in 2007, a joint analysis between GE Healthcare and the Mayo Clinic reported the amounts paid for uterine fibroid procedures including absence from work and disability. This further illustrates the reduced cost burden associated with image-guided nonsurgical alternatives for symptomatic uterine fibroids, compared to hysterectomy and myomectomy [30], as shown in Figure 19.1.

19.7.5 For Some Patients, the Only Option

In the minds of many patients with benign conditions such as fibroids, the treatment choice is not between surgery and an image-guided minimally invasive procedure. The choice is between a conservative management approach of watchful waiting or active surveillance, and image-guided therapy. Many women also do not want to have surgery to their uterus to retain potential for future fertility or for cultural reasons.

There is evidence to show that women are seeking minimally invasive alternatives to hysterectomy motivated by a trend towards later child bearing and desire to minimize recovery time [31]. In an evaluation of women undergoing UAE for fibroid symptoms, women with symptomatic fibroids waited an average of 5 years and consulted with an average of three gynecologists before undergoing UAE [23]. In a prospective study of 146 women who got a hysterectomy due to fibroids, 36% chose hysterectomy due to no alternative treatment being available [32]. In a survey about factors that influenced patient decision to choose uterine artery embolization, the top factors included: desire to avoid adverse effects of other treatments (90%), anticipated prolonged recovery from surgery (83%), and avoiding surgery (71%) [33].

The reasoning for avoiding or delaying surgery may also be due to cultural beliefs. In a study involving 30 African American women, results indicated that there were negative connotations associated with hysterectomy. Women chose to delay the procedure until they had no choice. The impact on self-esteem and perception of African American men were cited as reasons [34].

It is a misconception to believe that patients who choose the "do-nothing" watchful-waiting approach and who postpone treatment are not a burden to healthcare economics. These patients will require visits to the doctor for abnormal bleeding, urinary and sexual problems, and pelvic pain, as well as drugs for hormonal regulation or pain relief, which cost a lot of money. Patients with fibroids may also need to spend more on feminine hygiene products as a result of their symptoms.

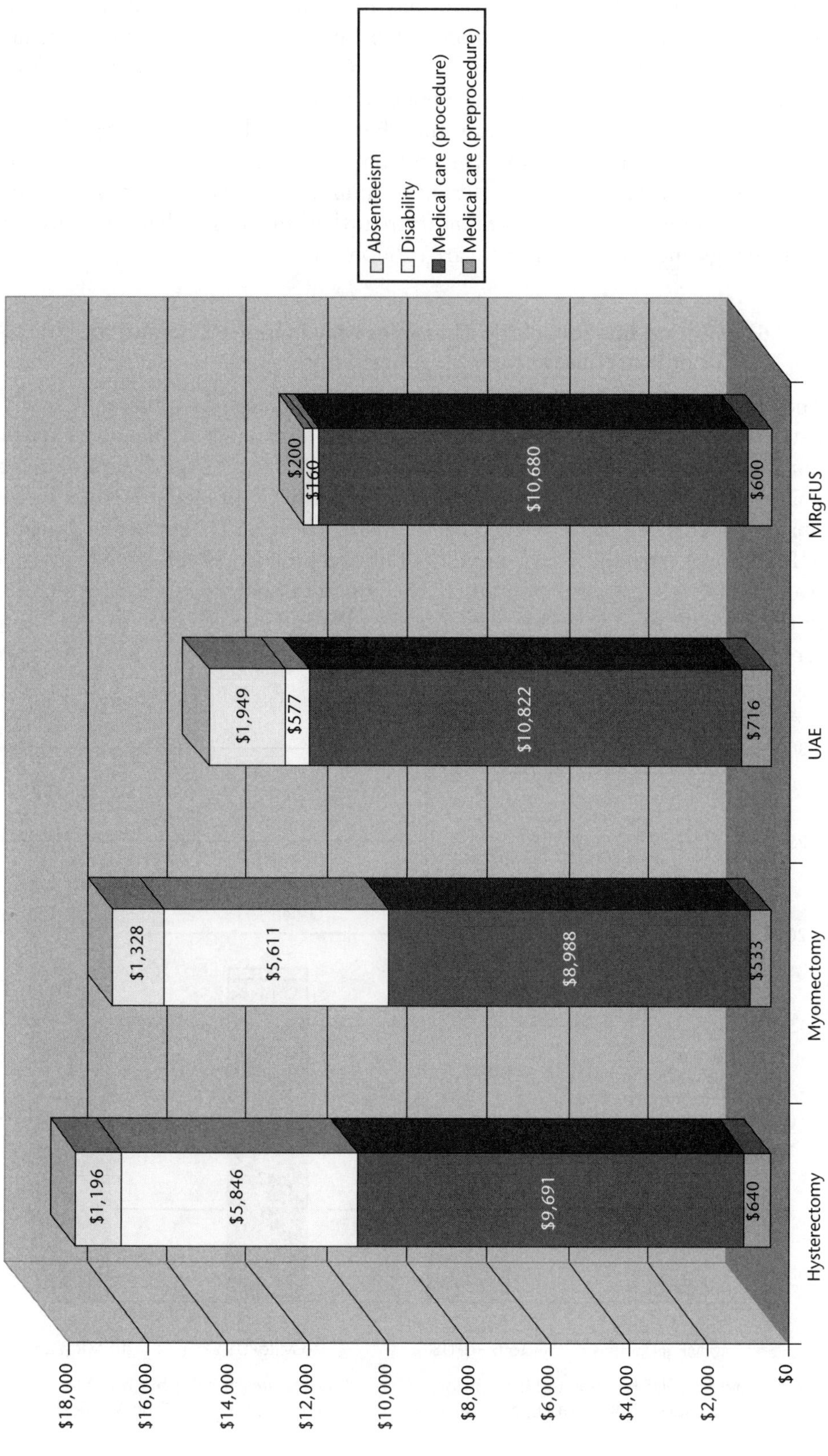

Figure 19.1 Total costs of fibroid procedures, with UAE and MRgFUS being image guided treatments. (*From:* [30]. © 2007 G. Carls et al. Reprinted with permission.)

Furthermore, since fibroid symptoms may have an effect on a woman's self-esteem and mood, treatments for depression and lost productivity as a result can be taxing. Due to the large prevalence of fibroids, even just 1 to 2 missed days of work per patient due to fibroid symptoms is a huge economic burden.

Prolonged treatment also means that the fibroid will have proliferated, and having a larger fibroid may exclude women from some of the lesser invasive procedures available. The emergence and offering of minimally invasive image-guided procedures for women to be more willing to treat their fibroids earlier will only lead to cost savings and improved healthcare economics.

19.7.6 Offering Image-Guided Therapies May Increase Demand for Other Procedures

The introduction of a new image-guided treatment at a medical center may entice new patients, and as such, the center may see an influx of patients. An unexpected positive outcome arose at a Japanese hospital that started offering MRgFUS as a noninvasive image-guided therapy for fibroid patients. At Itabashi Chuo Medical Center in Tokyo, fibroid patients who came to their center increased by 600% in the first 2 years that MRgFUS was introduced. The number of fibroid procedures performed increased by over 300%, as shown in Figure 19.2. The amount of hormonal therapy quadrupled in the 2 years after the system was installed. Patients would come to Itabashi to be screened for MRgFUS, but not all patients were suitable for the procedure, so the

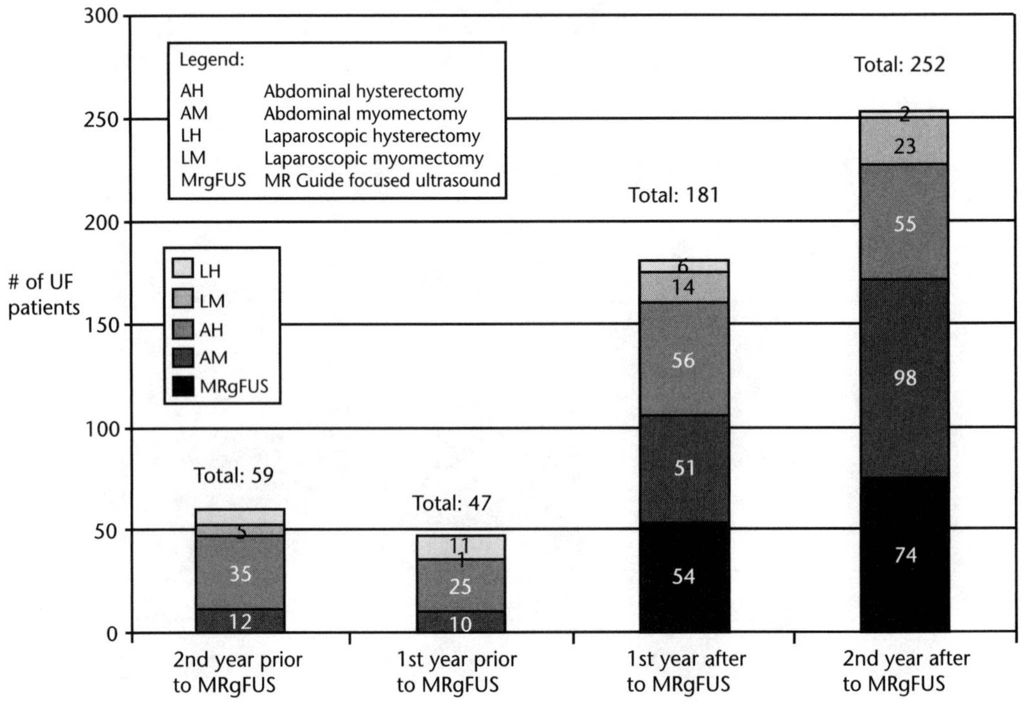

Figure 19.2 How MRgFUS has affected the number of fibroid procedures at Itabashi Chuo Medical Center, Tokyo. (Courtesy of Yutaka Morita, M.D., and Tetsuya Nakamura, M.D., Itabashi Chuo Medical Center.)

number of invasive and minimally invasive surgeries increased significantly by 170%. The Ob/Gyn department saw their revenue increase by 24% excluding income from obstetrics. More gynecologists had to be hired to cover the workload.

It is reasonable to believe that patients would rather go to a center that offers a complete array of treatment options rather than one that offers a limited selection. Patients may feel that the physicians are truly recommending the best procedure for them.

Another impact that novel image-guided therapies bring to centers that adopt them are the number of referrals. The successful treatment of a fibroid patient with MRgFUS may lead to their friends and families coming to the center for other medical needs. In fact, the number of patients who were referred to Itabashi Chuo Medical Center has significantly increased. Before installing the MRgFUS the Ob/Gyn department received 30 referrals per month. This increased to 110 per month (70% originating from outside Tokyo) according to Tetsuya Nakamura, M.D., at the Itabashi Chuo Medical Center in Tokyo, Japan.

19.8 Image-Guided Therapy Is Changing Healthcare

19.8.1 Imaged-Guided Therapy Results in an Increased Demand for Imaging

An increase in the number of image-guided therapy procedures will inevitably result in a concomitant increase in the demand for imaging. For image-guided therapy procedures, images are needed not just for diagnosis but also for guiding the procedure and to determine treatment outcome as well.

This phenomenon is evident in MRgFUS procedures. Patients who are considering a MRgFUS treatment first need to obtain an MRI screening examination to determine eligibility for the procedure. In applications such as uterine fibroids, a MRI exam is traditionally not prescribed to visualize fibroids. Diagnostic ultrasound images usually provide sufficient information for the gynecological surgeon to count, locate, and measure fibroids in the uterus. However, certain criteria for MRgFUS patient selection require the use of MRI. Parameters such as fibroid vascularity, the presence and degree of calcifications or degeneration, and heterogeneity of fibroid tissue are visible solely on magnetic resonance images.

The increase in utilization of high-resolution imaging technologies such as MRI can be of benefit to the patient, as physicians are able to diagnose conditions better than with palpation, ultrasound imaging, or a diagnosis based on symptoms. For example, a patient who presented herself as having uterine fibroids was determined to have a leiomyosarcoma (uterine cancer tumor) after MRI screening for MRgFUS [35].

There is also an economic benefit for MRI centers in that more patients will be seeking scans to determine eligibility for MRgFUS. A proprietor of an MRI center will be able to profit from not just the image-guided treatment, but the patients coming to be prescreened for the procedure. These patients may also come back for a follow-up scan to ensure the treatment was efficacious. While paying the capital cost of the MRI equipment, center owners will be looking at many avenues to generate a return on their investment. One method to increase the time that a MRI unit is in use is by offering image-guided therapies.

19.8.2 Procedures Need to Be Efficient and Cost-Effective

The downside of image-guided therapies such as MRgFUS, however, is that the procedure time can be lengthy. Currently, it can take up to 3 hours to treat a fibroid measuring 10 cm with focused ultrasound. The MRI center must be able to generate sufficient revenue that is greater than the opportunity cost of performing routine imaging scans. If a center is able to perform four routine MRI scans in 3 hours, and receive $1,500 for each scan, they need to be able to receive at least $6,000 for the MRgFUS procedure.

Hence, the efficiency of the procedure, both from a technological and a clinical practice perspective, is crucial to the cost-effectiveness of an image-guided technology which affects hospitals and imaging centers' decision to adopt and purchase an image-guided technology. The opportunity cost of tying up an imaging system to perform image-guided therapy plays a large role in determining the overall cost of the procedure to patients and insurance providers alike. Companies developing these technologies need to be diligent in ensuring procedure time is well aligned with the price that patients and insurers are willing to pay for the procedure after imaging time is taken into consideration.

19.8.3 A Multidisciplinary Approach

The successful implementation of image-guided therapy relies on the availability of a multidisciplinary team of physicians, and their willingness to collaborate. The emergence of such novel therapies will result in a paradigm shift away from the traditional "roles" and "specialties" of physicians.

Radiologists may be more involved with teaching other disciplines about reading and interpreting MRI or CT images, and provide patient candidacy and treatment recommendations for image-guided treatments. As an example, radiologists may be collaborating with urologists and radiation oncologists to determine if image-guided focused ultrasound or radiation therapy or a combination of both would be best suited for a prostate cancer patient.

Radiologists are also finding themselves involved with more minimally invasive procedures rather than just prescribing imaging and reading films. They are often involved with treating tumors using image-guided embolization and percutaneous ablation techniques.

However, the path to collaboration is not without hurdles. Surgeons may feel threatened that procedures in the surgical arena will be taken over by image-guided alternatives performed by interventional radiologists. This dilemma can be illustrated by observing what transpired when UAE was first introduced. The gynecologists were surgically trained physicians who had patients in need of fibroid treatments, and the interventional radiologists would have to rely on referrals from gynecologists to have patients suitable for treatment. However, a gynecologist may be hesitant to refer patients for this procedure since they would lose the professional fee that they would charge for performing surgeries such as hysterectomies or myomectomies. It came down to patients self-educating themselves and demanding UAE that persuaded gynecologists to become more knowledgeable of the procedure and work with the interventional radiologists [36, 37].

With the emergence of image-guided tumor treatments, many interventional radiologists and radiation oncologists are finding themselves treating cancer patients. However, cancer patients have traditionally sought medical oncologists as their primary physicians who seek out a complete treatment plan for their cancer care, from advice and diagnosis to treatment and follow-up. As such, it is important for radiologists to not only foster a positive relationship with medical oncologists, but equally crucial for their image-guided therapies to be efficacious and durable. Imagine a medical oncologist who refers a patient to an interventional radiologist for a MRgFUS treatment of a bone tumor. The likelihood of future referrals would be dependant on the success of the first treatment. The medical oncologist may work together with the interventional radiology to see how the MRgFUS treatment fits into the cancer treatment plan—whether as primary, secondary, or a combination treatment.

In fact, as the collaboration between interventional radiologists and oncologists continues to grow, a new field has emerged: interventional oncology. At an annual meeting of the World Conference of Interventional Oncology (WCIO), image-guided therapies comprised many of the sessions and talks (www.wcio2008.com). To further illustrate the trend in collaboration between specialties, the European division known as European Congress of Interventional Oncologists (ECIO) is trying to entice medical oncologists to join. Their offer for the 2008 meeting: an interventional radiologist can bring their referring oncologist to the meeting for free, all expenses paid (www.ecio2008.org, incentive program).

Technologists' roles will also change as image-guided therapies require new techniques such as simulations of therapy plans and dose regimens, image processing techniques, and the localization and targeting of treatment. With advances in imaging technology, traditional evaluations of biopsied tissue may even evolve into real-time evaluation of treatment outcome as imaging modalities such as magnetic resonance spectroscopy become validated as accurate means of diagnosis.

As image-guided treatments become more prevalent in cancer care, radiologists and imaging specialists will have more interaction with medical oncologists and pathologists as well. Imaging modalities may be used to aid in the diagnosis of disease and progression of cancer, as well as guide the treatment of the tumor. Physicians will be working more closely with bioengineers and physicists in developing cutting edge systems that combine imaging and therapy. Bioengineering programs around the world have implemented special courses and study tracks in image-guided therapy. For example, the medical imaging and image-guided therapy program at the University of Washington offers research opportunities in subjects such as advanced processing for image-guided therapies, image-guided drug delivery and ablation, and 3D ultrasonic angiography.

This partnership and collaboration between physicians of various disciplines will only benefit patients. Many cancer therapies are now emerging as a multimodality approach. Hospitals pride themselves on being able to offer a team of specialists dedicated to a customized treatment plan for a patient, rather than the traditional method of assigning multiple patients to a physician. The emergence of image-guided treatments has fostered such cooperation, and as physicians and patients are discovering the socioeconomic benefits associated with such collaboration, image-guided therapies are bound to continue to improve and thrive.

Looking again at the Gamma Knife as a perfect example of image-guided therapy, the treatment plan is designed by a team of skilled neurosurgeons, radiation oncologists, and radiation physicists. Each of these specialists contributes their knowledge and expertise to program computer software which conforms the radiation dose precisely to the size and shape of the targeted lesion.

19.9 Conclusions

Image-guided therapies offer patients less invasive treatments with fewer complications, less hospital utilization, and shorter recovery times while maintaining efficacy. These procedures are adopted and outcomes are achievable through physician awareness, education, and training. For procedures to be practiced widely, they must make economic sense. The socioeconomic benefits of image-guided therapies are changing the landscape of healthcare, from the way hospitals are designed to how physicians are collaborating.

References

[1] Tan, T. C., and P. M. Black, "Sir Victor Horsley (1857–1916): Pioneer of Neurological Surgery," *Neurosurgery*, Vol. 50, No. 3, March 2002, pp. 607–611.

[2] Golombeck, K., et al., "Maternal Morbidity After Maternal-Fetal Surgery," *Am. J. Obstet. Gynecol.*, Vol. 194, No. 3, March 2006, pp. 834–839.

[3] http://www.oispine.com, accessed November 7, 2008.

[4] Fox, S., and L. Rainie, "Vital Decisions: How Internet Users Decide What Information to Trust When They or Their Loved Ones Are Sick," *The Pew Internet & American Life Project*, May 22, 2002.

[5] Nelson, H., et al., "A Comparison of Laparoscopically Assisted and Open Colectomy for Colon Cancer. The Clinical Outcomes of Surgical Therapy Study Group," *N. Engl. J. Med.*, Vol. 350, 2004, pp. 2050–2059.

[6] SCAI/SVMB/SVS Writing Committee, "SCAI/SVMB/SVS Clinical Competence Statement on Carotid Stenting: Training and Credentialing for Carotid Stenting—Multispecialty Consensus Recommendations," *Vasc Med.*, Vol. 10, No. 1, February 2005, pp. 65–75.

[7] Seymour, N. E., et al., "Virtual Reality Improves Operating Room Performance: Results of a Randomized Double-Blind Study," *Ann. Surg.*, Vol. 236, 2002, pp. 458–464.

[8] Spies, J. B., and D. Sacks, "Credentials for Uterine Artery Embolization," *J. Vasc. Interv. Radiol.*, Vol. 15, 2004, pp. 111–113.

[9] Spies, J. B., et al. "Outcome of Uterine Embolization and Hysterectomy for Leiomyomas: Results of a Multicenter Study," *Am. J. Obstet. Gynecol.*, Vol. 191, No. 1, 2004, pp. 22–31.

[10] Regan, J. J., H. Yuan, and P. C. McAfee, "Laparoscopic Fusion of the Lumbar Spine: Minimally Invasive Spine Surgery. A Prospective Multicenter Study Evaluating Open and Laparoscopic Lumbar Fusion," *Spine*, Vol. 24, 1999, pp. 402–411.

[11] Catane, R., et al., "MR-Guided Focused Ultrasound Surgery (MRgFUS) for the Palliation of Pain in Patients with Bone Metastases—Preliminary Clinical Experience," *Ann. Oncol.*, Vol. 18, No. 1, January 2007, pp. 163–167.

[12] Hinshaw, J. L., and F. T. Lee, Jr., "Image-Guided Ablation of Renal Cell Carcinoma," *Magn. Reson. Imaging Clin. N. Am.*, Vol. 12, No. 3, August 2004, pp. 429–447.

[13] Fergany, A., "Current Status and Advances in Nephron-Sparing Surgery," *Clin. Genitourin Cancer*, Vol. 5, No. 1, June 2006, pp. 26–33.

[14] Uzzo, R. G., and A. C. Novick, "Nephron Sparing Surgery for Renal Tumors: Indications, Techniques and Outcomes," *J. Urol.*, Vol. 166, No. 1, July 2001, pp. 6–18.

[15] Atwell, T. D., et al., "Percutaneous Cryoablation of 40 Solid Renal Tumors with US Guidance and CT Monitoring: Initial Experience," *Radiology*, Vol. 243, No. 1, April 2007, pp. 276–283.

[16] Mogami, T., et al., "Percutaneous MR-Guided Cryoablation for Malignancies, with a Focus on Renal Cell Carcinoma," *Int. J. Clin. Oncol.*, Vol. 12, No. 2, April 2007, pp. 79–84.

[17] Issa, N., et al., "Nephrogenic Systemic Fibrosis and Its Association with Gadolinium Exposure During MRI," *Cleve. Clin. J. Med.*, Vol. 75, No. 2, February 2008, pp. 95–97, 103–104.

[18] Cogliandolo, A., et al., "Results of Laparoscopic and Open Splenectomy for Nontraumatic Diseases," *Surg. Laparosc. Endosc. Percutan. Tech.*, Vol. 11, No. 4, August 2001, pp. 256–261.

[19] Pessaux, P., et al., "Laparoscopic Versus Open Cholecystectomy: A Prospective Comparative Study in the Elderly with Acute Cholecystitis," *Surg. Laparosc. Endosc. Percutan. Tech.*, Vol. 11, No. 4, August 2001, pp. 252–255.

[20] Sarli, L., et al., "Simultaneous Repair of Bilateral Inguinal Hernias: A Prospective, Randomized Study of Open, Tension-Free Versus Laparoscopic Approach," *Surg. Laparosc. Endosc. Percutan. Tech.*, Vol. 11, No. 4, August 2001, pp. 262–267.

[21] Lepine, L. A., et al., "Hysterectomy Surveillance—United States, 1980–1993," *Mor. Mortal. Wkly. Rep. CDC Surveill. Summ.*, Vol. 46, No. 4, 1997, pp. 1–15.

[22] Becker, E. R., et al., "Inpatient Surgical Treatment Patterns for Patients with Uterine Fibroids in the United States, 1998–2002," *J. Natl. Med. Assoc.*, Vol. 97, No. 10, 2005, pp. 1336–1342.

[23] Pron, G., et al., "Ontario Uterine Fibroid Embolization Collaboration Group. The Ontario Uterine Fibroid Embolization Trial. Part 1. Baseline Patient Characteristics, Fibroid Burden, and Impact on Life," *Fertil. Steril.*, Vol. 79, No. 1, January 2003, pp. 112–119.

[24] Pron, G., et al., "Tolerance, Hospital Stay, and Recovery After Uterine Artery Embolization for Fibroids: The Ontario Uterine Fibroid Embolization Trial," *J. Vasc. Interv. Radiol.*, Vol. 14, No. 10, 2003, pp. 1243–1250.

[25] Al-Fozan, H., et al., "Cost Analysis of Myomectomy, Hysterectomy, and Uterine Artery Embolization," *Am. J. Obstet. Gynecol.*, Vol. 187, No. 5, November 2002, pp. 1401–1404.

[26] Goodwin, S. C., et al., "Uterine Artery Embolization Versus Myomectomy: A Multicenter Comparative Study," *Fertil. Steril.*, Vol. 85, No. 1, 2006, pp. 14–21.

[27] Hehenkamp, W. J., et al., "Pain and Return to Daily Activities After Uterine Artery Embolization and Hysterectomy in the Treatment of Symptomatic Uterine Fibroids: Results from the Randomized EMMY Trial," *Cardiovasc. Intervent. Radiol.*, Vol. 29, No. 2, March–April 2006, pp. 179–187.

[28] Tempany, C. M., "From the RSNA Refresher Courses: Image-Guided Thermal Therapy of Uterine Fibroids," *Radiographics*, Vol. 27, No. 6, November–December 2007, pp. 1819–1826.

[29] Stewart, E. A., et al., "Clinical Outcomes of Focused Ultrasound Surgery for the Treatment of Uterine Fibroids," *Fertil. Steril.*, Vol. 85, No. 1, January 2006, pp. 22–29.

[30] Carls, G. S., et al., "What Does Surgical Treatment for Uterine Fibroids Really Cost?" *ACOG 2007.*

[31] Stewart, E. A., "Uterine Fibroids," *Lancet*, Vol. 357, No. 9252, January 27, 2001, pp. 293–298.

[32] Carlson, K. J., B. A. Miller, and F. J. Fowler, Jr., "The Maine Women's Health Study: II. Outcomes of Nonsurgical Management of Leiomyomas, Abnormal Bleeding, and Chronic Pelvic Pain," *Obstet. Gynecol.*, Vol. 83, No. 4, April 1994, pp. 566–572.

[33] Nevadunsky, N. S., et al., "Women's Decision-Making Determinants in Choosing Uterine Artery Embolization for Symptomatic Fibroids," *J. Reprod. Med.*, Vol. 46, No. 10, October 2001, pp. 870–874.

[34] Augustus, C. E., "Beliefs and Perceptions of African American Women Who Have Had Hysterectomy," *J. Transcult. Nurs.*, Vol. 13, No. 4, 2002, pp. 296–302.

[35] Samuel, A., et al., "Avoiding Treatment of Leiomyosarcomas: The Role of Magnetic Resonance in Focused Ultrasound Surgery," *Fertil. Steril.*, November 15, 2007.

[36] Arleo, E. K., J. Pollak, and M. G. Tal, "Changing Trends in Gynecologists' Opinions of Uterine Artery Embolization for Fibroids: The Patient's Perspective," *J. Vasc. Interv. Radiol.*, Vol. 14, No. 12, December 2003, pp. 1559–1561.

[37] Plaskos, N. P., and J. R. Kachura, "Survey of Gynecologists' and Interventional Radiologists' Opinions of Uterine Fibroid Embolization," *Can. Assoc. Radiol. J.*, Vol. 57, No. 3, June 2006, pp. 140–146.

About the Editors

Shahram Vaezy is an associate professor in the Department of Bioengineering at the University of Washington in Seattle. He holds a B.S. in electrical engineering and a Ph.D. in bioengineering, both from the University of Washington.

Vesna Zderic is an assistant professor in the Department of Electrical and Computer Engineering at the George Washington University in Washington, D.C. She holds a B.S. in electrical engineering from the University of Belgrade in Serbia and a Ph.D. in bioengineering from the University of Washington.

List of Contributors

Fernando J. Bianco, Jr.
Columbia University
Division of Urology
Mt. Sinai Medical Center
4306 Alton Road, 3rd Floor
Miami Beach, FL 33140
United States
fb2271@columbia.edu

Arthur H. Chan
InSightec, Inc.
4851 LBJ Freeway
Dallas, TX 75244
United States
arthurc@insightec.com

Isaac A. Chang
U.S. Food and Drug Administration
10903 New Hampshire Avenue
Bldg 62, Room 1108
Silver Spring, MD 20993
United States
isaac.chang@fda.hhs.gov

Rajiv Chopra
Sunnybrook Health Sciences Centre
2075 Bayview Avenue, Room C7 36A
Toronto, ON M4N 3M5
Canada
rajiv.chopra@sunnybrook.ca

Michael C. Dobelbower
Department of Radiation Oncology
University of Alabama
1824 6th Ave. S.
Birmingham, AL 35294
United States
mdobelbower@uabmc.edu

Ralph R. Dobelbower
Department of Radiation Oncology
University of Toledo Medical Center
3000 Arlington Avenue
MS1151
Toledo, OH 43614
United States
ralph.dobelbower@utoledo.edu

Theodore J. Dubinsky
Department of Radiology
Body Imaging
University of Washington Medical Center
1959 Pacific Street
Seattle, WA 98195
United States
tdub@u.washington.edu

Victor Frenkel
Radiology and Imaging Sciences
Clinical Center
National Institutes of Health
10 Center Drive
Bethesda, MD 20892
United States
vfrenkel@cc.nih.gov

Christos S. Georgiades
Division of Vascular and Interventional Radiology
Johns Hopkins Hospital
600 N. Wolfe Street
Baltimore, MD 21287
United States
cgeorgi@jhmi.edu

Jean-Francois Geschwind
Division of Vascular and Interventional Radiology
Johns Hopkins Hospital
600 N. Wolfe Street
Baltimore, MD 21287
United States
jfg@jhmi.edu

David E. Goertz
Sunnybrook Health Sciences Centre
2075 Bayview Avenue
Toronto, ON M4N 3M5
Canada
goertz@sri.utoronto.ca

Riadh Habash
School of Information Technology and Engineering
University of Ottawa
800 King Edward Avenue
Ottawa, ON, K1N 6N5
Canada
rhabash@site.uottawa.ca

Dieter Haemmerich
Medical University of South Carolina
Division of Pediatric Cardiology
165 Ashley Avenue
MSC 915
Charleston, SC 29425
United States
haemmer@musc.edu

Allan Haynes
Department of Surgery
Texas Tech University School of Medicine
3601 4th Street
Lubbock, TX 79430
United States
tres.haynes@ttuhsc.edu

Kullervo Hynynen
Department of Medical Biophysics
University of Toronto
Sunnybrook Health Sciences Centre
2075 Bayview Avenue
Toronto, ON M4N
Canada
khynynen@sri.utoronto.ca

Matthew Kay
Department of Electrical and Computer Engineering
Department of Pharmacology and Physiology
The George Washington University
801 22nd Street NW
Washington, D.C. 20052
United States
phymwk@gwu.edu

Orpheus Kolokythas
Department of Radiology
Body Imaging
University of Washington Medical Center
1959 Pacific Street
Seattle, WA 98195
United States
orpheus@u.washington.edu

David Larson
Department of Radiation Oncology
University of California San Francisco
505 Parnassus Ave., L-08
San Francisco, CA 94143
United States
dlarson@radonc.ucsf.edu

Daniel F. Leotta
Applied Physics Laboratory
University of Washington
1013 NE 40th Street
Seattle, WA 98105
United States
leotta@u.washington.edu

Lijun Ma
Department of Radiation Oncology
University of California San Francisco
505 Parnassus Ave., L-08
San Francisco, CA 94143
United States
ma@radonc17.ucsf.edu

Marco Mercader
Division of Cardiology
Medical Faculty Associates
2150 Pennsylvania Avenue, NW
Washington, D.C. 20037
United States
mmercader@mfa.gwu.edu

Keyvan Moghissi
Yorkshire Laser Centre
The UK Medical Laser Centre
Woodlands Avenue
Goole
E. Yorkshire
DN14 6RX
United Kingdom
kmoghissi@yorkshirelasercentre.org

E. Ishmael Parsai
University of Toledo Health Science Campus
Department of Radiation Oncology
3000 Arlington Avenue
Toledo, OH 43614
United States
e.parsai@utoledo.edu

T. Joshua Pfefer
U.S. Food and Drug Administration
10903 New Hampshire Avenue
Bldg. 62, Room 1222
Silver Spring, MD 20993
United States
joshua.pfefer@fda.hhs.gov

Arjun Sahgal
Department of Radiation Oncology
The Princess Margaret Hospital and Sunnybrook Health Sciences Centre
610 University Avenue
Toronto, Ontario, M5G2M9
Canada
arjun.sahgal@sunnybrook.ca

David F. Schaeffer
Department of Pathology
Faculty of Medicine
The University of British Columbia
899 West 12th Avenue
Vancouver, BC V5Z1M9
Canada
david.schaeffer@web.de

Charles H. Scudamore
Department of Surgery
Faculty of Medicine
The University of British Columbia
855 West 10th Avenue
Vancouver, BC V5Z 1L7
Canada
charles.scudamore@vch.ca

Dean K. Shibata
Department of Radiology
Neuroradiology
University of Washington Medical Center
1959 Pacific Street
Seattle, WA 98195
United States
shibatad@u.washington.edu

Mika Sinanan
Department of Surgery
University of Washington
1959 Pacific Street
Seattle, WA 98195
United States
mssurg@u.washington.edu

Mark Stringer
The Institute of Microwaves and Photonics
University of Leeds
Yorkshire Laser Centre
The UK Medical Laser Centre
Woodlands Avenue
Goole E. Yorkshire
DN14 6RX
United Kingdom
m.r.stringer@leeds.ac.uk

May Tsao
Department of Radiation Oncology
Sunnybrook Health Sciences Centre
2075 Bayview Avenue
Toronto, Ontario, M4N 3M5
Canada
may.tsao@sunnybrook.ca

Shahram Vaezy
Department of Bioengineering
University of Washington
1705 NE Pacific Street
Seattle, WA 98195
United States
adasi@u.washington.edu

Bill H. Warren
Department of Radiology
Body Imaging, University of Washington Medical Center
1959 Pacific Street
Seattle, WA 98195
United States
bhwarren@u.washington.edu

Jason Zara
Department of Electrical and Computer Engineering
The George Washington University
801 22nd Street NW
Washington, D.C. 20052
United States
jzara@gwu.edu

Vesna Zderic
Department of Electrical and Computer Engineering
The George Washington University
801 22nd Street NW
Washington, D.C. 20052
United States
zderic@gwu.edu

Index

D

I

N

O

P

Q

R

T